PEDIATRIC SECRETS

Second Edition

RICHARD A. POLIN, MD
Professor of Pediatrics
University of Pennsylvania School of Medicine
Department of Pediatrics, Division of Neonatology
Children's Hospital of Philadelphia
Philadelphia, Pennsylvania

MARK F. DITMAR, MD
Chief, Section of General Pediatrics
Norwalk Hospital
Norwalk, Connecticut
Assistant Clinical Professor of Pediatrics
Yale University School of Medicine
New Haven, Connecticut

HANLEY & BELFUS, INC./ Philadelphia
MOSBY/ St. Louis • Baltimore • Boston • Carlsbad • Chicago • London
Madrid • Naples • New York • Philadelphia • Sydney • Tokyo • Toronto

Publisher: HANLEY & BELFUS, INC.
             Medical Publishers
             210 South 13th Street
             Philadelphia, PA 19107
             (215) 546-7293; 800-962-1892
             FAX (215) 790-9330

North American and worldwide sales and distribution:

             MOSBY
             11830 Westline Industrial Drive
             St. Louis, MO 63146

In Canada: Times Mirror Professional Publishing, Ltd.
             130 Flaska Drive
             Markham, Ontario L6G 1B8
             Canada

Library of Congress Cataloging-in-Publication Data

Polin, Richard A. (Richard Alan). 1945-
    Pediatric Secrets / Richard A. Polin, Mark F. Ditmar. – 2nd ed.
       p.   cm. – (The Secrets Series®)
    Includes bibliographical references and index.
    ISBN 1-56053-171-1 (alk. paper)
    1. Pediatric–Examinations, questions, etc.   I. Ditmar, Mark F.
  II. Title.   III. Series.
    [DNLM: 1. Pediatrics–examination questions.   WS 18.2 P768p 1996]
RJ48.2.P65 1996
  618.92' 00076–dc20
  DNLM/DLC
  for Library of Congress   96-29336
                                                                   CIP

PEDIATRIC SECRETS, 2nd edition   ISBN 1-56053-171-1

Last digit is the print number: 9 8 7 6 5 4 3 2 1

In Memoriam

This book is dedicated to the memory of
Drs. David Cornfeld and Edward Charney

THE FAR SIDE By GARY LARSON

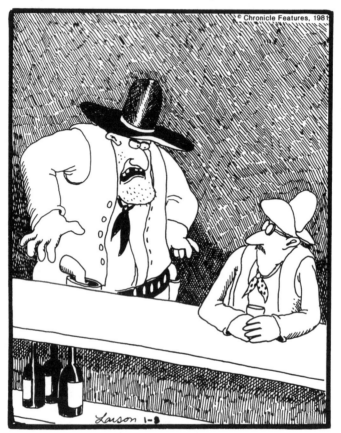

"I asked you a question, buddy . . . What's the square root of 5,248?"

CONTENTS

CONTRIBUTORS

JoAnn Bergoffen, M.D.
Division of Genetics, Permanente Medical Group, San Jose, California

Gerard T. Berry, M.D.
Professor of Pediatrics, University of Pennsylvania School of Medicine, Philadelphia; Children's Hospital of Philadelphia, Philadelphia, Pennsylvania

Peter M. Bingham, M.D.
Assistant Professor of Neurology and Pediatrics, University of Pennsylvania School of Medicine, Philadelphia; Children's Hospital of Philadelphia, Philadelphia, Pennsylvania

Nathan J. Blum, M.D.
Assistant Professor of Pediatrics, University of Pennsylvania School of Medicine, Philadelphia; Division of Child Development and Rehabilitation, Children's Seashore House, Philadelphia, Pennsylvania

Anthony Chang, M.D.
Assistant Professor of Pediatrics and Surgery, University of Southern California School of Medicine, Los Angeles, California; Medical Director, Cardiac Intensive Care Unit, Children's Hospital, Miami, Florida

Edward B. Charney, M.D. (deceased)
Professor of Pediatrics, University of Pennsylvania School of Medicine, Philadelphia; Division of Child Development, Department of Pediatrics, Children's Hospital of Philadelphia, Philadelphia, Pennsylvania

Robert Ryan Clancy, M.D.
Professor of Neurology and Pediatrics, University of Pennsylvania School of Medicine, Philadelphia; Senior Neurologist, Children's Hospital of Philadelphia, Philadelphia, Pennsylvania

Bernard J. Clark, III, M.D.
Associate Professor of Pediatrics, University of Pennsylvania School of Medicine, Philadelphia; Associate Cardiologist, Division of Cardiology, Department of Pediatrics, Children's Hospital of Philadelphia, Philadelphia, Pennsylvania

Alan R. Cohen, M.D.
Professor of Pediatrics, University of Pennsylvania School of Medicine, Philadelphia; Chief, Division of Hematology, Children's Hospital of Philadelphia, Philadelphia, Pennsylvania

Richard S. Davidson, M.D.
Associate Professor of Orthopaedics, University of Pennsylvania School of Medicine, Philadelphia; Department of Orthopaedic Surgery, Children's Hospital of Philadelphia, Philadelphia, Pennsylvania

Mark F. Ditmar, M.D.
Chief, Section of General Pediatrics, Norwalk Hospital, Norwalk, Connecticut; Assistant Clinical Professor of Pediatrics, Yale University School of Medicine, New Haven, Connecticut

Alan E. Donnenfeld, M.D.
Associate Professor of Obstetrics and Gynecology, Thomas Jefferson University School of Medicine, Philadelphia; Pennsylvania Hospital, Philadelphia, Pennsylvania

John P. Dormans, M.D.
Assistant Professor of Orthopaedics, University of Pennsylvania School of Medicine, Philadelphia; Children's Hospital of Philadelphia, Philadelphia, Pennsylvania

Stephen D. Douglas, M.D.
Professor of Pediatrics, University of Pennsylvania School of Medicine, Philadelphia; Chief, Section of Immunology, Children's Hospital of Philadelphia, Philadelphia, Pennsylvania

Andrew H. Eichenfield, M.D.
Assistant Professor of Pediatrics, Mt. Sinai School of Medicine, New York, New York

Lawrence F. Eichenfield, M.D.
Chief, Pediatric Dermatology, Children's Hospital and Health Center, San Diego; Assistant Professor of Pediatrics and Medicine (Dermatology) and Chief, Division of Pediatric Dermatology, University of California, San Diego, School of Medicine, San Diego, California

John W. Foreman, M.D.
Professor, Department of Pediatrics, and Chief, Division of Pediatric Nephrology, Duke University School of Medicine, Durham, North Carolina

Daniel E. Hale, M.D.
Associate Professor of Pediatrics, University of Texas Health Sciences Center at San Antonio, San Antonio, Texas

Mary Catherine Harris, M.D.
Associate Professor of Pediatrics, University of Pennsylvania School of Medicine, Philadelphia; Children's Hospital of Philadelphia, Philadelphia, Pennsylvania

David B. Haslam, M.D.
Instructor, Department of Pediatrics and Molecular Microbiology, Washington University School of Medicine, St. Louis, Missouri

Bruce P. Himelstein, M.D.
Assistant Professor of Pediatrics, University of Pennsylvania School of Medicine, Philadelphia; Division of Oncology, Children's Hospital of Philadelphia, Philadelphia, Pennsylvania

Fred M. Henretig, M.D. M.D.
Associate Professor of Pediatrics, University of Pennsylvania School of Medicine, Philadelphia; Division of Emergency Medicine, Medical Director, Poison Control Center, Children's Hospital of Philadelphia, Philadelphia, Pennsylvania

Paul J. Honig, M.D.
Professor of Pediatrics and Dermatology, University of Pennsylvania School of Medicine, Philadelphia; Division of Dermatology, Department of Pediatrics, Children's Hospital of Philadelphia, Philadelphia, Pennsylvania

Ellen B. Kaplan, M.D.
Chief, Section of Pediatric Pulmonology, Department of Pediatrics, Hackensack University Medical Center, Hackensack, New Jersey

Lorraine E. Levitt Katz, M.D.
Senior Fellow, Department of Pediatrics, Division of Endocrine, University of Pennsylvania School of Medicine, Philadelphia; Children's Hospital of Philadelphia, Philadelphia, Pennsylvania

Beverly Lange, M.D.
Professor of Pediatrics, University of Pennsylvania School of Medicine, Philadelphia; Division of Oncology, Children's Hospital of Philadelphia, Philadelphia, Pennsylvania

Jane M. Lavelle, M.D.
Assistant Professor of Pediatrics, University of Pennsylvania School of Medicine, Philadelphia; Division of Emergency Medicine, Children's Hospital of Philadelphia, Philadelphia, Pennsylvania

Chris A. Liacouras, M.D.
Assistant Professor of Pediatrics, University of Pennsylvania School of Medicine, Philadelphia; Director of Endoscopy, Division of Gastroenterology and Nutrition, Children's Hospital of Philadelphia, Philadelphia, Pennsylvania

Mark R. Magnusson, M.D., Ph.D.
Clinical Assistant Professor of Pediatrics, University of Pennsylvania School of Medicine, Philadelphia; Children's Hospital of Philadelphia, Philadelphia, Pennsylvania

Peter J. Marro, M.D.
Assistant Professor of Pediatrics, University of Vermont College of Medicine, Burlington, Vermont; Division of Neonatology, Maine Medical Center, Portland, Maine

Jeffrey E. Ming, M.D., Ph.D.
Fellow, Division of Human Genetics and Molecular Biology, Children's Hospital of Philadelphia, Philadelphia, Pennsylvania

Carlos R. Perez, M.D.
Assistant Professor of Pulmonary Medicine, University of Cincinnati College of Medicine, Children's Hospital Medical Center, Cincinnati, Ohio

David A. Piccoli, M.D.
Associate Professor of Pediatrics, and Section Chief, Division of Pediatric Gastroenterology and Nutrition, University of Pennsylvania School of Medicine, Philadelphia; Senior Physician, Children's Hospital of Philadelphia, Philadelphia, Pennsylvania

Richard A. Polin, M.D.
Professor of Pediatrics, University of Pennsylvania School of Medicine, Philadelphia; Department of Pediatrics, Division of Neonatology, Children's Hospital of Philadelphia, Philadelphia, Pennsylvania

Linda G. Rabinowitz, M.D.
Associate Professor of Pediatrics and Dermatology, Medical College of Wisconsin, Milwaukee, Wisconsin

Wayne Rackoff, M.D.
Assistant Professor of Pediatrics, Albert Einstein College of Medicine, Bronx; Associate Director, Division of Neonatology, Montefiore Medical Center, Bronx, New York

Claudio Ramaciotti, M.D.
Assistant Professor of Pediatrics, University of Texas Southwestern Medical Center, Dallas, Texas

Joseph W. St. Geme, III, M.D.
Assistant Professor of Pediatrics and Molecular Microbiology, Washington University School of Medicine, St. Louis; St. Louis Children's Hospital, St. Louis, Missouri

Carlos Vega-Rich, M.D.
Assistant Professor of Pediatrics, Albert Einstein College of Medicine; Director of Newborn Services, and Director, Affiliation and Transport Program, Jack D. Weiler Hospital of the Albert Einstein College of Medicine, Bronx, New York

Robert W. Wilmott, M.D.
Associate Professor of Pediatric Pulmonology, and Director, Department of Pulmonary Medicine, Allergy, and Clinical Immunology, University of Cincinnati College of Medicine, Children's Hospital Medical Center, Cincinnati, Ohio

Elaine H. Zackai, M.D.
Professor of Pediatrics/Genetics, University of Pennsylvania School of Medicine, Philadelphia; Director, Clinical Genetics Center, Children's Hospital of Philadelphia, Philadelphia, Pennsylvania

PREFACE TO THE FIRST EDITION

Medical school and residency are arduous and exhausting runs of discovery. It is through constant questioning and reappraisal that patient care is improved. Never should the spirit of inquiry be discouraged or curiosity be repressed, for according to a Chinese proverb: "He who asks a question may be a fool for five minutes, but he who does not ask a question remains a fool forever."

The transition from the beginnings of medical school to clerkships and residency is made more difficult because it is a transition from the written to the oral tradition. The relatively passive approach of lectures, notes, and textbooks is replaced in large part by vigorous give-and-take question and answer exchanges on rounds, in seminars, and even during exams. Depending on the point of view, the exchanges can be illuminating, intimidating, or constipating. Even in this age of computers, it is unlikely that the emphasis on the didactic oral tradition will lessen.

The purpose of this pediatric text is to address the questions that are commonly posed in the daily routine of a teaching hospital, in this case Children's Hospital of Philadelphia. Most of the questions were submitted by housestaff and University of Pennsylvania medical students. The questions represent a wide spectrum of topics—from basic pathophysiology to general pediatric principles to practical management issues. Many of the questions have no right or wrong answer. However, we hope that points discussed in areas of controversy will stimulate efforts on the part of the reader to develop an ongoing appreciation of and interest in changing approaches to pediatric care.

We are indebted to the chapter authors for their diligent participation in the project; to Deborah H. Schaible, PharmD, for her editorial assistance; to Linda Belfus and Jack Hanley for their exceptional editorial expertise and tireless good nature in the conception and evolution of this book; to Carol Miller for her dedication and grace in preparation of the manuscript; to the Children's Hospital housestaff and medical students for their enthusiasm in times of fatigue; and to the hospital housekeeping department for not tearing down the illegal "Pediatric Secrets" question boxes posted on each floor.

PREFACE TO THE SECOND EDITION

In this second edition, we have tried to incorporate many of the suggestions received regarding chapter organization and topic selection. As with the first edition, many questions have no simple right or wrong answer. These shades of grey for issues from newborns to adolescents continue to provide texture to the science and art of pediatrics.

A brief note on style. We tried to follow the trend to minimize the use of possessives in medical nomenclature (e.g., Hodgkin disease instead of Hodgkin's disease, etc.).

We are grateful to the chapter authors for their perseverance and flexibility over time; to publisher Linda Belfus for her insightful comments and boundless patience; and to Nina Ditmar for her editorial assistance and sense of humor.

Sadly, since the first edition, Drs. David Cornfeld and Edward Charney of the Children's Hospital of Philadelphia passed away. Both were instrumental in the evolution of this book, with Dr. Charney contributing to the Behavior and Development section. Both were gifted educators and first-rate physicians with unique perspectives. They continue to be greatly missed. We dedicate this book to their memory.

Richard A. Polin, M.D.
Mark F. Ditmar, M.D.

1. ADOLESCENT MEDICINE

Mark F. Ditmar, M.D.

CLINICAL ISSUES

1. What are the most common causes of death in adolescents?

Eighty percent of deaths in 15–19-year olds and 60% of deaths in 10–14-year olds are due to injuries. On any given day in the United States, about 23 teenagers are killed in motor vehicle crashes, 6 are victims of homicide, and 6 take their own lives.

2. Name the four major risk factors associated with injuries to adolescents.

1. Use of **alcohol** while engaged in activities (e.g., driving, swimming)—20% of all adolescent deaths are alcohol-related car crashes.

2. Failure to use **safety devices** (e.g., seat belts, motorcycle or bicycle helmets)—Seat belt use among adolescents is the lowest of any age group (30–50%).

3. Access to **firearms**—50% of deaths of black male teenagers and 20% of deaths of white male teenagers are due to firearms, primarily handguns.

4. **Athletic** participation—Most injuries are reinjuries, highlighting the importance of proper rehabilitation.

Elster AB, Kuznets NJ (eds): AMA Guidelines for Adolescent Preventive Services (GAPS). Baltimore, Williams & Wilkins, 1994, pp 29–40.

3. What should be considered in the differential diagnosis of major depression in the adolescent?

Alcohol abuse, substance abuse, cocaine or stimulant withdrawal, endocrinopathies, medication side effects, occult malignancies, primary sleep disorders, prodrome of schizophrenia, and adjustment disorder.

4. What causes chronic fatigue syndrome in teenagers?

The chronic fatigue syndrome is characterized by persistent or recurrent symptoms of fatigue, sore throat, mild cognitive dysfunction, and myalgias lasting at least 6 months. Most patients fitting this description are young adults, primarily females. Despite extensive virologic, immunologic, and psychiatric evaluations in these patients, a unifying cause has not been determined. Although the illness usually presents abruptly with a profound debilitating fatigue and various nonspecific constitutional symptoms following a viral-type illness, it does not appear to be a "postviral" syndrome. Epstein-Barr virus-associated infectious mononucleosis should be ruled out. A high percentage of patients do have psychologic illness, especially depression. Research is hindered by lack of uniform criteria for diagnosis in children and adolescents.

Carter BD, et al: Case control study of chronic fatigue in pediatric patients. Pediatrics 95:179–186, 1995.

5. At what age do teenagers reach expected adult hematologic parameters?

In general, girls reach adult values at age 12, and boys 2 years later at age 14. Sexual maturity rating is also helpful, as most achieve adult values when they reach Tanner stage II–III.

6. How do you evaluate a breast lump noted by a teenage girl on self-examination?

Although the incidence of cancerous lesions is extremely low in adolescents, it is not zero, and breast lumps do require careful follow-up. **Fibrocystic changes** (i.e., proliferation of stromal and epithelial elements, ductal dilatation, cyst formation) are common in later adolescence and are characterized by variations in size and tenderness with menstrual periods. The most common

1

tumor (up to 95%) is a **fibroadenoma**, which is a firm discrete smooth mass usually found later-ally. Other causes of masses include lipomas, hematomas, abscesses, and, rarely, **adenocarci-noma** (especially if a bloody nipple discharge is present).

If a mass is noted, its size, location, and other characteristics should be documented and reevaluated over the next one to three menstrual periods. A persistent or slowly growing mass should be evaluated with **fine-needle aspiration**. **Ultrasound** can be helpful in distinguishing cystic from solid masses. **Mammography** is a very poor tool for identifying distinct pathologic lesions in teenagers because the dense breast tissue of adolescents makes interpretation difficult.

Neinstein LS: Review of breast masses in adolescents. Adolesc Pediatr Gynecol 7:119–129, 1994.

7. What causes should be considered in a teenage girl with galactorrhea?

1. Drug-induced—including oral contraceptives, amphetamines, cocaine, marijuana, opi-ates, phenothiazines, reserpine, methyldopa
2. Pregnancy-associated—postabortion or postmiscarriage (may persist up to 3 months), postpartum (if term delivery, may persist up to 1 year)
3. Malignancy—including pituitary adenoma (more likely if serum prolactin is very ele-vated), hypothalamic craniopharyngioma, hypothalamic infiltrative disease (e.g., histiocytosis, sarcoidosis)
4. Hypothyroidism
5. Chronic renal disease (in part due to delayed clearance of prolactin)
6. Chest wall factors—nipple manipulation, surgery, herpes zoster

8. What is the most common cause of chronic pelvic pain in adolescents without a history of pelvic inflammatory disease?

Endometriosis. This condition results from implantation of endometrial tissue at ectopic lo-cations within the peritoneal cavity. The pain is both noncyclic (may occur with intercourse or defecation) and cyclic (often most severe just before menses) and poorly controlled by an-tiprostaglandin medications or oral contraceptives. Intermenstrual bleeding is common. Although adult women classically have tender nodules noted in the posterior vaginal fornix and along the uterosacral ligaments, nodularity is rare in adolescents, which often masks clinical diagnosis. Definitive diagnosis is by laparoscopy and biopsy.

Emans SJH, Goldstein DP: Pediatric and Adolescent Gynecology, 3rd ed. Boston, Little, Brown & Co., 1990, pp 278–289.

9. Why should you ask teenage girls about their cola consumption?

High consumption of carbonated cola beverages (and low milk intake) appears to be associ-ated with increased likelihood of fractures in teenage girls. Data are emerging that development of osteoporosis in women in later life may be strongly influenced by bone changes beginning as early as the teenage years. Thus, simple nutritional changes, such as decreasing carbonated cola intake, may be valuable.

Wyshak G, Frisch RE: Carbonated beverages, dietary calcium, the dietary calcium/phosphorus ratio, and bone fractures in girls and boys. J Adolesc Health 15:210–215, 1994.

10. Discuss the typical clinical picture in teenagers with psychosomatic musculoskeletal pain.

In one large study, 75% were female, the median age was 13 years, and the median duration of symptoms was 1 year. Multiple sites of pain were common, and hyperesthesia occurred in 45%. Nearly all maintained a cheerful affect when complaining of severe pain. Two types of fam-ilies were seen. One was cohesive, stable, and organized but intolerant of separation and auton-omy. The other was chaotic and emotionally unsupportive with high levels of conflict. Nearly all responded favorably to intensive physical and occupational therapy along with individual or family psychotherapy.

Sherry DD, et al: Psychosomatic musculoskeletal pain in children: Clinical and psychological analyses of 100 children. Pediatrics 88:1093–1099, 1991.

11. Should an athlete be allowed back into a game following a concussion?

A general rule is that an athlete who has had any period of unconsciousness or confusion with amnesia following head trauma should not be allowed to return to the event on that day. If there is initial confusion that is not accompanied by amnesia or loss of consciousness (grade 1 concussion), return is permitted if frequent neurologic and mental status evaluations at rest and after exertion (over a 20-minute period) are normal. A second grade 1 concussion in the contest mandates removal without return.

Colorado Medical Society: Guidelines for the Management of Concussion in Sports. Denver, Colorado Medical Society, 1991.

12. Which teenagers get "stingers"?

Most commonly, football players. Stingers, also called burners, are traumatic injuries to the brachial plexus (brachial plexus neuropraxia). They usually result from a head-on collision, as in tackling, which stretches or compresses the brachial plexus with resultant arm pain (such as stinging or burning), paresthesia, or weakness. Although typically transient, recurrent stingers suggest cervical spine pathology.

13. What diagnoses require mandatory disclosure regardless of issues of confidentiality?

In most states:

• Notification to child welfare authorities under state child-abuse (physical and sexual) reporting laws

• Notification to law enforcement officials of gunshot and stab wounds

• Warning from a psychotherapist to a reasonably identifiable victim of a patient's threat of violence

• Notification to parents or other authorities if a patient represents a reasonable threat to himself or herself (i.e., suicidal ideation)

14. What techniques can increase compliance in the adolescent?

- Simplify the regimen
- Discuss potential side effects
- Educate the patient
- Enlist cooperation
- Make the patient responsible
- Use praise liberally
- Avoid confrontation
- Work together with the parents without giving them complete control

15. When can adolescents give their own consent for medical care or procedures?

Teenagers who are married, parents themselves, members of the armed forces, living apart from their parents, or high school graduates may fit the definition of an emancipated or "mature minor." However, that definition varies from state to state. For certain services, many states waive the legal requirement of emancipation, and any individual under age 18 may obtain services without parental permission. These include care for sexually transmitted diseases, contraception services, pregnancy-related care, substance abuse treatment, mental health services, and treatment for rape or sexual assault.

English A: Overcoming obstacles to adolescent care: Legal issues. Adolesc Med State Art Rev 2:429–436, 1991.

16. How does the "HEADSS" system assist in adolescent interviewing?

This mnemonic, devised at the Children's Hospital of Los Angeles, allows a systematic approach to multiple health issues and risk factors affecting teenagers.

H —Home (living arrangements, family relationships)
E —Education (school issues, employment)
A —Activities (friends, exercise, television time)
D —Drugs (personal use, peer use)
S —Sex (orientation, contraception, abuse)
S —Suicide (ideation)

EATING DISORDERS

17. What types of dieting raise concern for the development of an eating disorder?
Dieting that is associated with:
• Decreasing weight goals
• Increasing criticism of the body
• Increasing social isolation
• Amenorrhea or oligomenorrhea
Woodside DB: A review of anorexia nervosa and bulimia nervosa. Curr Probl Pediatr 25:69, 1995.

18. How is the diagnosis of anorexia made?
Anorexia nervosa constitutes a spectrum of psychological, behavioral, and medical abnormalities. The 1994 DSM-IV criteria list four components:
1. Internal fear of becoming obese not diminished by weight loss
2. Distortion of body image ("feeling" fat when emaciated)
3. Refusal to maintain body weight over age/height minimum
4. Amenorrhea in postmenarchal females

19. What are good and bad prognostic indicators for recovery from anorexia?
Good: Early age at onset, high educational achievement, improvement in body image after weight gain.
Poor: Late age at onset, continued overestimation of body size, self-induced vomiting or bulimia, laxative abuse, male.

20. What hormonal features are seen in anorexia nervosa?
Amenorrhea is seen in most cases of anorexia nervosa due to hypothalamic/pituitary dysfunction. Twenty-five percent of affected girls experience amenorrhea before significant weight loss occurs, suggesting the psychological effect on physiology. **Symptoms suggestive of hypothyroidism,** such as constipation, cold intolerance, dry skin, bradycardia, and hair or nail changes, are common. Thyroid studies, however, have relatively normal results, except for a low triiodothyronine (T_3) and increased reverse T_3 (rT_3), a less active isomer. The T_3/rT_3 reversal is also seen in conditions associated with weight loss, possibly indicating it is a physiologic means of adapting to a lower energy state. Other abnormalities include a loss of diurnal variation in cortisol, diminished plasma catecholamine levels, normal or increased growth hormone levels, and a flattened glucose tolerance curve.

21. Describe the psychologic profile of a typical patient with anorexia nervosa.

• Distorted body image	• Overwhelming sense of ineffectiveness
• Poor self-esteem	• Distrustful nature
• Depression	• Self-destructive behavior
• Overachiever, perfectionist	• Difficulty in concentrating
• Strong-willed, determined nature	• Irritability
• Uncommunicative behavior	• Obsessive thoughts about food, eating, and body shape

From Nussbaum MP: Anorexia nervosa. In McAnarney ER, et al (eds): Textbook of Adolescent Medicine. Philadelphia, W.B. Saunders, 1992, p 537; with permission.

22. What causes sudden death in anorectics?
The chronic emaciation affects the myocardium. Anorectics develop depressed cardiovascular functions and an altered conduction system. ECG changes are common, including bradycardia, decreased QRS amplitudes, prolonged QT intervals, and nonspecific ST-segment changes. These ECG changes often occur without underlying electrolyte abnormalities. The arrhythmogenic potential is heightened if electrolytes (specifically potassium) are distorted by excessive vomiting or laxative abuse. Sudden death is likely due to the culmination of chronic myocardial injury in emaciated patients (> 35–40% below ideal weight) with resultant failure and dysrhythmia.

23. How is the diagnosis of bulimia nervosa made?

Bulimia nervosa is a syndrome of voracious, high-caloric overeating and subsequent forced vomiting (by gagging or ipecac) and/or other purging methods (e.g., laxatives, diuretics), often done during periods of frustration or psychological stress. Its incidence is much higher than that of anorexia nervosa, and males are rarely involved. The diagnosis is made by **history**.

24. List the medical complications of bulimia nervosa.

Electrolyte abnormalities: hypokalemia, hypochloremia, and metabolic alkalosis. The hypokalemia can cause a prolonged QT interval and T-wave abnormalities.

Esophageal: acid reflux with esophagitis and (rarely) Mallory-Weiss tear

Cardiac: Use of ipecac can result in cardiomyopathy (due to a toxic effect of one of its principal components, the alkaloid emetine).

CNS: Neurotransmitters can be affected, causing changes in perceptions of satiety.

Miscellaneous: enamel erosion, salivary gland enlargement, cheilosis, and knuckle calluses (signs of recurrent vomiting)

25. How do anorexia nervosa and bulimia nervosa differ?

ANOREXIA NERVOSA	BULIMIA NERVOSA
Vomiting or diuretic/laxative abuse uncommon	Vomiting or diuretic/laxative abuse
Severe weight loss	Less weight loss; avoidance of obesity
Slightly younger	Slightly older
More introverted	More extroverted
Hunger denied	Hunger pronounced
Eating behavior may be considered normal and a source of self-esteem	Eating behavior is egodystonic
Sexually inactive	Sexually active
Obsessional fears with paranoid features	Histrionic features
Amenorrhea	Menses irregular or absent
Death from starvation/suicide	Death from hypokalemia/suicide

From Shenker IR, Bunnell DW: Bulimia nervosa. In McAnarney ER, et al (eds): Textbook of Adolescent Medicine. Philadelphia, W.B. Saunders, 1992, p 545; with permission.

26. What modalities are used to treat eating disorders?

1. **Nutritional rehabilitation**—Very large caloric intakes (e.g., 3000–4000 kcal/day) may be needed to achieve adequate gain. Controversy exists regarding strict versus lenient inpatient protocols. Routine use of appetite stimulants, nasogastric feedings, or hyperalimentation is not recommended.

2. **Medication**—Prokinetic agents (e.g., cisapride, domperidone) are used to minimize postprandial bloating. Antidepressants, including serotonin-specific reuptake inhibitors, are more commonly used in bulimia nervosa.

3. **Psychotherapy**, including family therapy

Woodside DB: A review of anorexia nervosa and bulimia nervosa. Curr Probl Pediatr 25:67–89, 1995.

27. Name the three features constituting the "female athlete triad."

Disordered eating, amenorrhea, and **osteoporosis**. These three distinct yet interrelated disorders are often seen in active girls and young women. All female athletes are at risk for developing this triad, with 15–60% of female athletes demonstrating abnormal weight-control behaviors. Diagnosis is based on history, physical examination, and laboratory evaluation. The basic lab workup should include urine hCG, TSH, prolactin, FSH, LH, testosterone, DHEA-S, and progesterone challenge test. Ongoing counseling is often indicated, as well as nutritional and hormonal intervention. Treatment commonly includes calcium supplements and oral contraceptives.

28. What are the risk factors for obesity in teenagers?

1. Socioeconomic status: Generally, higher socioeconomic status confers a higher likelihood of obesity. This trend is maintained in adulthood for boys but reverses in late adolescence for girls.

2. Parental/sibling obesity: Significantly correlates with the likelihood of obesity.

3. Race: More common among whites than blacks.

4. Family size: Obesity decreases as family size increases and has the greatest prevalence among single children.

5. Television viewing: Increased TV viewing debatably correlates with the likelihood of obesity.

6. Childhood status: Obese children are more likely to become obese teenagers.

Bandini LG: Obesity and the adolescent. Adolesc Med State Art Rev 3:459–471, 1992.

29. Which is a better tool to estimate body fat in an adolescent—body mass index (BMI) or triceps skinfold?

BMI (weight in kg/height in m²) above the 85th percentile has been used to define obesity. However, it can be elevated in individuals with large frames ("big-boned") who are overweight but not overfat.

Triceps skinfold (TSF) correlates better with percent body fat and total body fat in adolescents. A TSF >85% for age, sex, and race is the most widely accepted criterion for obesity. Of note, a problem with the TSF is the variability of technique, which limits the reproducibility of results.

30. Do obese children and adolescents become obese adults?

Only 25–50% in most tracking studies have become obese adults, but in some studies it has ranged as high as 75%. The most important risk factors for persistence of obesity are later age of onset and increased severity of obesity at any age. The problem is very significant and worsening. For the period from 1988–1991, 11% of children and adolescents were > 95th percentile for weight; 22% were > 85th percentile.

Dietz WH, Robinson TN: Assessment and treatment of childhood obesity. Pediatr Rev 14:337–343, 1993.

Troiano RP, et al: Overweight prevalence and trends for children and adolescents. Arch Pediatr Adolesc Med 149:1085, 1995.

31. What cardiac risk factors are present in obese adolescents?

Elevated triglycerides, elevated total cholesterol, decreased HDL cholesterol, hypertension, diminished maximum work capacity, and strong family history of coronary artery disease. The incidence of these associations is not small. In one study, 97% of obese adolescents had at least three risk factors present.

Becque MD, et al: Coronary risk incidence of obese adolescents: Reduction by exercise plus diet intervention. Pediatrics 81:605–612, 1988.

32. What is the long-term outlook for the obese teenager?

Obesity in adolescence is associated with medical, economic, and social consequences. Obese teenagers, especially females, have lower levels of school completion, lower rates of marriage, lower household incomes, and higher rates of poverty. Even if weight corrections occur later, the early obesity is associated with increased atherosclerotic heart disease in men and women, with colorectal cancer and gout in men, and with arthritis in women.

Gortmake SL, et al: Social and economic consequences of overweight in adolescence and young adulthood. N Engl J Med 327:1008–1012, 1992.

Must A, et al: Long-term morbidity and mortality of overweight adolescents: A follow-up of the Harvard Growth Study of 1922 to 1935. N Engl J Med 327:1350–1355, 1992.

33. Are fat distribution measurements of any prognostic value in adolescents?

In adults, the distribution of body fat rather than percent excess of body fat seems to be a better indicator of potential morbidity. For example, when the waist-hip circumference ratio is measured, an adult with a higher ratio (increased abdominal fat or "android" habitus) has a higher frequency of hypertension, diabetes, and hyperlipidemia compared with an equally obese individual with a lower ratio (increased pelvic fat or "gynecoid" habitus). However, prospective long-term data are not available to indicate whether fat distribution measurements have any prognostic significance in adolescents.

MENSTRUAL DISORDERS

34. What is the difference between primary and secondary amenorrhea?

Primary amenorrhea: no onset of menses by age 16, or within 3 years of onset of secondary sex characteristics, or within 1 year of Tanner V breast/pubic hair development

Secondary amenorrhea: no menses for 3 months after previous establishment of regular menstrual periods

35. What causes primary amenorrhea?

The key feature in the differential diagnosis is whether the amenorrhea is associated with the development of secondary sex characteristics.

Amenorrhea without secondary sex characteristics

Chromosomal or enzymatic defects (e.g., Turner syndrome, chromosomal mosaics, 17α-hydroxylase deficiency)

Congenital absence of uterus

Gonadal dysgenesis (with elevated gonadotropins)

Hypothalamic-pituitary abnormalities (with diminished gonadotropins)

Amenorrhea with secondary sex characteristics

Dysfunction of hypothalamic release of GnRH (e.g., stress, excessive exercise, weight loss, chronic illness, polycystic ovary disease, medications, hypothyroidism)

Abnormalities of pituitary gland (e.g., tumor, empty sella syndrome)

Ovarian dysfunction (e.g., irradiation, chemotherapy, trauma, viral infection, autoimmune inflammation)

Abnormalities of genital tract (e.g., cervical agenesis, imperforate hymen, testicular feminization with absent uterus)

Pregnancy

36. How can estrogen influence be evaluated on vaginal or cervical smears?

Vaginal smear: In patients with normal estrogen, 15–30% of cells are superficial (small pyknotic nuclei with large cytoplasm), and the remainder are intermediate (larger nuclei with visible nucleolus, but still with a predominant cytoplasm). If parabasal cells are noted (nuclear: cytoplasmic ratio of $\geq$ 50:50), relative estrogen deficiency should be suspected.

Cervical smear: Cervical mucus is smeared onto a glass slide and allowed to dry. If a fern pattern appears, estrogen is normal (since salts crystallize only if estrogen is unopposed by progesterone). No fern pattern occurs in the second half of menses after ovulation due to the presence of progesterone. Absence of ferning in pregnancy is also due to higher progesterone levels.

37. What is the value of a progesterone challenge test in a patient with amenorrhea?

If bleeding ensues within 2 weeks after the administration of oral medroxyprogesterone (10 mg daily for 5 days) or intramuscular progesterone in oil (50–100 mg), the test is positive. This indicates that the endometrium has been primed by estrogen and that the pituitary-hypothalamic-ovarian axis and outflow tract are functioning.

38. A 14-year-old girl has Tanner III features and monthly abdominal pain but no onset of menstrual flow. What is the likely diagnosis?

An anatomic abnormality of the vagina (e.g., imperforate hymen or transverse vaginal septum) or cervix (e.g., agenesis).

39. An obese 16-year-old has oligomenorrhea, hirsutism, and an elevated LH/FSH ratio. What condition is likely?

Polycystic ovary syndrome. This disorder is characterized by the triad of amenorrhea/ oligomenorrhea, hirsutism, and obesity which begins during puberty. In these individuals, there is an apparent gonadotropin-dependent, functional ovarian hyperandrogenism with elevated LH (or LH:FSH ratio > 3:1) and insulin resistance. A dysregulation of ovarian synthesis of androgens and estrogen is likely. With administration of GnRH, levels of 17-hydroxyprogesterone uniquely rise without evidence of a steroidogenic block.

Franks S: Polycystic ovary syndrome. N Engl J Med 333:853–861, 1995.

40. What constitutes excessive menstrual bleeding in an adolescent?

As a rule, most menstrual periods do not last > 8 days, do not occur more frequently than every 21–40 days, and are not associated with > 80 ml of blood loss. The quantitation can be difficult, as pad or tampon numbers correlate poorly with total blood loss. Blood clots or a change in pad number appears to have more reliability. Suspicion of excessive loss should prompt an evaluation of hematocrit and/or reticulocyte count.

41. How common are anovulatory menstrual periods in adolescents?

Anovulatory cycles (and with them, an increased likelihood of irregular periods) occur in 50% of adolescents for up to 2 years after menarche and in up to 20% after 5 years (the rate in adults). Anovulatory cycles result in unopposed estradiol production which can cause (1) breakthrough bleeding at varying intervals due to insufficient hormone to support a thickened endothelium, and (2) heavy and prolonged menstrual flow due to lack of progesterone. However, most anovulatory menstrual cycles are normal because the intact negative feedback loop (rising estradiol lowers FH and LSH which, in turn, lower estradiol) does not allow prolonged elevated estrogen with endometrial proliferation.

42. Describe the evaluation for a patient with dysfunctional uterine bleeding.

Dysfunctional uterine bleeding is abnormal bleeding in the absence of structural pelvic pathology. It remains a diagnosis of exclusion. Depending on the age of the patient and history of sexual activity, the following studies should be considered:

• Speculum exam for evidence of trauma, vaginal foreign body, DES-induced adenosis
• Bimanual exam for ovarian mass, uterine fibroid, signs of pregnancy or pelvic inflammatory disease
• Pap smear for cervical dysplasia
• Pregnancy test
• Serum prolactin
• Thyroid function tests
• Coagulation studies (especially for von Willebrand disease)

43. Can the timing of abnormal uterine bleeding help identify the most likely cause?

Abnormal bleeding at the normal time of cyclic shedding
Blood dyscrasia (especially von Willebrand disease)
Endometrial pathology (e.g., submucous myoma, intrauterine device)

Abnormal bleeding at any time in the cycle, but normal cycles
Vaginal foreign body
Trauma
Endometriosis
Infection
Uterine polyps
Cervical abnormality (e.g., hemangioma)

Noncyclic bleeding or abnormal cyclic bleeding (< 21 days or > 45 days, usually associated with anovulatory cycles)
Physiologic (especially in early adolescence)
Polycystic ovary disease
Psychosocial pathology
Excessive exercise
Endocrine disorders
Adrenal/ovarian tumors
Ovarian failure

Adapted from Kozlowski K, et al: Adolescent gynecologic conditions presenting in emergency settings. Adolesc Med State Art Rev 5:65, 1993; with permission.

44. How should dysfunctional uterine bleeding be managed?

Management depends on the estimated blood loss as determined by hemoglobin (Hb) concentration and signs of orthostatic hypotension:

1. **No acute hemorrhage, no anemia**
   Expectant management, consider oral contraceptive
   Use of menstrual calendar
   Begin iron supplementation
2. **No acute hemorrhage, mild anemia** (Hb 10–12 gm/dl)
   Oral contraceptive: potent progestin (e.g., norgestrel/ethinyl estradiol) or cyclic
      medroxyprogesterone (e.g., 10 mg for 5–7 days every 35–40 days) with change to
      a less potent progestin when flow is lighter
   Begin iron supplementation
3. **No acute hemorrhage, moderate anemia** (Hb < 10 gm/dl)
   Oral contraceptive: high-dose estrogen (50 µg)–potent progestin combination, since
      severe bleeding may have left little endometrium on which the progestin can act
   Begin iron supplementation
4. **Acute hemorrhage, significant anemia** (Hb 7–9 gm/dl), no orthostatic changes
   Oral contraceptive: high-dose estrogen (50 µg)–potent progestin combination every
      6 hrs for 2 days tapered over 1 wk, with longer-term use likely (after estrogen tapered)
   Consider hospitalization if bleeding is severe
   Clotting studies due to higher likelihood of underlying coagulopathy
5. **Acute hemorrhage, severe anemia** (< 7 gm/dl), orthostatic changes
   Hospitalize for high-dose estrogen intravenously (e.g., 25 mg every 4 hrs for 24 hrs)
      with concurrent oral high-dose progestin
   Consider transfusion
   Unresponsive bleeding may require dilatation and curettage
   Clotting studies

45. Why is dysmenorrhea more common in later adolescence than in early adolescence?

Dysmenorrhea occurs almost entirely with ovulatory cycles. Menses shortly after the onset of menarche is usually anovulatory. With the establishment of more regular ovulatory cycles after 2–4 years, primary dysmenorrhea becomes more likely.

46. In a teenager with dysmenorrhea, what factors suggest an underlying identifiable pathologic problem rather than primary dysmenorrhea?

Primary dysmenorrhea is painful menses without identifiable pelvic pathology and accounts for the vast majority of cases in teenagers. However, underlying pathology is more likely if any of the following conditions is present: menorrhagia (excessive volume or duration of menses); intermenstrual bleeding; pain at times other than menses (suggesting endometriosis); increasing severity of pain with subsequent menses (suggesting outflow obstruction); or abnormal uterine shape on exam (suggesting uterine malformation).

47. Compare the mechanism of action of the two most effective types of treatment for pronounced primary dysmenorrhea.

Prostaglandin inhibitors: evidence strongly supports a key role for prostaglandins in pain production (especially $PGF_2\alpha$ and $PGE_2\alpha$). Naproxen, ibuprofen, and mefenamic acid are all effective. Side effects of indomethacin and phenylbutazone limit their use. Aspirin is no more effective than placebo.

Oral contraceptives: OCs act by reducing endometrial growth, which limits total production of endometrial prostaglandin. Ovulation is suppressed which also minimizes pain. A 30–35 µg combined estrogen-progestin pill is preferred. After 4–6 months, OCs may be stopped and symptoms reassessed if the need for contraception is not an issue.

Polaneczky MM, Slap GB: Menstrual disorders in the adolescent: Dysmenorrhea and dysfunctional uterine bleeding. Pediatr Rev 13:83–87, 1992.

SEXUAL DEVELOPMENT

48. What are the ranges of normal in the stages of pubertal development in boys?

Dr. James Tanner in 1969–70 categorized the progression of stages of puberty, dividing pubertal development in boys into pubic and genital development. Nearly all boys begin puberty with testicular enlargement, followed in about 6 months by pubic hair and then about 6–12 months later by phallic enlargement. For boys, puberty lasts on average 3.5 years.

Tanner Stages of Sexual Maturation in Boys

STAGE	DESCRIPTION	MEAN AGE	AGE RANGE 5–95%
	Pubic Hair		
I	None	—	—
II	Countable; straight; increased pigmentation and length; primarily at base of penis	12	10–14
III	Darker; begins to curl; increased quantity	13	11.25–15
IV	Increased quantity; coarser texture; covers most of pubic area	13.75	12–15.75
V	Adult distribution; spread to medial thighs and lower abdomen	14.5	13–17.5
	Genital Development		
I	Prepubertal	—	—
II	Testicular enlargement (> 4 ml volume); slight rugation of scrotum	11.5	9.5–13.75
III	Further testicular enlargement; penile lengthening begins	12.5	10.25–14.5
IV	Testicular enlargement continues; increased rugation of scrotum; increased penile breadth	13.25	11.25–15.5
V	Adult	14.25	12.5–17

49. What are the ranges of normal in the stages of pubertal development in girls?

Tanner divided pubertal development in girls according to pubic hair and breast development. About 85% of girls begin puberty with initiation of breast enlargement, while 15% have axillary hair as the first sign. Menarche usually occurs about 18–24 months after the onset of breast development. For girls, the duration of puberty is longer than boys and averages 4.5 years.

Tanner Stages of Sexual Maturation in Girls

STAGE	DESCRIPTION	MEAN AGE	AGE RANGE 5–95%
	Pubic Hair		
I	None	—	—
II	Countable; straight; increased pigmentation and length; primarily on medial border of labia	11.25	9–13.5
III	Darker; begins to curl; increased quantity on mons pubis	12	9.5–14.25
IV	Increased quantity; coarser texture; labia and mons well covered	12.5	10.5–15
V	Adult distribution with feminine triangle and spread to medial thighs	14	12–16.5
	Breast Development		
I	None	—	—
II	Breast bud present; increased areolar size	11	9–13
III	Further enlargement of breast; no secondary contour	12	10–14
IV	Areolar area forms secondary mound on breast contour	13	10.5–15.5
V	Mature; areolar area is part of breast contour; nipple projects	15	13–18
Menarche		12.8	11–14.5

50. At what Tanner stage does the female and male adolescent growth spurt begin?

In females, the maximum growth spurt typically occurs at Tanner stage IV (usually around age 12.25). In boys, it also occurs at Tanner stage IV (usually around age 13.5).

51. How has the average age of menarche changed in the United States over the past century?

Since 1950, the average age has been 12.8 years. In 1877, the average age was 14.75 years and a downward trend of about three months per decade began. This decline has been attributed to an improved standard of living with reduced levels of both undernutrition and strenuous physical exercise (two factors which delay menarche).

Wyshak G, Frisch RE: Evidence for a secular trend in age of menarche. N Engl J Med 306:1033–1035, 1982.

52. When do boys develop the ability to reproduce?

The average age of spermarche (as demonstrated by the presence of spermatozoa in first morning urine) is 13.3 years. Unlike in girls in whom menarche follows the peak height velocity, in boys spermarche occurs before the growth spurt.

53. When is delayed sexual development a concern?

The first easily recognizable sign of puberty in most females is a breast bud, which occurs at a mean age of 11 years. In boys, it is testicular enlargement, which on average begins at 11.5 years. Evaluation should be considered in girls with no breast development by 13 years or no menarche by 15 years and in boys with no testicular enlargement by age 14. By statistical definition, this is 3% of teenagers.

54. Why should you test the sense of smell in a teenager with delayed puberty?

Kallmann syndrome is characterized by a defect in GnRH with resultant gonadotropin deficiency and hypogonadism. Maldevelopment of the olfactory lobes occurs, with resultant anosmia or hyposmia. Less commonly, cleft palate, congenital deafness, and color blindness can occur. These patients require hormonal therapy to achieve puberty and fertility.

55. Which tests do you consider in a boy or girl with delayed puberty?

If history or physical examination do not suggest an underlying cause (e.g., anorexia nervosa), tests should include LH, FSH, testosterone (male), and bone age. These tests will help categorize the condition as hypergonadotropic (implying possible gonadal defects, androgen insensitivity, or enzyme defects) or hypogonadotropic (implying constitutional delay or primary hypothalamic-pituitary problems).

Further testing is predicated on the results of these initial tests. For example, a 14½-year-old male with a bone age of 11.5 and a total testosterone of 23 ng/dl (normal prepubertal level is < 10) will probably begin to show outward evidence of puberty within the next few months. Therefore, no further studies are warranted. On the other hand, if this boy had a bone age of 12.5, testosterone < 10 ng/dl, and no elevation of LH and FSH, specific testing of the hypothalamic-pituitary axis is indicated.

56. Can puberty be safely accelerated?

In some teenagers, more commonly boys, the constitutional delay in puberty has significant psychological effects. Studies have shown that in **boys**, puberty can be accelerated without any compromise in expected adult height. In boys aged > 14 with plasma testosterone levels of < 10 nmol/L, testosterone enanthate, 50–100 mg IM, can be given monthly for 4–6 months. Treatment for **girls** who are constitutionally-delayed is less well studied. Conjugated estrogen, 0.3 mg (e.g., Premarin), or ethinyl estradiol (5–10 μg) daily for 2–3 months has been used in females aged > 13 without breast buds.

57. When do lesbians and gay males begin to personalize homosexuality?

During adolescence. For this reason, health providers need to be sensitive not to assume sexual identities during their interactions with teenagers.

Friedman RC, Downey JI: Homosexuality. N Engl J Med 331:923–930, 1994.

SEXUALLY TRANSMITTED DISEASES

58. How does the prevalence of sexually transmitted diseases (STDs) in adolescents compare with that in adults?

Among sexually active individuals, adolescents have a **higher likelihood** than adults of being infected with an STD. About 25% of adolescents will contract at least one STD by the time of high school graduation. Reasons for the increased susceptibility include:

1. Cervical ectropion: *Neisseria gonorrhoeae* and and *Chlamydia trachomatis* more readily infect columnar epithelium, and the adolescent ectocervix has more of this type of epithelium than does that of an adult.

2. Cervical metaplasia in the transformation zone (from columnar to squamous epithelium) is more susceptible to human papillomavirus infection.

3. Less frequent use of barrier methods of contraception

59. What is considered the most common STD in teenagers?

Human papillomavirus (HPV) affects 20–40% of sexually active adolescent females. More than 60 HPV types have been identified, with variable presentations including anogenital condyloma acuminatum and cervical infection which may lead to cervical dysplasia. In the latter infection, the association of HPV with the potential for cervical carcinoma increases the urgency of screening for HPV in sexually active teenagers. Visualization of anogenital warts can be enhanced by wetting the area with 3–5% acetic acid (vinegar), which whitens the lesions. HPV is also a cause of non-sexually transmitted disease, including deep plantar warts, palmar warts, and common warts.

60. Is the presence of an ectropion noted on pelvic exam a concern?

An ectropion is the outward rolling of a margin. A cervical ectropion is the extension of the erythematous columnar epithelium from the os onto the duller, pink cervix. It is a relatively common finding in adolescents. However, large ectropions extending to the vaginal wall or abnormal cervical shape can be associated with diethylstilbestrol (DES) exposure in utero or chronic cervicitis.

61. Which teenage girls should have Pap smears done?

Although carcinoma is rare in teenagers, cervical dysplasia is not. This is due in large part to the widespread acquisition of HPV, of which a number of subtypes are rapidly oncogenic. All females who are sexually active and/or ≥ 18 years of age should have at least an annual Pap test. Because the false-negative rate of the test can be up to 30%, those teenagers at particularly high risk (e.g., multiple sexual partners, recurrent STDs) should be considered for more frequent testing.

62. How can you minimize the chance of a false-negative Pap smear?

1. Lubricate the speculum with warm water only (avoid lubricating gels)

2. Obtain endocervical specimen with cytobrush rather than cotton-tipped swab for greater collection of cells

3. Fix slides immediately to avoid drying artifacts

4. Paired cervical smears increase the yield (but also the cost)

63. Which teenagers should have colposcopic evaluation?

1. Abnormal Pap smear

2. Condyloma acuminatum in the patient or partner

3. High-risk sexual behavior (e.g., multiple sexual partners with little or no barrier-method contraception)

64. Describe the appearance of condylomata acuminata.

Condylomata acuminata (anogenital warts) are soft, fleshy, wet, polypoid or pedunculated papules that appear in the genital and perianal area. They may coalesce and take on a cauliflower appearance.

65. How do you treat condylomata acuminata and HPV infection?

A common approach is 20% podophyllin resin in benzoin applied carefully and washed off completely in 3–6 hours, but failure rates can be > 50%. Other approaches include liquid nitrogen, 85% trichloroacetic acid, topical 5-fluorouracil, alpha-interferon, and ablative therapy.

66. A sexually active 17-year-old woman with adnexal and right-upper-quadrant (RUQ) tenderness likely has what condition?

Fitz-Hugh–Curtis syndrome. This is a perihepatitis caused by gonococci or, less commonly, chlamydiae. It should be suspected in any patient with pelvic inflammatory disease (PID) who has RUQ tenderness. It may be mistaken for acute hepatitis or cholecystitis. The pathophysiology is felt to be direct spread from a pelvic infection along the paracolic gutters to the liver, where inflammation develops and capsular adhesions form (the so-called "violin string" adhesions seen on surgical exploration). If RUQ pain persists despite treatment for PID, ultrasonography should be done to rule out a periphepatic abscess.

67. A teenage girl develops migratory polyarthritis, fever, and scattered petechial lesions several days prior to menses. What condition should be suspected?

Gonococcal-arthritis-dermatitis syndrome (GADS). Following a migratory polyarthritis or polyarthralgia, the arthritis settles in one or two large joints. The patient then develops painful tenosynovitis over the tendon sheaths, in addition to a characteristic crop of embolic skin lesions over the trunk and extremities. Diagnosis is confirmed by culturing gonococci from blood, synovial fluid, and/or oral, rectal, or genitourinary sites.

68. What are the clinical criteria for pelvic inflammatory disease?

All three of the following must be present:

  History of lower abdominal pain and presence of abdominal tenderness, with or without rebound tenderness
  Tenderness with motion of the cervix and uterus
  Adnexal tenderness

Plus one or more of the following:

  Temperature ≥ 38°C
  White blood cell (WBC) count ≥ 10,500/mm^3
  Erythrocyte sedimentation rate > 15 mm/hr
  Evidence of *Neisseria gonorrhoeae* and/or *Chlamydia trachomatis* in endocervix: Gram stain from the endocervix positive for gram-negative intracellular diplococci or a monoclonal-directed smear positive for *Chlamydia* (or similar rapid tests) or > 5 WBCs/oil immersion field on Gram stain of endocervical discharge
  Pelvic abscess or inflammatory complex on bimanual examination or by sonography
  Purulent material (WBCs present) from peritoneal cavity by culdocentesis or laparoscopy

From Chacko MR, Woods CR: Gynecologic infections in childhood and adolescence. In Feigin RD, Cherry JD (eds): Pediatric Infectious Diseases, 3rd ed. Philadelphia, W.B. Saunders, 1992, p 536; with permission.

69. What are the sequelae of pelvic inflammatory disease (PID)?

Twenty-five percent of patients who have had PID will have one or more major sequelae of the disease, including:

  1. Tubo-ovarian abscess—approximately 20% of all adolescents with PID
  2. Recurrent infection
  3. Chronic abdominal pain—may include exacerbated dysmenorrhea and dyspareunia related to pelvic adhesions, which occur in approximately 20% of patients with PID
  4. Ectopic pregnancy—risk is increased 7–10-fold
  5. Infertility—up to 15% after 1 episode of PID, 35% after 2 episodes, and 50% after ≥ 3 episodes

Paradise JE, Grant L: Pelvic inflammatory disease in adolescents. Pediatr Rev 13:216–223, 1992.

70. Why should adolescents with PID be hospitalized for intravenous antibiotics?

1. Aggressive IV therapy may limit tubal scarring, thus lowering likelihood of infertility or ectopic pregnancy (particularly in nulliparous teenagers with first-episode PID).

2. High risk of tubo-ovarian abscess (up to 20%), with potential for acute rupture and surgical emergency, warrants frequent clinical evaluations.

3. Clinical diagnosis is often in error (up to one-third of cases of "clinical" PID are not verifiable by laparoscopy).

4. Compliance by teenagers on outpatient therapy is notoriously lax.

71. Does the risk of PID vary with the type of contraception used?
Decreased risk
   Condom
   Diaphragm (or other barrier method) with spermicide
   Oral contraceptives (which thicken cervical mucus, providing more of a barrier to bacteria
      and sperm)
Increased risk
   Intrauterine device
   McCormack WM: Pelvic inflammatory disease. N Engl J Med 330:115–119, 1994.

72. When do STDs occur in relation to menses?

Gonorrhea is much more likely to present during menstruation. Of patients with gonorrhea, 85% develop symptoms during the first 7 days of menses, compared with only 33% with chlamydia infection.

73. How are the genital ulcer syndromes differentiated?

Genital ulcers may be seen in herpes simplex, syphilis, chancroid, lymphogranuloma venereum, and granuloma inguinale (donovanosis). Herpes and syphilis are the most common, and granuloma inguinale is very rare. Although there is overlap, clinical distinction is as follows:

Differentiation of Genital Ulcer Syndromes

	HERPES SIMPLEX	SYPHILIS (PRIMARY, SECONDARY)	CHANCROID	LYMPHOGRANULUM VENEREUM (LGV)
Agent	Herpes simplex virus	*Treponema pallidum*	*Haemophilus ducreyi*	*Chlamydia trachomatis*
Primary lesions	Vesicle	Papule	Papule-pustule	Papule-vesicle
Size (mm)	1-2	5–15	2–20	2–10
Number	Multiple, clusters (coalesce ±)	Single	Multiple (coalesce ±)	Single
Depth	Superficial	Superficial or deep	Deep	Superficial or deep
Base	Erythematous, nonpurulent	Sharp, indurated, nonpurulent	Ragged border, purulent, friable	Varies
Pain	Yes	No	Yes	Yes
Lymphadenopathy	Tender, bilateral	Nontender, bilateral	Tender, unilateral, may suppurate, unilocular fluctuance	Tender, unilateral, may suppurate, multilocular fluctuance

From Shafer MA: Sexually transmitted disease syndromes. In McAnarney ER, et al (eds): Textbook of Adolescent Medicine. Philadelphia, W.B. Saunders, 1992, p 708; with permission.

74. What is the value of oral acyclovir in the treatment of genital herpes infections in immunocompetent hosts?
   • Useful mainly in primary episode of disease
   • Lessens duration of pain and itching

- Lessens number of new lesions
- Hastens crusting of old lesions
- Shortens viral shedding (and thus may shorten period of contagion)
- Delays and reduces frequency of recurrences while on therapy

Acyclovir appears to be safe when used in adults for up to 3 years, but long-term studies of its toxicity have not been done. Thus, chronic administration should not be used for prophylaxis in individuals who have mild disease. Topical therapy also provides similar benefits for individuals with primary disease. However, it does not reduce the frequency of recurrences and is less effective for symptoms of recurrent disease.

75. What is a treatment regimen for genital herpes?

For the first episode, oral acyclovir is given at a dose of 200 mg five times a day for 10 days. For recurrent genital herpes, early therapy with oral acyclovir is given at a dose of 200 mg five times a day for 5 days. Suppressive therapy (400 mg twice daily) is indicated in patients with > 6 episodes/year or in patients with < 6 episodes if severe (lasting ≥ 3 weeks).

76. How are the three most common causes of postpubertal vaginitis clinically distinguished?

- Candidal vaginitis: vulvar itching and erythema, vaginal discharge (thick, white, curdlike)
- Trichomonas vaginitis: vulvar itching and erythema, vaginal discharge (gray, yellow-green, frothy; rarely malodorous)
- Bacterial vaginosis: minimal erythema, vaginal discharge (malodorous; thin white discharge clings to vaginal walls)

77. How does the vaginal pH help indicate the cause of a vaginal discharge?

Ordinarily, the vaginal pH of a pubertal girl is < 4.5 (compared with 7.0 in prepubertal girls). If the pH is > 4.5, infection with *Trichomonas* or bacterial vaginosis should be suspected.

78. How does evaluation of the vaginal discharge help distinguish the three?

	Candidal Vaginitis	Trichomonas Vaginitis	Bacterial Vaginosis
pH	≤ 4.5	≥ 5.0	≥ 5.0
KOH prep	Mycelia pseudohyphae	Normal	Fishy odor (Pos. "whiff" test)
NaCl prep	Few WBCs	Many WBCs Motile trichomonads	Few WBCs Clue cells

79. What are "clue cells"?

Clue cells are vaginal epithelial cells to which are attached many bacteria. This gives the cell a stippled appearance when viewed in a normal saline preparation. Clue cells are characteristic, but not diagnostic, of bacterial vaginosis.

80. What is the etiology of bacterial vaginosis?

Formerly called nonspecific, gardnerella, or haemophilus vaginitis, bacterial vaginosis is the replacement of normal vaginal lactobacilli with a variety of bacteria, including *Gardnerella vaginalis*, genital mycoplasmas, and anaerobic species. *G. vaginalis* can be found in small numbers in up to 30% of nonsexually active adolescents, so vaginal cultures are of limited value.

81. What is the most common STD in sexually active teenage males?

Urethritis, both gonococcal and nongonococcal. Nongonococcal urethritis, particularly that due to *Chlamydia trachomatis*, is more common and is often asymptomatic. Other less common causes of nongonococcal urethritis include *Ureaplasma urealyticum, Trichomonas vaginalis*, herpes simplex, human papillomavirus, and yeast.

82. How should asymptomatic, sexually active teenage males be screened for urethritis?

Although the most exact screening method is to obtain urethral swabs for culture or antigen testing, this method is considered invasive and not cost-effective. Since *Chlamydia trachomatis* is the most common cause of asymptomatic urethritis, a recommended strategy is to obtain 15 ml of unspun first-void urine and test it for leukocyte esterase (a dipstick test for the presence of WBCs). If positive, more specific studies (e.g., enzyme immunoassay, direct fluorescent antibody, or culture) can be done for *C. trachomatis* on spun urine or a urethral swab. This approach is about 70% sensitive. Generally, unless a precise STD exposure is known, studies for gonorrhea are not done because this organism is more commonly associated with symptoms (dysuria or penile discharge).

Shafer MA, et al: Evaluation of urine-based screening strategies to detect *Chlamydia trachomatis* among sexually active asymptomatic males. JAMA 270:2065–2070, 1993.

SUBSTANCE ABUSE

83. What are the four types of alcohol and drug use by teenagers?
1. Experimental—weekend beer or marijuana use at parties
2. Recreational—weekday use and progression to harder drugs, liquor
3. Problematic—daily use; personality changes noted; difficulties at school and with family
4. Addictive—most time under the influence of drugs or alcohol; frequent legal problems

84. When should drug users be referred for professional evaluation and counseling?

Referral or more extensive evaluation depends on the age and development of the adolescent. At any age, the recreational, problematic, or addictive user warrants professional intervention. The younger adolescent may also benefit from evaluation at the experimental stage, if only in an effort to postpone such behavior.

85. Should an adolescent be screened for drug abuse without his or her consent?

This is an area of contention. The official position of the American Academy of Pediatrics is that testing not be done without consent in a competent older adolescent, even if a parent wishes otherwise. Others have argued that a teenager's right to privacy and confidentiality does not supersede potential risks of serious damage from drug abuse, particularly if there is strong clinical suspicion or parental concerns. The legal ramifications are evolving and vary from state to stage. In 1995, the U.S. Supreme Court ruled that random drug testing of high school athletes was legal.

86. A teenager who is being screened for drug abuse submits a suspicious urine specimen for testing. How can you tell if it is urine?
- pH should be 4.6–8.0.
- Temperature should range between 90.5 and 98.6°F (32.5–37°C).
  Urine submitted at body temperature will exceed 90.5°F (32.5°C) for 15–20 minutes. If the temperature is below this level in first 4 minutes, the specimen should be considered suspect.
- Urine creatinine concentration should exceed 0.2 mg/ml.
- Urine specific gravity should be not < 1.003.

87. How long do illicit drugs remain detectable in urine specimens?

There is variability depending on a patient's hydration status and method of intake, but as a rule, metabolites can be detected after ingestion as follows:

Amphetamines	48 hrs	Marijuana	3 days for light smoker
Barbiturates (short acting)	24 hrs		21–27 days for heavy smoker
Benzodiazepines	3 days	Morphine	48 hours
Cocaine	2–3 days	Phencyclidine	3 days for casual use
			8 days for heavy use

Of note, most urine screens are very sensitive and may detect drugs up to 99% of the time in concentrations established as analytic cutoff points. However, the screens can be much less specific, sometimes with false-positive rates up to 35%. Therefore, second tests utilizing the analytic methodology most specific for the suspected drug should be used.

AAP Task Force on Substance Abuse: Substance Abuse: A Guide for Health Professionals. Elk Grove Village, IL: American Academy of Pediatrics, 1988, p 55.

88. What factors increase the likelihood of teenage alcohol and/or drug abuse?

1. Peer use
2. School problems (school failure, poor school achievement)
3. Psychologic problems (rebelliousness, early antisocial behavior)
4. Age at first experimentation (particularly age < 15 yrs associated with later drug use)

89. What types of drinking behavior are concerning for the development of alcoholism in teenagers?

Patterns of drinking: drinking before going to a party, morning drinking to overcome a hangover, frequent loss of control with drinking, drinking at school, drinking more than peers, mixing of drugs with alcohol to achieve a stronger high

Drinking-related behaviors: marked personality changes while drinking, development of blackouts or temporary amnesia, drinking-related arrests, drinking-related fights, guilt about drinking

Werner MJ, Adger HA: Early identification, screening and brief intervention for adolescent alcohol use. Arch Pediatr Adolesc Med 149:1241–1248, 1995.

90. What is the genetic predisposition of alcoholism?

A male child of an alcoholic father is four times more likely to become an alcoholic. If a monozygotic twin is an alcoholic, the likelihood of the other twin becoming an alcoholic is 55%; for dizygotic twins, it is 25%.

91. Which type of substance abuse is more common in younger adolescents than older adolescents?

Inhalants. Up to 20% of 8th graders in some surveys report recent use of inhalants, compared with about 15% of 12th graders. A variety of inhalants are abused, including aliphatic hydrocarbons (e.g., gasoline, butane in cigarette lighters), aromatic hydrocarbons (e.g., benzene and toluene in glues and acrylic paints), alkyl halides (e.g., methylene chloride and trichloroethylene in paint thinners and spot removers) and ketones (e.g., acetone in nail polish remover).

Henretig F: Inhalant abuse in children and adolescents. Pediatr Ann 25:47–52, 1996.

92. What are the toxicities of chronic marijuana use?

Pulmonary: Decreased pulmonary function. Compared to cigarette smoke, marijuana smoke contains more carcinogens and respiratory irritants and produces higher carboxyhemoglobin levels and greater tar deposition. Long-term studies will determine if there is a link between chronic marijuana smoke exposure and lung cancer.

Endocrine: Associated with decreased sperm count and motility. May interfere with hypothalamic/pituitary function and increase likelihood of anovulation. Antagonizes insulin, which may affect diabetic management.

Behavioral: Short-term memory impairment, interference with learning, possible "amotivational syndrome"

Brown RT, Coupey SM: Illicit drugs of abuse. Adolesc Med State Art Rev 4:321–325, 1993.

93. Teenagers who report the use of "peace pills," "angel dust," or "gorilla biscuits" are likely referring to what illicit drug?

Phencyclidine (PCP). Related to the anesthetic drug ketamine, PCP is categorized as an hallucinogen. It should be considered as a possible cause if a teenager presents with a distorted thought process and signs of nystagmus, hypertension, ataxia, and miotic pupils.

94. Describe the possible clinical picture and management strategy for acute cocaine intoxication.

Presentation and Management of Acute Cocaine Intoxication

	CLINICAL FEATURES	MANAGEMENT
Cardiovascular	Chest pain, tachycardia, hypertension, dysrhythmias	Phenytoin or cardioversion for dysrhythmias; nitroprusside or labetalol for hypertension
Respiratory	Tachypnea leading to apnea	Ventilatory support as needed; naloxone if concurrent opiate use is suspected
Neurologic	Mydriasis, hyperreflexia, seizures, coma, flaccid paralysis	Diazepam or lorazepam for seizures
Metabolic	Acidosis, hyperthermia	Aggressive treatment of acidosis; cooling blanket
Psychiatric	Euphoria, anxiety, panic, suicidal or homicidal behavior	Careful observation; possible benzodiazepine therapy

Farrar HC, Kearns GL: Cocaine: Clinical pharmacology and toxicology. J Pediatr 115:665–675, 1989.

95. List the potential side effects of anabolic steroids.

Endocrine: in males—testicular atrophy, oligospermia, gynecomastia; in females—hirsutism, masculinization
Musculoskeletal: premature epiphyseal closure
Dermatologic: acne, alopecia, temporal hair recession
Hepatic: impaired excretory function with cholestatic jaundice, elevated LFTs peliosis hepatitis (a form of hepatitis in which hepatic lobules have microscopic pools of blood), benign and malignant tumors
Cardiovascular: hypertension, decreased HDL cholesterol, increased LDL cholesterol
Psychologic: aggressive behavior, mood swings, increased libido

Bagatell CJ, Bremner WJ: Androgens in men—Uses and abuses. N Engl J Med 334:707–714, 1996.
Johnson MD: Steroids. Adolesc Med State Art Rev 2:79–92, 1991.

96. If a teenager is using anabolic steroids, what is the risk of other substance abuse?

The use of anabolic steroids is associated with a wide range of illicit substance abuse (especially cocaine and marijuana), alcohol and tobacco use (both cigarettes and smokeless tobacco), and the use of shared needles. If a teenager is suspected of anabolic steroid use, the likelihood of abuse of other compounds should be considered.

Durant RH, et al: Use of multiple drugs among adolescents who use anabolic steroids. N Engl J Med 328:922–926, 1993.

97. What are the risks of smokeless tobacco?

Due to the decreased gingival blood flow caused by nicotine, chronic ischemia and necrosis can occur. Chronic use results in gingival recession and inflammation, periodontal disease, and oral leukoplakia (a premalignant change). The risk of oral and pharyngeal cancer is increased. Although more commonly used by males, smokeless tobacco used by pregnant females may be associated with low-birthweight infants and premature birth. Smokeless tobacco, as with cigarettes, is also addictive.

98. What impact does cigarette advertising have on adolescents?

Approximately 3 million adolescents smoke a total of 1 billion packs of cigarettes yearly. The average age of their first cigarette is 14.5 years, and of these, nearly 70% are regular smokers by age 18. While peer influences are significant factors, advertising plays a major role. In 1993, the three most heavily advertised brands were Marlboro, Camel, and Newport. These three were also the brands smoked by > 85% of surveyed adolescents.

CDC: Changes in the cigarette brand preferences of adolescent smokers—United States, 1989–1993. MMWR 43:577–581, 1994.

99. How does nicotine withdrawal present in teenagers?

Nicotine withdrawal can occur abruptly, within 2 hours of last use, peaking at 24 hours and persisting for weeks. Symptoms include a strong desire for nicotine, irritability, frustration, anger, anxiety, depression, difficulty in concentrating, restlessness, increased appetite, headache, and GI disturbances. Signs include decreased heart rate, weight gain, slow waves on electroencephalogram, decreased catecholamine levels, decreased metabolic rates, and alteration of REM sleep patterns.

Nicotine is a reinforcing and addicting drug, and in teenagers (as in adults), attempts at discontinuing cigarettes have multiple physiologic consequences. Therefore, in addition to behavior-modifying techniques, pharmacologic treatments (e.g., nicotine replacement patches) should be considered.

Miller NS, Cocores JA: Nicotine dependence: Diagnosis, chemistry, and pharmacologic treatments. Pediatr Rev 14:275–279, 1993.

TEENAGE MALE DISORDERS

100. How common is gynecomastia in teenage boys?

As many as 75% of boys aged 12–14.5 years have some breast development. In about 25%, it lasts for > 1 year, and in 7%, for > 2 years. It occurs most commonly during Tanner genital stage II–III and usually consists of subareolar enlargement (breast bud). It may be unilateral or bilateral. The breast bud may be tender, indicating recent rapid growth of tissue. Obese boys often have breast enlargement due to the deposition of adipose tissue, and differentiation from gynecomastia (true breast budding) is sometimes difficult.

101. Why does gynecomastia occur so commonly?

Early in puberty, production of estrogen (a stimulator of ductal proliferation) increases relatively faster than that of testosterone (an inhibitor of breast development). This slight imbalance causes the breast enlargement. In obese teenagers, the enzyme aromatase, found in higher concentrations in adipose tissue, converts testosterone to estrogen.

102. What drugs are associated with gynecomastia?

   C: Calcium-channel blockers: verapamil, nifedipine
   H: Hormonal medications: anabolic steroids, oral contraceptives
   E: Experimental/illicit drugs: marijuana, heroin, amphetamines, methadone
   S: pSychoactive drugs: phenothiazines, tricyclic antidepressants, diazepam
   T: Testosterone antagonists: spironolactone, ranitidine, cimetidine, ketoconazole

103. What other entities besides drugs are associated with gynecomastia?

The overwhelming majority of cases of gynecomastia in adolescent males occur as part of normal pubertal development. In addition to drugs, other causes include:

- Recovery from chronic disease
- Inadequate androgen production—Klinefelter syndrome, testicular failure, isolated LH deficiency (fertile eunuch)
- Excess estrogen production—feminizing tumors (usually adrenal)
- Pseudo-gynecomastia—carcinoma of the breast, neurofibromatosis, hemangiomas, lipomas, abscess, bruise
- Other—pituitary tumor, testicular tumor, hypo- or hyperthyroidism, liver disease

Braunstein GD: Gynecomastia. N Engl J Med 492:490–495, 1993.

104. Which boys with gynecomastia warrant further evaluation?
  • Prepubertal boys
  • Pubertal-age boys with little or no virilization and small testes
  • Hepatomegaly or abdominal mass palpated
  • Child with CNS complaints
Evaluations may include testing for hypothalamic or pituitary disease, feminizing tumors of the adrenal or testes, and genetic abnormalities (e.g., Klinefelter syndrome). Of note, although breast cancer is nearly reportable if it occurs in boys and is extremely rare in men (0.2%), in patients with Klinefelter syndrome, the rate increases to 3–6%.

105. What treatment options are available for developmental gynecomastia?
Treatment usually depends on the amount of breast tissue present and the degree of psychological problems that this causes. There are three primary options:
    1. Reassurance. Explanation of the process and expected resolution usually suffices for most adolescents. They should be told that resolution can take up to 24 months.
    2. Medications. These may include antiestrogens (clomiphene citrate, tamoxifen), aromatase inhibitors (testolactone), non-aromatizable androgens (dihydrotestosterone), and weak androgens (danazol).
    3. Surgery. This should be done by a plastic surgeon who has experience in breast reduction.

106. What are the clinical manifestations of testicular torsion?
Testicular torsion in adolescents usually presents with acute-onset hemiscrotal pain that radiates to the groin and lower abdomen. Nausea and vomiting are common, but fever is rare. The testis is acutely tender and swollen and may be high-riding. The cremasteric reflex is absent. Many patients report previous episodes of severe acute scrotal pain. Radionuclide imaging of the scrotum with Tc-99m pertechnetate and/or color Doppler ultrasound demonstrates low or absent blood flow and can be helpful in equivocal cases. However, testis salvage depends on timely restoration of blood flow, and obtaining such studies should not delay a highly suspect case from surgical exploration. The spermatic cord sometimes can be untwisted manually, giving temporary relief, but surgical exploration is still required for fixation to prevent recurrence. Both testes may be secured since the underlying suspension defect is often bilateral.

107. How is testicular torsion clinically differentiated from other causes of the acute painful scrotum?
Epididymitis: Usually slower in onset; pain initially localized to epididymis, but as inflammation spreads, whole testis may become painful; not usually associated with vomiting; pain does not usually radiate to the groin; usually associated with dysuria, pyuria, and discharge; often caused by *Neisseria gonorrhoeae* and *Chlamydia trachomatis;* history of STDs is suggestive; unusual in prepubertal boys and in nonsexually active teenagers
Orchitis: Usually slower in onset; often systemic symptoms (nausea, vomiting, fever, chills) secondary to diffuse viral infection; in mumps, occurs about 4–6 days after parotitis; bilateral involvement more common
Torsion of appendix testis: Sudden onset of pain; localized tender nodule at upper pole (often with bluish discoloration); nausea and vomiting uncommon
Incarcerated hernia: Acute onset; pain not localized to hemiscrotum; usually palpable inguinal mass; testes not painful; symptoms and signs of bowel obstruction (vomiting, abdominal distension, guarding, rebound tenderness)

108. How does the Prehn sign help distinguish between epididymitis and testicular torsion?
Classically, relief of pain with elevation of the testis (negative Prehn sign) is associated with epididymitis, while persistent pain (positive Prehn sign) is more indicative of testicular torsion. However, there is considerable overlap, and this relatively nonspecific sign should be interpreted in the context of other signs and symptoms.

109. If complete testicular torsion has occurred, how long before irreversible changes develop?

Irreversible changes develop in 4–6 hours. However, it is clinically impossible to distinguish partial from complete torsion, and thus duration of symptoms should not be used as a gauge for determining viability. Duration of symptoms does correlate with abnormal testicles on follow-up examination, underscoring the need for prompt diagnosis. Two-thirds of patients with testicles salvaged between 12 and 24 hours after the onset of symptoms have palpable evidence of testicular atrophy on follow-up, compared with only 10% when the diagnosis is made in < 6 hours.

110. What is the most frequent solid cancer in older adolescent males?

Testicular cancer. The most common type is a seminoma which, if detected when confined to the testicle (stage I), has a cure rate of up to 97% with orchiectomy and radiation. Although its overall effectiveness is debated, most authorities recommend that all adolescent males be taught testicular self-examination so that irregularities or changes in size can be noted early.

111. What is the significance of a varicocele in a teenager?

A varicocele is an enlargement of the veins of the spermatic cord which results in a boggy enlargement ("bag of worms") of the upper scrotum. About 15% of boys aged 10–15 years have a varicocele, and in 2%, the varicoceles are very large. Most are asymptomatic. Longitudinal studies of adolescents show that large varicoceles may interfere with normal testicular growth and result in decreased spermatogenesis. Surgical correction can prevent the progressive damage. If a varicocele is very large, causing pain, or associated with asymmetric testicular volume, surgical referral is advisable.

Kass EJ, Reitelman C: Adolescent varicocele. Urol Clin North Am 22:151–159, 1995.

112. On which side do varicoceles more commonly occur?

The left side. The left spermatic vein drains into the left renal vein, and the right spermatic vein drains into the inferior vena cava. These hemodynamics favor higher left-sided pressures, which predispose to left-sided varicoceles.

113. An adolescent who boasts of his overpowering "hircismus" is likely in need of what corrective action?

Both a dictionary and a shower. Hircismus is offensive axillary odor.

TEENAGE PREGNANCY

114. How common is teenage pregnancy in the United States?

About 1 in 10 girls and young women under age 20 years become pregnant each year (about 1 million pregnancies). The likelihood that an adolescent will become pregnant before age 20 is about 1 in 4. Up to 90% are unplanned. About 50% of pregnancies progress to delivery, 35% are terminated by abortion, and 15% end by miscarriage.

115. If a teenager has been pregnant once, how likely is she to become pregnant again during her teenage years?

Repeat adolescent pregnancy is common. Up to 30% become pregnant again within 1 year, and 25–50% during the second year. Factors associated with a likely second teen pregnancy include age < 16 years at first conception, boyfriend > 20 years, school dropout, below expected grade level at the time of first pregnancy, welfare dependency after the first pregnancy, complications during the first pregnancy, and departure from the hospital without birth control.

Stevens-Simon C, White MM: Adolescent pregnancy. Pediatr Ann 20:322–331, 1991.

116. What are the risks for infants of teenage mothers?

Teenage mothers have a disproportionately increased risk of having babies who are low-birth-weight, premature, or small-for-gestational age. In addition, infant mortality is two to three times greater for infants of teenage mothers. Studies conflict as to whether these risks are due to inherent biologic difficulties with pregnancy at a young age or due to sociodemographic factors associated with teenage pregnancy (e.g., poverty, inadequate prenatal care).

Fraser AM, et al: Association of young maternal age with adverse reproductive outcomes. N Engl J Med 332:1113–1117, 1995.

117. How soon after conception will a urine pregnancy test be positive?

Human chorionic gonadotropin (hCG) is a glycoprotein (with α and β subunits) produced by trophoblastic tissue. Urine levels of 25 mIU/ml are detectable by the most sensitive methods (i.e., radioimmunoassay or enzyme immunoassay to the β subunit) by about 7 days after fertilization. Although many home pregnancy tests can detect these low levels, some are less sensitive and detect levels of hCG of around 1500 mIU/ml. This occurs on average about 3 weeks after fertilization (or 1 week after the missed menstrual period).

118. In what setting should ectopic pregnancy be suspected?

Amenorrhea with unilateral abdominal or pelvic pain and irregular vaginal bleeding is ectopic pregnancy until proved otherwise. Sequential hCG levels can help in determining an ectopic from an intrauterine pregnancy. Ordinarily, the doubling time is hCG levels is about 48 hours. In ectopic pregnancy, there is significant lag. Other causes of lag include missed abortion and spontaneous abortion. Abdominal or transvaginal ultrasound is also useful in diagnosis. Laparoscopy may be necessary if the diagnosis remains unclear.

119. What is the mechanism of action of oral contraceptive pills (OCPs)?

1. Interference with hypothalamic GnRH, with suppression of pituitary FSH and LH and subsequent lack of ovulation
2. Changes in cervical mucus, with less volume, but thicker and more tenacious, acting as a barrier to sperm
3. Histologic changes in endometrium, with atrophy and decreased glycogen content, affecting implantation

120. List the absolute contraindications to OCP use.

• History of thromboembolic disease (e.g., thrombophlebitis, stroke)
• Abnormal liver function
• Estrogen-dependent neoplasia
• Breast cancer
• Undiagnosed vaginal or uterine bleeding
• Pregnancy

121. After OCPs are discontinued, how long is amenorrhea likely to persist?

OCPs suppress the hypothalamic-pituitary axis, and this suppression can continue for a few months following discontinuation. If amenorrhea continues for > 6 months, secondary causes of amenorrhea should be sought.

122. What is the risk to the fetus if a teenager is pregnant and is begun inadvertently on OCPs?

The most common risk is masculinization of female infants, which occurs rarely (< 1%) but especially with the use of OCPs with higher concentrations of progestational agents. The development of pseudohermaphroditism is not a problem. Maternal use of the OCPs is associated with higher bilirubin levels in the newborn. Suspected (but unproven) associations have included congenital heart disease (e.g., transposition of the great arteries, ventricular septal defects, tetralogy of Fallot), CNS malformations, and limb reduction anomalies.

123. Is there an association between urinary tract infections and certain contraceptives?

Use of the diaphragm and spermicide with nonoxynol-9 appear to be significant risk factors.

124. What oral treatment is effective for emergency postcoital contraception (e.g., rape)?

The most commonly used "morning-after" pill is Ovral (50 μg ethinyl estradiol, 0.5 mg norgestrel) which is given as two tablets at the time of evaluation and two tablets 12 hours later. It is most effective when given within 72 hours of intercourse. Mifepristone (RU486) is as effective as the estrogen-progesterone combination and is associated with fewer side effects.

Glasier A, et al: Mifepristone (RU 486) compared with high-dose estrogen and progestogen for emergency postcoital contraception. N Engl J Med 327:1041–1044, 1992.

125. Describe the implantable (Norplant) and injectable (Depo-Provera) methods of contraception.

Both are progestin-only contraceptive methods with extended duration, which minimizes problems with compliance. **Norplant** (levonorgestrel), following surgical implantation, provides contraception for 5 years. Side effects include menstrual irregularities (prolonged bleeding, irregular bleeding, intermenstrual spotting) and weight gain (usually secondary to increased appetite). Amenorrhea is common in the first year but diminishes with time. The devices may be visible under the skin, and surgical removal can be difficult and associated with scarring. Its effect is reversible immediately upon surgical removal, with relatively rapid return of fertility.

Depo-Provera (depot medroxyprogesterone acetate), following intramuscular injection, provides contraception for 3 months. Menstrual irregularities and weight gain are common, with amenorrhea being very common. Following discontinuation, there may be a prolonged period of infertility (up to 24 months).

126. In evaluating a teenager, what is the progression of cervicouterine changes that suggest pregnancy?

4–6 wks	Softening of the lower uterine segment (Hegar's sign) and softening of the cervix (Goodell's sign)
6 wks	Vagina and cervix assume a bluish hue (Chadwick's sign)

Uterine size changes

Nongravid	Lemon
8 wks	Tennis ball or orange
10 wks	Baseball
12 wks	Softball or grapefruit (unless uterus retroflexed)
>12 wks	Palpable above the symphysis
16 wks	Palpable between the symphysis and umbilicus
20 wks	Level of the umbilicus

TEENAGE SUICIDE

127. How commonly do adolescents attempt suicide?

About 2000 teenagers die from suicide each year, but data on the frequency of attempts are hampered by underreporting. For each death by suicide, there are an estimated 50–200 attempts that fail, placing the number of attempts between 250,000–1,000,000 in the United States. Suicidal ideation alone occurs in up to 25% of adolescents.

128. Who are more likely to attempt suicide, males or females?

Up to nine times as many females as males attempt suicide. However, males (particularly white males) are much more likely to succeed, due in large part to the choice of more lethal methods (especially firearms). Females more commonly try ingestions or wrist slashing.

129. What are the most common major stressors of teenagers?

1. Failing grades in school
2. Increasing arguments between parents
3. Serious family illness or death

4. Failing relationship with boyfriend or girlfriend

5. Problem with sibling(s)

Green JW, et al: Stressful life events and somatic complaints in adolescents. Pediatrics 75:19–22, 1985.

130. Which adolescents are at increased risk for suicide?

1. History of previous attempts, especially those involving very lethal methods and those within the past 2 years (1–10% of failed suicides will be successful in future attempts)

2. Signs of major depression (fatigue, sadness, loss of appetite, sleep irregularities)

3. Substance abuse (up to 25% of victims aged 18–24 years have blood alcohol levels ≥ 0.10%)

4. Family history of psychiatric problems, including suicide

5. Personal history of "acting out" behavior (delinquency, truancy, sexual promiscuity)

131. What types of teenagers commit suicide?

Four broad categories occur:

50%:   Teenagers, especially males, with a long history of school and behavioral problems, fighting at school and with parents, and impulsiveness

20–25%: Anxious, perfectionistic, rigid teenagers performing well at school ("model children")

20–25%: Depressed girls

1–2%:   Psychotic adolescents

Strasburger VC, Brown RT: Adolescent Medicine. Boston, Little, Brown, 1991, p 423.

132. Which adolescents who have attempted suicide should be hospitalized?

Although many programs admit all patients, even if medically stable, those adolescents with failed attempts who strongly should be considered for inpatient evaluation include:

• All with recurrent attempts

• Evidence of psychosis or persisting pervasive wish to die

• Method other than ingestion (e.g., jumping, use of firearm, attempted asphyxiation by hanging or carbon monoxide inhalation)

• Attempt at remote location (with less likelihood of discovery)

• Inadequate home, social, and supervisory situation

2. BEHAVIOR AND DEVELOPMENT

Nathan J. Blum, M.D., Mark F. Ditmar, M.D., and Edward B. Charney, M.D.

ATTENTION DEFICIT HYPERACTIVITY DISORDER

1. According to DSM-IV criteria, how is attention deficit hyperactivity disorder (ADHD) classified?

In 1994, the *Diagnostic and Statistical Manual of Mental Disorders* (DSM-IV) established new criteria for the diagnosis of ADHD. Symptoms of inattention, hyperactivity, and impulsivity must have lasted for > 6 months and be inconsistent with developmental level. These symptoms have to involve more than one setting and result in significant social or school impairment. It classified ADHD as a single disorder of various subtypes: predominantly inattentive, predominantly hyperactive-impulsive, and combined. A category for milder symptoms was also established. To meet the diagnostic criteria, some symptoms must have begun before age 7.

2. What are risk factors for ADHD?

In community samples, ADHD occurs three times more frequently in males than females. CNS disorders, such as cerebral palsy, epilepsy, Tourette syndrome, and learning disabilities, may be predisposing factors. There is an increased incidence of ADHD in first-degree relatives of individuals with a history of ADHD. There is also an increased incidence of substance abuse, conduct disorder, learning disabilities, depression, and antisocial personality disorder in families of ADHD children.

Roizen NJ, et al: Psychiatric and developmental disorders in families of children with attention deficit hyperactivity disorder. Arch Pediatr Adolesc Med 150:203–208, 1996.

3. Do any disorders frequently coexist in patients with ADHD?

Oppositional defiant disorder	30–60%
Specific developmental disorders (e.g., academic skills disorders, language and speech disorders, motor skills disorders)	20–60%
Conduct disorder	20–30%
Anxiety disorders (e.g., separation anxiety disorder, avoidant disorder, overanxious disorder)	20–30%
Mild mental retardation	3–10%
Other neurologic disorders	< 10%

Wender E: Hyperactivity. In Parker S, Zuckerman B (eds): Behavioral and Developmental Pediatrics. Boston, Little, Brown & Co., 1995, p 187.

4. What conditions can mimic ADHD?

Pervasive developmental disorders (i.e., autism and autistic-like disorder)
Major affective disorders (e.g., recurrent depression, bipolar disease, cyclothymia)
Stress reactions (e.g., post-traumatic stress disorder)
Hyperthyroidism or hypothyroidism
Iron deficiency anemia
Lead toxicity
Hearing loss
Seizure disorder (e.g., absence seizures)

Wender E: Hyperactivity. In Parker S, Zuckerman B (eds): Behavioral and Developmental Pediatrics. Boston, Little, Brown & Co., 1995, p 190.

5. Should children with ADHD have thyroid testing routinely done?

In 1993, considerable publicity was generated with the report of a large group of children with ADHD and generalized resistance to thyroid hormone (GRTH) due to genetically inherited abnormal thyroid hormone receptors. All had normal or elevated thyroid-stimulating hormone (TSH) and elevated triiodothyronine (T_3) and thyroxine (T_4) due to peripheral resistance. However, this entity is very rare. A subsequent prospective study of 277 children with ADHD found 5% with thyroid abnormalities compared to 1% of the general population. Surprisingly, hypothyroidism was more common than hyperthyroidism (despite the hyperactivity). None had GRTH. It is unclear if treatment alleviated symptoms. At present, routine testing of thyroid function for ADHD remains of unproven utility, but it should be considered if a child has stigmata of hyper- or hypothyroidism, an enlarged thyroid gland on exam, or a family history of thyroid disease.

Hauser P, et al: Attention deficit-hyperactivity disorder in people with generalized resistance to thyroid hormone. N Engl J Med 328:997–1001, 1993.

Weiss RE, et al: Attention deficit-hyperactivity disorder and thyroid function. J Pediatr 123:539–545, 1993.

6. What is the most commonly used method of evaluating ADHD symptoms?

Rating scales, of which the Conners' Behavior Rating Scale is probably the most common. It consists of a 28-item teacher-rating scale and a 48-item parent-rating scale that assess adults' judgments of a child's functioning in home and school settings. Originally developed to provide a means of assessing the effects of various medications on behavior, they are now used in screening for hyperactivity, inattention, and conduct problems in children aged 3–17. It is one of a number of rating scales used in clinical and research work with ADHD.

Barbaresi WJ: Primary-care approach to the diagnosis and management of attention-deficit hyperactivity disorder. Mayo Clin Proc 71:463–471, 1996.

7. How effective are medications for ADHD?

Stimulant medications (methylphenidate [Ritalin], amphetamines, pemoline) result in improvement in 70–80% of affected children. Some children who do not respond to one stimulant will respond to another. The primary benefits occur in improving attention deficiencies and, to a lesser extent, in diminishing hyperactivity. Benefits in cognition are more controversial. Stimulants appear to work by altering the neurochemical balance of monoamines (e.g., norepinephrine, dopamine) in the CNS. Short-term side effects, such as sleep disturbances and decreased appetite, are common but are usually amenable to dose adjustment. Precipitation of Tourette syndrome may occur. Long-term side effects are under study but may include reduction of both height and weight growth.

8. Is a positive response to stimulant medication diagnostic of ADHD?

A positive response is not diagnostic because (a) children without symptoms of ADHD given stimulants demonstrate positive responses in sustained and focused attention, and (b) observer bias (i.e., parent or teacher) can be considerable. Thus, many experts recommend a placebo-controlled trial when stimulant medication is used.

9. What are the side effects of Ritalin?

The most common side effects are decreased **appetite, insomnia, headaches,** and **abdominal pain**. Growth delay, while reported, is rarely seen with the current dosage recommendations. Dysphoria and rebound effects (worsening of behavior as the medication wears off) may necessitate stopping the medication in some patients. The medication may cause reversible exacerbations of tics in some patients, while in others the onset of tics after treatment is begun may be the first sign of a chronic motor tic disorder or Tourette syndrome.

Barkley RA, et al: Side effects of methylphenidate in children with attention deficit hyperactivity disorders: A systemic placebo-controlled evaluation. Pediatrics 86:184–192, 1990.

10. Is the Feingold diet of any value in the treatment of ADHD?

Dr. Benjamin Feingold hypothesized in the early 1970s that hyperactivity in children was due to the ingestion of low-molecular weight chemicals, such as salicylates and artificial additives for color and flavor. He recommended a diet devoid of these substances and claimed up to a 50% improvement in children on such a diet. Few controlled studies, however, have been able to demonstrate such an effect.

11. Does sugar make children hyperactive?

Although it would be gratifying if complex behavioral problems could be attributable solely or in large measure to dietary causes, this has not been shown to be the case. In a double-blind controlled trial involving excessive dietary intakes of sucrose or aspartame (Nutrasweet), no adverse behavioral or cognitive changes were noted.

Wolraich ML, et al: Effect of sugar on behavior or cognition in children. JAMA 274:1617–1621, 1995.

12. Is there evidence for an organic basis for ADHD?

The evidence is inconclusive. Some findings that suggest an organic basis include:

1. Xenon cerebral blood flow studies have demonstrated decreased blood flow in the striatal and posterior periventricular regions. Flow was increased to these regions by administration of methylphenidate.

2. Positron emission tomography (PET) scanning of parents of ADHD children have shown decreased glucose metabolism in the left frontal and parietal regions.

3. Methylphenidate is an agonist of norepinephrine and dopamine, suggesting a role for these neurotransmitter systems in ADHD.

13. Do children with ADHD become adults with ADHD?

Of those diagnosed with ADHD as children, approximately 70% continue to have symptoms as adolescents and up to 30% have ADHD as adults. During adolescence, 25–50% of teenagers with ADHD will engage in antisocial behaviors. As adults, 20–30% will be diagnosed with antisocial personality disorder, a rate 5–10 times that found in control groups. Those who develop antisocial personality disorder are at high risk for criminal behavior and substance abuse. Those with persistent symptoms in the absence of antisocial personality disorder do not seem to have a significant degree of functional impairment in the workplace and may have very successful careers.

Klein RG, Mannezza S: Long-term outcome of hyperactive children: A review. J Am Acad Child Adolesc Psych 30:383–387, 1991.

BEHAVIOR PROBLEMS

14. What are the most common types of behavioral problems in children?

1. Problems of daily routine (e.g., food refusal, sleep abnormalities, toilet difficulties)
2. Aggressive-resistant behavior (e.g., temper tantrums, aggressiveness with peers)
3. Overdependent-withdrawing behavior (e.g., separation upset, fears, shyness)
4. Hyperactivity
5. Undesirable habits (e.g., thumb-sucking, head banging, nail biting, playing with genitals)
6. School problems

Chamberlin RW: Prevention of behavioral problems in young children. Pediatr Clin North Am 31:332, 1984.

15. At what age does continued use of transitional objects or security blankets become abnormal?

Use of transitional objects varies with age and between cultures. Their use is common in toddlers and decreases during the preschool years. While most school-aged children do not use transitional objects during the day, a study of over 900 seven-year-olds in New Zealand found the 13% still had strong attachments to a transitional object at bedtime.

16. Is physical injury a concern in children with head banging?

Although a common problem occurring in 5–15% of normal children, head banging rarely results in physical injury, and then usually in autistic or otherwise developmentally abnormal children. Normal children often show signs of bliss as they bang away. The activity usually resolves by 4 years of age. It may resume spontaneously during national board exams.

17. What is the difference between a "blue" breathholding spell and a "white" breathholding spell?

Actually, there are far more similarities than differences. Both are syncopal attacks occurring commonly in children ages 6 month to 4 years, peaking between ages 1½ and 3. The **blue** or cyanotic spell is more common. Distraught crying is provoked by physical or emotional upset, causing anger or frustration. Sudden apnea ensues, followed by cyanosis, opisthotonus, rigidity, and later loss of tone. Brief convulsive jerking may occur. The episode lasts from 10–60 seconds. A short period of sleepiness may ensue. The **white** or pallid spell is similar except for skin color. These children on testing demonstrate increased responsiveness to vagal maneuvers. This parasympathetic hypersensitivity may cause cardiac slowing, diminished cardiac output, and diminished arterial pressure, resulting in a pale appearance.

18. When should a diagnosis of seizure disorder be considered rather than a breathholding spell?

1. Precipitating event is minor or nonexistent.
2. History of no or minimal crying or breathholding.
3. Episode lasts > 1 minute.
4. Period of postepisode sleepiness lasts > 10 minutes.
5. Convulsive component of episode is prominent and occurs before cyanosis.
6. Occurs in child < 6 months or > 4 years old.

19. Does thumb-sucking vary with race and culture?

Yes. Various studies found that 45% of American children < 4 years of age suck their thumbs (boys and girls equally) compared with 30% of Swedish children, 17% of Indian children, and 1% of Eskimo children. Eskimo children probably don't need to suck their thumbs because they are usually carried in their mothers' backpacks with a bottle close at hand. Most thumb-sucking stops spontaneously by age 4.

Curzon ME: Dental implications of thumb sucking. Pediatrics 54:196, 1974.

20. When does prolonged thumb-sucking warrant intervention?

If thumb-sucking persists beyond 4–5 years (or when permanent teeth begin to erupt), treatment is usually indicated. Treatment commonly has two components: application of a substance with an unpleasant taste at frequent intervals (such products are commercially available), or modification with positive reinforcement (small rewards) given when a child is observed not sucking his or her thumb. Occlusive dental appliances are generally not recommended. Persistent thumb-sucking after eruption of permanent teeth can lead to malocclusion.

21. A 10-month-old infant who is demonstrating frequent self-gagging behavior has what likely diagnosis?

Rumination syndrome is a rare disorder characterized by the regurgitation and reswallowing of food. It typically occurs in infants between 2 and 12 months of age after a period of normal feeding. The infant may be noted to be gagging himself or herself with the tongue or hand while alone. A chaotic family situation often exists. If gastrointestinal pathology has been eliminated as a cause of the problem, treatment consists of increasing family interaction and instituting antireflux measures (e.g., thickened feedings).

22. When should "toilet training" be started?

When the child is physically and emotionally ready. The physical prerequisite of neurologic maturation of bladder and bowel control usually occurs between 1 and 3 years of age. The child's emotional readiness is often influenced by his or her temperament, parental attitudes, and parent-child interactions. The "potty chair" should be introduced sometime between 2 and 3 years of age. Most children will achieve daytime bladder and bowel control by 3½ years.

23. Are girls or boys toilet-trained earlier?

On average, girls are toilet-trained earlier than boys. With regard to most other developmental milestones in the first years of life, however, there do not seem to be significant sex differences (e.g., in walking or running, sleep patterns, or verbal ability). Girls do show more rapid bone development.

24. When is masturbation in a child considered pathologic?

Masturbation, or the rhythmic self-manipulation of the genital area, is considered a normal part of sexual development. In some situations, however, masturbation may be a sign of sexual abuse, CNS abnormalities, or psychological pathology. These behaviors are of special concern in children above ages 5 or 6.

Normal	*Needs Further Assessment*
Occasional	Frequent, compulsive
Discreet, private	No regard for privacy
Not preferred over other activity or play	Often preferred over other activity or play
No physical symptoms or signs	Produces genital discomfort, irritation, or physical signs
External stimulation of genitalia only	Involves penetration of the genital orifices
	Includes bizarre practices or rituals

From Haka-Ikse K, Mian M: Sexuality in children. Pediatr Rev 14:402, 1993; with permission.

25. When is a child's laughter nothing to sneer at?

Pathologic laughter is that which occurs without a stimulus, is not in response to the environmental surroundings, and has no associated emotional feelings. Causes can include Angelman syndrome, gelastic epilepsy, multiple sclerosis, Wilson disease and mood-altering drugs (e.g., hallucinogens, alcohol, benzodiazepines, nitrous oxide).

Nirenberg SA: Normal and pathologic laughter in children. Clin Pediatr 30:630–632, 1991.

CRANIAL DISORDERS

26. How many fontanels are present at birth?

Although there are 6 fontanels present at birth (2 anterior lateral, 2 posterior lateral, 1 anterior, and 1 posterior), only 2 (the anterior and posterior fontanels) are usually palpable on physical examination.

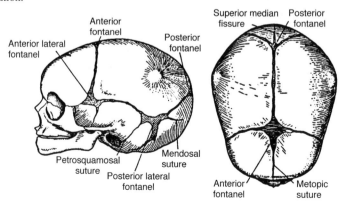

The cranium at birth, showing major sutures and fontanels. No attempt is made to show molding or overlapping of bones, which sometimes occurs at birth. (From Silverman FN, Kuhn JP (eds): Caffey's Pediatric X-ray Diagnosis, 9th ed. St. Louis, Mosby, 1993, p 5; with permission.)

27. When does the anterior fontanel close?

Usually between 10 and 14 months of age. However, it may not be palpable as early as 3 months, or it may remain open until 18 months of age.

28. Which conditions are associated with premature or delayed closure of the fontanel?

Premature closure: Microcephaly, high calcium/vitamin D ratio in pregnancy, craniosynostosis, hyperthyroidism, or it may be a normal variant.

Delayed closure:

Skeletal disorders	Chromosomal abnormalities	Other conditions
Acondroplasia	Down syndrome	Athyrotic hypothyroidism
Aminopterin-induced	Trisomy 13 syndrome	Hallermann-Streiff
syndrome	Trisomy 18 syndrome	syndrome
Alpert syndrome	Malnutrition	
Cleidocranial dysostosis	Progeria	
Hypophosphatasia	Rubella syndrome	
Kenny syndrome	Russell-Silver syndrome	
Osteogenesis imperfecta		
Pyknodysostosis		
Vitamin D deficiency rickets		

29. When is an anterior fontanel too big?

The size of the fontanel can be calculated using the formula: (length + width) / 2, where length = anterior-posterior dimension and width = transverse dimension. Although there is wide variability in the normal size range of the anterior fontanel, designation of normal upper limits is helpful in identifying disorders in which a large fontanel may be a feature (e.g., hypothyroidism, hypophosphatasia, skeletal dysplasias, increased intracranial pressure). Of note, the **posterior** fontanel normally is fingertip size or smaller in 97% of full-term newborns.

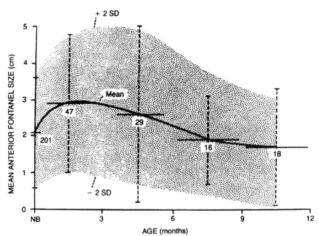

Mean anterior fontanel size ± 2 SD during the first postnatal year. Beyond the newborn period (NB), the data are averaged at 3-month intervals with the number of individuals in each group indicated. (From Popich GA, Smith DW: Fontanels: Range of normal size. J Pediatr 80:749, 1982; with permission.)

30. Name the types of primary craniosynostosis.

Craniosynostosis is the premature fusion of various cranial suture lines, resulting in ridging of the sutures, asymmetric growth, and deformity of the skull. Suture lines (with resultant disorders listed in parentheses) include sagittal (scaphocephaly or dolichocephaly), coronal (brachycephaly), unilateral coronal or lambdoidal (plagiocephaly), and metopic (trigonocephaly). Multiple fused sutures can result in a high and pointed skull (oxycephaly or acrocephaly).

Normocephaly Dolichocephaly Trigonocephaly Plagiocephaly Plagiocephaly Brachycephaly

From Gorlin RJ: Craniofacial defects. In Oski FA, et al (eds): Principles and Practice of Pediatrics, 2nd ed. Philadelphia, J.B. Lippincott, 1994, p 508; with permission.

31. What is the most common type of primary craniosynostosis?
Sagittal (60%). Coronal synostosis accounts for 20% of cases.

32. What causes craniosynostosis?
Most cases of isolated craniosynostosis have no known etiology. Primary craniosynostosis may be observed as part of craniofacial syndromes, including Apert, Crouzon, and Carpenter syndromes. Secondary causes can include abnormalities of calcium and phosphorus metabolism (e.g., hypophosphatasia, rickets), hematologic disorders (e.g., thalassemia), mucopolysaccharidoses, and hyperthyroidism. Inadequate brain growth, as in microcephaly, can lead to craniosynostosis.

33. Which syndrome of craniosynostosis most commonly has exophthalmos as a constant finding?
Crouzon syndrome. In this syndrome, the craniosynostosis is associated with midface hypoplasia and shallow orbits. This leads to prominent ocular proptosis and associated hypertelorism, strabismus, and exposure conjunctivitis.

34. What conditions are associated with skull softening?
- Cleidocranial dysostosis
- Craniotabes
- Lacunar skull (associated with spina bifida, major CNS anomalies)
- Osteogenesis imperfecta
- Multiple wormian bones (associated with hypothyroidism, hypophosphatasia, chronic hydrocephalus)
- Rickets

35. What is the significance of craniotabes?
In this condition, abnormally soft, thin skull bones buckle under pressure and recoil like a ping-pong ball. It is best elicited on the parietal or frontal bones and is often associated with rickets in infancy. It may also be seen in hypervitaminosis A, syphilis, and hydrocephalus. Craniotabes may be a normal finding during the first 3 months of life.

36. Which imaging study is preferable in the evaluation of microcephaly, CT or MRI?
MRI has superior ability to:
1. Differentiate gray and white matter
2. Identify abnormalities of neuronal migration, sulcation, and gyration
3. Identify patterns of myelin deposition or demyelination
4. Provide greater details of the basal ganglia, brainstem, and cerebellum

DeMyer W: Microcephaly, micrencephaly, megalocephaly, and megalencephaly. in Swaiman K (ed): Pediatric Neurology. St. Louis, Mosby-Year Book, 1994, pp 205–218.

37. In addition to careful sequential charting of head circumference, what other features on history or examination should raise suspicion for the later development of microcephaly?
  • Infants up to age 6 months whose chest circumference exceeds head circumference (unless infant is very obese)
  • Delayed developmental milestones
  • Neurologic abnormalities (e.g., seizures, spasticity)
  • Marked backward slope of forehead (seen in familial microcephaly)
  • Occipital flattening not related to positioning
  • Early closure of anterior fontanel
  • Significantly prominent suture lines
  Moe PG, Seay AR: Neurologic and muscular disorders. In Hay WW, et al (eds): Current Pediatric Diagnosis and Treatment, 12th ed. Norwalk, Appleton & Lange, 1995, p 750.

38. What are the three main general causes of macrocephaly?
  1. **Increased intracranial pressure:** from dilated ventricles (e.g., progressive hydrocephalus of various causes), subdural fluid collections, intracranial tumors, benign increased intracranial pressure (i.e., pseudotumor cerebri) from various causes
  2. **Thickened skull:** cranioskeletal dysplasias (e.g., osteopetrosis), various anemias
  3. **Megalencephaly** (enlarged brain): familial, syndromic (e.g., Sotos syndrome), storage diseases, leukodystrophies, neurocutaneous disorders (e.g., neurofibromatosis)

DENTAL DEVELOPMENT AND DISORDERS

39. When do primary and secondary teeth erupt?
  Mandibular teeth usually erupt first. The central incisors appear by 5–7 months, with approximately 1 new tooth per month thereafter until 23–30 months, at which time the second molars (and thus all 20 primary or deciduous teeth) are in place. Of the 32 secondary teeth, the central incisors erupt first between 5 and 7 years, and the third molars are in place by 17–22 years.

40. What is the significance of natal teeth?
  Although the first primary tooth usually erupts by 6–12 months of age, occasionally teeth are present at birth (natal teeth) or erupt within 30 days after birth (neonatal teeth). When x-rays are taken, 95% of natal teeth are primary incisors and 5% are supernumerary teeth or extra teeth. Very sharp teeth which can cause tongue lacerations and very loose teeth which can be aspirated should be removed. Females are affected more commonly than males, and the prevalence is 1:2000–3500. Most cases are familial and without consequence, but natal teeth can be associated with genetic syndromes, including the Ellis–van Creveld and Hallermann-Streiff syndromes.

41. How common is congenital absence of teeth?
  Congenital absence of primary teeth is very rare, but up to 25% of individuals may have absence of one or more third molars, and up to 5% may have absence of another secondary or permanent tooth (most commonly the maxillary lateral incisors and mandibular second premolar).
  Abrams RB, Mueller WA: Oral medicine and dentistry. In Hay WW, et al (eds): Current Pediatric Diagnosis and Treatment, 12th ed. Norwalk, Appleton & Lange, 1995, p 447.

42. What are mesiodentes?
  These are peg-shaped supernumerary teeth, occurring in up to 5% of individuals, which most commonly are situated in the maxillary midline. They should be considered for removal because they interfere with the eruption of permanent incisors.

43. What constitutes the 32 permanent teeth?
  Upper and lower central incisors, lateral incisors, cuspids, first bicuspids, second bicuspids, first molars, second molars, third molars.

44. What is a ranula?

A large **mucocele**, usually bluish, painless, soft, and unilateral, that occurs under the tongue. Most self-resolve. If large, surgical marsupialization can be done. If recurrent, excision may be needed.

45. What causes tooth discoloration?

COLOR	CAUSE	COLOR	CAUSE
Generalized		*Localized*	
Bluish-brown	Dentinogenesis imperfecta	Yellow	Trauma
Yellow	Amelogenesis imperfecta		Chromogenic bacteria
	Tetracycline ingestion	Gray	Trauma
Reddish-brown	Porphyria	Black/blackish-	Trauma
	Fluorosis	brown	Liquid iron supplements
Blue/bluish-green	Rh incompatibility		Tobacco
			Tea or other foods
Brown	Tetracycline ingestion		Chromogenic bacteria
Gray	Tetracycline ingestion	Pink	Internal resorption

From Kula K: Dental problems. In Oski FA, et al (eds): Principles and Practice of Pediatrics, 2nd ed. Philadelphia, J.B. Lippincott, 1994, p 864; with permission.

46. Where are Epstein's pearls located?

These white, superficial, mobile nodules, usually midline and often paired, are present on the hard palate in many newborns. They are keratin-containing cysts that are asymptomatic, do not increase in size, and usually exfoliate spontaneously within a few weeks.

47. How does fluoride minimize the development of dental caries?

1. Topical fluoride from toothbrushing is thought to increase remineralization of enamel.

2. Bacterial fermentation of sugar into acid plays a major role in the development of caries, and fluoride inhibits this process.

3. As teeth are developing, fluoride incorporates into the hydroxyapatite crystal of enamel, making it less soluble and less susceptible to erosion.

48. Should fluoride supplements be given with or without food?

Fluoride absorption is reduced by 30–40% in infants when it is given with formula. Thus, the recommendation is to give fluoride on an empty stomach.

49. How long should fluoride supplementation be continued?

Fluoride supplementation should continue until 14–16 years of age, when the third molar crowns are completely calcified.

50. How effective are dental sealants in preventing cavities?

Dental sealants may reduce the development of caries by up to 80% when compared to rates in untreated teeth. Although fluoride acts primarily by protecting smooth surfaces, dental sealants (commonly bisphenol A and glycidyl methacrylate) act by protecting the pits and fissures of the surface, especially in posterior teeth. Reapplication may be needed every 2 years. As a preventive dental procedure, it is relatively underutilized.

51. Which children are susceptible to periodontitis?

The periodontium consists of the gingiva, alveolar bone, and periodontal ligament that connects the two. Periodontitis is the triad of hypertrophied gingiva, loose teeth (due to loss of alveolar bone), and purulent exudate. It is rare in children but may be seen in adolescents with chronically poor periodontal hygiene. Juvenile periodontitis is a disease of rapid alveolar bone loss due to colonization by bacteria pathogenic to the periodontium. It is mainly seen in children with disorders of neutrophil function (e.g., Chediak-Higashi syndrome, cyclic neutropenia).

52. How common is gingivitis in children?

Gingivitis is extremely common, affecting nearly 50% of children. The disorder is usually painless and is manifested by bluish-red discoloration of gums, which are swollen and bleed easily. *The cause:* bacteria in plaque deposits between teeth. *The cure:* improved dental hygiene and daily flossing.

DEVELOPMENTAL ASSESSMENT

53. When do the primitive reflexes in a neonate become extinct?

Primitive or developmental reflexes are normally present at birth and should be extinct by about 6 months of age. Some of these reflexes include Moro, palmar grasp, rooting, and tonic neck. Abnormalities in these reflexes include an asymmetric response, absence of expected response, sustained obligatory response, or persistence beyond age 6 months.

54. What three primitive reflexes, if persistent beyond 4–6 months, can interfere with the development of midline activities and the ability to roll and sit?

Moro reflex: Sudden neck extension results in extension, abduction, and adduction of upper extremities with flexion of fingers, wrists, and elbows.

Asymmetric tonic neck reflex: In a calm supine infant, turning of the head laterally results in relative extension of the arm and leg on the side to the turn and flexion of both on the side away from the turn (the "fencer" position).

Tonic labyrinthine reflex: In an infant being held suspended in the prone position, flexion of the neck results in shoulder protraction and hip flexion, while neck extension causes shoulder retraction and hip extension.

55. In evaluating the development of premature infants, what correction factor should be used?

Although most agree that some correction factor for prematurity should be used when assessing development, there is not a definite answer to how much correction is indicated or for how long. In general, it is probably appropriate to make a correction during the first year of life by subtracting the number of months the child is premature from the chronologic age. For example, an 8-month-old infant who was 3 months premature should be "scored" on a developmental test as if he or she was 5 months old. Between 1 and 2 years of age, the amount of correction gets a bit cloudy, and an appropriate compromise appears to be 50% correction factor. For example, the 18-month-old infant who was 2 months premature should be "scored" as if the chronologic age was 17 months. Most agree that there should not be any correction for prematurity after 2 years of age.

56. When can an infant "taste"?

Taste is present at birth, and infants demonstrate a definite preference for sweetness over saltiness or plain water.

57. When do the Landau, propping, and parachute reflexes develop?

These are postural responses that normally appear in the middle part of the first year of life (following the disappearance of various primitive reflexes) and coincide with volitional movement.

Landau reflex: When an infant is held in ventral (prone) suspension, the head, spine, and legs extend. Appearance is usually at 3–6 months and disappearance at around 12 months.

Lateral propping reflex: A sitting baby, when pushed sideways, will extend the arms to prevent a fall. It usually appears around 7 months.

Parachute reflex: An infant held prone by the waist over a surface and lowered with the head downward will extend the arms and legs as a form of protection. This usually appears at 7–9 months.

58. Name the major developmental landmarks for motor skills during the first 2 years of life.

Developmental Landmark	Months
Major gross motor	
Steadiness of head when placed in supported position	1–4
Transfers objects from hand to hand	5–7
Sits without support for > 30 sec	5–8
Cruises or walks holding on	7–13
Stands alone	9–16
Walks alone	9–17
Walks up stairs with help	12–23
Major fine motor	
Grasp	2–4
Reach	3–5
Transfers objects from hand to hand	5–7
Fine pincer grasp with index finger and thumb apposition	9–14
Spontaneous scribbling	12–24

59. Do infant walkers promote physical strength or development of the lower extremities?

No evidence supports this claim. In fact, infant walkers may delay crawling. Most importantly, up to 35% of infants who use walkers sustain an injury requiring medical attention. The most serious involve falling down unprotected stairs and can result in death. The American Academy of Pediatrics has recommended a ban on the manufacture and sale of mobile infant walkers.

AAP Committee on Injury and Poison Control: Injuries associated with infant walkers. Pediatrics 95:778–780, 1995.

60. What behavioral patterns of early infancy are suspicious for a possible cognitive handicap?

Poor responsiveness to touch, poor eye contact during feeding, diminished spontaneous activity, decreased alertness to voice, irritability, slow feeding. These are particularly worrisome in the setting of higher risks, such as prematurity or early-onset seizures.

Crocker AC, Nelson RP: Major handicapping conditions. In Levine MD, et al (eds): Developmental-Behavioral Pediatrics. Philadelphia, W.B. Saunders, 1983, p 760.

61. How predictive are standardized developmental screening tests?

In general, the predictive validity of developmental screening tests is poor. However, children with developmental quotients (developmental age/chronologic age) < 0.5 are at high risk for having a developmental disability, while the outcome for children with developmental quotients > 0.5 is more variable.

The Denver Developmental Screening test is the most widely used. It is scored as normal, questionable, or abnormal. The abnormal score on the original Denver Developmental Screening Test was criticized for having poor sensitivity in detecting developmental disabilities, but it has recently been revised as the Denver II. The Denver II may have better sensitivity but worse specificity than the original Denver test.

62. At what ages do children learn to copy geometric figures?

A child's ability to copy geometric patterns (also called Gesell figures) is an indicator of fine motor control and visual-perceptual abilities. After a child is shown a figure and asked to copy it, accomplishment of the task correlates with problem-solving abilities that are age-related. Significant delay can indicate a problem in vision, attention or neuromuscular control.

3 yrs—copies circle   7 yrs—copies vertical diamond
4 yrs—copies cross   8 yrs—copies "Red Cross" symbol
4½ yrs—copies square   9 yrs—copies cylinder
5 yrs—copies triangle   11 yrs—copies cube
6 yrs—copies horizontal diamond

63. When does a child learn to button-up clothing?

By 3 years of age, approximately 50% of children can button. About 90% can do so by 4 years. In these days of Velcro, it is important to ascertain that the child has had adequate opportunities to practice the technique. Inability to button by age 4 raises concerns about delays in fine motor skills.

64. What is the value of the Goodenough-Harris drawing test?

This "draw-a-person" test is a screening tool used to evaluate a child's cognition and intellect, visual perception, and visual-motor integration. The child is asked to draw a person, and a point is given for each body part drawn with pairs, such as legs (considered 1 part). An average child aged 4¾ will draw a person with 3 parts, and most children by 5¼ years will draw a person with 6 parts.

65. What are Erikson's eight life-cycle crises of psychosocial development?

1. Trust vs mistrust (infancy)
2. Autonomy vs shame and doubt (early childhood)
3. Initiative vs guilt (early childhood)
4. Industry vs inferiority (school-age)
5. Identity vs confusion (adolescents)
6. Intimacy vs isolation (young adults)
7. Generativity vs stagnation (middle age)
8. Integrity vs despair (old age)

Erikson believed that psychodevelopment involves a healthy resolution, balance, or problematic persistence of these alternatives as each stage of life is reached.

Erikson E: Childhood and Society. New York, W.W. Norton, 1950.

66. Do twins develop at a rate comparable to infants of single birth?

Twins exhibit significant verbal and motor delay in the first year of life. The difficulty lies not in the lack of potential but in the relative lack of individual stimulation. In general, children who are more closely spaced in a family have slower acquisition of verbal skills. Twins with significant language delay or with excessive use of "twin language" (language understood only by the twins themselves) may be candidates for interventional therapy.

Groothius JR: Twins and twin families. Clin Perinatol 12:467–468, 1985.

67. At what age do children develop handedness?

Usually by 18–24 months. The hand preference is usually fixed after 5 years of age. Handedness before 1 year of age may be an early sign of cerebral palsy, with the infant demonstrating decreased use of a compromised upper extremity.

68. What percentage of children are left-handed?

Various studies put the prevalence at between 7 and 10%. However, in former premature infants without cerebral palsy, the rate increases to 20–25%. While antecedent brain injury has been hypothesized to account for this increase in prevalence of left-handedness, studies of unilateral intraventricular hemorrhage and handedness have not demonstrated a relationship. Of note, animals such as mice, dogs, and cats show paw preferences, but in these groups, 50% prefer the left paw and 50% the right paw.

Marlow N, et al: Laterality and prematurity. Arch Dis Child 64:1713–1716, 1989.

69. As children, why were George Bush and Bill Clinton more likely than most to spend time in an emergency room?

Both are left-handed. Left-handedness in children has been shown to be a risk factor for unintentional injury. Other evidence supports the association of left-handedness with developmental disorders (e.g., dyslexia, stuttering, mental retardation, autism) and immune-related diseases (e.g., atopic dermatitis, autoimmune diseases, allergic rhinitis, asthma).

Graham CJ, et al: Left-handedness as a risk factor for unintentional injury in children. Pediatrics 92:823–826, 1993.

LANGUAGE DEVELOPMENT AND DISORDERS

70. Which is usually said first, "mama" or "dada"?

Between 10 and 15 months of age, most children start producing their first clearly identifiable words, and often they are reduplicated syllables, such as "dada," "baba," or "mama." Most infants usually say "dada" first.

71. What are average times for development of expressive and receptive language milestones?

Expressive	Receptive
Social smile—2 mos	Alerts to voice—1 mo
Babbles—6 mo	Orients to voice—4 mos
Dada/mama (nonspecific)—8 mos	Understands "no"—9 mos
Dada/mama (specific)—10 mos	Follows one-step command with gesture—12 mos
First word—11 mos	Knows one body part—18 mos
4–6 words—16 mos	Follows two-step command—24 mos
2-word phrases—21 mos	Follows prepositional commands—3 yrs
Plurals—3 yrs	

72. How does the development of speech normally progress?

Early vocalization (ages 1–4 mos): Vowel and consonant sounds are formed in the back of the mouth, such as those in the words "coo" and "gurgle."

Babbling (ages 3–15 mos): Babbling consists of clear vowel and consonant sounds in which a rising and falling pattern of voice pitch can be heard. As the child begins to mimic the intonation and sound patterns of those around him or her, the babbled sounds will seem to occur in sentence-like sequences. This is referred to as jargon.

Acquisition of true speech (18–50 mos): As opposed to babbling, where there is an almost infinite number of sequential combinations of sounds, true speech consists of a limited number and combination of sounds.

Stabilization of articulation skills (50–80 mos): Normal children may still have articulation errors involving sounds such as *s, sh, z,* and *ch,* and distortions of sounds *l* or *r.*

73. Do deaf infants babble?

Yes. Babbling begins at about the same time in deaf and hearing infants, but deaf infants stop babbling without the normal progression to meaningful communicative speech.

74. At what age does a child's speech become intelligible?

Intelligibility increases by about 25% per year. A 1-year-old has about 25% intelligibility, a 2-year-old 50%, a 3-year-old 75%, and a 4-year-old 100%. Significantly delayed intelligibility should prompt more extensive language evaluation.

75. What are the warning signs of delayed language development?

Danger Signals of Speech-Language Problems in Preschool Children

By 6 mos	No response or inconsistent response to sound or voice
By 9 mos	No response to his/her name
By 12 mos	Stopped babbling or did not babble yet
By 15 mos	Does not understand and respond to "no" and "bye-bye"
By 18 mos	No words other than "mama/dada"
By 2 yrs	No two-word phrases
After 2 yrs	Still jargons or echoes excessively
By 2½ yrs	Speech that is not intelligible to family
By 3 yrs	No simple sentences
By 3½ yrs	Speech that is not intelligible to strangers
By 4 yrs	Consistent articulation errors (besides *r, s, l, th*)
By 5 yrs	Sentence structure is awkward
After 5 yrs	Noticeable, persistent dysfluency (stuttering)
By 6 yrs	Unusual confusions, reversals, or word-finding problems in connected speech
After 7 yrs	Any speech errors
Any age	Any persistent hypernasality or hyponasality, monotone pitch, or hoarseness of voice

From Schwartz ER: Speech and language disorders. In Schwartz MW, et al (eds): Pediatric Primary Care: A Problem-Oriented Approach, 2nd ed. Chicago, Year Book Medical Publ., 1990, p 696; with permission.

76. Which children should be considered for a formal hearing test?
1. Parental concern that the child does not hear normally. (This is listed first because although it is often the most reliable early sign of hearing problems, it unfortunately is often overlooked by the pediatrician.)
2. Birth weight < 1500 gm
3. Family history of childhood hearing impairment
4. Delay in acquisition of language and/or speech
5. Congenital perinatal infection (e.g., cytomegalovirus, rubella, herpes, toxoplasmosis, syphilis)
6. Anatomic malformations involving the head or neck (i.e., microtia, micrognathia, cleft palate)
7. Hyperbilirubinemia at level exceeding indications for exchange transfusion
8. Bacterial meningitis
9. Severe birth asphyxia
10. Other developmental disabilities (i.e., mental retardation, cerebral palsy)
Vohr BR, Maxon AB: Screening infants for hearing impairment. J Pediatr 128:710–714, 1996.

77. What do ELMS, CLAMS, REEL, and PPVT have in common?
All are screening tests that can be used for in-office screening when language delay is suspected: Early Language Milestone Scale (ELMS), Clinical Linguistic and Auditory Milestone Scale (CLAMS), Bzoch-League Receptive Emergent Language (REEL) Scale, and the Peabody Picture Vocabulary Test (PPVT). Failure on one of these tests should prompt referral for an audiologic and cognitive assessment. Major conditions in the differential diagnosis for a child with significant language delay include hearing impairment or deafness, mental retardation, or autism.
Coplan J, Gleason JR: Quantifying language development from birth to 3 years using the Early Language Milestone Scale. Pediatrics 86:963–971, 1990.

78. Should all newborns be screened for hearing impairment?

A controversial issue. The National Institutes of Health (NIH) recommended in 1993 that all newborns be screened by a device that measures otoacoustic emissions (OAEs). OAEs are acoustic echoes from the cochlea when a sound is introduced into the external auditory canal. Abnormal results warrant testing using the more specific auditory brainstem response, which uses scalp electrodes to determine responses to broad-band auditory stimuli.

The NIH recommendation was made to identify hearing disability (as early as possible). Such disability occurs in 1.5/1,000 children, but testing only those children with high-risk criteria (see Question 76) identifies only 50% of infants with hearing impairment. The recommendation for universal screening has been criticized because of the poor specificity and poor positive-predictive value of abnormal test results in the newborn period as well as unclear cost-benefit analyses.

Eilers RE, Berlin C: Advances in early detection of hearing loss in infants. Curr Probl Pediatr 25:60–66, 1995.

79. What causes flat tympanograms?

Tympanometry is an objective measurement of the compliance of the tympanic membrane and the middle ear compartment that involves varying the air pressure in the external ear canal from approximately –200 to +400 mm H_2O while measuring the reflected energy of a simultaneous acoustic tone (often 220 Hz). A normal tracing looks like an inverted V with the peak occurring at an air pressure of 0 mm H_2O, indicating a functionally normal external canal, an intact tympanic membrane, and a lack of excess of middle ear fluid. Flat tympanograms occur with perforation of the tympanic membrane, occlusion of the tympanometry probe against the wall of the canal, obstruction of the canal by a foreign body or impaction by cerumen, or large middle ear effusion.

Hayden GF, Lambert PR: Ear, nose and throat procedures. In Lohr JA (ed): Pediatric Outpatient Procedures. Philadelphia, J.B. Lippincott, 1991, p 92.

80. A toddler with a bifid uvula and hypernasal speech likely has what condition?

Velopharyngeal insufficiency with a possible submucosal cleft palate. The velum, or soft palate, moves posteriorly during swallowing and speech, separating the oropharynx from the nasopharynx. Velopharyngeal insufficiency exists when this separation is incomplete, as may occur after cleft palate repair or following adenoidectomy (usually transient). In severe cases, nasopharyngeal regurgitation of food may occur. In milder cases, the only manifestation may be hypernasal speech. If a bifid uvula is present, one should palpate the palate carefully for the presence of a submucous cleft. Furthermore, the soft palate is often short in these children, creating the insufficiency.

81. Which infants with "tongue-tie" should have surgical correction?

"Tongue-tie," or partial ankyloglossia, is the restriction of mobility of the tongue due to a short or thickened lingual frenulum. In theory, partial ankyloglossia can interfere with breast-feeding and speech. The vast majority of infants, particularly those who can extend the tip of the tongue past the lips, accommodate and eventually develop normal lingual mobility. Indications for surgical correction are imprecise, but children with persistent speech problems after 2–4 years should be considered.

82. How do cluttering and palilalia differ from stuttering?

Cluttering is speech so rapid that it is often intelligible. There is repetition and omission of sounds, syllables, and whole words. Unlike stuttering, cluttering may benefit from advising a child to consciously slow his or her speech. **Palilalia** is intelligible speech in which whole words or phrases are repeated rapidly. This can be associated with neurologic diseases such as pseudobulbar palsy or Tourette syndrome.

83. What advice should be given to parents whose child stutters?

Stuttering is a common characteristic of the speech of preschool children. However, the vast majority of children do not persist with stuttering beyond 5 or 6 years of age. Preschoolers at increased risk for persistence of stuttering include those with a positive family history of stuttering and those with anxiety-provoking stress related to talking. A child older than 5 or 6 years who stutters should be referred to a speech-language pathologist for assessment and treatment. The pediatrician can help guide parents of children < 5 years of age with stuttering by making the following suggestions:

    1. Do not give the child directives about how to deal with his or her speech (e.g., "slow down" or "take a breath").

    2. Provide a relaxed, easy speech model in your own manner of speaking to the child.

    3. Reduce the need/expectations for the child to speak to strangers, adults, or authority figures or to compete with others (such as siblings) to be heard.

    4. Listen attentively to the child with patience and without showing concern.

    5. Seek professional guidance if speech is not noticeably more fluent in 2–3 months.

Schwartz ER: Speech and language disorders. In Schwartz MW et al (eds): Pediatric Primary Care: A Problem-Oriented Approach, 2nd ed. Chicago, Year Book Medical Publ., 1990, pp 699–700.

84. List the three major features of autism.

Autism is a behaviorally defined developmental disorder. Children diagnosed with this disorder must have significant problems in three areas:

    1. Impaired social interactions, such as failure to make eye contact or show interest in interacting with others

    2. Absent or abnormal speech and language development

    3. Narrow range of interest and stereotyped or repetitive response to objects

Although most children with autism also have mental retardation, about 25% have an IQ > 70.

American Psychiatric Association: Diagnostic and Statistical Manual of Mental Disorders, 4th ed. Washington, D.C., APA, 1994.

85. Which behaviors of children should arouse suspicion of possible autism?

    1. Avoidance of eye contact during infancy

    2. Relating to only part of a person's body (i.e., lap) rather than to whole person

    3. Failure to acquire speech or speech acquisition in an unusual manner, such as echolalia (repeating another person's speech)

    4. Repetition of TV commercials and singing out of context and without communicative purpose

    5. Spending long periods of time in repetitive activities and fascination with movement (i.e., spinning records, dripping water)

    6. Interest in small visual details or patterns

    7. Unusual abilities, such as early letter and number recognition

    8. Early reading with minimal comprehension

86. Is there a biochemical or neurologic basis for autistic behavior?

General consensus is that the early hypothesis that autism resulted from parental coldness, rejection, or mishandling is incorrect. The current belief is that autistic behavior arises from neurodevelopmental dysfunction of the CNS. Unfortunately, neither the biochemical basis nor the anatomic abnormality for autism is known.

87. The parents complain that their daughter has poor communication skills, decreased social interaction, marked periodic breathing, and loss of purposeful hand movements. What diagnosis should be suspected?

Rett syndrome. This neurodegenerative disorder of unclear etiology affects girls exclusively. After a normal birth and early infancy, developmental arrest begins around 7–18 months of age, followed by severe decline of cognitive skills and loss of purposeful hand movements. Profound dementia, microcephaly, ataxia, spastic paraparesis, seizures, and characteristic hand-wringing and respiratory stereotypies develop progressively. Often confused with autism, Rett syndrome is established on clinical grounds.

MENTAL RETARDATION

88. Define mental retardation.

Mental retardation is characterized by "significantly subaverage intellectual functioning existing concurrently with related limitations in two or more of the following applicable adaptive skill areas":

Communication	Self-care	Home living
Social skills	Community use	Self-direction
Health and safety	Functional academics	Leisure
Work		

Mental retardation manifests before age 18.

American Association on Mental Retardation: Mental Retardation: Definition, Classification, and Systems of Support. Washington, D.C., AAMR, 1992.

89. How is the intelligence quotient (IQ) determined?

Mental age divided by chronologic age times 100. It is important to note that IQ is not a static phenomenon but can be changed significantly, depending on the developmental environment.

90. How is intelligence classified with IQ scores?

130+	Very superior
120–129	Superior
110–119	High average
90–109	Average
80–89	Low average
70–79	Borderline
50–69	Mild mental retardation
35–49	Moderate mental retardation
20–34	Severe mental retardation
<20	Profound mental retardation

91. What features can indicate cognitive problems in infants and young children?

In younger infants and toddlers, fine motor and especially language development are the usual best correlates of cognitive achievement. As the child ages, the various milestones can be evaluated. Significant sequential delay should warrant referral for formal developmental testing to evaluate the possibility of mental retardation.

2–3 mos	Not alerting to mother with special interest
6–7 mos	Not searching for dropped object
8–9 mos	No interest in peek-a-boo
12 mos	Does not search for hidden object
15–18 mos	No interest in cause-and-effect games
2 yrs	Does not categorize similarities (e.g., animals vs vehicles)
3 yrs	Does not know own full name
4 yrs	Cannot pick shorter or longer of two lines
4½ yrs	Cannot count sequentially
5 yrs	Does not know colors or any letters
5½ yrs	Does not know own birthday or address

First LR, Palfrey JS: The infant or young child with developmental delay. N Engl J Med 330:478–483, 1994.

92. What findings in a child with mental retardation should prompt a cranial MRI?

- Cerebral palsy or motor asymmetry
- Abnormal head size or shape
- Craniofacial malformation
- Loss or plateau of developmental skills
- Multiple somatic anomalies
- Neurocutaneous findings
- Seizures
- IQ < 50

Palmer FB, Capute AJ: Mental retardation. Pediatr Rev 15:473–479, 1994.

93. Worldwide, what is the most common preventable cause of mental retardation?

Iodine deficiency leads to maternal and fetal hypothyroxinemia during gestation, which causes brain developmental injury. Severe endemic iodine deficiency can cause cretinism (characterized by deaf-mutism, severe intellectual deficiency, and often hypothyroidism) and may occur in 2–10% of isolated world communities. Moderate iodine deficiency, even more common, leads to milder degrees of cognitive impairment.

Xue-Yi C, et al: Timing of vulnerability of the brain to iodine deficiency in endemic cretinism. N Engl J Med 331:1739–1744, 1994.

PSYCHIATRIC DISORDERS

94. What is the prevalence of childhood psychiatric disorders?

Overall, 17–22% of children aged 4–20 in community samples are diagnosed with a specific psychiatric disorder. The most common disorders are:

Attention deficit hyperactivity disorder (4–10%)   Separation anxiety (3–5%)
Oppositional disorder (5–10%)   Overanxious disorder (2–5%)
Conduct disorder (1–5%)   Depression (2–6%)

Costello EJ: Developments in child psychiatric epidemiology. J Am Acad Child Adolesc Psychiatry 28:836–841, 1989.

95. If a parent has an affective disorder, what is the likelihood that an offspring will have similar problems?

Twenty to 25% of these children will develop a major affective disorder, and as many as 40–45% will have a psychiatric problem.

96. How do manic disorders differ in children and adolescents?

Rare in children, mania may present as irritability, agitation, emotional lability, hyperactivity, and distractability. Children may also have pressured speech. More common in adolescents, mania presents with symptoms similar to those in adults: elated mood, flight of ideas, pressured speech, sleeplessness, bizarre behavior, delusions of grandeur, paranoia, or euphoria. Transient mood disturbances common in adolescence must be distinguished from a true mood disorder.

97. Describe the essential features of a conversion reaction in children.

A conversion reaction is the presence of symptoms (suggestive of a physical disorder) that cannot be explained by a known physical disorder and instead are thought to be an expression of psychologic conflict or need, particularly in settings of anxiety or depression. The child cannot be intentionally producing the symptoms, as in malingering. Chronic abdominal or chest pain, headaches, fainting spells, and other symptoms may be be manifestations of a conversion reaction.

98. What ritualistic behaviors are common in children with obsessive-compulsive disorder (OCD)?

The most common rituals involve excessive cleaning, repeating gross motor rituals (e.g., going up and down stairs), and repetitive checking behaviors (e.g., checking that doors are locked or that homework is correct). Obsessions most commonly deal with fear of contamination. Symptoms tend to wax and wane in severity, and the specific obsessions or compulsions change over time. Most children attempt to disguise their rituals. Anxiety and distress that interfere with school or family life can occur when children fail in efforts to resist the thoughts or activities. Counseling and serotonin-reuptake-inhibiting medications (clomipramine, fluoxetine, sertraline, paroxetine) can be beneficial.

99. What distinguishes a conduct disorder from an oppositional defiant disorder?

Both are disruptive behavior disorders of childhood and early adolescence. **Conduct disorder** is the more serious disorder in that it is diagnosed when the child's behaviors violate the rights of others (e.g., assault) or major societal norms (e.g., stealing, truancy, fire setting). Children with conduct disorder are at risk for developing the antisocial personality disorder of adults. **Oppositional defiant disorder** is characterized by recurrent negativistic, defiant behaviors toward authority figures.

100. How are organic and psychiatrically based psychoses differentiated?

Psychosis is the manifestation of marked abnormalities in mental functions with diminished grasping of reality and can present in a variety of ways, including disoriented thought, rapidly fluctuating moods, or violent behavior. **Organic psychosis** refers to abnormal behavior and mentation that has a known underlying cause (e.g., illicit drugs). **Psychiatrically based psychosis** does not have an identifiable cause and includes diagnoses such as childhood and adolescent schizophrenia, and severe manic-depressive illness.

	Organic Psychosis	*Psychiatrically Based Psychosis*
Onset	Acute	Insidious, previous episodes
Premorbid state	Normal (history of substance abuse)	Poor social, sexual development
Mental status	Depressed sensorium	Normal sensorium
Orientation	Disoriented	Usually normal
Memory	Recent memory loss	Usually normal
Vital signs	Abnormal (tachycardia, fever)	Usually normal
Hallucinations	Visual, tactile, olfactory	Auditory
Response to therapy	Dramatic	Less dramatic

PSYCHOSOCIAL FAMILY ISSUES

101. How prevalent is divorce in the United States?

Between 1960 and 1980, the incidence of divorce in the United States doubled. By some estimates, nearly 40% of children born in the mid-1980s will experience the divorce of their parents, and by the year 2000, one-third of children will be living in a divorced or remarried family.

102. How do children of different ages vary in their response to parental divorce?

Preschool (ages 2½–5): Most likely to show regression in developmental milestones (e.g., toilet training); increased separation anxiety; sleep disturbances; preoccupation with fear of abandonment; demanding with remaining parent; aggressive with siblings and peers.

Early school-age (6–8): Most likely to demonstrate open grieving; preoccupied with fear of rejection and of being replaced; torn by guilt because of conflicting loyalties.

Later school-age (ages 9–12): More likely to demonstrate profound anger at one or both parents; more likely to distinguish one parent as the culprit causing the divorce; deterioration in school performance and peer relationships; sense of loneliness and powerlessness.

Adolescents: Significant potential for acute depression and even suicidal ideation; acting-out behavior (substance abuse, truancy, sexual activity); self-doubts about own potential for marital success.

Wallerstein JS: Separation, divorce, and remarriage. In Levine MD, et al (eds): Developmental-Behavioral Pediatrics, 2nd ed. Philadelphia, W.B. Saunders, 1992, pp 136–146.

103. What issues continue to affect children following a parental divorce?

- Continued fighting
- Abandonment by one parent
- Continued litigation over custody and visitation
- Emotional/mental disturbances in parents
- Diminished parenting
- Poor relationships with step-parents
- Little support from outside nuclear family
- Economic hardships

From Wallerstein JS: Separation divorce, and remarriage. In Levine MD, et al (eds): Developmental-Behavioral Pediatrics, 2nd ed. Philadelphia, W.B. Saunders, 1992, p 137; with permission.

104. What are the increased risks for children living with an alcoholic parent?

Approximately 1 of 8 children live with a parent with a past or current drinking problem. These children and adolescents are more likely to live in homes of stress, violence, permissiveness, poor communication, neglect, and undersocialization. They have increased risks of mental health problems (e.g., depression), behavioral problems (e.g., attention deficit hyperactivity disorder), abuse, delinquency, and the development of addiction problems.

Macdonald DI, Blume SB: Children of alcoholics. Am J Dis Child 140:750–754, 1986.

105. What is the "vulnerable child syndrome"?

The vulnerable child syndrome is characterized by excessive parental concern about the health and development of their child. It usually occurs after a medical illness in which the parents are understandably upset or worried about the health of their child (e.g., prematurity, congenital heart disease). However, this concern persists despite the child's recovery. Problems of the syndrome can include pathologic separation difficulties for parent and child, sleep problems, overprotectiveness, and overindulgence. Children are at risk for behavior, school, and peer relationship problems.

106. What are the signs of sibling deprivation in the presence of a child with a chronic illness?

Depression, rebellion, undue hypochondria, envy.

107. Is a child aware of his own fatal illness?

Many studies have demonstrated that even young children are cognizant that a medical condition is life-threatening and experience increased levels of anxiety and isolation compared to children with nonfatal illnesses.

108. How does the cognitive understanding of death evolve?

Toddler (< 3 yrs):	Death as separation, abandonment, or change
Preschool (3–6 yrs):	Prelogical thought with magical and egocentric beliefs that child may be responsible for death; death as temporary and reversible
School-age (6–11 yrs):	Concrete logical thinking; death as permanent and universal but due to a specific illness or injury rather than as a biologic process; death something that occurs to others
Adolescence (12+ yrs):	Abstract logical thinking; more complete comprehension of death; death as a possibility for self

Siegel BS: Bereavement and loss. In Parker S, Zuckerman B (eds): Behavioral and Developmental Pediatrics. Boston, Little, Brown, & Co., 1995, pp 343–347.

109. How should children be punished?

There is no one right way to punish a child, but there are wrong ways. Punishment should teach children that a specific behavior was wrong, but it should not be a mechanism for parents or others to vent their anger or frustration at the child. To meet these goals, punishment should be consistent and relatively brief, carried out in a calm manner as soon as possible after the infraction. Time-out from ongoing activity and removal of privileges are two punishment techniques that can be used. Corporal punishment is not recommended as it is too often used by parents to vent their anger and teaches that hitting is an appropriate response when one is angry at another person.

110. How valid is the proverb "spare the rod and spoil the child" as a defense for corporal punishment?

The actual biblical proverb (Proverbs 13:24) reads, "He who spares the rod hates his son, but he who loves him is careful to discipline him." While the proverb has often been used as a justification for spanking, in actuality it does not refer to specific discipline strategies but rather the need for love and discipline. In addition, the rod may refer to the shepherd's staff, which was used to guide, rather than hit, sheep. Most developmental authorities advise against corporal punishment as a means of discipline.

Carey TA: Spare the rod and spoil the child: Is this a sensible justification for the use of punishment in child rearing? Child Abuse Negl 18:1005–1010, 1994.

111. Should adopted children be informed of their adoption?

In general, yes. It should not occur as a one-time event, but increasing information can be given over time. Most preschool children will not understand the process or meaning of adoption, and for them disclosure should be guided by what the child wants to know. School-age children should be aware of their adoption and feel comfortable discussing it with their parents.

112. What are the consequences of being a "latchkey" child?

The term refers to the millions of children < age 18 who are in unsupervised care after school due to families where one or two parents work. Because of the enormous variability of circumstance, the consequences may be positive (e.g., increased maturity, self-reliance) or negative (e.g., isolation, feelings of neglect). Increased after-school programs may minimize negative consequences.

113. What are the effects of heavy television watching in children?

The extent of television viewing by children in the United States is enormous, with average daily viewing being 3–4 hours. TV viewing ranks as the #1 waking activity of the American child. Schorr has summarized seven principal effects:
1. Increased aggressive behavior and acceptance of violence
2. Difficulty in distinguishing between fantasy and reality
3. Distorted perceptions of reality (i.e., consumerism, extent of violence, role of minorities)
4. Trivialization of sex and sexuality
5. Increased passivity and disengagement
6. Negative effects on cognitive learning
7. Loss of time and potential to inform and teach "prosocial" behavior

From Schorr LB: Environmental deterrents: Poverty, affluence, violence and television. In Levine MD, et al (eds): Developmental-Behavioral Pediatrics. Philadelphia, W.B. Saunders, 1983, p 207, with permission.

SCHOOL PROBLEMS

114. Define learning disability.

About 5% of school-aged children (boys twice as often as girls) are diagnosed with a learning disability. A learning disability is defined most commonly as "a disorder in one or more of the basic psychological processes involved in understanding or using language, written or spoken, which may manifest itself in an imperfect ability to listen, think, speak, read, write, spell, or to do mathematical calculations." The term does not include children who have learning problems which are primarily the result of visual, hearing, or motor handicaps, mental retardation, emotional disturbance, or environmental, cultural, or economic disadvantage.

Shapiro BK, Gallico RP: Learning disabilities. Pediatr Clin North Am 40:491–490, 1993.

115. Is there a standard classification for learning disabilities?

There is no universally accepted classification, and in fact, nearly 100 studies on the classification of learning disabilities have been done since 1963. One common scheme divides children between **auditory-linguistic** (verbal) learning disability and **visual-spatial** (nonverbal) learning disability.

116. How is dyslexia defined?

The World Federation of Neurology defines dyslexia as a disorder manifested by difficulty in learning to read despite conventional instruction, adequate intelligence, and sociocultural opportunity. It is diagnosed by finding a significant discrepancy between reading achievement and IQ test scores. Letter or number reversals (95 read as 59), while common in children with poor reading skills, are neither necessary nor sufficient to make a diagnosis of dyslexia.

117. How is dyslexia treated?

There is no cure for dyslexia. Appropriate management requires a multidisciplinary team effort involving educators, psychologists, and pediatricians. Counseling is helpful in teaching both the child and parent to deal with the frustrations of a learning disability. Medical interventions should be directed at the optimal management of any associated illnesses or disabilities (visual, hearing, motor). Attention deficits frequently coexist, and medical management should be considered. Other treatments that have been advocated for children with dyslexia include visual training (ocular muscle or tracking exercises), tinted or colored lenses, and sensory-motor integration therapy. No good evidence supports the efficacy of these treatments.

118. What laboratory studies are indicated in the evaluation of a child with school failure?

In children with school failure, hearing and vision should be routinely screened. Psycho-educational evaluation for learning disabilities and IQ measurement should be strongly considered. Most children will not need other specific laboratory tests, with the possible exception of lead screening. The history and physical exam should be used to direct the evaluation. The routine use of electroencephalography, CT scan, MRI, and blood chemistries is not helpful.

119. What are the two types of school refusal?

1. *Anxiety-related:* fearful of separation from parents; insecure; more commonly has school phobia with specific fears; girls affected more often than boys; usually good students.

2. *Secondary-gain type:* no anxiety about school; prefers ease and comfort of home; boys affected more often than girls; usually poor students.

Schmitt BD: School refusal. Pediatr Rev 8:99, 1986.

120. What is Public Law 94-142?

The Education for All Handicapped Children's Act was passed in 1975 and guarantees educational opportunities for disabled children. Originally implemented for those in need of "special education and related services," it has been expanded to apply to children whose chronic illnesses might keep them from school but do not require special education per se. The law mandates the development and implementation of an individualized education plan (IEP) to meet the child's special needs and that such plans be carried out in the "least restrictive environment." The law and revisions originally were for children ages 3–21, but legislation in 1986 (P.L. 99-457) added children birth to age 3 and expanded the early-intervention programs.

121. What is the value of early-intervention or stimulation programs for children with handicapping conditions?

Early-intervention programs vary dramatically in their duration, age at which the intervention begins, intensity, and type of intervention. Thus, a consensus on the outcome of early intervention services has not developed. For children with disabilities, the severity of the disability is the best predictor of outcome. Intensive and comprehensive early-intervention services may result in modest improvements in cognitive development, especially for children at environmental risk. However, the jury is still out. Distinguishing various advances attributable to intervention from those due to maturation alone is difficult.

Turnbull JD: Is early intervention beneficial for children with cerebral palsy? Am J Dis Child 17:54–59, 1993.

122. Is there a role for neurophysiologic retraining or orthomolecular medicine in developmental pediatrics?

Neurophysiologic retraining refers to a group of approaches for developmental disabilities in which it is felt that by stimulating specific sensory inputs or repeating specific motor patterns, the CNS can be retrained or recircuited. These include patterning and optometric visual training, which have been used in the treatment of mental retardation, cerebral palsy, and learning disabilities. However, the AAP (and other organizations) discourages its use, as controlled studies have failed to document significant improvements, and the demands placed on parents attempting these interventions are often extreme.

Orthomolecular medicine (coined by Linus Pauling in 1967) is based on the belief that the developmental and/or emotional disorders are due to deficiencies or abnormalities in the metabolism of specific vitamins or trace elements, which can be overcome by administering massive doses of the vitamin or trace element. Except for some rare inborn errors of metabolism, there is no evidence for the efficacy of this approach. Moreover, large doses of certain vitamins can have toxic side effects.

123. In a toddler or preschooler, what are clues to giftedness?

The entity of giftedness is controversial in developmental pediatrics, and its definition imprecise. Giftedness does not correlate solely with high IQ but instead has components of superior intellect, high levels of creativity, and exceptional task commitment. These are more difficult to assess in the younger child. However, early language development and early reading ability with comprehension are possible markers of superior cognitive abilities.

SLEEP PROBLEMS

124. What is the average daily sleep requirement by age?

Birth—16 hrs	4 yrs—11.5 hrs
6 mos—14.5 hrs	6 yrs—9.5 hrs
12 mos—13.5 hrs	12 yrs—8.5 hrs
2 yrs—13 hrs	18 yrs—8 hrs

125. How do the sleep-wake patterns of breastfed infants compare with non-breastfed infants?

Breastfed infants tend to sleep for shorter times and wake more frequently during the night. This may be related to the fact that gastric emptying is more rapid with breast milk than with formula.

126. Why is the supine sleeping position recommended for infants?

In countries (e.g., New Zealand, United Kingdom, Netherlands) that advocated the supine sleeping position as a preventive measure for sudden infant death syndrome (SIDS), there were dramatic decreases in the incidence of SIDS. Hypotheses on why the prone position is more dangerous for infants have included the potential for airway obstruction and the possibility of rebreathing carbon dioxide, particularly when soft bedding is used. Prone sleeping is still advocated for children with significant gastroesophageal reflux or potential airway problems in the supine position (e.g., those with small mandibles).

Willinger M: Sleep position and sudden infant death syndrome. JAMA 273:818–819, 1995.

127. Do infants sleep better prone or supine?

Although the supine position is recommended to minimize the chance of SIDS, infants sleep longer (by 16%), have fewer and shorter arousals (by 40%), and spend greater time in non-REM sleep (by 25%) in the prone position.

Kahn A, et al: Prone or supine body position and sleep characteristics in infants. Pediatrics 91:1112, 1993.

128. Does feeding infants cereal before bedtime promote their sleeping through the night?

It is important to have current references on hand when debating a knowledgeable grandmother because most will insist it is so. In truth, data remain conflicting. One randomized study found no evidence of a relationship between the introduction of cereal and the likelihood of sleeping through the night at age 3 weeks or 4 months, while another (Bamford et al) found increasing duration of sleep with the earlier introduction of solids.

Macknin ML, et al: Infant sleep and bedtime cereal. Am J Dis Child 143:1066–1068, 1989.
Bamford FN, et al: Sleep in the first year of life. Dev Med Child Neurol 32:718–724, 1990.

129. How much do babies normally cry each day?
In Brazleton's oft-quoted 1962 study of 80 infants, it was found that at 2 weeks of age, the average crying time was nearly 2 hours per day, increasing to nearly 3 hours at 6 weeks and then declining to about 1 hour at 12 weeks.
Brazelton TB: Crying in infancy. Pediatrics 29:579–586, 1962.

130. What characterizes infantile colic?
Colic is excessive crying or fussiness, which occurs in 10–20% of infants, and is one of the most frequent problems encountered in early pediatric office visits. For study purposes, it is defined as paroxysms of crying in an otherwise healthy infant for > 3 hours/day on > 3 days/week. The typical picture is a baby (usually ages 2 wks to 3 mos) who screams continuously in the late afternoon or evening, often after feedings. The baby is nearly inconsolable, appears in pain, and frequently has a slightly distended abdomen with legs drawn up. Occasional temporary relief occurs if gas is passed.

The symptoms nearly always resolve by 3 months, but the problem can have repercussions, including early discontinuation of breastfeeding, multiple formula changes, heightened maternal anxiety and distress, diminished maternal-infant interaction, and increased risks for child abuse.
Lehtonen LA, Rautava PT: Infantile colic: Natural history and treatment. Curr Probl Pediatr 26:79–85, 1996.

131. Explain the origins of colic.
Studies have not revealed a unifying explanation for colic, but many theories have been proposed including:
Gastrointestinal: cow's milk protein intolerance, lactose intolerance, immature GI system with hyperperistalsis and excessive gas, faulty feeding techniques (especially overfeeding)
Hormonal (causing enterospasm): increased motilin levels, increased circulating serotonin, progesterone deficiency
Temperamental: difficult temperament, hypersensitivity to stimulation
Parental handling: inappropriate responses to a crying infant, heightened maternal anxiety
Parker S: Colic. In Parker S, Zuckerman B (eds): Behavioral and Developmental Pediatrics. Boston, Little, Brown, & Co., 1995, p 101–105.

132. Are any treatments useful for colic?
Treatment for possible GI causes, including dietary changes to eliminate cow's milk in the infant's or nursing mother's diet or use of simethicone to decrease intestinal gas, have yielded minimal positive benefit. Other medications, such as phenobarbital and diphenhydramine, are used empirically in clinical practice for severe cases of crying. They may be helpful due to their sedating qualities, but large double-blind studies have not been done and long-term use is not encouraged. Dicyclomine HCl had been used effectively in earlier decades for colic but was associated with apnea and is now contraindicated for infants. Interventions which increase vestibular stimulation (e.g., increased carrying, real or simulated automobile rides) have not been shown to be consistently beneficial. Parental counseling with regard to colic and the appropriate responses to crying has shown more success.
Carey WB: The effectiveness of parent counseling in managing colic. Pediatrics 94:333–334, 1994.

133. When do infants begin to sleep through the night?
By about 3 months of age, about 70% of infants (slightly more for bottlefed and slightly less for breastfed babies) will not cry or awaken their parents between midnight and 6 AM. By 6 months, 90% of infants fit this category.

134. How common is night waking in infancy?
Although infants in increasing percentages appear to sleep uninterrupted through the night in the first 6 months, videotaping reveals that nearly all will awaken at varying intervals but fall back to sleep on their own. Beginning at about 6 months, infants awaken and arouse their caretakers, and by 9 months, 20–50% may become problem wakers unable to fall asleep without help.

135. What do you tell parents to minimize the problem of night waking?

1. After a parental-child bedtime routine, place the infant in the sleep setting while awake (e.g., do not rock an infant to sleep).

2. Parent should not be present as the child falls asleep.

3. Gradually eliminate night feedings (infants by 6 months receive sufficient daytime nutrition to allow this).

4. Transitional objects (e.g., blanket, teddy bear, etc.) may minimize separation issues.

Adair R, et al: Reducing night waking in infancy: A primary care intervention. Pediatrics 899:585–588, 1992.

136. How do sleep patterns vary between an infant and an adult?

Parameter	Infant	Adult
Ratio of REM to non-REM	50:50	20:80
Periodicity of sleep states	50- to 60-min REM-non-REM cycle	90- to 100-min REM-non-REM cycle
Sleep onset state	REM sleep onset	Non-REM sleep onset
Temporal organization of sleep states	REM-non-REM cycles equally throughout sleep period	Non-REM stages III and IV predominant in first third of night; REM state predominant in last third of night

Of note, non-REM parasomnias are partial arousals from deep stage IV sleep and can include night terrors (*pavor nocturnus*), sleepwalking (somnambulism), sleeptalking (somniloquy), and possibly stage IV sleep-related enuresis. REM parasomnias include nightmares and REM behavior disorder (a rare disorder of vigorous, violent self-directed motor attacks).

From Anders TF: Nightmares and other sleep disturbances. In Hoekelman RA, et al (eds): Primary Pediatric Care, 2nd ed. St. Louis, Mosby 1992, p 718; with permission.

137. At what age do sleepwalking and sleeptalking occur?

Sleepwalking occurs most commonly between ages 5 and 10. As many as 15% of children aged 5–12 may have somnambulated once, and as many as 10% of 3-10-year-old children may sleeptalk regularly. The sleepwalking child is clumsy, noncommunicative, restless, and nonpurposeful. The episode is not remembered. Injury is common during this outing. Sleeptalking is monosyllabic and incomprehensible. Both conditions usually end before age 15. Severe cases may benefit from diazepam or imipramine therapy.

138. What is *pavor nocturnus*?

Pavor nocturnus (Latin for fear of the night) is more commonly known as **night terrors**. These are brief episodes of 30 seconds to 5 minutes in which a child sits up, screams, and appears aroused, often staring and sweating profusely. The child cannot be consoled, rapidly goes back to sleep, and does not recall the episode in the morning. Onset of night terrors in an older child or persistent multiple attacks may indicate more serious psychopathology.

139. What is the difference between night terrors and nightmares?

Nightmares are frightening dreams that occur during REM sleep, usually in the last half of the night, and may be readily recalled on awakening. The child is aroused without difficulty and usually consolable, but returning to sleep after a nightmare may be problematic. **Night terrors** occur in non-REM stage IV sleep, usually in the first third of the night, and cannot be recalled. The child is difficult to arouse and poorly consolable; however, the child will usually fall asleep easily if he or she has not been fully aroused.

Blum NJ, Carey WB: Sleep problems among infants and young children. Pediatr Rev 17:87–93, 1996.

140. How can night terrors be prevented?

Often, an explanation of the phenomenon to the parent, with emphasis on not awakening the child, is all that is needed. If stress or sleep deprivation coincide with the night terrors, then they should be addressed. If this is not successful, other approaches may be considered.

1. When night terrors occur at the same time each night, the parent may awaken the child 15 minutes before the anticipated event over a 7-day period and keep him or her awake for at least 5 minutes. This often disrupts the sleep cycle and results in resolution of the problem.

2. Rarely, for severe night terrors, a short course of diazepam will suppress REM sleep, reset the sleep cycles, and result in cessation of the problem.

Lask B: Novel and non-toxic treatment for night terrors. BMJ 297:592, 1988.

VISUAL DEVELOPMENT/DISORDERS

141. How good is a newborn infant's vision?

The visual perception system functions in a fairly complex manner at the time of birth, and as early as 36 hours after birth many infants can both discriminate a number of facial expressions and imitate them. The human face is the most preferred object of fixation in early infancy. The light sense is one of the most primitive of all visual functions and is present by the 7th fetal month.

142. When do binocular fixation and depth perception develop in children?

Binocularity of vision depends primarily on adequate coordination of the extraocular muscles and is normally established by 3–6 months of age. At about 6–8 months, early evidence of depth perception is seen, but it is still poorly developed. Depth perception becomes very accurate at 6 or 7 years and continues to improve through the early teens.

143. How does refractive capacity vary with age?

The newborn infant is typically slightly hyperoptic (far-sighted). The mild hyperopia actually increases slowly for about the first 8 years. Hyperopia then decreases gradually until adolescence, when vision is emmetropic (no refractive error). After 20 years, there is a tendency for myopia (near-sightedness).

144. What is normal visual acuity for children?

Birth–6 mos:	Improves from 20/400 to 20/80 gradually
6 mos–3 yrs:	Improves from 20/80 to 20/50
2–5 yrs:	Improves to 20/40 or better and a < 2-line difference between left and right eyes on visual charts
> 5 yrs:	20/30 or better and < 2-line difference between eyes on visual charts

It should be noted that almost 20% of the pediatric population require eyeglasses for correction of refractive errors prior to adulthood.

145. How common is physiologic anisocoria?

Anisocoria refers to unequalness in pupillary size, which is a relatively common condition. Up to 20% of individuals without any illness will have a difference > 0.4 mm in the size of their pupils.

146. Is heterochromia normal?

It can be. Heterochromia (different colored irises) can be familial, usually transmitted as an autosomal dominant trait. It is also seen in the Waardenburg syndrome (white forelock, congenital deafness, and partial albinism). However, changes in color can occur from trauma, hemorrhage, inflammation (uveitis, iridocyclitis), malignancy (retinoblastoma, neuroblastoma), or glaucoma.

147. How are the degrees of blindness classified?

The World Health Organization defines blindness as:

1. Visual impairment: Snellen visual acuity ≤ 20/60 (best eye corrected)
2. Social blindness: Snellen visual acuity ≤ 20/200 or a visual field ≤ 20°
3. Virtual blindness: Snellen visual acuity < 20/1200 or visual field ≤ 10°
4. Total blindness: No light perception.

148. Which children are at high risk for visual abnormalities?

- Prematurity (birth weight < 1250 gm)
- Family history of congenital ocular abnormality (e.g., cataract, retinoblastoma), strabismus, or amblyopia
- Maternal intrauterine or cervicovaginal infection or substance abuse
- Systemic condition with vision-threatening ocular manifestations

Trobe J: Physician's Guide to Eye Care. San Francisco, American Academy of Ophthalmology, 1993, p 19.

149. What separates pseudostrabismus from true strabismus?

Often a cause of unnecessary ophthalmologic referrals, **pseudostrabismus** is the appearance of ocular misalignment (usually esotropia) that occurs in children with a broad and flat nasal bridge and prominent epicanthal folds. The iris appears shifted to the midline with differing amounts of white sclera on each side. This is a common condition that may occur in up to 30% of newborns. No treatment is required. It may be distinguished from true esotropia, or **strabismus**, by observation of full extraocular movements, by symmetric reflections of a flashlight on the cornea from a distance of about 12 in (although this test as a measure of strabismus is more accurate in infants ≥ 6 months), and by normal visualization of red reflexes by direct ophthalmoscopy.

Infants do not focus well because the macula and fovea are poorly developed at birth. Therefore, it is not uncommon for infants occasionally to have an inward crossing of the eyes or for their eyes to be turned slightly outward to 10° or 15°. Persistent in-turning of the eyes for more than a few seconds or outward deviation > 10–15° requires ophthalmologic referral.

Romano PE: Vision/eye screening: Test twice and refer once. Pediatr Ann 19:359–367, 1990.

150. Name the four most common types of childhood strabismus.

Strabismus is the misalignment of the eyes with either an in-turning (esotropia), out-turning (exotropia), or up-turning (hypertropia) of one eye. Four types most commonly occur:

1. **Strabismus of visual deprivation:** occurs when normal vision in one or both eyes is disrupted by any cause. The most serious varieties occur with tumors (e.g., retinoblastoma). In children with ocular tumors, strabismus may be the presenting sign.

2. **Infantile** or **congenital esotropia:** occurs within the first few months of life, usually as an isolated conditions. Corrective surgery is usually required.

3. **Accommodative esotropia:** commonly occurs between ages 2 and 4 in very far-sighted (hyperopic) children. These children use extra lens accommodation because of their visual problems, leading to persistent convergence. Eyeglasses to correct the hyperopia usually correct the esotropia.

4. **Childhood exotropia:** appears between ages 2 and 5 as intermittent misalignment, often brought on by fatigue, visual inattention, or bright sunlight. There is a strong hereditary component. Surgery is often necessary after correction of refractive errors and elimination of any pathology that might have caused visual deprivation.

Trobe J: Physician's Guide to Eye Care. San Francisco, American Academy of Ophthalmology, 1993, p 157.

151. How does amblyopia develop?

Amblyopia, seen in 2% of American children, is decreased vision not correctable by glasses which occurs in the developing eye due to a variety of causes, including strabismus, anisometropia (large refractive errors between the eyes), congenital cataracts, corneal opacities, or ptosis. Until 9 years of age in children, the visual cortex responds to conflicting images from each eye by suppressing the information from one eye. If this suppression persists for long periods of time, a type of visual disuse atrophy occurs, and vision may be permanently lost despite later correction of the underlying ocular problem. Consequently, vigilant eye screening and ophthalmologic follow-up are important, beginning in the newborn period if abnormalities are noted at that time.

Stager DR, et al: Amblyopia and the pediatrician. Pediatr Ann 19:308–315, 1990.

152. What are the causes of cataracts in children?

33%: Maternal infection during pregnancy (rubella, rubeola, varicella, toxoplasmosis, cytomegalovirus, infectious mononucleosis, herpes simplex)

33%: Idiopathic, sporadic cases

25%: Familial (autosomal dominant with almost complete penetrance)

 9%: Miscellaneous, including associations with various syndromes (e.g., Down syndrome, Turner syndrome, Lowe oculocerebrorenal syndrome, Alport syndrome) and systemic diseases (e.g., galactosemia, galactokinase deficiency, diabetes mellitus)

Magramm I: Amblyopia: Etiology, detection and treatment. Pediatr Rev 13:7–14, 1992.

153. Describe the natural history of nasolacrimal duct obstruction.

Almost all (95%) resolve by 6 months and a few thereafter. Ophthalmologic referral in the first 6 months is usually unnecessary, unless there are multiple episodes of acute dacrocystitis or a large congenital mucocele. Most ophthalmologists advise referral between 6 and 13 months, because during this period simple probing of the duct is curative in 95% of patients. After 13 months, the cure rate by probing alone falls to 75%, and silicone intubation of the duct is often necessary.

Katowitz JA, Welsh M: Timing of initial probing and irrigation in congenital nasolacrimal duct obstruction. Ophthalmology 94:698–705, 1987.

154. How is color blindness inherited?

Color blindness typically involves variable loss of the ability to distinguish colors, especially red, green, and blue. The defects can be partial (anomaly) or complete (anopia). Defects in appreciating red or green color are transmitted in an X-linked recessive manner and affect up to 1% and 6%, respectively, of the male population. Blue color blindness is an autosomal dominant phenomenon and occurs in 0.1% of the population.

155. What visionary in pediatric medicine was also an Olympic gold medalist?

Dr. Benjamin Spock. At the Paris Olympics in 1924, he was a member of the Yale University rowing team that won the gold medal in the eight-oared shell with coxswain. His book, *The Common Sense Book of Baby and Child Care*, has helped many parents stay afloat and has sold over 25 million copies since its original publication in 1945.

3. CARDIOLOGY

Bernard J. Clark, III, M.D., Claudio Ramaciotti, M.D., and Anthony Chang, M.D.

CLINICAL ISSUES

1. Is mitral valve prolapse (MVP) always pathologic?

It's debatable, as some studies show that up to 13% of normal children have some degree of posterior leaflet prolapse on echocardiography. Probably, there is a spectrum of anatomic abnormalities, the most minor of which are a variation of normal. Those children with clinical features of mitral valve insufficiency constitute the pathologic category. Whenever auscultation reveals that classic finding of MVP, referral to a pediatric cardiologist is recommended. This allows evaluation of the child for possible accompanying cardiac abnormalities (e.g., secundum atrial septal defects) and confirmation of the diagnosis.

2. In what ways does MVP present in childhood?

Most MVPs are asymptomatic with a click or murmur heard on physical examination. Other possible presentations include palpitations, shortness of breath, dyspnea on exertion, chest pain, congestive heart failure, subacute bacterial endocarditis, and cerebrovascular accident. MVP is classified as primary or secondary. Secondary forms include:
- An associated systemic manifestation of connective tissue disease (Marfan syndrome, Ehlers-Danlos syndrome, pseudoxanthoma elasticum, osteogenesis imperfecta, Hurler syndrome)
- A reduction in left ventricular cavity size (ostium secundum, atrial septal defect, anorexia nervosa, Ebstein's anomaly)

MacMahon SW, et al: Clinical and epidemiologic issues in mitral valve prolapse: Proceedings of a National Heart, Lung, and Blood Institute Symposium. Am Heart J 113:1265–1332, 1987.

3. Do patients with MVP require prophylaxis against subacute bacterial endocarditis (SBE)?

The incidence of endocarditis in patients with MVP *and* systolic murmur is 1/2000 per annum. Three factors—**male gender, advanced age,** and the presence of **systolic murmur**—seem to be associated with an increased risk of endocarditis in patients with MVP. Thus only patients with MVP and systolic murmur (mitral regurgitation) should receive SBE prophylaxis.

4. Which cardiac conditions lead to Eisenmenger syndrome?

Eisenmenger syndrome refers to cardiac right-to-left or bidirectional shunting that results from the development of high pulmonary resistance due to obstructive pulmonary vascular disease. The resultant right-to-left shunting can cause chronic hypoxia with cyanosis, polycythemia, right ventricular hypertrophy, and congestive heart failure, depending on the size of the shunt. Congenital heart lesions that have high systemic-to-pulmonary (left-to-right) flow, such as ventricular septal defect, atrioventricular canal defects, and patent ductus arteriosus, can progressively cause pathologic changes in pulmonary arterioles and arteries with medial and intimal thickening. These changes eventually become irreversible, and the shunt direction changes. Eisenmenger syndrome then results.

5. A child with a chronic cyanotic heart disease develops polycythemia. At what level should phlebotomy or partial exchange be considered?

As a consequence of cyanosis, younger patients develop iron-deficiency anemia, whereas older patients develop polycythemia. Polycythemia secondary to cyanosis can lead to CNS complications such as cerebrovascular accident and brain abscess. Phlebotomy or partial exchange is usually performed when hematocrit is > 60–65%.

6. What are the most common vascular rings and slings?

	Frequency	Symptoms	Treatment
"Complete" rings			
Double aortic arch	40%	Respiratory difficulty (onset < 3 mos) Swallowing dysfunction	Surgical division of a smaller arch
Right aortic arch with left ligamentum arteriosum	30%	Mild respiratory difficulty (onset > 1 yr) Swallowing dysfunction	Surgical division of ligamentum arteriosum
"Incomplete" rings			
Anomalous innominate artery	10%	Stridor and/or cough in infancy	Conservative management or surgical suturing of artery to the sternum
Aberrant right subclavian artery	20%	Occasional swallowing dysfunction	Usually no treatment necessary
Vascular sling or anomalous left pulmonary artery (LPA)	Rare	Wheezing and cyanotic episodes since birth	Surgical division of anomalous LPA (from RPA) and anastomosis to the MPA

Adapted from Park MK: Cardiology for Practitioners, 3rd ed. St. Louis, Mosby-Year Book, 1995.

7. Describe the three main categories of cardiomyopathy in children.

1. **Dilated cardiomyopathy** is the most common and is the end stage of several processes, especially viral myocarditis. Most commonly, no specific cause is identified. Anatomically, the heart is normal, but both ventricles are dilated. Older children present with symptoms of congestive heart failure, including malaise, edema, weight gain, respiratory distress, and nocturia. Infants present with poor weight gain, feeding difficulty, and respiratory distress. In all pediatric age groups, a more acute presentation with shock can occur. Treatment includes inotropic support, diuretics, and afterload-reducing agents. In progressive forms, cardiac transplant is the only definitive treatment.

2. **Hypertrophic cardiomyopathy** *without* **LV outflow obstruction** is usually associated with systemic metabolic disease, particularly storage disease. Pompe disease (glycogen storage disease type II) and some deficiencies of mitochondrial enzymes are prototypical. Patients may present either gradually with failure to thrive or acutely in shock. Cardiomegaly is a constant feature. Pompe disease may have associated hypoglycemia. Treatment generally includes inotropic support, diuretics, and dietary manipulation to treat the underlying metabolic problems.

3. **Hypertrophic cardiomyopathy** *with* **LV outflow obstruction** is also known by terms such as idiopathic hypertrophic subaortic stenosis (IHSS) or asymmetric septal hypertrophy. Of these patients, 90% have a degree of LV outflow tract obstruction secondary to abnormal hypertrophy of the subaortic region of the intraventricular septum. Most are inherited in an autosomal dominant fashion. This cardiomyopathy is associated with ventricular dysrhythmias and sudden death. Treatment usually includes beta-blockers (e.g., propranolol) or calcium channel blockers (e.g., verapamil). Occasionally, surgical myomectomy of the obstructing portion of the septum is needed.

8. What are the cardiac causes of sudden death in young athletes?

Sudden death occurs because of ventricular fibrillation in the setting of myocardial or coronary abnormalities or primary rhythm disorders. The main structural causes are hypertrophic cardiomyopathy, anomalies of the coronary artery, Marfan syndrome, and arrhythmogenic RV dysplasia. Abnormal coronary arteries as a sequelae of Kawasaki syndrome may be a consideration. Prolonged QT syndrome and Wolff-Parkinson-White syndrome have also been implicated. Children with repaired congenital heart disease (especially aortic stenosis, tetralogy of Fallot, transposition of the great vessels, and Ebstein's anomaly) are at higher risk for sudden death.

Despite the notoriety of sudden death (especially in professional or college athletes), it should be noted that sudden death is rare in younger athletes. Of the approximately 5 million high schoolers who participate in athletics each year, only 25 (or 1/200,000) die of atraumatic causes during sports.

Liberthson RR: Current concepts: Sudden death from cardiac causes in children and young adults. N Engl J Med 334:1039–1044, 1996.

Rowland TW: Sudden unexpected death in sports. Pediatr Ann 21:189–195, 1992.

9. How can the preparticipation sports physical identify patients at risk for sudden death?

History

1. Some common causes of sudden death may be associated with preceding symptoms of exertional chest discomfort, dizziness or prolonged dyspnea with exercise, syncope, or palpitations.

2. Family history of cardiovascular disease at an early age or sudden death. For example, although 40% of cases of hypertrophic cardiomegaly are sporadic, 60% are inherited in an autosomal dominant fashion.

3. History of seizures may be associated with prolonged QT syndrome.

Physical exam

1. Marfanoid features: tall and thin habitus, hyperextensible joints, pectus excavatum, click and murmur suggestive of MVP.

2. Pathologic murmurs, particularly a systolic murmur that increases with expiration and standing or decreases with squatting and is associated with an increased LV impulse (e.g., hypertrophic cardiomyopathy) or one associated with a suprasternal thrill (e.g., valvular aortic stenosis).

3. Dysrhythmia present.

McCaffrey FM, et al: Sudden cardiac death in young athletes. Am J Dis Child 145:177–183, 1991.

10. In which patients is syncope more likely to be of a cardiac nature?

Syncope is suspicious for a cardiac cause if it includes:

1. Sudden onset without any prodromal period of dizziness or imminent awareness
2. Syncope during exercise
3. Complete loss of awareness and muscle tone so that fall results in injury, usually head trauma
4. History of palpitations or abnormal heartbeat prior to event
5. Very fast or very slow heart rate after event
6. Family history of sudden death

Cardiac syncope can be caused by hypertrophic cardiomyopathy, congenital heart disease (although syncope is very rare as an initial presentation), and pathologic rhythm disturbances, including tachydysrhythmias (especially in Wolff-Parkinson-White and prolonged QT syndrome) and bradydysrhythmias (especially in sick sinus syndrome and heart block).

Gersony WM: The older child and adolescent with chest pain, mitral valve prolapse, syncope. In Gessner IH, Victoria BE (eds): Pediatric Cardiology: A Problem Oriented Approach. Philadelphia, W.B. Saunders, 1993, pp 147–154.

11. Can tilt-table testing help in evaluating children with unexplained syncope?

One of the causes of syncope in children and adolescents is neurally mediated hypotension and bradycardia. This condition goes by various names, including vasovagal neuroregulatory syncope, neurocardiogenic syncope, or vasodepressor syncope. In this syncope, individuals who experience an orthostatic challenge may paradoxically respond with a decreased heart rate and increased peripheral vasodilation, which results in recurrent syncope. Tilt-table testing can identify those individuals with this abnormal physiologic response.

Samoil D, et al: Head-upright tilt table testing in children with unexplained syncope. Pediatrics 92:426–430, 1993.

12. Which clinical and laboratory findings are suggestive of transient myocardial ischemia in a neonate?

Transient myocardial ischemia is usually encountered in a term infant with a history of hypoxic stress. Respiratory difficulty and signs of congestive heart failure (e.g., tachycardia, cardiomegaly,

and a gallop rhythm) are frequently present. A systolic murmur due to tricuspid or mitral regurgitation is also a common finding. The severity of the clinical picture may vary from mild to circulatory
shock. The ECG frequently demonstrates features of subendocardial ischemia with generalized
flattening of T waves and ST-segment depression. During recovery, abnormal Q waves may also be
observed. On echocardiography, decreased ventricular shortening and Doppler findings of mitral
and/or tricuspid regurgitation occur. Serum levels of creatinine kinase (MB fraction) are characteristically elevated, particularly in the presence of tricuspid regurgitation. The uptake of thallium by
the myocardium may be abnormal but usually normalizes within 1–2 months.

13. How valuable is the pediatric autopsy?

As diagnostic technology has developed, the percentage of autopsies performed has declined
in both adult and pediatric medicine. However, in one review of autopsies of 193 children, 10%
of cases revealed an unexpected finding that, had it been known, might have changed management with possibilities of cure or significantly prolonged survival. Another 18% had unexpected
major findings that would not have changed management.

Stambouly JJ, et al: Correlation between clinical diagnoses and autopsy findings in critically ill children. Pediatrics 92:248–251, 1993.

CONGENITAL HEART DISEASE

14. What are the proven etiologies for congenital heart disease (CHD)?

Only a small percentage of cases have identifiable causes:

• Primary genetic factors (e.g., chromosomal abnormalities or single gene abnormalities)	10%
• Environmental factors (e.g., chemicals, drugs such as isotretinoin, viruses such as rubella, and maternal disease)	3–5%
• Genetic-environmental interactions (i.e., multifactorial)	85%

15. What prenatal maternal factors may be associated with cardiac disease in the neonate?

Prenatal Historical Factor	Associated Cardiac Defect
Diabetes mellitus	LV outflow obstruction (asymmetric septal hypertrophy, aortic stenosis), D-transposition of great arteries, ventricular septal defect
Lupus erythematosus	Heart block, pericarditis, endomyocardial fibrosis
Rubella	Patent ductus arteriosus, pulmonic stenosis (peripheral)
Alcohol abuse	Pulmonic stenosis, ventricular septal defect
Trimethadione usage	Ventricular septal defect, tetralogy of Fallot
Lithium usage	Ebstein's anomaly
Aspirin abuse	Persistent pulmonary hypertension syndrome
Coxsackie B infection	Myocarditis

From Gewitz MH: Cardiac disease in the newborn infant. In Polin RA, Yoder MC, Burg FD (eds): Workbook
in Practical Neonatology, 2nd ed. Philadelphia, W.B. Saunders, 1993, p 271; with permission.

16. In a cyanotic newborn, how can you distinguish primary pulmonary parenchymal disease from CHD?

The **hyperoxia test**. The infant is placed in 100% oxygen, and an arterial blood gas is obtained. A PaO$_2$ > 100 mmHg is usually achieved in infants with primary lung disease, whereas a
PaO$_2$ < 100 mmHg is characteristic of heart disease. Unfortunately, the hyperoxia test does not usually distinguish children with cyanotic heart disease from those with persistent pulmonary hypertension (PPHN). To distinguish between these entities, 100% O$_2$ is administered while the patient is
gently hyperventilated. If the PaO$_2$ rises above 100 mmHg, the diagnosis is more likely to be PPHN.

17. During the first day of life, which congenital heart lesions commonly present with cyanosis?

Independent pulmonary and systemic circulations (severe cyanosis)
   Transposition of great arteries with an intact ventricular septum
Inadequate pulmonary blood flow (severe cyanosis)
   Tricuspid valve atresia
   Pulmonary valve atresia with intact ventricular septum
   Tetralogy of Fallot
   Ebstein's anomaly of the tricuspid valve
Admixture lesions (moderate cyanosis)
   Total anomalous pulmonary venous return
   Victoria BE: Cyanotic newborns. In Gessner IH, Victoria BE (eds): Pediatric Cardiology: A Problem Oriented Approach. Philadelphia, W.B. Saunders, 1993, p 101.

18. In the patient with suspected heart disease, what bony abnormalities seen on a chest x-ray increase the likelihood of CHD?

- Hemivertebrae, rib anomalies—associated with tetralogy of Fallot, truncus arteriosus, VACTERL syndrome
- 11 ribs—seen in Down syndrome
- Skeletal chest deformities (scoliosis, pectus excavatum, narrow AP diameter)—associated with Marfan syndrome, mitral valve prolapse
- Bilateral rib notching—coarctation of the aorta (usually older children)

19. How do pulmonary vascular markings on a chest x-ray help in the differential diagnosis of a cyanotic newborn with suspected cardiac disease?

In a moderate or severely cyanotic newborn with findings suggestive of anatomic heart disease, the chest x-ray may help to differentiate the types of congenital heart defects. The increase or decrease in pulmonary vascular markings is indicative of pulmonary blood flow:

Decreased pulmonary markings
   Ebstein's anomaly
   Pulmonary atresia or severe stenosis
   Tetralogy of Fallot
   Tricuspid atresia, severe stenosis or insufficiency
Increased pulmonary markings
   Total anomalous pulmonary venous return
   Transposition of great arteries

20. What ECG and chest x-ray findings are considered characteristic for various congenital heart malformations?

ECG
- Left axis deviation—atrial septal defect (primum), endocardial cushion defect, tricuspid atresia
- Wolff-Parkinson-White—Ebstein's anomaly, L-transposition of great arteries
- Complete heart block—L-transposition of great arteries, polysplenia

Chest x-ray
- Boot-shaped heart—tetralogy of Fallot or tricuspid atresia
- Egg-shaped heart—transposition of great arteries
- "Snowman"—total anomalous pulmonary venous return

21. Which are the ductal-dependent cardiac lesions?

- Ductal-dependent pulmonary blood flow
   Critical pulmonic stenosis
   Pulmonary atresia with intact ventricular septum
   Tricuspid atresia

- Ductal-dependent systemic blood flow
    - Aortic arch interruption
    - Coarctation of the aorta
    - Hypoplastic left heart syndrome

22. Which types of CHD are associated with right aortic arch?

Tetralogy of Fallot with pulmonary atresia (pseudotruncus arteriosus)	50%
Truncus arteriosus	35%
Classic tetralogy of Fallot	25%
Double outlet right ventricle	25%
Single ventricle	12.5%

Crowley JJ, et al: Telltale small signs of congenital heart disease. Radiol Clin North Am 31:573–582, 1993.

23. Which genetic syndromes are most commonly associated with CHD?

Syndrome	Patients with CHD	Predominant Heart Defect(s)
Down	50%	ECD, VSD, TOF
Turner	20	CoA
Noonan	65	PS, ASD, ASH
Marfan	60	MVP, AoAn, AR
Trisomy 18	90	VSD, PDA
Trisomy 13	80	VSD, PDA
DiGeorge	80	IAA-B, TA
Williams	75	SVAS, peripheral PS

AoAn = aortic aneurysm; AR = aortic regurgitation; ASD = atrial septal defect; ASH = asymmetric septal hypertrophy; CoA = coarctation of the aorta; ECD = endocardial cushion defect; IAA-B = interrupted aortic arch, type B; MVP = mitral valve prolapse; PDA = patent ductus arteriosus; PS = pulmonic stenosis; SVAS = supravalvular aortic stenosis; TA = truncus arteriosus; TOF = tetralogy of Fallot; VSD= ventricular septal defect.
From Frias JL: Genetic issues of congenital heart defects. In Gessner IH, Victoria BE: Pediatric Cardiology: A Problem Oriented Approach. Philadelphia, W.B. Saunders, 1993, p 238; with permission.

24. Which infants with CHD should be evaluated for other anomalies?

In the evaluation of the newborn with heart disease, several known associations between CHD and other anomalies should be considered, especially for the patient with more complex disease. Syndromes such as CHARGE or VACTERL may first be detected by the presence of heart disease and one other anomaly. More subtle is the now-known association between conotruncal defects—including tetralogy of Fallot, truncus arteriosus, and interrupted aortic arch—and deletion in chromosome 22. Some of these patients may have DiGeorge syndrome or velo-cardio-facial syndrome, but others may have only subtle palatal dysfunction. For this reason, patients with conotruncal cardiac defects should undergo screening for deletions in chromosome 22, and if found, these patients should be referred to a geneticist for special testing and evaluation.

25. Why does the ductus arteriosus close after birth?

Patency of the ductus arteriosus in the neonate is regulated by the opposing actions of oxygen (constrictor) and prostaglandin E_2 (dilator). In addition, several mediators (bradykinin, acetylcholine histamine, and 5-hydroxytryptamine) have been demonstrated to constrict the ductus in vitro. Most of these substances, however, are not active in vivo. Permanent closure is brought about by destruction of the endothelium and proliferation of the subintimal layers. Ultimately, connective tissue is formed which seals the lumen.

26. Describe the clinical manifestations of a patent ductus arteriosus.

- Tachypnea and tachycardia
- Bounding pulses
- Hyperdynamic precordium
- Systolic murmur or systolic and diastolic murmur
- Wide pulse pressures
- Labile oxygenation
- Apnea

27. When should indomethacin be administered to newborns with a PDA?

Indomethacin is effective in closing a PDA within the first 10 days of life and may be most effective during the first 24–48 hours of life. Indomethacin is indicated in preterm infants with a hemodynamically significant PDA, defined as one in which there is deteriorating respiratory status (e.g., tachypnea, apnea, CO_2 retention, increased ventilatory support, failure to wean ventilatory support) or evidence of congestive heart failure. For infants < 1000 gm, indomethacin treatment should be initiated at the first sign of a clinical PDA. An asymptomatic murmur will develop into a large hemodynamically significant shunt in 80% of these babies. Infants > 1000 gm have a higher rate of spontaneous closure, and only 30% will develop a hemodynamically significant shunt. For these infants, a PDA murmur may be followed, without treatment, but therapy should be initiated as soon as symptoms of a significant shunt occur.

Clyman RI: Recommendations for the postnatal use of indomethacin: An analysis of four separate treatment strategies. J Pediatr 128:601–607, 1996.

28. How often does a PDA reopen after indomethacin therapy?

Reopening following successful closure with indomethacin occurs in approximately 25% of infants (33% of infants < 1000 gm). The ductus is more likely to reopen when indomethacin therapy is initiated beyond the first week of life. In most cases, permanent constriction does not occur after a single dose; second and third doses are recommended 12 and 36 hours following the initial one. Of note, the response to indomethacin does not, in general, depend on the peak concentration or duration of therapy. Recurrence is also independent of the initial concentrations or duration of administration. The rate of reopening is the same whether the drug is given continuously for 36 hours or over 5–7 days.

29. When should the ductus arteriosus be surgically ligated?

Surgical ligation is generally indicated in infants who have failed two courses of medical management, including indomethacin. In infants in whom indomethacin is contraindicated (e.g., BUN > 30 mg/dl, creatinine > 1.8 mg/dl, platelet count < 60,000/mm³, evidence of bleeding diathesis) and decompensation has occurred secondary to the PDA, surgical ligation should be performed.

30. Does phototherapy increase the incidence of PDA in premature infants?

In vitro studies have demonstrated that exposure of isolated ductal rings to light resulted in photorelaxation and prevention of constriction despite stimulation with oxygen. While a significant reduction in the incidence of PDA with shielding of the chest wall from phototherapy has been reported in premature infants, the use of shielding remains very controversial and should not be used routinely.

31. How do an ostium primum and an ostium secundum defect differ?

A variety of atrial septal defects exist, categorized in large part by their location. Defects may be isolated to the septum itself or may extend into the ventricles (e.g., endocardial cushion defects). An **ostium secundum** is an isolated defect that involves a persistently enlarged opening at the fossa ovalis, which is approximately in the center of the septum. An **ostium primum** defect is located more inferiorly and is part of an atrioventricular canal defect, often in association with a regurgitant mitral valve.

32. How do the presentations of VSD and ASD differ?

Ventricular septal defect: The child with a small VSD usually presents with a systolic murmur in the first few days of life, frequently before discharge from the nursery. These infants do not have signs related to the cardiovascular system, and spontaneous closure occurs in most. In an infant with a large VSD, signs indicative of congestive heart failure generally appear at 4–8 weeks of age, as the pulmonary vascular resistance drops and pulmonary blood flow increases. Congestive heart failure can occasionally be seen at 1–2 weeks of age in infants with large shunts in whom vascular resistance falls more quickly.

Atrial septal defects: Most children with an isolated ASD are not diagnosed until they are of school age. The majority are totally asymptomatic at the time of diagnosis. About 10–15%

of infants with an ASD demonstrate signs of congestive heart failure during the first months of life. The congestive heart failure is due to a large left-to-right shunt and increased pulmonary blood flow and is often associated with failure to thrive or recurrent lower respiratory infections.

33. What occurs during a "tet spell"?

Tet spells are cyanotic and hypoxic episodes that occur in patients with classic tetralogy of Fallot (TOF), in children with TOF with pulmonary atresia, and in those with complex anatomy and TOF "physiology" (such as double-outlet right ventricle with pulmonary stenosis). The specific cause is usually uncertain, but episodes are characterized by a **decrease** in systemic vascular resistance and an **increase** in pulmonary vascular resistance and pulmonary outflow tract narrowing. Increased right-to-left shunting results in progressive cyanosis and hypoxia. While most episodes are self-limited and last < 30 minutes, a prolonged tet spell can lead to stroke or death. Anemia may be a predisposing factor.

34. How do you prevent a "tet spell" from becoming trouble?

1. Patient should assume a squatting or knee-chest position to increase systemic vascular resistance.
2. Supplemental oxygen should be given.
3. Morphine, 0.1 mg/kg IM or IV (exact mechanism of action unclear but may relate to both sedation and pulmonary vascular dilation).
4. If prolonged, $NaHCO_3$, 1.0 mEq/kg IV.
5. If prolonged, phenylephrine, 50–100 μg/kg IV bolus, or propranolol, 0.1 mg/kg IV.
6. If prolonged, volume expansion.
7. Whether brief or prolonged, a calm physician.

35. After what age does a presumed peripheral pulmonic stenosis murmur deserve more detailed study?

The murmur of peripheral pulmonic stenosis, a low-intensity systolic ejection murmur heard frequently in newborns, is due to the relative hypoplasia as well as the acute angle of the branching of pulmonary arteries in the early newborn period. This murmur usually persists until 3–6 months of age.

36. What should parents be told about the risk of recurrence for common heart defects?

Recurrence risks for cardiovascular anomalies vary from 1–3% and are usually higher with the more common lesions (e.g., the recurrence risk for VSD is 3%, higher than the 1% recurrence risk for Ebstein's anomaly). The risk of CHD in pregnancies after the birth of one affected child is about 1–4%. With 2 affected first-degree relatives, the risk is tripled; with 3, the family may be considered "type C," in which recurrence risk may be even higher than that in mendelian inheritance.

CONGESTIVE HEART FAILURE

37. Identify the clinical signs and symptoms associated with congestive heart failure (CHF) in children.

They may be grouped into three categories (* = often seen in infants):

1. **Signs of impaired myocardial performance:** cardiomegaly,* tachycardia,* gallop rhythm, cold extremities or mottling, pulsus paradoxus and pulsus alternans, growth failure,* sweating*
2. **Signs of pulmonary congestion:** tachypnea,* wheezing, rales, cyanosis, dyspnea, cough
3. **Signs of systemic venous congestion:** hepatomegaly,* neck vein distention, peripheral edema

38. What acid-base changes are associated with CHF?

Mild CHF—respiratory alkalosis, as a result of tachypnea (stimulation of J receptors by increasing pulmonary edema)

Moderate or severe CHF—respiratory acidosis, as a consequence of pulmonary edema and reduced compliance, and metabolic acidosis, as a result of decreased tissue perfusion

39. In infancy, how does the likely cause of CHF vary by age?

At birth	• Hypoplastic left heart syndrome
	• Severe birth asphyxia (hypoxia + acidosis)
	• Volume overload lesions
	Severe tricuspid or pulmonary insufficiency
	Large systemic AV fistula
First week	• PDA in small premature infants
	• Transposition of great arteries
	• Hypoplastic left heart syndrome (with more favorable anatomy)
	• Total anomalous pulmonary venous return, particularly with pulmonary venous obstruction
	• Others:
	Systemic AV fistula
	Critical aortic or pulmonic stenosis
1–4 wk	• Coarctation of the aorta (preductal, with associated anomalies)
	• Critical aortic stenosis
	• Large left-to-right shunt lesions (VSD, PDA) in premature infants
	• All other lesions listed above
4–6 wk	• Some left-to-right shunt such as complete AV canal defect
6 wk–4 mo	• Large VSD
	• Large ASD
	• Others (e.g., anomalous left coronary artery from the pulmonary artery)

From Park MK: Pediatric Cardiology for Practitioners, 3rd ed. St. Louis, Mosby, 1995; with permission.

40. If a patient develops CHF and cardiomegaly but no murmur is heard, what is the differential diagnosis?

Newborns
• Myocarditis
• Cardiomyopathy secondary to asphyxia, hypoglycemia, or hypocalcemia
• Glycogen storage disease (Pompe disease)
• Cardiac dysrhythmia
    Paroxysmal supraventricular tachycardia
    Congenital heart block
    Atrial flutter and/or fibrillation
• Arteriovenous malformations, e.g., CNS (vein of Galen)
• Sepsis
Outside newborn period
• Myocardial diseases
    Endocardial fibroelastosis
    Myocarditis (viral or idiopathic)
    Glycogen storage disease (Pompe disease)
• Coronary artery diseases resulting in myocardial insufficiency
    Anomalous origin of LCA from pulmonary artery
    Collagen disease (periarteritis nodosa)
    Kawasaki syndrome (mucocutaneous lymph node syndrome)
    Calcification of coronary artery
    Medial necrosis of coronary artery
• CHD with severe heart failure
    Coarctation of the aorta in infants
    Ebstein's anomaly

41. When should afterload reduction be used in children?

In settings of low cardiac output (CO) due to myocardial dysfunction with increased peripheral vascular resistance (cool extremities and poor capillary refill) and pulmonary congestion,
afterload reduction can decrease overall cardiac work and myocardial O_2 consumption while increasing CO and oxygen delivery. It is best used to aid a failing heart in the immediate postoperative period but also may be of value in children with chronic ventricular dysfunction and
those with mitral and/or aortic regurgitation or systemic-to-pulmonic shunts. Agents can be used
that preferentially dilate arterioles (e.g., hydralazine), veins (e.g., sodium nitroprusside), or both
(e.g., captopril and other ACE inhibitors). As a rule, arteriolar vasodilators tend to increase CO,
and venous dilators tend to lessen pulmonary congestion. Afterload reduction may be of little
use in shock states due to causes other than myocardial failure. If the blood pressure remains
unacceptably low (i.e., unstable shock), there is no role for afterload reduction. Volume replacement and inotropic support should first be used. Afterload reduction may also be of little benefit
in the "warm phase" of septic shock when CO is actually increased and there is peripheral
vasodilation.

DIAGNOSTIC STUDIES AND PROCEDURES

42. What are normal pressures and saturations as measured in cardiac catheterizations?

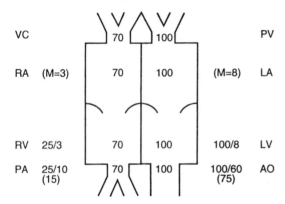

Normal pressure and oxygen saturation
values in children. AO, aorta; LA, left
atrium; LV, left ventricle; PA, pulmonary
artery; PV, pulmonary veins; RA, right
atrium; RV, right ventricle; VC, vena
cava. (From Stromberg D: Cardiac catheterization. In Taeusch HW, et al (eds):
Pediatric and Neonatal Tests and Procedures. Philadelphia, W.B. Saunders,
1996, p 242; with permission.)

43. What is the significance of the Qp/Qs ratio?

Qp/Qs is the ratio of pulmonary blood flow (Qp) to systemic blood flow (Qs), thus quantifying the amount of left-to-right shunt. (It is 1:1 in a normal heart). A quick way of estimating
Qp/Qs is to take the difference of O_2 saturations of aorta and superior vena cava (SVC), and
divide this by the difference of O_2 saturations in the pulmonary vein and artery (assuming the
pulmonary vein to be 99% saturated):

$$Qp/Qs = (Ao\ sat - SVC\ sat)/PV\ sat - PA\ sat$$

44. How is shortening fraction calculated by echocardiography?

$$(LVED - LVES/LVED) \times 100$$

where LVED = left ventricular end-diastolic dimension, and LVES = left ventricular end-systolic
dimension. The normal range is 28–38%.

45. Is echocardiography helpful in diagnosing a patent ductus arteriosus?

With the use of high-resolution, two-dimensional echocardiography, PDA is detectable in
90% of cases. This sensitivity increases to 100% with the addition of pulsed Doppler to detect reversal of blood flow in the descending aorta during diastole. Nevertheless, the *clinical* assessment

of a preterm infant with a PDA is generally adequate to guide therapeutic decisions. When the diagnosis of PDA is in doubt, the echocardiogram can help to confirm the diagnosis.

46. What are the indications for endomyocardial biopsy (EMB)?
1. Cardiac transplant rejection—EMB is still the most reliable technique for diagnosing rejection, even though cyclosporine has altered biopsy findings.
2. Doxorubicin cardiotoxicity—EMB is the most sensitive method for determining the extent of myocardial injury. This had lead to a decrease in deaths due to cardiomyopathy-related CHF.
3. Other potential uses for EMB: myocarditis, glycogen storage disease, cardiac tumors, and rheumatic carditis.

47. When is exercise testing indicated in a child?
Exercise testing is generally performed on children ≥ 4 years of age since coordination and cooperation are needed for the treadmill or bicycle ergometer.
Indications
• Diagnosis of exercise-induced symptoms, such as syncope, chest pain, or palpitations
• Evaluation of patients with known or suspected dysrhythmias; usually tachydysrhythmias or ectopy
• Evaluation of exercise tolerance, especially postoperatively
• Assessment of potential myocardial ischemia, as in LV outflow tract obstruction, cardiomyopathies, or coronary artery diseases
• Assessment of blood pressure responses, especially in coarctation of the aorta
Contraindications
• Active inflammatory cardiac disease
• Acute heart failure
• Critical cardiac outflow obstruction
• Known ischemic disease with angina
• Severe pulmonary vascular disease
• Severe hypertension
• Serious rhythm disturbance
Graham TP, et al: Recommendations for use of laboratory studies for pediatric patients with suspected or proven heart disease. Circulation 72:207, 443A–450A, 1987.

48. Name the most common indication in children for a pacemaker.
Symptomatic bradycardia. Bradycardia may be due to a variety of reasons, including complete heart block, sick sinus syndrome, or the use of cardiac medications that cause bradycardia (e.g., propranolol). Other indications include the use of ventricular pacemakers to better control certain types of ventricular dysrhythmias, such as those due to prolonged QT syndrome.

49. Explain the code system used to describe pacemakers.
The most commonly used code for pacemakers remains the 3-letter code. The first letter refers to the chamber being paced (**V**entricle, **A**trium, **D**ual), the second to the chamber being sensed (**V**entricle, **A**trium, **D**ual), and the third to the mode of action (**I**nhibit, **T**rigger, n**O**—nothing). Thus, a **VVI** unit indicates a paced ventricle and sensing of spontaneous ventricular activity that can inhibit the pacer. A **VAT** unit senses atrial activity to trigger the ventricle.

50. What methods can be used to diagnose neonatal pulmonary hypertension (PH)?
• Absolute measurements only by right-heart catheterization
• Likely PH if echocardiography demonstrates right-to-left shunting across patent foramen ovale or ductus arteriosus
• Likely PH if the preductal oxygen saturation (e.g., right radial artery) is higher than a simultaneously recorded postductal value (e.g., umbilical artery)
Of note, PH is usually accompanied by tricuspid regurgitation, which can be identified as a regurgitant jet seen on Doppler analysis.

ECG AND DYSRHYTHMIAS

51. What are the developmental changes in the pediatric ECG during childhood?
   1. Lengthening of most, but not all, intervals: P wave duration, PR interval, and QRS duration (an exception is QTc interval).
   2. Decrease in RV forces with increasing age: R in V_1 and S in V_6 decrease in magnitude (axis shifts as well from +75° to +180° in a newborn to –15° to +110° in an adolescent).

52. How does an ECG in the neonate differ from that in an older child or adult?
   While the mass of the two ventricles is similar at midgestation, RV growth is greater during the third trimester. The ECG during the newborn period normally reflects RV dominance. As a consequence, the QRS complex shows a tall R in V_1–V_2 and a deep S wave on V_5–V_6. The leftward sectors are small. The normal newborn also has a rightward QRS axis of +135° to +180° (normal adult, 0° to +90°) and a normal heart rate of 100–140 bpm.

53. What are the most helpful clues for diagnosing right ventricular hypertrophy by ECG in a newborn?
   1. Pure R wave (with no S wave) in V_1 > 10 mm
   2. R in V_1 > 25 mm or R in aVR > 8 mm
   3. A qR pattern in V_1 (also present in 10% of normal newborns)
   4. Upright T in V_1 after 3 days of age
   5. RAD > +180°

54. Describe the ECG abnormalities associated with potassium and calcium imbalances.

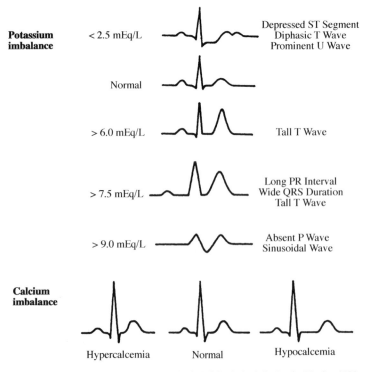

Potassium imbalance	< 2.5 mEq/L	Depressed ST Segment, Diphasic T Wave, Prominent U Wave
	Normal	
	> 6.0 mEq/L	Tall T Wave
	> 7.5 mEq/L	Long PR Interval, Wide QRS Duration, Tall T Wave
	> 9.0 mEq/L	Absent P Wave, Sinusoidal Wave
Calcium imbalance	Hypercalcemia Normal Hypocalcemia	

From Park MK, Guntheroth WG: How to Read Pediatric ECGs, 3rd ed. St. Louis, Mosby, 1992, pp 106–107; with permission.

56. What is the corrected QT interval (QT_C)?

The QT interval represents the time required for ventricular depol
tion. It spans the onset of the QRS complex to the end of the T wave. Th
heart rate, but after about 6 months, it does not vary with age. The QT
ferences. As a rule, a prolonged QT_C interval is diagnosed when the QT $_C$ ᴗ..

$$QT_C = QT \text{ (in sec)} / \sqrt{RR \text{ (in sec)}}$$

57. What causes a prolonged QT interval?

Congenital long QT syndrome
- Hereditary form
   Jervell-Lange-Nielsen syndrome (associated with deafness)
   Romano-Ward syndrome
- Sporadic type

Acquired long QT syndrome
- Drug-induced
   Antidysrhythmic agents (esp. quinidine, procainamide)
   Phenothiazines
   Tricyclic antidepressants
   Lithium
- Metabolic/electrode abnormalities
   Hypocalcemia
   Very-low-energy diets
- CNS and autonomic nervous system disorders (esp. after head trauma or stroke)
- Cardiac disease
   Myocarditis
   Coronary artery disease
- Short QT interval
   Hypercalcemia
   Digitalis effect

58. How abnormal are premature atrial contractions (PACs)?

Premature atrial beats are usually benign, with two exceptions:
1. Infants < 1 year old have a small risk of developing supraventricular tachycardia or atrial flutter if PACs occur frequently.
2. In children on digoxin, PACs may be an early sign of digoxin toxicity.

59. How does paroxysmal atrial tachycardia differ from physiologic sinus tachycardia?

1. Persistent ventricular rate of > 180 bpm
2. Fixed or almost fixed RR interval on ECG
3. Abnormal P-wave shape or axis or absent P waves
4. Little change in heart rate with activity, crying, or breathholding

60. Name the common causes of atrial flutter and fibrillation in childhood.

- Intra-atrial surgery (Mustard, ASD repair)
- Congenital heart disease (Ebstein's anomaly)
- Heart disease with dilated atria (AV valve regurgitation)
- Idiopathic with an otherwise normal heart
- Cardiomyopathy
- Wolff-Parkinson-White syndrome
- Sick sinus syndrome
- Myocarditis
- Digoxin

**,hen are isolated premature ventricular contractions (PVCs) acceptable in the other-
⌐ healthy school-aged child?**
1. ECG intervals, especially QT_C, are normal.
2. No paired or multiform PVCs or "R-on-T" phenomena
3. No evidence of myocarditis, cardiomegaly, or ventricular tumor
4. No history of drug use
5. Electrolytes and glucose are normal.
and *especially* if
6. PVCs decrease with exercise

62. Name the common causes of supraventricular tachycardia.
1. Idiopathic (with a structurally normal heart)
2. CHD (preoperative): Ebstein's anomaly, L-transposition of great arteries, single ventricle
3. CHD (postoperative): atrial surgery
4. Drugs: sympathomimetics (cold medications, theophylline, beta-agonist)
5. Infections: myocarditis or fever
6. Others: Wolff-Parkinson-White syndrome, hyperthyroidism

63. How do you differentiate aberrancy from ventricular tachycardia?
Aberrancy occurs when a supraventricular impulse reaches the AV node or His bundle prematurely and finds only one bundle branch excitable and the other refractory. This results in a
QRS complex resembling a bundle branch block. Premature wide QRS complexes due to aberrancy (vs. one due to a PVC) may be identified by the following five characteristics:
1. The mean ventricular rate is relatively fast.
2. There is QRS variability (in morphology).
3. There is variation of the coupling interval.
4. There is no attempt at a compensatory pause.
5. It is not associated with AV dissociation.
A widened QRS complex could also be due to bundle branch blocks, pre-excitation syndrome
(Wolff-Parkinson-White), intraventricular blocks (such as metabolic disturbance), or pacemakers.

**64. What vagal maneuvers are used to treat paroxysmal supraventricular tachycardia
(PSVT) in children?**
Vagal stimulation slows conduction in the atria and AV node and prolongs refractoriness of
the sinus and AV nodes, interrupting reentrant tachycardias.
Infants
1. Placement of an ice-soaked wet washcloth or rubber cloth filled with crushed ice over
forehead and nose for up to 30 sec
2. Insertion of rectal thermometer
3. Gagging with tongue blade
Older children, adolescents
1. Above methods
2. Unilateral carotid massage
3. Valsalva maneuver (abdominal straining while holding breath)
4. Headstand with support
In general, Valsalva maneuver and carotid massage are not effective for children under age 4.
Eyeball pressure is not recommended because it has been associated with retinal injury.
Kaminer SJ, Strong WB: Cardiac arrhythmias. Pediatr Rev 15:437–439, 1994.

65. Other than vagal maneuvers, what treatments are used acutely in managing PSVT?
If a patient's clinical condition has deteriorated rapidly, synchronized direct-current (DC)
cardioversion is indicated. However, this is rarely used in pediatrics. **Digoxin** is ordinarily *not*

used in acute situations because of its delayed onset of action (3–6 hours). **Adenosine** has replaced **verapamil** as the first drug of choice. An initial bolus of 50 μg/kg will exert an effect in 10–20 sec by blocking conduction through the AV node. If ineffective, the dose can be increased in increments of 50–100 μg/kg every 1–2 min up to 300 μg/kg. Adenosine has a very short half-life (< 10 sec) and minimal side effects (e.g., minor flushing, headache, dyspnea). Because it may provoke or exacerbate bronchospasm, it is relatively contraindicated in asthmatics.

66. How is Wolff-Parkinson-White (WPW) syndrome diagnosed on ECG?

A short PR interval and delta wave (slurring of the QRS upstroke) are characteristic of WPW. An A-V bypass tract can cause early ventricular depolarization (pre-excitation) and may result in supraventricular tachycardia. In infants and younger children with rapid heart rates, the delta wave may not be evident. Additional clues suggestive of WPW include:

1. No Q wave in left chest leads
2. PR interval < 100 msec
3. Left axis deviation
4. QRS duration of > 80 msec

Perry JC, et al: Clues to the electrocardiographic diagnosis of subtle Wolff-Parkinson-White syndrome in children. J Pediatr 117:871–875, 1990.

67. Which children are candidates for transcatheter ablation techniques for supraventricular tachycardia (SVT)?

For children with frequent or intermittently symptomatic SVT, digoxin and beta-blockers are the first line of therapy. Second-line agents include various antidysrhythmics (e.g., flecainide, propafenone, amiodarone) and calcium channel blockers (e.g., verapamil). In transcatheter ablation, a high-frequency alternating electrical current is applied to endocardial tissue. This results in a destructive thermal lesion directly at the focus of abnormal electrical activity or accessory pathway. Ablation therapy is used most commonly in children with dysrhythmias refractory to medical management and in those with life-threatening symptoms or possible lifelong medication requirements.

Villain E: Drugs and ablation in the treatment of supraventricular tachyarrhythmias in children. Curr Opin Pediatr 5:606–610, 1993.

INFECTIOUS AND INFLAMMATORY DISORDERS

68. How many blood cultures should be obtained to rule out subacute bacterial endocarditis?

Three separate blood cultures should be obtained. In 10–30% of children, the first two cultures may be negative. The timing of blood cultures in relation to fever has been found to be unimportant, but the use of multiple sites may decrease the likelihood of mistaking a contaminant for the true etiologic agent.

69. Why might properly collected blood cultures be negative in the setting of clinically suspected bacterial endocarditis?

1. The bacterial endocarditis may be right-sided.
2. Prior antibiotic use
3. Nonbacterial infection: fungal (e.g., aspergillus, candida) or unusual organism (e.g., rickettsia, chlamydia)
4. Unusual bacterial infection: slow-growing organisms or anaerobes
5. Lesions are mural, nonvalvular (less likely to be hematogenously seeded)
6. Nonbacterial thrombotic endocarditis (sterile platelet–fibrin thrombus formations following endocardial injury)
7. Incorrect diagnosis

Starke JR: Infectious endocarditis. In Feigin RD, Cherry JD (eds): Textbook of Pediatric Infectious Diseases, 3rd ed. Philadelphia, W.B. Saunders, 1992, p 332.

70. Which cardiac lesions are most at risk for bacterial endocarditis?

- Tetralogy of Fallot
- Patent ductus arteriosus
- Aortic stenosis
- Pulmonic stenosis
- Ventricular septal defect
- D-transposition of the great arteries
- AV canal defect

71. How reliable is the echocardiogram for diagnosing subacute bacterial endocarditis (SBE)?

Although the yield of echocardiography for diagnosing SBE is low, the likelihood of a positive finding is increased under certain conditions: indwelling catheters, prematurity, immunosuppressed patients on antibiotics, and evidence of peripheral embolization. SBE is still a clinical and laboratory diagnosis (physical examination and blood cultures, respectively) and *not* an "echocardiographic" diagnosis. A negative study does not rule out SBE.

72. How do Osler nodes and Janeway lesions differ?

Both types of lesions are noted in individuals with bacterial endocarditis. Pain is a key discriminator. **Osler nodes** are painful, tender nodules found primarily on the pads of the fingers and toes. **Janeway lesions** are painless, nontender, hemorrhagic nodular lesions seen on the palms and soles, especially on thenar and hypothenar eminences. Both lesions are rare in children with endocarditis.

Farrior JB, Silverman ME: A consideration of the differences between a Janeway's lesion and an Osler's node in infectious endocarditis. Chest 20:239–243, 1976.

73. When should myocarditis be suspected?

The presentation of myocarditis can be variable, ranging from subclinical to rapidly progressive CHF. It should be considered in any patient who presents with unexplained heart failure, particularly if there is tachycardia out of proportion to fever, grunting respirations with relatively clear lungs to auscultation (in early CHF), a quiet precordium, and hepatomegaly.

74. What conditions are associated with the development of myocarditis?
Infections
   Bacterial: diphtheria
   Viral: coxsackie B (most common), coxsackie A, HIV, echoviruses, rubella
   Mycoplasmal
   Rickettsial: typhus
   Fungal: actinomycosis, coccidioidomycosis, histoplasmosis
   Protozoal: trypanosomiasis (Chagas' disease), toxoplasmosis
Inflammatory
   Kawasaki syndrome, systemic lupus erythematosus, rheumatoid arthritis
Chemical/physical agents
   Radiation injury
   Drugs: doxorubicin
   Toxins: lead
   Animal bites: scorpion, snakes

75. When should steroids be given to a child with myocarditis?

The use of steroids in myocarditis is controversial. Some authorities feel that the use of steroids may inhibit interferon synthesis and increase viral replication. If the inflammatory process is secondary to rheumatic disease, however, steroids may be indicated.

76. A child visiting from Mexico presents with unilateral eye swelling and new-onset acute CHF. What is a likely diagnosis?

Acute myocarditis due to **Chagas' disease** (American trypanosomiasis). Seen in 25–50% of patients in endemic areas with early Chagas' disease, Romaña's sign is unilateral, painless, violaceous, palpebral edema often accompanied by conjunctivitis. The swelling occurs near the bite site of the parasitic vector, the *Triatoma* bug. Chagas' disease, a protozoan infection, is the most common cause of acute and chronic myocarditis in Central and South America.

77. What are the common clinical symptoms and signs of pericarditis?

Symptoms: chest pain, fever, cough, palpitations, irritability, abdominal pain, decreased feeding

Signs: friction rub, pallor, pulsus paradoxus, muffled heart sounds, neck vein distention.

78. Describe the possible infectious causes of pericarditis in a child.

Purulent
1. Bacterial: *Staphylococcus aureus, Haemophilus influenzae,* streptococci, *Neisseria meningitidis, Streptococcus pneumoniae,* anaerobes, *Francisella tularensis, Salmonella,* enteric bacilli, *Pseudomonas, Listeria, Neisseria gonorrhoeae, Actinomyces, Nocardia*
2. Tuberculosis
3. Fungal: histoplasmosis, coccidioidomycosis, aspergillosis, candidiasis, blastomycosis, cryptococcosis

Viral
1. Coxsackie virus B
2. Other: influenza A and B, mumps, echoviruses, adenoviruses, infectious mononucleosis, hepatitis viruses, measles, cytomegalovirus

Other
1. Rickettsial: typhus, Q fever
2. Mycoplasma: *Mycoplasma pneumoniae*
3. Parasitic: *Entamoeba histolytica,* echinococcus
4. Spirochetal: syphilis, leptospirosis
5. Chlamydial: psitticosis
6. Protozoal: toxoplasmosis

From Pinsky WW, et al: Infectious endocarditis. In Feigin RD, Cherry JD (eds): Textbook of Pediatric Infectious Diseases, 3rd ed. Philadelphia, W.B. Saunders, 1992, p 378; with permission.

79. What are noninfectious causes of pericarditis?

• Postpericardiotomy syndrome
• Rheumatic fever
• Connective tissue disorders: juvenile rheumatoid arthritis, systemic lupus erythematosus, dermatomyositis, periarteritis nodosa
• Trauma: blunt or penetrating
• Metabolic: uremia, myxedema
• Hypersensitivity: serum sickness, pulmonary infiltrates with eosinophilia, Stevens-Johnson syndrome, drugs (hydralazine, procainamide, chemotherapy)
• Neoplasm: leukemia, metastatic
• Postirradiation

From Pinsky WW, et al: Infectious endocarditis. In Feigin RD, Cherry JD (eds): Textbook of Pediatric Infectious Diseases, 3rd ed. Philadelphia, W.B. Saunders, 1992, p 378; with permission.

80. How do ECG findings in myocarditis and pericarditis differ?

Myocarditis: A prolonged PR intervals is seen in conditions of myocardial inflammation. Other findings include flattened ST segments and flattened or inverted T waves in leads 2–3 aVF and V_{5-7}. Voltages in V_{5-7} may or may not be increased and can occasionally be decreased. The QRS complex can be widened. Dysrhythmias, including premature ventricular contractions, second-degree AV block, and premature atrial contractions, may be present.

Pericarditis: The classic finding is decreased voltage, but this may not always be seen. The ST-T wave abnormalities, if present, can be indistinguishable from those seen in myocarditis. Elevated ST segments may be observed.

81. What are the principal diagnostic criteria for Kawasaki syndrome?

The mnemonic **My HEART** may be helpful:

M   Mucosal changes, especially oral and upper respiratory; dry and chapped lips; "strawberry tongue"

H   Hand and extremity changes, including reddened palms/soles, edema, desquamation from fingertips and toes (later)

E   Eye changes, primarily a bilateral conjunctival injection without discharge

A   Adenopathy, usually cervical, often unilateral, of at least 1.5 cm in diameter

R   Rash, usually a truncal exanthem without vesicles or crusts

T   Temperature elevation, often to 104° or above, lasting for > 5 days

The presence of fever and at least 4 of the other 5 features are needed for the classic diagnosis. However, cases of atypical Kawasaki's have been reported which feature < 5 of the criteria accompanied by the typical coronary artery changes. A high index of suspicion is important as Kawasaki syndrome has replaced acute rheumatic fever as the leading cause of identifiable acquired heart disease in children in the United States.

82. Why should all children with Kawasaki syndrome receive gammaglobulin therapy?

IV gammaglobulin has been demonstrated to decrease the incidence of coronary artery abnormalities in children with Kawasaki syndrome. Additionally, fever and laboratory indices of inflammation resolve more quickly after treatment. Early trials used a dose of 400 mg/kg/day for 4 consecutive days. More recent studies demonstrate that a single infusion over 12 hours of 2 mg/kg is at least as effective as the 4-day regimen in preventing aneurysms and is better at hastening defervescence.

At present, there is no reliable means of predicting which children with Kawasaki syndrome will develop coronary artery abnormalities. Therefore, all children with Kawasaki syndrome should receive parenteral gammaglobulin. The efficacy of this therapy has not been evaluated in children who have been ill for > 10 days. However, treatment in this situation is reasonable if the child remains symptomatic.

83. Is aspirin therapy of benefit in children with Kawasaki syndrome?

By itself, high-dose aspirin (80–100 mg/kg/day divided every 6 hours) is effective in decreasing the degree of fever and discomfort in patients during the acute stages of illness up to about 14 days. Serum salicylate levels of 15–25 mg/dl should be sought. It is unclear if high-dose aspirin has an additive effect in decreasing the incidence of coronary artery abnormalities when used in conjunction with gammaglobulin. It may be that aspirin is most beneficial when administered in low dose after resolution of fever, due to its effects on platelet aggregation and and prevention of the thrombotic complications seen in children with Kawasaki syndrome. Therefore, aspirin in low dose (3–5 mg/kg/day) is advised for about 6–8 weeks. If a follow-up echocardiogram at that time reveals no coronary abnormalities, therapy is usually discontinued. If abnormalities are present, therapy is continued indefinitely.

84. When are corticosteroids indicated in the treatment of Kawasaki syndrome?

Despite an early report that methylprednisolone decreased the incidence of cardiac abnormalities in children with Kawasaki syndrome, subsequent evaluations have failed to confirm this finding. In fact, in some studies, the incidence of coronary artery abnormalities has actually increased in children who received prednisone versus placebo. As a result, steroids are presently contraindicated in the treatment of this disease.

85. What causes Kawasaki syndrome?

Despite considerable progress in understanding the pathogenesis of this syndrome, the inciting agent remains undiscovered. Toxic agents, such as mercury and lead, and allergic and immunologic causes have been studied as potential causative factors. Numerous case reports and clinical series report infectious agents associated with Kawasaki syndrome, including rickettsiae, *Klebsiella pneumoniae, Escherichia* sp., parainfluenza virus, Epstein-Barr virus, retrovirus,

Propionibacterium acnes, retroviruses, and toxic shock syndrome toxin 1 (TSST-1) staphylo-cocci. The association between Kawasaki syndrome and shampooing or spot-cleaning rugs or carpets has been studied, as well as the importance of mites.

Melish ME: Kawasaki syndrome. Pediatr Rev 17:153–162, 1996.

86. How do the clinical stages of Kawasaki syndrome correlate with the arterial pathologic changes?

Kawasaki Syndrome: Disease Phases, Complications, and Degree of Arteritis

	ACUTE (1–11 DAYS)	SUBACUTE (11–21 DAYS)	CONVALESCENT (21–60 DAYS)	CHRONIC (? YEARS)
Clinical findings	Fever, conjunctivitis, oral changes, extremity changes, irritability	Irritability persists; prolongation of fever may occur; normalization of most clinical findings; palpable aneurysms may develop	Most clinical findings resolve; aneurysmal dilation of peripheral vessels may persist; conjunctivitis may persist	—
Arterial correlates	Perivasculitis, vasculitis of capillaries, arterioles, and venules; inflammation of intima of medium and larger arteries	Aneurysms, thrombi, stenosis of medium-sized arteries, panvasculitis, and edema of vessel wall; myocarditis less prominent	Vascular inflammation decreases	Scar formation; intimal thickening

From Hicks RV, Melish ME: Kawasaki syndrome. Pediatr Clin North Am 33:1115–1175, 1986; with permission.

87. How is Kawasaki syndrome distinguished from measles?

These two entities can have a large degree of clinical overlap, and in countries where measles is more prominent, the need for clinical distinction is not rare. As a rule, the conjunctivitis of Kawasaki syndrome is nonexudative; in measles, it is exudative. Koplik spots seen in measles are discrete oral lesions, whereas in Kawasaki syndrome the mucosal erythema is more diffuse. The rash of measles usually begins on the face and hairline; in Kawasaki syndrome on the trunk and extremities. In measles, a low total WBC count and ESR are the norm, whereas both are usually elevated in Kawasaki syndrome.

88. What factors are most strongly associated with the development of coronary artery disease in patients with Kawasaki syndrome?
1. Duration of fever > 16 days
2. Recurrence of fever after an afebrile period of ≥ 48 hours
3. Dysrhythmias (other than first-degree heart block)
4. Cardiomegaly
5. Male gender
6. Age < 1 year

PHARMACOLOGY

89. How valuable are digoxin levels?

Digoxin levels may not be helpful in children because of the presence of endogenous digoxin-like immunoreactive substances (DLIS), which cross-react with immunoassay antibodies to digoxin. Also, in children, the concentration of digoxin is much higher in the myocardium than in the plasma. Digoxin levels may be helpful, however, in older children (especially in presence of dysrhythmias).

90. How long before oral digoxin begins to work?

Oral digoxin reaches peak plasma levels 1–2 hours after administration, but a peak "hemodynamic" effect is not evident until 6 hours after administration (vs. 3 hours for IV digoxin).

91. An infant with Wolff-Parkinson-White (WPW) syndrome and supraventricular tachycardia (SVT) is given digoxin, and the attending cardiologist is dismayed. Why?

Digoxin can enhance conduction through a bypass tract while slowing conduction through the AV node. Ventricular fibrillation has been reported in infants with WPW treated with digoxin. This effect is believed to be due to enhanced conduction down the bypass tract. For this reason, propranolol has replaced digoxin as the drug of choice in the treatment of infants with SVT and WPW.

92. What are the indications for prostaglandin E_1 (PGE_1) in the neonate?

PGE_1 is indicated in cardiac lesions with ductal dependent blood flow to either the pulmonary circulation (e.g., pulmonary atresia with intact ventricular septum, tricuspid atresia with intact ventricular septum, critical pulmonary stenosis) or systemic circulation (e.g., critical coarctation of the aorta, interrupted aortic arch, hypoplastic left heart syndrome). In infants with *suspected CHD* in whom a specific diagnosis is not known (e.g., prior to transport to a tertiary care center), PGE_1 is clinically indicated in cases of profound cyanosis ($PaO_2 < 25$ mmHg), poor perfusion, and/or metabolic acidosis.

93. What are the major side effects of PGE_1?

Apnea, pyrexia, cutaneous flushing, seizures, hypotension, bradycardia/tachycardia.

94. Are there any conditions during the newborn period in which PGE_1 use is contraindicated?

PGE_1 maintains the patency of the ductus arteriosus and is usually most effective in infants < 96 hours of age. The use of PGE_1 may have *adverse* physiologic effects under certain situations:

1. Transposition of the great arteries with a restrictive atrial septal defect
2. Tetralogy of Fallot without a patent ductus arteriosus
3. Total anomalous pulmonary venous return
4. Persistent pulmonary hypertension of the newborn

95. What are the side effects of indomethacin in the neonate?

1. Mild but usually transient renal dysfunction
2. Hyponatremia
3. Hypoglycemia
4. Platelet dysfunction producing a prolonged bleeding time
5. Occult blood loss from gastrointestinal tract
6. Spontaneous perforation of the intestine

96. How do alpha, beta, and dopaminergic receptors differ?

Alpha—in vascular smooth muscle; cause vasoconstriction

$Beta_1$—in myocardial smooth muscle; increase inotropic (contractile force) and chronotropic (cardiac rate) effect

$Beta_2$—in vascular smooth muscle; cause vasodilation

Dopaminergic—in renal and mesenteric vascular smooth muscle; cause vasodilation

97. How do relative receptor effects differ by drug type?

Drug	Alpha	$Beta_1$	$Beta_2$	Dopaminergic
Epinephrine	+++	+++	+++	0
Norepinephrine	+++	+++	+	0
Isoproterenol	0	+++	+++	0
Dopamine	0 to +++ (dose-related)	++ to +++ (dose-related)	++	+++
Dobutamine	0 to +	+++	+	0

Effect of medication: 0 = none, + = small, ++ = moderate, +++ = large.

For dopamine, at low doses (2–10 µg/kg/min), dopaminergic effects predominate. At high doses (5–20 µg/kg/min), increased alpha and beta effects are seen. At very high doses (> 20 µg/kg/min), a markedly increased alpha effect with decreased renal and mesenteric blood flow occurs. For dobutamine, beta$_1$ inotropic effects are more pronounced than chronotropic effects.

98. How are emergency infusions for cardiovascular support prepared?

Catecholamine	Mixture	Dose
Isoproterenol Epinephrine Norepinephrine	0.6 mg × body wt (in kg), added to diluent to make 100 ml	1 ml/hr delivers 0.1 µg/kg/min
Dopamine Dobutamine	6 mg × body wt (in kg), added to diluent to make 100 ml	1 ml/hr delivers 1 µg/kg/min

PHYSICAL EXAMINATION

99. Which cardiac conditions accentuate or diminish the intensity of the first heart sound?

The intensity of the S$_1$ depends mainly on the position of the mitral leaflets at the time when the left ventricle begins to contract. The loudness is greatest in situations that cause wide separation of the leaflets at the beginning of systole: short PR interval, left-to-right shunts, tachycardia, short cycle lengths in atrial fibrillation, mitral stenosis with mobile cusps, high-output states, and mobile left atrial myxoma. Fibrosis or calcification of the mitral valve cusps cause a faint S$_1$, as does bradycardia and first-degree AV block.

100. In what settings can an abnormal second heart sound be auscultated?
1. Widely split S$_2$
   - Prolonged right ventricular (RV) ejection time:
     RV volume overload—atrial septal defect, partial anomalous pulmonary venous return
     RV pressure overload—mild pulmonary stenosis
     RV conduction delay—right bundle branch block
   - Shortened left ventricular (LV) ejection time
     Early aortic closure—mitral regurgitation
2. Single S$_2$
   - Presence of only one semilunar valve—aortic or pulmonary atresia, truncus arteriosus
   - P2 not audible—tetralogy of Fallot, transposition of great arteries, pulmonary stenosis, pulmonary hypertension
   - A2 delayed—severe aortic stenosis
   - May be normal in a newborn
3. Paradoxically split S$_2$ (A2 follows P2): present in severe aortic stenosis, left bundle branch block, pulmonary hypertension
4. Loud P2
   - Pulmonary hypertension
   - Dilation of nonhypertensive pulmonary artery, as in atrial septal defect

101. When can S3 and S4 be considered a normal finding during a pediatric cardiac examination?

An S$_3$, or "ventricular"gallop, occurs early in diastole. It is usually benign but can be abnormal in children with dilated ventricles and decreased compliance (as in CHF). An S$_4$, or "atrial" gallop, occurs late in diastole. It is usually abnormal in children (although it can be normal in an older adult).

102. What are the possible etiologies of an ejection click?

An ejection click occurs at the onset of ventricular ejection, follows S_1, and is best heard at the base of the heart. Possible etiologies include:

1. Stenosis of semilunar valves: aortic stenosis or pulmonary stenosis (not infundibular or supravalvular PS)
2. Dilation of great arteries: tetralogy of Fallot (dilated aorta), truncus arteriosus, hypertension, or coarctation of the aorta
3. Mitral valve prolapse (produces midsystolic click)
4. Other (rare): cardiac tumors, atrial septal aneurysms, and dissecting aortic aneurysms

103. How can the likelihood of finding mitral valve prolapse (MVP) on auscultation be increased?

In MVP, the leaflets of the mitral valve apparatus billow into the left atrium. The characteristic midsystolic click of MVP may represent the snapping of the chordae tendineae or redundant portions of the cusps themselves. The crescendo, late systolic murmur represents mitral insufficiency. Maneuvers that *decrease LV* size and volume (and thus increase the relative size of the leaflets) increase the likelihood of hearing the click or murmur. These include the straining phase of a Valsalva maneuver, inspiration, and change from a supine to sitting position or from a squatting to standing position. The left lateral decubitus position may also be facilitative.

104. What is the difference between pulsus alternans and pulsus paradoxus?

Pulsus alternans is a pulse pattern in which there is alternating (beat-to-beat) variability of pulse strength due to decreased ventricular performance (sometimes seen in CHF).

Pulsus paradoxus indicates an exaggeration of normal reduction of systolic blood pressure during inspiration. Associated conditions include cardiac tamponade (effusion or constrictive pericarditis), respiratory illness (asthma or pneumonia), and myocardial disease affecting wall compliance (endocardial fibroelastosis or amyloidosis).

105. How is pulsus paradoxus measured?

To measure a pulsus paradoxus, determine the systolic pressure by noting the first audible Korotkoff sound. Then, retake the blood pressure by raising the manometer pressure to at least 25 mmHg higher than the systolic pressure, and allow it to fall slowly. Stop as soon as the first sound is heard. Note that the sound disappears during inspiration. Lower the pressure slowly and note when all pulsed beats are heard. The difference between these two pressures is the pulsus paradoxus. Normally, in children, there is an 8–10 mmHg fluctuation in systolic pressure with different phases of inspiration.

106. As a screening tool for coarctation of the aorta, how effective is palpation of femoral pulses?

It is likely more valuable in asymptomatic older children than in asymptomatic infants, although it is much more commonly performed in the newborn period. In infants, a patent ductus arteriosus may provide blood flow to the lower extremities, bypassing a severe coarctation. Upper and lower pulses may be equal. A differential cyanosis (lower extremities more cyanotic than upper extremities) may be noted. However, as the ductus closes, signs of respiratory distress and cardiac failure may develop. In older children, coarctation usually manifests as a suspicious murmur or hypertension rather than CHF. It is vital to remember to check pulses in those settings. Simultaneous palpation of upper and lower extremity pulses is important. If collaterals have developed, a delay in pulse rather than diminished volume may be noted.

107. What is the differential diagnosis for a systolic murmur in each auscultatory area?

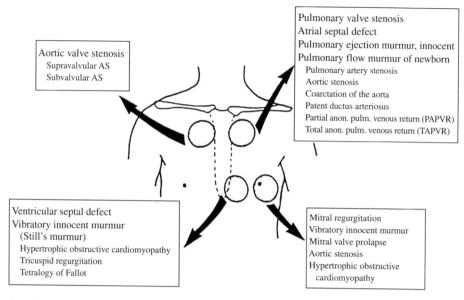

Systolic murmurs audible at various locations. Less common conditions are shown in smaller type. From Park MK: Pediatric Cardiology for Practitioners, 3rd ed. St. Louis, Mosby-Year Book, 1995, with permission.

108. What are the most common innocent murmurs?

Type (Timing)	Description of Murmur	Age Group
Classic vibratory murmur (Still's murmur) (systolic)	Maximal at MLSB or between LLSB and apex Grade 2–3/6 Low-frequency vibratory, "twanging string," groaning, squeaking, or musical	3–6 yr Occasionally in infancy
Pulmonary ejection murmur (systolic)	Maximal at ULSB Early to midsystolic Grade 1–3/6 in intensity Blowing in quality	8–14 yr
Pulmonary flow murmur of new-born (systolic)	Maximal at ULSB Transmit well to left and right chest, axillae, and back Grade 1–2/6 intensity	Premature and full-term newborns Usually disappears by 3–6 mos of age
Venous hum (continuous)	Maximal at right (or left) supra- and infraclavicular areas Grade 1–3/6 intensity Inaudible in supine position Intensity changes with rotation of head and compression of jugular vein	3–6 yr
Carotid bruit (systolic)	Right supraclavicular area and over carotids Grade 2–3/6 in intensity Occasional thrill over a carotid artery	Any age

MLSB, mid-left sternal border; LLSB, lower-left sternal border; ULSB, upper-left sternal border.

109. What features are suggestive of a pathologic murmur?
- Diastolic murmurs
- Pansystolic murmurs
- Late systolic murmurs
- Very loud murmurs
- Murmurs associated with a thrill
- Continuous murmurs
- Associated cardiac abnormalities (e.g., asymmetric pulses, click, abnormal splitting)

McCrindle BW, et al: Cardinal clinical signs in the differentiation of heart murmurs in children. Arch Pediatr Adolesc Med 150:169–174, 1996.

Rosenthal A: How to distinguish between innocent and pathologic murmurs in childhood. Pediatr Clin North Am 31:1229–1240, 1984.

110. If a murmur is detected, what noncardiac factors suggest that the murmur is pathologic?

1. Evidence of growth retardation (most commonly seen in murmurs with large left-to-right shunts)

2. Associated dysmorphic features (e.g., valvular disease in Hurler syndrome, Noonan syndrome)

3. Exertional blueness, pallor, or dyspnea, especially if associated with minor exertion such as climbing a few stairs (may be sign of early CHF)

4. Short feeding times and volumes in infants (may be sign of early CHF)

5. Syncopal or presyncopal episodes (may be seen in hypertrophic cardiomyopathy)

6. History of IV drug abuse (risk factor for endocarditis)

7. Maternal history of diabetes mellitus (associated with asymmetric septal hypertrophy, VSD, d-transposition), alcohol use (associated with pulmonic stenosis and VSD), other medications

8. Family history of congenital heart disease

SURGERY

111. Name the major shunt operations for congenital heart disease (CHD).

Shunt operations between a systemic artery and pulmonary artery are used to improve oxygen saturation in patients with cyanotic CHD and diminished pulmonary blood flow. Veno-arterial shunts which connect a systemic vein and the pulmonary artery are also used for similar purposes.

1. The **Blalock-Taussig** shunt consists of an anastomosis between a subclavian artery and the ipsilateral pulmonary artery. The subclavian artery can be divided, and the distal end anastomosed to the pulmonary artery (classic BT shunt), or a prosthetic graft can be interposed between the two arteries (modified BT shunt).

2. The **Waterston** shunt is an anastomosis between the ascending aorta and right pulmonary artery.

3. The **Potts** shunt is an anastomosis between the descending aorta and left pulmonary artery.

4. The **Glenn** anastomosis is a connection between the distal right pulmonary artery and the superior vena cava, which is ligated below the site of the anastomosis.

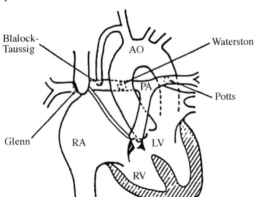

From Park MK: Pediatric Cardiology for Practitioners, 3rd ed. St. Louis, Mosby-Year Book, 1995; with permission.

112. Which factors are associated with more favorable outcomes with the Fontan procedure?

The Fontan procedure, initially done in 1971 for tricuspid atresia, establishes a direct continuity between the systemic venous channels (right atrium/superior vena cava/inferior vena cava) and pulmonary arteries. It thus bypasses the need for a functioning ventricle to pump blood to the lungs and also minimizes the need for conduits and valves. Favorable outcomes are more likely if:

1. Pulmonary artery pressure is normal
2. Pulmonary vascular resistance is normal
3. Pulmonary arteries are of adequate size
4. End-diastolic pressure is low
5. Lesion is tricuspid atresia

Adapted from Park MK: Pediatric Cardiology for Practitioners, 3rd ed. St. Louis, Mosby-Year Book, 1995; with permission.

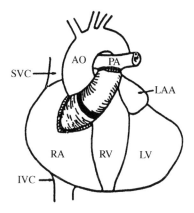

113. For which congenital heart disorder is the "switch operation" done?

Transposition of the great arteries (TGA). Also known as the Jatene operation, the procedure involves reimplantation of the coronary arteries, bisection of the pulmonary artery and aorta, and resuturing of the two great vessels into their correct anatomic positions. This operation, first done in 1976, has become the treatment of choice for TGA over others which use intra-atrial baffles to redirect blood along more proper anatomic paths (i.e., Senning and Mustard procedures). These baffles are associated with much higher incidences of RV failure and dysrhythmias.

114. What are the indications for surgical repair of ASD and VSD?

Ventricular septal defect: Infants with a large VSD refractory to medical therapy, causing failure to thrive and/or repeated lower respiratory tract infections, should be referred for surgery. Pulmonary hypertension is another indication for surgery. In older children with normal pulmonary artery pressure, but with pulmonary blood flow near or equal to twice systemic blood flow, surgical closure is advised.

Atrial septal defect: Symptomatic infants with an ASD should undergo surgery at the time of diagnosis. Surgical results usually are excellent. Asymptomatic children should be scheduled for repair during the first 5 years of life.

115. Is there any surgical therapy for hypoplastic left heart syndrome (HLHS)?

Two surgical options are available: **heart transplantation** and the **Norwood procedure**. In HLHS, severe underdevelopment of the left ventricle, mitral valve, aortic valve, and ascending aortic arch occurs. Newborns usually develop signs of severe CHF.

The **Norwood procedure**, reported initially in 1983, is performed in three stages. In *stage 1*, the proximal main pulmonary artery is transected, and with additional homograft material, it is used to help rebuild the aorta. This creates a univentricular systemic pumping chamber and changes the physiology from aortic atresia to pulmonic atresia. The distal main pulmonary artery is oversewn, and a systemic-to-pulmonary shunt placed between the innominate artery and right pulmonary artery to correct pulmonary flow. *Stage II* (performed at about age 6 weeks) seeks to regulate pulmonary blood flow by changing to a bidirectional Glenn anastomosis (superior vena cava to distal right pulmonary artery). One to 2 years later, a Fontan procedure (Stage III) is performed (right atrium to pulmonary artery) which ultimately separates the venous and arterial sides. Long-term survival is significantly better with heart transplantation, but donor shortages are major problems and 20–30% of infants die awaiting transplant.

116. What is the long-term prognosis for heart transplantation in infancy and childhood?

Survival statistics have improved dramatically over the last 5 years with the use of newer and safer immunosuppressive agents such as cyclosporine and FK506. However, children who receive transplanted hearts are at increased risk for recurrent infection, accelerated coronary artery disease, and lymphoproliferative syndromes in association with Epstein-Barr infection. Current 5-year survival rates vary between 70–85%.

117. What are the most common cardiothoracic postoperative syndromes?

1. Postcardiotomy syndrome—arteritis in the mesenteric circulation, causing abdominal pain (2–8 days after surgery).

2. Postpericardiotomy syndrome—immunologic phenomenon leading to pericardial effusion, causing chest pain and vomiting (2–3 weeks following surgery).

3. Postperfusion syndrome—cytomegalovirus infection causing fever and splenomegaly (3–6 weeks following surgery).

4. Hemolytic anemia syndrome—trauma to red cells leading to fever, jaundice, and hepatomegaly (1–2 weeks following surgery).

4. DERMATOLOGY

Lawrence F. Eichenfield, M.D., Paul J. Honig, M.D., and Linda G. Rabinowitz, M.D.

ACNE

1. Does chocolate aggravate outbreaks of acne?

According to controlled studies, no. However, it is not worth forcing a patient to eat chocolate just to prove a point. If a patient says that chocolate makes the acne worse, take him or her at face value.

2. How do a "blackhead" and a "whitehead" differ histopathologically?

Both lesions are produced by obstruction and distention of the sebaceous follicle with sebum and cellular debris. When the follicular contents tent the overlying skin but are not exposed to the atmosphere, a **whitehead** occurs. If the contents project out of the follicular opening, oxidation of the exposed mass of debris produces a color change and a **blackhead**.

3. Explain the pathophysiologic basis for the treatment of acne.

Therapy of acne is directed toward several abnormalities seen in the sebaceous follicles of patients. The lining cells of the follicular channel do not desquamate, which leads to obstruction of the sebaceous follicle. Debris and sebum are trapped, and the bacteria responsible for acne (*Propionibacterium acnes*) replicate. Low-molecular-weight particles produced by this organism attract white blood cells, which insinuate through the follicular wall. Following ingestion of *P. acnes*, the white blood cell releases enzymes that rupture the follicular wall. Once the contents of the follicle are emptied into the dermis, an inflammatory response is triggered (including activation of the complement cascade), resulting in inflammatory lesions (papules, pustules, and cysts). Retinoic acid cream is used to unstick the follicular cells that form the lining of the follicle. Obstruction is therefore prevented. Topical and systemic antibiotics reduce the concentration of bacteria responsible for the acne process.

4. What are the principles of topical acne therapy?

1. Never apply a topical medication to wet skin! (wait ½ hour after washing)
2. Dispense no more than a pea-sized amount of medication onto the finger.
3. Gently spread medication over all acne-prone areas (not just to each active comedome or pimple).
4. Wash finger that was in contact with medication.
5. Warn patients of possible side effects:
   Benzoyl peroxide—1 in 10 have allergic reaction and get fiery red skin
   Tretinoin (Retin A) cream—erythema and peeling are normal initially; marked redness and severe stinging are not! Since tretinoin thins the skin, use of a sunscreen is mandatory!
6. Don't apply lotions, creams, makeups, or other potions that are comedogenic.

5. Can systemic antibiotics be given to children with severe acne?

Absolutely! Acne can leave permanent scars (cosmetic and psychological), and prolonged courses of erythromycin, tetracycline, or related drugs may be required to prevent a negative outcome. Patients have been on these antibiotics for > 5 straight years without ill effects.

6. When is the use of oral isotretinoin indicated in teenagers with acne?

Isotretinoin, which is 13-*cis*-retinoic acid (Accutane), is most appropriately used for nodulocystic acne, acne conglobata, or severe scarring acne that has been unresponsive to standard modes of treatment (including topical or systemic antibiotics and topical retinoin).

7. List the common side effects and toxicities of oral isotretinoin.

Side effects: Dry skin, dry mucous membranes, epistaxis, pruritus, alopecia, curly hair, paronychia, dry eyes, conjunctivitis

Toxicities: Fetal anomalies (Accutane embryopathy), dysmorphogenesis, hepatic injury with increased liver enzymes, pseudotumor cerebri, depression

8. What is acne fulminans?

The acute onset of numerous inflamed, painful, ulcerated, and crusted acne lesions in association with fever, chills, malaise, weight loss, and musculoskeletal pain (polyarthralgia). Individuals may have leukocytosis, increased sedimentation rate, anemia, hematuria, and osteolytic lesions. Unlike acne conglobata, which occurs more frequently in females, most patients with acne fulminans are males. Comedones are absent in contrast to acne conglobata. Although no known etiology has been determined, immune complexes are thought to be involved. Prednisone is the drug of choice.

CLINICAL ISSUES

9. What is the characteristic rash of hepatitis B virus infection?

Circulating immune complexes contribute to the pathogenesis of cutaneous manifestations of hepatitis B. The most common cutaneous associations are urticaria and Gianotti-Crosti syndrome (papular acrodermatitis of childhood).

Urticaria, or "hives," may be the major feature of the prodrome of hepatitis B. The rash may precede the arthralgias and icterus and may last several days; it may also be maculopapular or petechial.

Gianotti-Crosti syndrome consists of nonpruritic, erythematous, 1–5-mm papules arranged symmetrically on the face, buttocks, and extremities. The lesions erupt over a few days and do not become confluent (remember, the trunk is spared!). They may last for 3 weeks; lymphadenopathy may persists for months. This rash is classically associated with anicteric hepatitis, which develops at the same time as the rash or weeks later. The association is more common in Europe, where hepatitis B Adw serotype is more common than in the U.S., where the Ayw serotype predominates. Other viruses, such as Epstein-Barr virus, may also be associated with these cutaneous findings.

10. Describe the characteristic clinical picture of erythema nodosum.

A prodrome of fever, chills, malaise, and arthralgia may precede the typical skin findings. Crops of red to blue tender nodules appear over the anterior shins. Lesions may be seen on the knees, ankles, thighs, and, occasionally, lower extensor forearms and face. They may evolve through a spectrum of colors that resemble a bruise. Often, the changes are misdiagnosed as cellulitis or secondary to a traumatic event.

11. What infectious and noninfectious conditions are associated with erythema nodosum?

Infectious	Noninfectious
Group A β-hemolytic streptococci	Sarcoidosis
Tuberculosis	Ulcerative colitis
Yersinia	Regional ileitis
Coccidioidomycosis	Hodgkin disease
Histoplasmosis	Lymphosarcoma
North American blastomycosis	Leukemia
Psittacosis	Behçet syndrome
Lymphogranuloma venereum	Sulfonamides
Ornithosis	Halogens
Cat-scratch fever	Contraceptives
Measles	

12. What is the most effective way to treat warts?

The mode of therapy depends on the type and number of warts, location on the body, and age of the patient. No matter what treatment is used, warts can always recur; there are no absolute cures. The major goal is to remove warts without residual scarring. Of course, a major option is no treatment at all because most warts self-resolve in 1–2 years.

Flat warts	Liquid nitrogen (lightly)
	Topical tretinoin cream
	Cantharidin, if not facial
Filiform warts	Liquid nitrogen
	Curettage and electrodesiccation
Common warts	Liquid nitrogen
	Cantharidin
	Salicylic acid preparations
	Curettage and electrodesiccation, if solitary
Plantar warts	Salicylic acid preparations, including 40% plaster
	Liquid nitrogen (gently)
	Cantharidin
	Curettage and electrodesiccation (may scar)
	Podophyllin (concentration and contact time can be varied)

Some dermatologists also use intralesional bleomycin for recalcitrant warts, carbon-dioxide and pulsed-dye lasers, topical formaldehyde or glutaraldehyde, and other chemical mixtures. In some case reports, oral cimetidine has been effective, perhaps due to its immunomodulatory activity.

Siegfried EC: Warts on children: An approach to therapy. Pediatr Ann 25:79–90, 1996.

13. How should you treat impetigo?

This should be a simple answer, but the changing epidemiology of impetigo demands more attention. In past years, impetigo was mostly due to streptococcal infection (except for bullous impetigo, which was staphylococcal). Now, *Staphylococcus aureus*, primarily penicillinase-producing, appears to be the predominant organism in nearly all impetigo.

Consequently, treatment usually requires medication active against both group A streptococcus and *S. aureus*. These include cephalosporins and dicloxacillin. Erythromycin may be considered, although staphylococcal resistance is increasing. Topical mupirocin (Bactroban) applied three times daily is equivalent in efficacy to systemic antibiotics for most impetigo. Systemic antibiotics are usually indicated for extensive lesions, failure of topical remedies, and outbreaks among multiple family members, daycare attendees, or athletic teams.

14. Should the honey-colored crusts of impetigo be soaked and removed to facilitate healing?

While local custom may say otherwise, vigorous scrubbing does not seem to help.

15. Does treatment of streptococcal skin infections prevent post-streptococcal glomerulonephritis?

No study has ever demonstrated that treatment of impetigo or pyoderma prevents possible renal complications in the index case. Clearly, acute rheumatic fever does not occur following the skin infections, and glomerulonephritis is limited to a few serotypes, especially 49, 55, 57, and 60, which appear to be less prevalent in recent years. However, treatment lessens the likelihood of contagious spread to other hosts who may be susceptible to renal complications.

Of note, glomerulonephritis occurs about 7–21 days after the onset of the skin infection. Serum antistreptolysin (ASO) titers, which are elevated after streptococcal pharyngeal infections, are usually not elevated following skin infections. Therefore, to confirm the diagnosis of an antecedent skin infection, antihyaluronidase (AHT) and anti-DNase B are more appropriate titers to obtain.

16. What dermatologic sign starts from scratch?

Dermographism occurs when the skin is stroked firmly with a pointed object. The result is a *red line*, followed by an *erythematous flare*, which is eventually followed by a *wheal*. This "triple response of Lewis" usually occurs within 1–3 minutes. Dermographism (or skin writing) is an exaggerated triple response of Lewis and is seen in patients with urticaria. The tendency to be dermographic can appear at any age and may last for months to years. The cause is often unknown. White dermographism is seen in patients with an atopic diathesis, in whom the red line is replaced by a white line without a subsequent flare and wheal.

17. Do geographic tongues vary in the northern and southern hemispheres?
Alas, more research awaits. Geographic tongue refers to the benign condition in which denudations of the filiform papillae on the lingual surface occur, giving the tongue the appearance of a relief map. The patterns change over hours and days, and the histopathology resembles that of psoriasis. The patient is usually asymptomatic. No treatment is effective or necessary since self-resolution is the rule. Etiology in any hemisphere is unknown.

ECZEMATOUS DISORDERS

18. What is the usual distribution of rash in eczema?
Infant: Cheeks, trunk and extensor surfaces of extremities, knees and elbows
Child: Neck, feet, and antecubital and popliteal fossae
Older child: Neck, hands and feet, antecubital and popliteal fossae

19. Describe the five key battle plans to treat atopic dermatitis.
Atopic dermatitis is a chronic disorder for which there is no cure. (This must be explained to parents, who often expect that once their child is clear, he or she will remain clear.) Despite the chronicity of this skin condition, measures can be taken to reduce pruritus, hydrate the skin, reduce inflammation, control infection, and protect the skin from irritants and "triggers." Note that specific treatment plans may vary among physicians.
1. *Reduce pruritus.* This is crucial! It is important to break the itch-scratch cycle and to prevent new lesions from forming. Oral antihistamines should be used and titrated as needed to control itching. Some children may need higher than the recommended doses of Atarax and Benadryl.
2. *Hydrate the skin.* Emollients (Vaseline, Eucerin, Cetaphil, Nivea cream) prevent evaporation of moisture via occlusion and are best applied right after bathing, when the skin is maximally hydrated. Frequent bathing can actually dry out the skin, so bathing should be limited to 2–3 times per week. Room humidifiers may also be beneficial.
3. *Reduce inflammation.* Topical steroids are invaluable as anti-inflammatory agents and can hasten clearing of eruptions that are erythematous (inflamed). Medium-strength corticosteroids can be used on areas other than the face and perineum; low-strength steroids (such as 1% hydrocortisone) may be used in these thin-skinned areas.
4. *Control infection.* Superinfection with *Staphylococcus aureus* is extremely common. Skin can be cultured and sensitivities obtain. Erythromycin and cephalosporins are the usual antibiotics of choice for infected atopic dermatitis. Resistance to erythromycin occurs frequently.
5. *Avoid irritants.* Gentle soaps and shampoos should be used; wool should be avoided; tight garments may help minimize the "itchy" feeling; consider furniture, carpeting, pets, and dust mites as possible irritants and/or trigger factors.

20. Do soaps or clothes make any difference in atopic dermatitis?
Soaps: Less drying, nondetergent soaps, such as Dove, Tone, and Caress, are better than more drying soaps such as Ivory. Other mild soaps include Cetaphil, Purpose, Aveeno, and Basis; the latter is a superfatted soap.
Clothing: Avoid woolen clothes—the fibers can irritate the skin and trigger the itch-scratch cycle. If woolens must be used, they should be lined. Soft fibers are the least irritating and itchy (cotton jerseys).

21. Is there a genetic basis for atopic dermatitis?

Although specific genetic information is lacking, it has been strongly suggested that an individual's genotype determines whether he or she will develop atopic dermatitis. Many children with atopic dermatitis have a family history of atopy. If one parent has an atopic diathesis, 60% of offspring will be atopic; if two parents do, 80% of children are affected. Monozygotic twins are often concordant for atopic disease.

22. Are there consistent immunologic alterations in children with atopic dermatitis?

Humoral changes include elevated IgE levels and a higher-than-normal number of positive skin tests (type I cutaneous reactions) to common environmental allergens. Cell-mediated abnormalities have been found only during acute flares of the dermatitis. These include mild to moderate depression of cell-mediated immunity, a 30–50% decrease in lymphocyte-forming E-rosettes, decreased phagocytosis of yeast cells by neutrophils, and chemotactic defects of polymorphonuclear and mononuclear cells.

23. In the land of medicolinguistics, what is the difference between eczema and atopic dermatitis?

The term *eczema* derives from the Greek word *exzein*, to erupt—*ex* (out) plus *zein* (to boil). To most physicians, eczema is synonymous with atopic dermatitis, a chronic skin disease manifested by intermittent skin eruption. **Eczema** is primarily a morphologic term used to describe an erythematous, scaling, inflammatory eruption with itching, edema, papules, vesicles, and crusts. There are other "eczematous eruptions" (nummular eczema, allergic contact dermatitis), but "garden variety" eczema is certainly the most common.

Atopic dermatitis is a broader allergic tendency with multiple dermal manifestations mostly secondary to pruritus. Jacquet stated that atopic dermatitis is an "itch that rashes, not a rash that itches." Its manifestations are dry skin, chronic and recurrent dermatitis, low threshold to pruritus, hyperlinear palms, eyelid pleats (Dennie lines), pityriasis alba, and keratosis pilaris, among others.

24. What other skin conditions may mimic atopic dermatitis?

- Seborrheic dermatitis
- Contact dermatitis
- Xerotic eczema (dry skin)
- Nummular eczema
- Scabies
- Langerhans cell histiocytosis
- Immunologic disorders (e.g., Wiskott-Aldrich syndrome)
- Metabolic disorders (e.g., phenylketonuria)

25. What features help to differentiate seborrheic from atopic dermatitis in infancy?

	SEBORRHEIC DERMATITIS	ATOPIC DERMATITIS
Color	Salmon	Pink, red (if inflamed)
Scale	Yellowish, greasy	Whiter, nongreasy
Age	Infants < 6 mos or adolescents	May begin at 2–12 mos and continue through childhood
Itching	Not present	May be severe
Distribution	Face, postauricular scalp, axillae and groin	Cheeks, trunk, and extensors of extremities
Associated features	None	Dennie pleats, allergic shiners, palmar creases
Lichenification (thickening of skin with exaggerated skin markings)	None	May be prominent
Response to topical steroids	Rapid	Slower

26. How should parents cope with cradle cap?

Seborrheic dermatitis of the scalp in infancy presents as a scaly rash on the scalp and may spread to the forehead, eyes, ears, eyebrows, nose, and back of head. It appears in the first few months of life and generally resolves in several weeks to a few months. Treatment consists of frequent shampooing with baby shampoo, use of an antiseborrheic shampoo, and removal of thick scales with mineral oil or petrolatum with gentle scrubbing. Occasional refractory cases respond to topical corticosteroid lotion. Seborrheic dermatitis is rare after 6 months of age and before adolescence.

27. Name the common varieties of diaper dermatitis.

Common Varieties of Diaper Dermatitis

	LOCALIZATION	SYMPTOMS	CHARACTERISTICS
Generic	Abdomen, thighs, buttocks, spares deep folds	Minimal	Moderate erythema, poorly marginated, dry, wrinkled skin
Candidal	Involves deep folds—may spread to entire diaper area	Moderate— substantial	Satellites, bright red *erosions*
Noduloulcerative	Prominent anterior parts, thigh, penis, scrotum, labia	Minimal	2–4-cm *firm* nodules with central ulcer; no cellulitis or adenopathy
Impetigo	Any site, but not usually the deep folds	Minimal	Usually blisters rupture rapidly, leaving thin scale/crust; spreads rapidly to sites not covered by diaper
Infantile seborrheic dermatitis	Large confluent anterior surface of groin—usually spares posterior diaper area	None	Sharply marginated bright red plaques and satellites; no erosions—rapidly spreads to face, scalp, extremities, and other flexures
Intertrigo	Deep folds; slight white or yellow exudate	None— moderate	Diffuse margins; no satellites; mild erythema

From Rasmussen J: Diaper dermatitis. Pediatr Rev 6:77–82, 1984; with permission.

28. Are cloth diapers "better" than disposables?

There is no clear answer here, though there are parties who would swear by one or the other. Some studies have shown (1) a decreased incidence of diaper rash with disposable diapers, and (2) a documented decrease in skin moisture and incidence of rash with superabsorbent diapers. The adjective "better" implies a value judgment, and other factors such as cost, environmental impact, and convenience must be considered.

29. Are topical steroid/antifungal preparations useful for treating children with diaper dermatitis?

Diaper dermatitis is usually classified as either irritant dermatitis or candidal dermatitis. Irritant diaper dermatitis responds well to mild topical corticosteroids (due to their anti-inflammatory properties) and a topical barrier such as zinc oxide ointment. Candidiasis of the diaper area responds well to topical antiyeast preparations; sometimes, an oral anticandidal medication is also necessary. In both types of diaper dermatitis, frequent diaper changes, exposure to air, and avoidance of excessive moisture are helpful. Combination preparations containing both antifungal and corticosteroid medications are not recommended to treat diaper dermatitis, as the strength of the steroid molecule in these products is usually too high for use in the diaper area.

30. What is the differential diagnosis of dermatoses of the feet in children?

The seven wonders of the foot: (1) juvenile plantar dermatosis, (2) allergic contact dermatitis, (3) tinea pedis, (4) scabies, (5) psoriasis, (6) granuloma annulare, and (7) plantar warts.

31. Which dietary deficiencies may be associated with an eczematous dermatitis?
Zinc, biotin, essential fatty acids, histidine, and protein (kwashiorkor).

32. Describe the cutaneous manifestations of Langerhans cell histiocytosis.

Clinical Feature	Examples
Rash in "seborrheic" distribution	Scalp, postauricular folds, diaper area, trunk
Biologically aggressive process	Petechiae, purpura, vesicles or bullae, erosions with crusting, ulceration, nodules, atrophy
Failure to respond to mild topical therapies for seborrheic dermatitis	Frequent shampooing, 1% hydrocortisone
Characteristic histopathology	Infiltrate with atypical histiocytes, electron microscopic identification of Birbeck granule, cytochemical markers for Langerhans cell histiocytes

From Williams ML: Differential diagnosis of seborrheic dermatitis. Pediatr Rev 7:207, 1986; with permission.

33. How does the vehicle used in a dermatologic preparation affect therapy?
In general, **acute lesions** (moist, oozing) are best treated with aqueous, drying preparations. **Chronic, dry lesions** fare better when a lubricating, moisturizing vehicle is used. As a rule, any vehicle that enhances hydration of the skin enhances percutaneous absorption of topical medications (most of which are water-soluble). Thus, in preparations of equal concentration, the potency relationship is ointment > cream > gel > lotion.

Drying vehicles
Lotion: A suspension of powder in water. Therapeutic powder remains after aqueous phase evaporates. Useful in hairy areas, particularly the scalp.
Gel: Transparent emulsion that liquifies when applied to skin. Most useful in acne preparations and tar preparations for psoriasis.
Pastes: Combination of powder (usually cornstarch) and ointment which is stiffer than ointment

Moisturizing vehicles
Creams: Mixture of oil in a water emulsion. More useful than ointments when environmental humidity is high and in naturally occluded areas. Less greasy than ointment.
Ointments: Mixture of water in an oil emulsion. Also has an inert petroleum base. Longer lubricating effect than cream.

FUNGAL INFECTIONS

34. How do the features of tinea capitis vary by cause?

Organisms Responsible for Tinea Capitis

FEATURE	M. canis	T. tonsurans
Source	Cats and dogs	Other children
Fluorescence	Yellow-green	None
Contagious	Not very	Yes, very
Hair loss	Yes	Yes
Kerion	Yes	Yes
Children infected	Rural and suburban	Urban
Clinical patterns	Thickened hairs	Black-dot, dandruff-like, or multiple areas of alopecia

Adapted from Weston WL, Lane AT: Color Textbook of Pediatric Dermatology. St. Louis, Mosby, 1991, p 57; with permission.

35. Is a Wood's lamp helpful in screening for tinea capitis?

In 1930, yes. In the late 1990s, no. The reason is the changing epidemiology of tinea. Previously, more cases were caused by *Microsporum canis*, which fluoresces yellow-green with Wood's light. Now, more cases are caused by *Trichophyton tonsurans*, which does not fluoresce. In certain scenarios, a Wood's lamp can be helpful, but as a screening tool, it is not.

36. Why is topical therapy alone insufficient for tinea capitis?

The dermatophytes (i.e., fungi) that cause tinea can thrive deep in the hair shaft beyond the reach of topical therapy alone. Recommended therapy is a combination of oral griseofulvin, 15–20 mg/kg/day, of the microsize preparation in two divided doses, which is given with milk or ice cream to facilitate absorption, and biweekly shampooing with 2.5% selenium sulfide to decrease the spread of spores.

37. How should children receiving griseofulvin for tinea capitis be monitored?

The incidence of hepatitis or bone marrow suppression from griseofulvin in children is rare. Children who are undergoing an acute course of treatment (6–8 weeks) do not need obligatory blood counts or LFTs. However, a history of hepatitis or its risk factors would warrant a pretreatment evaluation of liver function and intermittent monitoring. For those rare cases in which griseofulvin is going to be used for > 2 months, one should consider obtaining complete blood counts and LFTs on an every-other-month basis.

38. Is a kerion a bacterial or fungal entity?

A kerion is a fluctulant and tender mass that occurs in some cases of tinea capitis. Occipital or posterior cervical lymph nodes are often enlarged. A kerion is felt to be primarily an excessive inflammatory response to tinea, and thus initial treatment consists of antifungal agents, principally griseofulvin and selenium sulfide shampoo. However, bacterial cultures of kerions will demonstrate *Staphylococcus aureus* or a mixture of gram-negative bacteria in two-thirds of cases. Since most kerions resolve without antibiotics, the role of these bacteria in the pathogenesis is unclear. Short courses of oral steroids are indicated in those lesions that are exquisitely painful.

Honig PJ, Caputo GL, et al: Microbiology of kerions. J Pediatr 123:422–424, 1993.

39. What puts the "versicolor" in tinea versicolor?

A very common superficial disorder of the skin, tinea versicolor is caused by the fungus *Pityrosporum orbiculare* (also known as *Malassezia furfur*). It presents as multiple macules and patches, with fine scales, over the upper trunk, arms, and occasionally the face and other areas. Lesions may be hypo- or hyperpigmented, appearing lighter than tanned skin in the summer and relatively darker in winter—thus "versatile" in color. Diagnosis can be confirmed by KOH preparation of a scraping from involved skin, which has characteristic fungal hyphae and a grape-like spore pattern referred to as "spaghetti and meatball" appearance. Wood's light will also display fluorescence (yellow-brown).

40. What is the treatment for tinea versicolor?

1. Selenium sulfide suspension (2.5% concentration) applied over the affected area overnight multiple times during the first week, with decreasing frequency over the ensuing weeks.

2. Topical antifungal creams (these can be expensive).

3. Oral ketoconazole is effective in adults in a single one-time dose and may be considered for use in older adolescents, although side effects may occur.

There are reports that this fungus causes central-line sepsis in neonates on hyperalimentation. So interest in this fungus isn't only skin deep.

41. After the sneaker is removed, how do you distinguish between "shoe dermatitis" and "athlete's foot"?

Allergic contact dermatitis (shoe dermatitis) involves the dorsa of the toes and distal third of the foot. The rash is red, scaly, and vesicular. KOH preparations of scrapings are negative.

In **tinea pedis** (athlete's foot), redness and scaling occur primarily on the instep or entire weight-bearing surface, with maceration between the toes. The nails may be yellowed and thickened. The KOH preparation is positive for hyphae. Tinea pedis is very uncommon in prepubertal children.

HAIR AND NAIL ABNORMALITIES

42. What causes alopecia in children?

Some hair loss is due to disorders of the hair itself—follicles, sebaceous glands, growing phase, etc. Others are secondary to diseases of the scalp. A useful approach is to classify loss by pattern (diffuse vs localized) and time of presentation (congenital vs acquired):

Congenital localized	**Congenital diffuse**
Sebaceous epidermal nevi	Hair shaft abnormalities
Melanocytic nevi	Trichorrhexis nodosa
Hemangiomas	Pili torti
Lymphangiomas	Trichorrhexis invaginata
Aplasia cutis	(Netherton syndrome)
Incontinentia pigmenti	Menkes' syndrome
Focal dermal hypoplasia	Trichoschisis
Chondrodysplasia punctata	Loose anagen syndrome
Intrauterine trauma (e.g., scalp electrodes)	Genetic syndromes
Infection (e.g., herpes, gonococcal)	(e.g., ectodermal dysplasia)
Acquired localized	**Acquired diffuse**
Alopecia areata	Telogen effluvium
Tinea capitis	Anagen effluvium
Traumatic scarring (e.g., trichotillomania)	Proximal trichorrhexis nodosa
Seborrheic dermatitis	Lamellar ichthyosis
Androgenic alopecia	Acrodermatitis enteropathica
Langerhans cell histiocytosis	Endocrinopathies
Neonatal lupus	(e.g., hypothyroidism)
Acne keloidalis	
Linear scleroderma	

Adapted from Datloff J, Esterly NB: A system for sorting out pediatric alopecia. Contemp Pediatr 3:53–56, 1986; with permission.

43. Are most hairs growing or resting?

Most infants and children have about 90% of scalp hair in the growing (anagen) and about 10% in the resting (telogen) state. On average, a single scalp hair will grow for about 3 years, rest for 3 months, and then, upon falling out, is replaced by a new growing hair.

44. What is the likely diagnosis in a child who develops diffuse hair loss 3 months after major surgery?

Telogen effluvium. This is a diffuse pattern of hair loss that occurs when a large number of scalp hairs convert from the anagen (growing) to the telogen (resting) phase. It may be associated with significant illness or fever, surgery, large weight loss, or severe emotional distress. The diagnosis is likely if there is a diffuse nature to the hair loss, a lack of scalp skin changes, and a characteristic microscopic pattern of the hair roots. Anagen hairs have pigmented cores and roots of a bulbous nature which are larger than the hair shaft. Often, the external root sheath is visible. In telogen hairs, the external root sheath and core pigment are absent and the root of the hair is often narrower than the shaft. Anagen effluvium, the loss of growing hairs, is most commonly seen during radiation and chemotherapy in the treatment of cancer.

Weston WL, Lane AT: Color Textbook of Pediatric Dermatology. St. Louis, Mosby-Year Book, 1991, p 184.

45. What puzzling cause of asymmetric hair loss in a child will sometimes cause an intern to pull his or her hair out?

Trichotillomania is hair loss due to self-manipulation, such as rubbing, twirling, or pulling. Hair loss is asymmetric. The most common physical finding is unequal hair lengths in the same region without evidence of epidermal changes of the scalp. Parents often do not observe the causative behavior, and convincing them of the likely diagnosis may take some effort. Behavior modification, along with application of petroleum or oil to the hair to make pulling more difficult, is the treatment of choice. Rarely, a child will swallow the hair and develop vomiting because of the formation of a gastric trichobezoar (hairball).

46. Which dermatologic diseases are commonly associated with nail abnormalities?

Psoriasis:	Nail pitting, longitudinal ridging, onycholysis (separation of nail plate from nailbed at distal margin), thickening of the nailplate, oil spots (yellowish-red discolorations of the nailbed), yellowish-white subungual hyperkeratosis
Lichen planus:	Longitudinal grooves, rough surface, thinning of nailplate, pterygium formation, scarring and loss of nailplate.
Alopecia areata:	Nail pitting, often in a grid-like pattern
Darier disease:	Red and white longitudinal streaks, breaks at distal edges resulting in V-shaped notches, wedge-shaped subungual hyperkeratosis

47. How should ingrown toenails be managed?

Soaks, open-toed sandals, properly fitting shoes, topical or systemic antibiotics, incision and drainage, or surgical removal of the lateral portion of the nail may all be utilized. Control is obtained best by letting the nail grow beyond the free end of the toe. Dental floss wedged between the nail and the lateral nailfold may help to prevent the nailplate from cutting into the skin and setting up a foreign body reaction. Proper instruction on nail care, including straight rather than arc trimming, is mandatory.

48. Which pathogens are responsible for paronychia?

Acute paronychia (inflammation of the nailfold usually with abscess formation) is most commonly caused by *Staphylococcus aureus*. The proximal or lateral nailfolds become intensely erythematous and tender. If a collection of pus develops at this site, it should be incised and drained. The treatment of acute paronychia includes oral administration of antistaphylococcal antibiotics.

Chronic paronychia is caused most often by *Candida albicans*. Although rarely inflamed, there is edema of the nailfolds and separation of the folds from the nailplate. A bacterial culture may reveal a variety of gram-positive and gram-negative organisms. The management of chronic paronychia should include avoidance of hand contact with water as much as possible. In addition, anticandidal solutions or lotions are often helpful.

INFESTATIONS

49. How do lice differ?

There are three main types of lice that infest humans, feeding primarily on human blood and causing pruritus and excoriations.

1. **Pediculosis capitis** (head lice). *Pediculus capitis*, the smallest and most common of the three human lice, is an obligate human parasite. Spread occurs directly by contact with an infected individual or indirectly through use of shared combs, brushes, or hats. For unknown reasons, infestation is nearly 35 times more likely in whites than blacks.

2. **Pediculosis corporis** (body lice). *Pediculus humanus*, the largest (2–4 mm) of the three types, is usually associated with poor hygiene. It does not live on the body but instead in the seams of clothing. It can be a vector for other diseases, such as epidemic typhus, trench fever, and relapsing fever.

3. **Pediculosis pubis** (pubic lice). *Phthirus pubis* is also known as the crab louse because it is a broad insect with legs that look like claws. It is sometimes mistaken for a brown freckle. Acquisition is primarily through sexual contact.

50. Can prepubertal children acquire pubic lice?

Though a relatively common infestation in adolescents and adults, in whom it is acquired through sexual contact, pediculosis pubis can occur in prepubertal children. Because of its predilection for hairy, nonscalp regions, the eyelashes are the most common location. The pubic louse can be transmitted via contaminated items such as towels, but its discovery on a child should raise the suspicion of sexual abuse.

51. What types of treatment are available for head lice?

1. Permethrin (e.g., Nix): A synthetic pyrethroid applied as a 10-minute creme rinse. It has higher residual and ovicidal activity than lindane and no risk for neurotoxicity. It is the drug of choice.

2. Malathion, 0.5% (e.g., Ovide): Applied as an 8–12-hour lotion, it also has better ovicidal activity and less toxicity than lindane.

3. Lindane, 1% (e.g., Kwell): Applied as a 10-minute shampoo. Ovicidal activity is low and repeat application is necessary. Resistance has been reported. If improperly used (e.g., ingestion or prolonged use), neurotoxicity is possible, especially in infants.

4. Pyrethrins (e.g., RID, A-200, R&C): Natural plant extracts mixed with piperonyl butoxide. These are applied as 10-minute shampoos and have same ovicidal activity as Nix, but no residual activity.

52. Should parents nit pick?

Once an infestation of lice has been properly treated, the nits are not viable or contagious. School policies of requiring students to be free of nits prior to return have not been of benefit. However, style (and paranoia) may rule over science. Methods of nit removal include soaking the hair with 3–5% acetic acid (white vinegar) and applying a towel dampened with the same solution for 30–60 minutes, use of specially designed fine-toothed nit combs, and commercial nit-removal solutions.

One other nit note is that the female louse usually attaches the nits to the hair about 3–4 mm from the scalp. Measuring the distance of the nits from the scalp allows approximate dating of the initiation of the infestation. (Human hair grows about 1 cm/month).

53. How is a skin scraping for scabies done?

Since the highest percentage of mites are usually concentrated on the hands and feet, the webspaces between digits is the best place to look for the characteristic linear burrows. Moisten the skin with alcohol or mineral oil, scrape across the area of the burrow with a small rounded (e.g., #15) scalpel blade, and place the scrapings on a glass slide with a drop of KOH (or additional mineral oil if used) and a cover slip. Burrows, if unseen, can be more precisely localized by rubbing a washable felt-tip marker across the webspace and removing the ink with alcohol. If burrows are present, ink will penetrate through the stratum corneum and outline the site.

Rasmussen JE: Scabies. Pediatr Rev 15:110–114, 1994.

54. What treatment eliminates the scabies' babies?

While lindane has long been the standard treatment for scabies, 5% permethrin cream has shown increased effectiveness with decreased risk of neurotoxicity and thus is the drug of choice in infants and children. Crotamiton and sulfur are much less effective than either of these agents. Permethrin may be used in children over 2 months of age. It must be stressed that all family members and close contacts should be treated simultaneously.

Complete application of the cream from the neck to the toes at night with removal by bathing or showering in the morning (8–14 hrs) should be adequate treatment. Retreatment in 1 week may be considered. Thick crusting in debilitated and immunosuppressed individuals may protect the mites and prevent adequate therapy, so removal of these crusts is essential. Physicians must make patients aware of the fact that lesions and pruritus may linger for 1–2 weeks after effective therapy. One must be supportive during this time to prevent unnecessary retreatment by parents. Antihistamines and topical steroids may help control symptoms.

    Peterson CM, Eichenfield LF: Scabies. Pediatr Ann 25:97–100, 1996.

55. What was the first human disease whose cause had a precise identification?

    Scabies. The etiologic agent, *Sarcoptes scabiei*, was first identified in 1687. The itch for knowledge, it seems, initially was stronger than the thirst for knowledge.

NEONATAL CONDITIONS

56. What is the most common birthmark?

    A variety of birthmarks compete for this title, depending on race. "Salmon patches" (faint red, macular, erythematous stains), which are distended dermal capillaries on the glabella, eyelids, and the nape of the neck, are seen in 70% of white infants and 60% of black infants. Mongolian spots, blue-black macules found on the lumbosacral area and occasionally on shoulders and backs, are seen in 80–90% of oriental, black, and Native American babies. They are seen in ≤ 10% of white infants.

57. Should a newborn with a sharp red line down the center of the body prompt a call to the NICU?

    Not unless the caller wants to be red-faced. This is likely the "harlequin color" change, a relatively common entity seen in up to 10% of newborns, particularly premature infants. It consists of reddening of one side of the body with a sharp line of demarcation along the midline. The change occurs only when the child is lying on one side. The superior half is light, whereas the dependent half is dark and subfused. The cause is thought to be an imbalance in autonomic regulation of peripheral blood vessels. If the infant is flipped, the color pattern reverses. If the infant is placed prone or supine, the color change disappears.

58. What is the medical significance of cutis marmorata?

    Cutis marmorata is the bluish mottling of the skin often seen in infants and young children exposed to low temperatures or chilling. The reticulated marbling effect is due to dilated capillaries and venules causing darkened areas on the skin. This disappears with warming. Cutis marmorata is of no medical significance and no treatment is indicated. However, persistent cutis marmorata is associated with trisomy 21, trisomy 18, and Cornelia de Lange syndromes. There is also a congenital vascular anomaly, termed cutis marmorata telangiectatic congenita, that has persistent blue reticulate mottling of the skin.

59. A healthy infant with multiple reddish nodules most likely has what entity?

    Subcutaneous fat necrosis consists of sharply circumscribed, indurated nodular lesions usually seen in healthy term newborns and infants in the first few days to weeks of life. The stony hard areas of panniculitis are generally movable and slightly elevated, and the overlying skin is a reddish, violaceous color. While the cause is unknown, it is thought that obstetric trauma and pressure on bony prominences may contribute to the problem. The usual sites (cheeks, back, buttocks, arms, and thighs) are consistent with this. Histologically, the lesions display extensive inflammation in the subcutaneous tissue with large fat lobules. Most lesions are self-limiting and require no therapy. However, occasionally they may extensively calcify and spontaneously drain with subsequent scarring. Remember that significant hypercalcemia may be present in a small number of patients. Therefore, a serum calcium should be ordered whenever the disorder is suspected and rechecked periodically until the condition resolves.

60. What is the long-term outcome for the collodion baby?

    A collodion baby is the term used to describe babies born encased in a translucent membrane (like saran-wrap). Generally, this membrane heralds ichthyosis. Two-thirds of affected infants develop lamellar ichthyosis or, less frequently, X-linked ichthyosis, epidermolytic hyperkeratosis,

Netherton syndrome, or Conradi syndrome. However, many infants with collodion membranes also end up with normal skin.

61. Cutis aplasia of the scalp is commonly associated with which chromosomal abnormality?

Aplasia cutis congenita (congenital absence of the skin) presents on the scalp as solitary or multiple well-demarcated ulcerations or atrophic scars. Of variable depth, the lesions may be limited to epidermis and upper dermis or occasionally extend to the skull and dura. While most children with this lesion are normal, scalp cutis aplasia has been classically associated with **trisomy 13 syndrome**.

62. What is the appearance and distribution of transient neonatal pustular melanosis?

Consisting of small vesicopustular lesions, 3–4 mm in size, transient pustular melanosis occurs in almost 5% of black and < 1% of white newborns. It may be present at birth or appear shortly after birth. The lesions most often cluster on the neck, chin, palms, and soles, although they may occur on the face and trunk. They are easily ruptured and progress to brown pigmented macules and a fine collarette of scale. Transient neonatal pustular melanosis is a benign disorder without associated systemic manifestations.

63. Is erythema toxicum neonatorum really toxic?

Not in the least. Erythema toxicum is a common eruption composed of erythematous macules, papules, and pustules occurring in newborns usually in the first few days of life. The lesions may start as irregular, blotchy, red macules, varying in size from millimeters to several centimeters. They often develop into 1–3-mm, yellow-white papules and pustules on an erythematous base, giving a "flea-bitten" appearance. They occur all over the body except on the palms and soles, which are spared because the lesions occur in pilosebaceous follicles, which are absent on the palmar and plantar surfaces. The rash is less common in premature infants, with incidence proportional to gestational age and peaking at 41–42 weeks. While it may be seen at birth, it is most common in the first 3–4 days of life and is occasionally noted as late as 10 days of life. Erythema toxicum usually lasts 5–7 days and heals without pigmentation.

64. How is the diagnosis of erythema toxicum confirmed?

Erythema toxicum is often confused with a variety of other skin disorders, including impetigo neonatorum, herpes simplex, transient neonatal pustular melanosis, milia, or miliaria. The diagnosis can be confirmed by staining the contents of a pustule with Wright or Giemsa stain. Clusters of eosinophils confirm the presence of erythema toxicum.

65. How are the most common neonatal papular lesions distinguished?

	NEONATAL ACNE	MILIA	ERYTHEMA TOXICUM
Distribution	Face	Face +	Face +
Appearance	Papule or pustule	yellow or white papule	Yellow or white papule
Erythematous	+	—	+
Contents on smear	PMNs	Keratin + sebaceous material	Eosinophils
Incidence	Occasional	40–50% of term infants	30–50% of term infants
Course	Last several months	Disappear in 3–4 wks	Disappear in 2 wks

PMN, polymorphonuclear cells.

66. For academic purposes (and ICD-9-CM coding), is it possible to be more scientific about the diagnosis of "prickly heat"?

The scientific name for this condition is **miliaria rubra.** It is due to sweat retention, and its clinical morphology is determined by the level at which sweat is trapped. Sweat trapped at a superficial level produces clear vesicles without surrounding erythema (sudamina or crystallina); miliaria rubra (prickly heat, erythematous papules, vesicles, papulovesicles) is produced by sweat trapped at a deeper level; pustular lesions (miliaria pustulosa) and even abscesses (miliaria profunda) are produced with sweat retention at the deepest of levels (infants rarely develop these types). With the advent of air conditioning, miliaria rarely occurs in newborn nurseries.

PAPULOSQUAMOUS DISORDERS

67. What diseases are associated with the Koebner reaction?

Koebnerization is an isomorphic response in which skin lesions occur at sites of local injury. The mechanism is unknown. Of the more common dermatologic problems, the Koebner phenomenon is seen in **psoriasis, warts,** and **lichen planus** with characteristic linear arrangements often along the lines of scratching.

68. A skin scale that easily bleeds on removal is characteristic of what condition?

The appearance of punctate bleeding points after removal of a scale is the **Auspitz sign**. It is seen primarily in psoriasis and is related to the rupture of capillaries high in the papillary dermis near the skin surface.

69. What is the typical pattern of lesions in childhood psoriasis?

A bilaterally symmetrical pattern with a distinct predilection for scalp, knees, elbows, presacral, and genital regions. The classic lesions are either guttate (teardrop) or round, erythematous, well-demarcated plaques covered with a silvery white micaceous scale.

70. What percentage of children with psoriasis have nail involvement?

Although pitting is said to be seen less often in childhood psoriasis than in the adult form, it is more common than is realized. Approximately 80% of children with psoriasis demonstrate pitting of the nails. Other nail changes include onycholysis (separation of the nailplate from nailbed at distal margin) and thickening of the nailplate, often with white-yellow discoloration.

71. Which joints are classically involved in psoriatic arthritis?

The distal interphalangeal joints of the hands and feet. Juvenile psoriatic arthritis (in patients < 16 years old) often presents as an acute monoarthritis. Joint changes often precede the skin changes. Psoriatic arthritis is more common in patients who have severe psoriasis. Flares are unrelated to the skin condition.

72. Why are systemic corticosteroids contraindicated in childhood psoriasis?

Following the discontinuation of the steroids, a condition called psoriatic erythroderma may result. Fever and hypoalbuminemia may also occur.

73. What are the 8 Ps of lichen planus?

1. Papules—usually 2–6 mm in diameter, which often are seen linearly due to the Koebner reaction
2. Plaques—commonly generated from a confluence of papules with exaggerated surface markings of the overlying skin (Wickham's striae)
3. Planar—individual lesions, usually flat-topped
4. Purple—distinctly violaceous
5. Pruritic—often intensely itchy
6. Polygonal—borders of papules are often angulated
7. Penis—common site of involvement in children
8. Persistent—chronic with remissions and exacerbations up to 18 months

74. How is pityriasis rosea distinguished from secondary syphilis?

Often with difficulty. Both are primarily papulosquamous rashes. **Pityriasis rosea** classically consists of oval lesions which organize in parallel fashion on the trunk (the "Christmas tree" distribution) and are preceded in 40–80% of cases by a large annular erythematous lesion (herald patch). **Secondary syphilis** lesions occur 3–6 weeks after the chancre, and in comparison to pityriasis rosea, they have more involvement of the palms, soles, and mucous membranes and have accompanying lymphadenopathy. However, because atypical presentations are common, testing for syphilis should be considered in any sexually active individual who is diagnosed with pityriasis rosea.

PHOTODERMATITIS

75. Which conditions are associated with marked sun sensitivity?
Connective tissue disorders—systemic lupus erythematosus, dermatomyositis
Porphyrias—erythropoietic protoporphyria, hepatoerythrocytic porphyria
Photoallergic disorders—associated with PABA esters, perfumes, phenothiazines
Phototoxic disorders—associated with sulfonamides, tetracyclines, thiazides, coal-tar derivatives, psoralens (in plants such as limes and celery)
Syndromes—xeroderma pigmentosa, Bloom, Rothmund-Thomson

76. What is the appearance of polymorphous light eruption?
It is characterized by itchy red papules; plaques or papulovesicles appear several hours to days after UV light exposure. It can be diagnosed by phototesting (induction of lesions by intentional UV light exposure) and by skin biopsy. It is usually diagnosed by the classic history and exclusion of other photosensitivity disease.

77. Why are French perfumes and a summertime walk on the beach sometimes a bad mix?
A photocontact dermatitis may result with some very unusual tan lines. Berloque dermatitis (*berloque* is French for pendant, which some lesions can resemble) is an irregularly patterned hyperpigmentation of the neck due to photosensitization by furocoumarins (i.e., psoralens) in perfumes. It is caused by fragrances that contain oil of bergamot, an extract from the peel of an orange grown in southern France and Italy. Oil of bergamot contains 5-methoxypsoralen, which enhances the erythematous and pigmentary response of UVA light.

78. How do sunscreens work?
Sunscreens either form a physical barrier (zinc oxide) or absorb UVB (PABA) or block UVA (benzophenones). The SPF (sun protection factor) is the ratio of time it takes to develop erythema with sunscreen on the skin to the time it takes to develop erythema without a sunscreen applied. An SPF of 15 means a person can spend 15 times longer in the sun without burning. The lifetime incidence of squamous and basal cell carcinomas could be reduced by almost 80% if sunscreens (SPF 15 or higher) were used regularly during the first 18 years of life!

79. Are steroids effective in the treatment of severe sunburn?
Steroids may be useful in treating severe sunburn. A short course of prednisone (1–2 mg/kg/day) with tapering after 4–8 days may abort severe sunburn reactions and provide relief.

80. Is a child with sun sensitivity protected by sitting behind a window?
Yes and no, depending on the reason for the sensitivity. UV light is divided into 3 wavelength groups: UVC (200–290 nm), UVB (290–320 nm), and UVA (320–400 nm). UVC light is cytotoxic and can cause retinal injury, but fortunately it is almost completely absorbed by the ozone layer. UVB light causes sunburn, dermatologic flares of systemic lupus erythematosus, and with chronic exposure, skin cancer. UVA light (which is also emitted from the fluorescent lamps used in most schools) is responsible for psoralen and drug phototoxicity and porphyria flares. Windows block UVB light, but not UVA. Thus, children with the latter kinds of disorders would not be protected.

PIGMENTATION DISORDERS

81. What disorders of childhood are associated with areas of hypopigmentation?
Hypopigmentation is a decrease in pigmentation, not total absence of pigmentation (depigmentation). Conditions that feature hypopigmented lesions include tuberous sclerosis, tinea versicolor, pityriasis alba, hypomelanosis of Ito, leprosy, and postinflammatory hypopigmentation.

82. How should vitiligio be treated?

There is no entirely safe and effective therapy available for children with vitiligo. Treatment with potent topical corticosteroids may be helpful. PUVA (topical or oral administration of 8-methoxypsoralen followed by exposure to UVA light) has been useful in some adults and older children but should be used with caution, as long-term sequelae such as skin cancer and cataracts are possible. Special cover-up makeups, such as Dermablend or Covermark, can be matched exactly to the patient's skin color and are waterproof. They provide excellent coverage of the vitiliginous areas. In addition, use of sunscreens with an SPF of ≥ 15 is necessary to protect the depigmented areas of skin. Counseling and education are important, and psychiatric intervention may be needed.

83. What is piebaldism?

Also sometimes called partial albinism, piebaldism is an autosomal dominant condition characterized by congenital leukoderma of the scalp and/or face, often accompanied by a prominent white forelock. Occasionally, the depigmented skin occurs on the limbs or trunk. The etiology is unknown, but histologically, there is localized absence of melanocytes in the affected skin. The differential diagnosis includes vitiligo, which, in contrast, is acquired, progressive, and often symmetrical. Piebaldism should not be confused with albinism, which is not localized and typically includes ocular problems such as nystagmus.

84. What are the metabolic causes of hyperpigmentation?

- Hepatobiliary disorders
- Hemochromatosis
- Addison disease
- Hyperthyroidism
- Hypothyroidism
- Acromegaly
- Cushing syndrome
- Heavy metals (silver, gold, mercury)
- Drugs (thorazine, antimalarials)
- Fixed drug eruptions (phenolphthalein, barbiturates, busulfan, cyclophosphamide, aspirin, phenacetin, phenytoin, gold, arsenic, sulfur, tetracycline)
- Porphyria cutanea tarda, variegate porphyria
- Gaucher disease
- Niemann-Pick disease
- B_{12} deficiency
- Wilson disease
- Hyperparathyroidism

85. Why are Spitz nevi and malignant melanoma often confused?

The Spitz nevus can appear suddenly and grow rapidly. Histologically, it has many pleomorphic cells and mitotic figures which can be mistaken for malignancy. It actually was previously referred to as benign juvenile melanoma. Benign is the key word for this red to brown, dome-shaped papule, which usually appears on the face or extremity. Because malignant melanoma is rare in children, beware of the misdiagnosed Spitz nevus.

86. What are the clinical features of familial dysplastic nevus syndrome?

The syndrome, also known as the familial atypical mole syndrome (FAMS), is the term used for families who have acquired nevi that develop into melanoma. These nevi are 5–15 mm in diameter and are round to oval in shape. Furthermore, they have irregular and indistinct margins, exhibit variation in color within the same lesion, and have both macular and elevated components. They tend to occur in sun-protected areas.

87. In children with pigmented nevi, what factors increase the risk of melanoma?

Melanoma is rare during childhood. If there is a family history of melanoma or the child has a giant congenital nevus, the risk is greater. Estimated risks vary for different sized congenital nevi. The projected lifetime risk for a melanoma developing in a small congenital nevus is 0.02%; for a giant nevus, 2–3%. Acquired nevi very rarely develop melanomas.

Ceballos PI, et al: Melanoma in children. N Engl J Med 332:656–662, 1995.

88. Who gets "mongolian spots"?

These are deep collections of spindle-shaped melanocytes typically found in infants on the buttocks and lumbosacral region and less frequently on the extremities, back, and shoulders. On rare occasions, they may be diffuse. Because of their depth, they appear blue-black or slate-gray. More commonly seen in dark-skinned individuals, occurrences are as follows: blacks (90–95%), native Americans (90%), Asians (80%), Latin (70%), and whites (10%). Most mongolian spots begin to fade by age 2 and disappear by age 10.

89. What are the characteristic findings of urticaria pigmentosa?
The characteristic lesions are red-brown, brown, yellow-brown, or yellow macules, papules, plaques, or nodules that have rippled surface (peau d'orange). The lesions are oval or round and frequently are mistaken for pigmented nevi or xanthoma. They vary in size from several millimeters to many centimeters. They occur on any portion of the skin surface but tend to concentrate on the trunk. The diagnosis is clinched by stroking the lesion, a maneuver which causes degranulation of the collection of mast cells, release of histamine, and urtication (Darier sign).

90. What is the differential diagnosis of yellow-brown or orange nodules in children?
- Benign cephalic histiocytosis
- Langerhans cell histiocytosis
- Juvenile xanthogranuloma
- Mastocytoma
- Urticaria pigmentosa
- Nevus lipomatosus
- Sebaceous nevus
- Spindle and epithelioid cell melanocytic nevus
- Xanthoma

Weston WL, Lane AT: Color Textbook of Pediatric Dermatology. St. Louis, Mosby-Year Book, 1991, p 151.

VASCULAR DYSPLASIAS

91. Describe the life history of hemangiomas.
The reason that watchful waiting should be the norm with these lesions is that 90–95% resolve spontaneously. However, parents should be told that hemangiomas may grow in the first 6–12 months before beginning to shrink. During this time, it is important to avoid the temptation of plastic surgery, cryotherapy, radiation therapy, or sclerosing agents, which can hasten resolution but lead to a higher likelihood of scarring. As a rule, 50% resolve by 5 years, 70% by 7 years, and 90% by 9 years. Even with the best management (i.e., doing nothing), residual skin changes, such as telangiectasias, pallor, atrophy, and skin redundancy may be present in 10–40% of patients.

92. When are systemic corticosteroids indicated in the treatment of cavernous or capillary hemangiomas?
While the approach to palpable hemangiomas generally involves observation over time, indications for systemic corticosteroids (prednisone, 2–4 mg/kg/day, tapered over 2–4 months) include:
1. Kasabach-Merritt syndrome with severe persistent thrombocytopenia (e.g., 40,000 platelet/mm³)
2. Lesions that interfere with normal physiologic functioning (breathing, hearing, eating, vision), especially periocular hemangiomas (to prevent ambylopia)
3. Recurrent bleeding, ulceration, or infection
4. A rapidly growing lesion that distorts facial features
5. High-output congestive heart failure

Wahrman JE, Honig PJ: Hemangiomas. Pediatr Rev 15:266–271, 1994.

93. If intralesional or systemic steroids fail in the treatment of hemangiomas with complications, what else may be of benefit?
1. Pulsed dye laser: May be used with other modalities; minimal scarring, but limited penetration (2 mm) restricts use to superficial lesions.
2. Interferon (alpha): Used subcutaneously, it may act by blocking endothelial cell motility and inhibit angiogenesis.
3. Cyclophosphamide: Because of systemic side effects, it is usually used for life-threatening hemangiomas with failure of other modalities.

94. Why is an infant with a hemangioma and new-onset thrombocytopenia so worrisome?

This can indicate the development of the Kasabach-Merritt syndrome, a condition of rapidly enlarging hemangiomas (usually cavernous) and progressive coagulopathy. Platelets are sequestered within the lesion(s), forming thrombi and consuming coagulation factors. Ecchymoses may develop initially around the hemangioma, but a disseminated coagulopathy with microangiopathic hemolytic anemia can result. Aggressive therapy (systemic steroids, alpha-interferon, and surgery) is frequently needed.

95. How do strawberry hemangiomas differ from post-wine stains?

Strawberry hemangiomas are superficial, palpable, vascular nevi that usually involute with time. Port-wine stains, sometimes called nevus flammeus or salmon patches, are flat vascular malformations that do not involute.

Strawberry hemangiomas	Port-wine stains
Palpable	Flat, macular
Common (up to 10% in children age < 1)	Less common (0.1–0.3%)
Often inapparent at birth (more visible at 2–52 wks)	Present at birth
Bright red	Pale pink to blue-red (darkens with age)
Well-defined borders	Borders variable
Predilection for head and neck (40–60%)	May be anywhere but increased percentage on head and face
Pathology: proliferating angioblastic endothelial cells with variable blood-filled capillaries	Pathology: dermal capillary dilation
90–95% involute spontaneously by age 9	No involution: may worsen with darkening and hypertrophy
Rapid growth phase	Proportionate growth (as child grows)
Suggested therapy: watchful waiting	Suggest therapy: flash lamp pulsed-dye laser in children

96. What is the clinical significance of lumbosacral hemangiomas?

Just like any other midline skin abnormality overlying the spine, one must rule out an underlying spinal defect with an MRI scan. It is especially important to rule out a tethered cord.

VESICULOBULLOUS DISORDERS

97. What is Nikolsky sign?

This sign demonstrates "epidermal fragility."

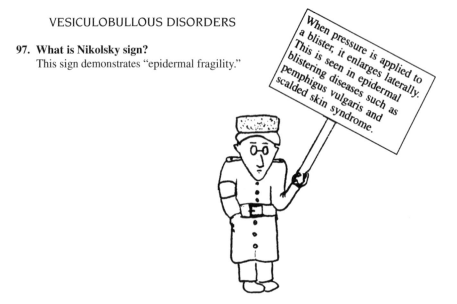

When pressure is applied to a blister, it enlarges laterally. This is seen in epidermal blistering diseases such as pemphigus vulgaris and scalded skin syndrome.

98. What is the differential diagnosis of epidermolysis in the neonate?

Epidermolysis is the separation of the epidermis from the skin, which can result in extensive areas of denudation. This characteristic is featured in staphylococcal scalded skin syndrome, epidermolytic hyperkeratosis (bullous ichthyosis), epidermolysis bullosa, and toxic epidermal necrolysis. In rare instances, candidiasis can have a similar presentation. Cultures, skin biopsies, immunofluorescence testing, and immunoelectron microscopy help confirm a diagnosis.

99. What are some of the associated findings of acquired epidermolysis bullosa (EB)?

This disorder is very similar to the inherited form of EB. It is seen first during adolescence or adulthood. Immunoelectron microscopy localizes the immune deposits below the basement membrane. Therefore the split is in a location similar to the dominantly inherited *dystrophic* form of EB. These patients blister following trauma. Scarring, milia formation, and nail dystrophy occur. Only the oral mucous membranes are involved. Other diseases associated with acquired EB and thought to be possible precipitants include amyloidosis, dermatitis herpetiformis, Ehlers-Danlos syndrome, impetigo, ingestions (arsenic, penicillamine, sulfonamides), inflammatory bowel disease, poison oak, porphyria, scarlet fever, and tuberculosis.

100. How are the varieties of epidermolysis bullosa inherited?

Disease	Inheritance	Other Designation	Location of Blister
Nonscarring			
Generalized EB simplex	Autosomal dominant	EB simplex	Epidermis
Localized EB simplex	Autosomal dominant	Recurrent bullous eruption of the hands and feet (Weber-Cockayne)	Epidermis
Junctional EB	Autosomal recessive	EB lethalis Herlitz disease	Basement membrane
Scarring			
Dystrophic EB	Autosomal dominant		Dermis
Dystrophic EB	Autosomal recessive		Dermis
Acquired EB			Dermis

From Honig PJ: Epidermolysis bullosa. Ostomy/Wound Manag 10:18–20, 1986; with permission.

101. When are steroids indicated in the treatment of erythema multiforme?

The use of steroids in erythema multiforme is controversial. In the vast majority of cases, the condition spontaneously remits. Glucocorticoids may help speed the resolution of some cases, but there are risks in their use, including immunosuppression and infection.

No Treatment	Consider Treatment
Eruption present ≥ 3 days	Eruptions present ≤ 2 days
> 20% skin denudation	< 20% skin denudation
Nontoxic	Toxic
Mucosal involvement: mouth only	Mucosal involvement: mouth plus other

From Eichenfield LF, Honig PJ: Blistering disorders in childhood. Pediatr Clin North Am 38:973, 1991; with permission.

102. What distinguishes erythema multiforme major versus minor?

Erythema multiforme is a hypersensitivity reaction to a variety of infections, drugs, and systemic diseases. Characteristic lesions are erythematous macules or papules, often mistaken for urticaria, with a central vesicle or bulla (termed target or iris lesions). Lesions may be present anywhere on the body, although commonly they are found symmetrically on extremities. Lesions of erythema multiforme remain for at least 1 week, unlike urticarial wheals, which disappear within hours. If the condition has minimal mucosal involvement or cutaneous denudation, it is **minor**. Widespread mucosal involvement, including ocular surfaces, and large surface desquamation connote **major**. Cutaneous erythema multiforme lesions and involvement of two or more mucosal surfaces may be termed Stevens-Johnson syndrome.

103. How is staphylococcal scalded skin syndrome (SSSS) differentiated from toxic epidermal necrolysis (TEN)?

Both are diffuse bullous diseases. SSSS develops after a localized staphylococcal infection with diffuse cutaneous disease caused by an exfoliative toxin. TEN is felt to be a hypersensitivity reaction, perhaps representing the most severe end of the spectrum of erythema multiforme.

Differentiation between SSSS and Ten

	SSSS	TEN
Etiology	Infectious; group II staphylococci	Immunologic; usually drug related
Morbidity/mortality	Low	High
Mucous membrane involvement	Rare	Frequent
Nikolsky sign	Present	Absent
Target lesions	Absent	Often present
Level of blister	Upper epidermis (below stratum corneum)	Subepidermal
Histopathology	No epidermal necrosis or dermal inflammation	Full-thickness epidermal necrosis; prominent perivascular dermal inflammation

Adapted from Roberts LJ: Dermatologic diseases. In Oski FA, et al (eds): Principles and Practice of Pediatrics, 2nd ed. Philadelphia, J.B. Lippincott, 1994, p 493; with permission.

104. When does the rash in poison ivy appear relative to exposure?

Poison ivy, or rhus dermatitis, is a typical delayed hypersensitivity reaction. The time between exposure and cutaneous lesions is usually 2–4 days. However, the eruption may appear as late as a week or more after contact (this explains why lesions continue to erupt after the initial "outbreak" of rash).

105. Are the vesicles in poison ivy contagious?

The contents of blisters do not contain the allergen. Washing the skin removes all surface oleoresin and prevents further contamination.

106. What disease should be considered if a child has chickenpox that is not resolving?

Mucha-Habermann disease. Another name for this disorder is **PLEVA** (pityriasis lichenoides et varioliformis). Generally speaking, the longer the name assigned to a particular dermatologic entity, the less likely a clear etiology has been established. Successive crops of papules appear which progress to form vesicles or necrotic centers. Frequently, the skin changes last a few weeks or months. At times, recurrences continue for several years. Other than chickenpox, this entity is often misdiagnosed as impetigo, vasculitis, or scabies. Rickettsialpox may even be considered. A skin biopsy clearly establishes the diagnosis (i.e., perivascular lymphocyte infiltrate with red blood cells migrating from the dermis to the epidermis). Sunlight, natural or artificial, alleviates the pruritus and skin changes. Oral erythromycin may help to clear the eruption.

5. EMERGENCY MEDICINE

Fred M. Henretig, M.D., Jane M. Lavelle, M.D., and Mark F. Ditmar, M.D.

CHILD ABUSE AND SEXUAL ABUSE

1. What is the most common cause of severe closed head trauma in infants < 1 year of age?
"Shaken baby" syndrome. Violent shaking of an infant can result in subdural hematomas, subarachnoid hemorrhages, and cerebral infarcts. The diagnosis is suggested by the lack of a corroborating mechanism of injury in the face of a severely symptomatic child. Physical examination may reveal retinal hemorrhages. Other signs of trauma are usually lacking. If a lumbar puncture is performed, the fluid may be bloody or xanthochromic. Diagnosis is confirmed by CT or MRI scanning. The prognosis is grim for an infant presenting in coma from this abuse: 50% die and nearly half of the survivors have significant neurologic sequelae.

2. What important historical and physical findings are indicators of child abuse?
Historical
1. Multiple previous hospital visits for injuries
2. History of untreated injuries
3. Cause of trauma not known or inappropriate for age or activity
4. Delay in seeking medical attention
5. History incompatible with injury findings
6. Parents unconcerned about injury or more concerned about unrelated minor problem (e.g., cold, headache)
7. History of abused siblings

Physical examination
1. Signs of general neglect, poor hygiene, or failure to thrive
2. Withdrawn or explosive personality
3. Burns, especially cigarette, or immersion burns on buttocks or perineum
4. Genital trauma or sexually transmitted infection
5. Signs of excessive corporal punishment (welts, belt or cord marks, bites)
6. Frenulum lacerations in young infants (associated with forced feeding)
7. Multiple lesions in various stages of resolution
8. Neurologic injury associated with retinal or scleral hemorrhages
9. Fractures suggestive of abuse

Kottmeier P: The battered child. Pediatr Ann 16:343–351, 1987.
Fontana V: The maltreatment syndrome of children. Pediatr Ann 13:740, 1984.

3. At what age is sudden and unexplained death unlikely to be caused by the sudden infant death syndrome (SIDS)?
Other causes (e.g., child abuse) should be considered in infants dying suddenly of unclear causes who are > 12 months. Deaths due to SIDS usually occur during the first year of life, and 90% of victims are < 7 months of age.

4. Which conditions with ecchymoses may be mistaken for child abuse?
Mongolian spots: Commonly mistaken for bruises, especially when they occur elsewhere than the classic lumbosacral area; unlike bruises, they do not fade with time.
Coagulation disorders: In 20% of cases of hemophilia, there is no family history of disease; bruising may be noted on unusual places in response to minor trauma.
Folk medicine: Southeast Asian practices of spoon rubbing (*quat sha*) or coin rubbing (*cao gio*) can produce ecchymoses; practice of cupping (inversion of heated cup on back) produces circular ecchymoses.

Ehlers-Danlos: Marked blood vessel fragility with easy bruising; suspect diagnosis if skin very hyperextensible.

Infectious/inflammatory: Multiple entities (such as erythema multiforme, Henoch-Schönlein purpura, meningococcemia) usually have other clinical features.

Dyes: Clothing dyes, especially from jeans, sometimes mimic bruising; easily removed by topical alcohol.

5. How do the color changes in an ecchymosis progress?

Visual aging of bruises is an inexact science with significant variability, but as a general rule:

0–1 day	Red/blue	8–10 days	Yellow/brown
1–5 days	Blue/purple	1.5–4 weeks	Resolution
5–7 days	Green/yellow		

Schwartz AJ, Ricci LR: How accurately can bruises be aged in abused children? Literature review and synthesis. Pediatrics 97:254–257, 1996.

6. How are fractures dated radiographically in children?

Following a fracture:

1–7 days	Soft-tissue swelling; fat and fascial planes blurred; sharp fracture line
7–14 days	Periosteal new bone formation as soft callus forms; blurring of fracture line; occurs earlier for infants, later for older children
14–21 days	More clearly defined (i.e., hard) callus forming as periosteal bone converts to lamellar bone
21–42 days	Peak of hard callus formation
≥ 60 days	Remodeling of bone begins with reshaping of deformity (up to 1–2 years)

If the timing of an injury does not correlate with the dating of a fracture, or if fractures at multiple stages of healing are present, child abuse should be suspected.

7. What fractures are suggestive of child abuse?

Spinal fractures, posterior and anterior rib fractures, skull fractures, metaphyseal chip fractures, and vertebral, femoral, pelvic, or scapular fractures. These are fractures that commonly result from twisting, throwing, and beating. Metaphyseal chip fractures are the result of the forceful jerking of an extremity. Anterior and posterior rib fractures occur with severe side-to-side compression of the thorax. They are almost never caused by CPR! The description and forcefulness of injury should be consistent with the fracture. One should be especially suspicious if such fractures occur in a child not yet walking.

Wissow LS: Child abuse and neglect. N Engl J Med 332:1425–1431, 1995.

8. When are burn injuries suspicious for child abuse?

Burn injuries account for about 5% of cases of physical abuse. As with other injuries, the description of the incident causing the burn should be consistent with the child's development and the extent and degree of the burn observed. The following types are suspicious for abuse:

Immersion burns: Sharply demarcated lines on the hands and feet ("stocking glove" distribution), buttocks, and perineum with a uniform depth of burn; the immersion of a child in a hot bath is classic.

Geographic burns: Burns usually of second or third degree in a distinct pattern, such as circular cigarette burns or steam iron burns.

Splash burns: Pattern with droplet marks projecting away from the most involved area.

9. How do you recognize Munchausen syndrome by proxy?

In this form of child abuse, adults inflict illness on a child or falsify symptoms in order to obtain medical care for a child. Features include:

1. Recurrent episodes of a confusing medical picture
2. Multiple diagnostic evaluations at medical centers ("doctor shopping")
3. Unsupportive marital relationship, often with maternal isolation

4. Compliant, cooperative, overinvolved mother
5. Higher level of parental medical knowledge
6. Parental history of extensive medical treatment or illness
7. Conditions resolve with surveillance of child in hospital
8. History of unexplained sibling death

Ludwig S: Child abuse. In Fleisher GR, Ludwig S (eds): Textbook of Pediatric Emergency Medicine, 3rd ed. Baltimore, Williams & Wilkins, 1993, p 1439.

10. How often is sexual abuse committed by an individual known previously by the child or adolescent?

75–80%. Relatives are the perpetrators in 50% of cases.

11. Following documentation of history and a careful physical exam, what evidence should be collected in suspected sexual abuse or assault of a postpubertal female?

If suspected history of sexual contact, loss of consciousness, or poor history:
1. Evidence of sexually transmitted disease (STD)
   • Gonococcal cultures of pharynx, vagina or cervix, and rectum
   • Chlamydial cultures of pharynx, vagina or urethra, and rectum
   • RPR or VDRL test for syphilis; if positive, confirm with specific antibody testing
   • Other studies for STDs if clinically suspected
2. Pregnancy testing if postmenarchal
3. Evidence of sexual contact, including 2–3 swabbed specimens from each area of assault for:
   • Sperm
   • Acid phosphatase (secreted by prostate and a component of seminal plasma)
   • P 30 (prostate glycoprotein present in seminal fluid)
   Blood group antigens
4. Evidence to document perpetrator
   • Foreign material on clothing
   • Suspected nonpatient hairs

12. How long does forensic evidence of sexual abuse persist after contact?

	Type of Evidence			
SITE	MOTILE SPERM	NONMOTILE SPERM	ACID PHOSPHATASE	P 30
Pharynx	0.5–6 hrs	6 hrs (?)	6 hrs (?)	Unknown
Rectum	0.5–8 hrs	24 hrs	24 hrs (?)	Unknown
Vagina	0.5–8 hrs	7–48 hrs	12–48 hrs	12–48 hrs
Clothing	< 0.5 hr	Up to 12 mos	Up to 3 yrs	Up to 12 yrs

Of note, lack of cervical mucus in prepubertal girls decreases survival of motile sperm. Data are very limited on pharyngeal persistence of nonmotile sperm and pharyngeal and rectal persistence of acid phosphatase. Both acid phosphatase and P 30 can persist indefinitely on clothing if it is kept dry and not washed.

From Reece RM: Child Abuse: Medical Diagnosis and Management. Philadelphia, Lea & Febiger, 1994, p 234; with permission.

13. What is the best predictor of *Neisseria gonorrhoeae* infection in children aged < 12 years examined for sexual abuse?

Vaginal or **urethral discharge**. Without evidence of discharge, the likelihood of a culture result being positive is near zero.

Sicoli RA, et al: Indications for *Neisseria gonorrhoeae* cultures in children with suspected sexual abuse. Arch Pediatr Adolesc Med 149:86–89, 1995.

14. If a patient is diagnosed with an infection caused by an STD-associated organism, how likely is sexual abuse the reason for acquisition?

Organism	Incubation	Sexual Abuse
Neisseria gonorrhoeae	2–7 days	Certain
Treponema pallidum (syphilis)	10–90 days (avg 3 wks)	Certain
Chlamydia trachomatis	Variable (min 1 wk)	Probable
Trichomonas vaginalis	4–20 days (avg 1 wk)	Probable
Herpes simplex virus, type II	2–14 days	Probable
Human papillomavirus (condyloma accuminatum)	Unknown; may range from 3 mos to several years	Possible
Hepatitis B	45–160 days (avg 120 days)	Possible
Herpes simplex virus, type I (genital location)	2–12 days	Possible
HIV	Variable (months to years)	Possible
Bacterial vaginosis (nonspecific vaginosis or Gardnerella-associated vaginosis)	Unknown	Uncertain
Ureaplasma urealyticum	10–20 days	Uncertain
Candida albicans	Unknown	Unlikely

All of these organisms can be acquired perinatally, complicating the diagnosis of sexual abuse in infants. As infants grow to prepubertal children, newly diagnosed acquisition of these organisms makes sexual abuse more likely.

American Academy of Pediatrics: Sexually transmitted diseases. In Peter G (ed): 1994 Red Book, 23rd ed. Elk Grove Village, IL, American Academy of Pediatrics, 1994.

Committee on Child Abuse and Neglect: Guidelines for the evaluation of sexual abuse in children. Pediatrics 87:254–260, 1991.

15. Is the size of the hymenal opening a helpful finding in the diagnosis of sexual abuse?

The hymenal opening is measured with a child in the supine, frog-leg position, and various studies have attempted to determine a size which most likely correlates with sexual abuse. The ranges have been from 4–10 mm, but variations in technique, positioning, and relative relaxation of the patient have limited the value of absolute numbers. In addition, there is considerable overlap in diameter between sexually abused and nonabused girls. Thus, the size of the hymenal opening should **not** be used as a diagnostic or confirmatory test, particularly as an isolated finding. More important in the exam is inspection for scarring and tears of the hymen and surrounding tissues.

Heger A, Emans SJ: Introital diameter as the criteria for sexual abuse. Pediatrics 85:222–223, 1990.

ENVIRONMENTAL EMERGENCIES

16. What cardiovascular changes occur as body temperature falls?

31–32° C: Elevated HR, cardiac output, and blood pressure; peripheral vasoconstriction and increased central vascular volume; normal ECG

32–28° C: Diminished HR, cardiac output, and blood pressure; ECG irregularities include PVCs, supraventricular dysrhythmias, atrial fibrillation, and T-wave inversion

< 28° C: Severe myocardial irritability; ventricular fibrillation, usually refractory to electrical defibrillation; often absent pulse or blood pressure; J waves on ECG

17. What are the hazards of externally rewarming a hypothermic patient too rapidly?

1. **Core temperature "afterdrop"**—External rewarming causes peripheral vasodilation and return of cold venous blood to the core.

2. **Hypotension**—Peripheral vasodilation increases total vascular space, and hypothermia is often a hypovolemic state because of cold-induced diuresis and cold-induced renal tubular and concentrating dysfunction in the setting of depressed myocardial function.

3. **Acidosis**—Lactic acid returns from the periphery, resulting in rewarming acidosis.

4. **Dysrhythmias**—Rewarming alters acid-base and electrolyte status in the setting of an irritable myocardium.

18. Why do victims of submersion usually suffer from heat loss and clinical hypothermia?
The thermal conductivity of water is 32 times greater than that of air.

19. Should the Heimlich maneuver be done as the first step in near-drowning resuscitation?
No. The Heimlich maneuver has no demonstrable effect in removing water from the lung or improving oxygenation. Because of laryngospasm, relatively small amounts of water are aspirated into the victim's lungs during drowning. Asphyxia results from cessation of respiration and obliteration of surfactant activity. The Heimlich maneuver may even be counterproductive. During the panic stage of drowning, the victim typically swallows a significant amount of water. Abdominal thrusts may cause regurgitation and complicate airway management.

20. Which causes greater harm to the lung in near-drowning victims, fresh water or salt water?
Salt water. Although as little as 2 ml/kg of fresh water can cause disruption of surfactant and alveolar instability with marked problems in oxygenation, the same amount of salt water causes even greater harm. While it does not denature surfactant (as fresh water does), salt water with its high osmolarity (greater than normal saline) causes an osmotic gradient that allows marked fluid accumulation and, in essence, overwhelms the surfactant. In practice, these differences have little clinical significance, as victims are at risk for hypoxemia and acute lung injury in both salt and fresh water drownings.

Thompson AE: Environmental emergencies. In Fleischer GR, Ludwig S (eds): Textbook of Pediatric Emergency Medicine, 3rd ed. Baltimore, Williams & Wilkins, 1993, pp 802–803.

21. What systems malfunction in heatstroke?
Heatstroke is a medical emergency of multisystem dysfunction caused by very high fever (usually $> 41.5°$ C). Profound CNS disturbance—confusion, seizures, loss of consciousness—is the hallmark of the condition. Other problems include (1) hypotension due to volume depletion, peripheral vasodilation, and myocardial dysfunction; (2) acute tubular necrosis and renal failure with marked electrolyte abnormalities; (3) hepatocellular injury and dysfunction; (4) abnormal hemostasis, often with signs of disseminated intravascular coagulation; and (5) rhabdomyolysis.

22. What is the "critical thermal maximum"?
$42°$ C. This is the body temperature at which cell death begins as physiologic processes unravel. Enzymes denature, lipid membranes liquefy, mitochondria misfire, and protein production fails.

23. Discuss the important considerations in the pulmonary and airway management of children with suspected smoke inhalation.
1. *How extensive are the signs of smoke inhalation?* Physical exam may reveal carbonaceous sputum, singed nasal hairs, facial burns, or pulmonary abnormalities. These make development of pneumonia more likely.

2. *Are there signs of impending airway obstruction due to mucosal injury and edema?* These include increasing respiratory distress, difficulty in handling secretions, or stridor.

3. *Are there signs of carbon monoxide poisoning and tissue hypoxia?* Possibilities include headache, confusion, irritability, visual changes, or other CNS abnormality. Their presence warrants aggressive oxygen therapy, including consideration of hyperbaric oxygen if available.

24. Which laboratory studies are needed in suspected carbon monoxide poisoning?
Blood carboxyhemoglobin (HbCO) level

0–1%	Normal (smokers may have up to 5–10%)
10–30%	Headache, exercise-induced dyspnea, confusion
30–50%	Severe headache, nausea, vomiting, increased HR and respirations, visual disturbances, memory loss, ataxia
50–70%	Convulsions, coma, severe cardiorespiratory compromise
> 70%	Usually fatal

Hemoglobin level—to evaluate correctable anemia
Arterial pH—to elevate acidosis
Urinalysis for myoglobin—Patients with CO poisoning are susceptible to tissue and muscle breakdown with possible acute renal failure resulting from renal deposition of myoglobin.

25. What are the key aspects in treatment of CO poisoning in children?
1. Very close monitoring
2. 100% oxygen until HbCO falls to 5%. The half-life of HbCO is 4 hours if the subject is breathing room (at sea level), 1 hour in 100% oxygen (at sea level), and < 1 hour in a hyperbaric oxygen chamber with 100% oxygen.
3. Correct metabolic acidosis, especially when pH < 7.2. Although correcting the acidosis shifts the oxyhemoglobin dissociation curve to the left, decreasing oxygen delivery to the tissues, a blood pH < 7.2 can compromise cardiac performance.
4. Refer for use of hyperbaric oxygen if: (a) history of coma, seizure, or abnormal mental status at the scene or in the emergency department; (b) persistent metabolic acidosis; (c) neonate; (d) pregnant woman; or (e) HbCO level > 25%, even if the patient is neurologically intact.

26. Why is carbon monoxide such a deadly toxin?
1. It is odorless and invisible and can overwhelm a patient without warning.
2. It is a product of partial combustion of nearly all fossil fuels, so it is ubiquitous in daily living, ranging from running cars to heating homes to barbecuing with charcoal.
3. Often misdiagnosed as flu-type illness because of subacute presentation of headache, dizziness, and malaise.
4. Nearly irreversible binding to hemoglobin (with affinity 200–300 times that of oxygen) which shifts the oxyhemoglobin dissociation curve to the left and changes its shape from sigmoidal to hyperbolic (with greatly diminished O_2 tissue release).
5. Strong binding to other heme-containing proteins, particularly in the mitochondria involving oxidative metabolism, leading to metabolic acidosis and cellular dysfunction (especially cardiac and CNS tissues).

27. If a victim of smoke inhalation has a severe and persistent metabolic acidosis despite therapy, what diagnosis should be suspected?
Cyanide poisoning. Hydrogen cyanide (HCN) gas results from the thermal decomposition of nitrogen-containing materials (e.g., polyurethane, silk, plastics). The short half-life of HCN (approximately 1 hour) can make the diagnosis difficult. In one study, elevated blood lactate levels ≥ 10 mmol/L correlated with toxic levels of blood cyanide when no other causes of acidosis existed. Many authorities recommend routine treatment for possible cyanide toxicity with sodium thiosulfate during the initial resuscitation of a fire victim. If the patient remains critically ill with coma, seizure, acidemia, and elevated lactate levels, treatment with sodium nitrate should be considered. Although this treatment detoxifies cyanide, it does result in the formation of methemoglobin, which decreases the O_2-carrying capacity of hemoglobin.

Baud FJ, et al: Elevated blood cyanide concentrations in victims of smoke inhalation. N Engl J Med 325:1761–1766, 1991.

28. What are the different degrees of burn injuries?

Classification of Burn Wounds

DEGREE	DEPTH	INCHES	CLINICAL APPEARANCE	CAUSE
1°	Epidermis	0.002	Dry, erythematous	Sunburn, scald
2°	Superficial dermis	0.02	Blisters, moist, erythematous	Scald, immersion, contact
	Deep dermis	0.035	White eschar	Grease, flash fire
3°	Subcutaneous	0.040	Avascular—white or dark, dry, waxy (yellow)	Prolonged immersion, flame, contact, grease, oil
4°	Muscle		Charred, skin surface cracked	Flame

From Coren CV: Burn injuries in children. Pediatr Ann 16:323–329, 1987.

29. How does the "rule of nines" apply in children?

The "rule of nines" is a device to estimate the extent of burns. For example, in adults, the entire arm is 9% of body surface area (BSA), the front of the leg is another 9%, etc. The resulting estimate of the extent of burns is particularly helpful in calculating fluid requirements. Correction for age is necessary with this formula because of differing body proportions. Of note, the surface of a patient's hand represents about 1% of BSA.

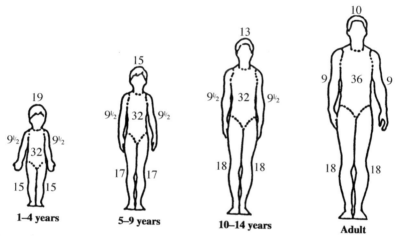

From Carajal HF: Burn injuries. In Behrman RE, et al (eds): Nelson Textbook of Pediatrics, 14th ed. Philadelphia, W.B. Saunders, 1992, p 235; with permission.

30. Which burn injuries require hospitalization?

- Second-degree burns covering > 10% of BSA
- Third-degree burns covering > 2% of BSA
- Significant burns involving hands, feet, face, or perineum
- Self-inflicted burns
- Burns resulting from child abuse
- Explosion, inhalation, or chemical burns (where other organ trauma may be involved)
- Significant burns in children with chronic metabolic or connective tissue diseases (in whom healing may be compromised with the increased risk of secondary infection)
- Significant burns in children younger than age 2 years

31. Why are alkali burns worse than acid burns of the eye?

Alkali burns are caused by lye, such as in Drano or Liquid Plumr, or by lime, or ammonia among others. They are characterized by **liquefaction necrosis**. They are worse than acid burns because the damage is ongoing. When spilled in the eye, acid is quickly buffered by tissue and limited in penetration by precipitated proteins; **coagulation necrosis** results, which is usually limited to the area of contact. Alkali, however, has a more rapid and deeper advancement, causing progressive damage at the cellular level by combining with membrane lipids. This underscores the importance of extended irrigation of the eyes, particularly in alkali burns.

32. How do the injuries produced by lightning and high-voltage wires differ?

Lightning consists of direct current (DC) of extremely high voltage (200,000 to 2 billion volts) delivered over milliseconds. In contrast, high-voltage wires deliver alternating current (AC) of lower voltage (rarely exceeding 70,000 V) over a longer period of time. Lightning exposure causes massive electrical countershock with asystole, respiratory arrest, and minimal tissue damage. High-voltage exposure causes ventricular fibrillation and deep tissue injury. Resultant muscle necrosis can lead to substantial myoglobin release and renal failure.

33. In electrical injury, is AC or DC more hazardous?

AC is more hazardous, especially at lower voltages which can cause ventricular fibrillation. Exposure to AC often results in tetanic contractions of the muscles, which prevent the victim from terminating contact and lead to greater tissue injury by prolonging exposure.

34. What are the major causes of anaphylaxis?

1. *Biologic agents:* antitoxins, blood transfusions, dextran plasma expanders, gamma globulin, other blood products
2. *Diagnostic agents:* iodinated contrast media
3. *Drugs:* antibiotics (penicillin, cephalosporins, sulfonamides, tetracycline), anesthetics (lidocaine), aspirin, chemotherapeutic agents (L-asparaginase)
4. *Exercise-induced*
5. *Foods:* eggs, milk, nuts (pecans, peanuts, walnuts), seafood/shellfish
6. *Food additives:* metabisulfite, monosodium glutamate
7. *Immunotherapy:* allergen extracts
8. *Insects:* Hymenoptera (bumble bee, fire ants, honey bee, hornet, wasp, yellow jacket)
9. *Latex:* gloves, urinary catheters, endotracheal tubes

35. What are the treatment options for a patient with anaphylaxis?

1. Proper patient positioning: recumbent position, elevation of lower extremities
2. Epinephrine: 1:1000, 0.01 ml/kg (max 0.3–0.5 ml) SC or IM every 10–20 min up to three times
3. Airway maintenance if laryngeal edema develops; may require nebulized use of racemic epinephrine, albuterol, or isoetharine
4. Supplemental oxygen as needed
5. Lessen urticaria or angioedema with IV diphenhydramine (H_1-receptor blocker) or ranitidine (H_2-receptor blocker)
6. Blood pressure maintenance with IV fluids, pressor agents
7. Relief of severe bronchospasm: IV aminophylline
8. Prevention of late-phase reactions: Hydrocortisone succinate, 5 mg/kg (max 250 mg), methylprednisolone 1 mg/kg (max 50 mg) IV every 6 hrs

Friday GA Jr: Insect stings. In Burg FD, Wald ER, Ingelfinger JR, Polin RA (eds): Current Pediatric Therapy, 15th ed. Philadelphia, W.B. Saunders, 1996, p 734.

36. How does one distinguish between poisonous and nonpoisonous snakes?

Preferably by turning the pages of *National Geographic*. North America has 41 groups of snakes, but nearly all of poisonous bites are caused by four groups: rattlesnakes, moccasins, copperheads, and coral snakes. Distinguishing features include:

1. Elliptical and vertically oriented pupils (in moccasins and copperheads) compared with round pupils (in nonpoisonous snakes)

2. Curved fangs that can fold against the palate
3. Triangular head contrasted with more oval-shaped head of harmless snakes
4. Bodies are more stout and sausage-like compared with slender bodies of harmless snakes
5. Distal tail scales arranged in a single row compared to the double-row scales of non-venomous snakes
6. Coral snakes with rings of yellow, red, and black with the red always touching the yellow but never the black. As the herpetologists sing: "Red touch yellow—kill a fellow/ Red touch black, a poison lack."

Roever JM: Snake Secrets. New York, Walker & Company, 1979, pp 39–43.

LACERATIONS

37. Which eyelid lacerations warrant ophthalmologic evaluation?
• Full-thickness lacerations
• Laceration involving the lid margin
• Deep lower-lid lacerations that may involve damage to the tear-drainage system
• Ptosis of the involved lid
• Significant tissue avulsion
• Associated eyeball injury

Levin AV: Eye trauma. In Fleisher GR, Ludwig S (eds): Textbook of Pediatric Emergency Medicine, 3rd ed. Baltimore, Williams & Wilkins, 1993, p 1205.

38. Which lacerations should be repaired by a surgeon?
• Large complex lacerations
• Stellate or flap lacerations
• Lacerations with questions of tissue viability
• Lacerations involving lip margins (vermilion border)
• Deep lacerations with nerve damage
• Lacerations that evoke intention tremors in the medical houseofficer

39. How many days should sutures remain in place?
In general, as the site of laceration proceeds, from head to toe, the length of time of suture placement increases: eyelids—3 days; face—5 days; trunk and upper extremities—7 days; and lower extremities—10 days.

40. When should a nerve injury be suspected in a finger laceration?
1. Abnormal testing of sensation (diminished pain or two-point discrimination)
2. Abnormal autonomic function (absence of sweat or lack of skin wrinkling after soaking in water)
3. Diminished range of motion of finger (may also indicate joint, bone, or tendon disruption)
4. Pulsating blood emerging from wound (on flexor aspect, nerve is superficial to digital artery and arterial flow implies nerve damage)

41. What should be done if nerve damage is suspected?
Immediate repair is not essential, and this is not a true emergency. Delayed nerve repair is very satisfactory, particularly in younger children. If an operating suite and personnel are not poised to proceed, skin closure can be done and the operation deferred. Care must be taken not to stop the arterial bleeding with a hemostat or other clamp, as this may further damage the nerve. Simple pressure, often for extended periods, generally suffices.

42. Which lacerations should not be sutured?
Lacerations at high risk for infection should be considered for healing by secondary intention or delayed primary closure. These include **cosmetically unimportant puncture wounds,**

human bites, lacerations involving mucosal surfaces (e.g., mouth, vagina), and wounds with a **high probability of contamination** (e.g., acquired in a garbage bin). Many authorities in the past recommended that wounds untreated for > 12 hours not be sutured. However, the type of wound and risk for infection are more important than any absolute time criterion. A clean knife laceration of 20 hours could be considered for closure.

43. Dog bites or cat bites: which are at greater risk for infection?

Generally, infection rates are higher in cat bites because of the greater likelihood of a puncture wound rather than a laceration injury. Additionally, *Pasteurella multocida*, the most common pathogen responsible for infection, is present in higher concentrations in cat bites. Wounds caused by cat and dog bites usually contain multiple other organisms, including *Staphylococcus aureus* and anaerobes. Vigorous high-pressure and high-volume irrigation with normal saline is key. Amoxicillin with clavulanic acid (Augmentin) is usually given prophylactically to individuals with cat bites or high-risk dog bites.

44. How is a human bite distinguished from a dog bite?

Human bites generally are crush injuries and crescent-shaped, while dog bites more commonly are tear injuries and triangular-shaped. The distance between the two main puncture sites (caused by the canines or cuspids) can be helpful. A distance > 3 cm suggests a human bite.

45. Antibiotic prophylaxis should be considered for which lacerations?

This is controversial, but a conservative set of guidelines would include:
1. Lacerations involving cartilaginous exposure of the nose or ear
2. Wounds of the perineum
3. "Dirty wounds" (trash sites, farm settings, gravel- or dirt-covered roads)
4. Cat bites (especially requiring resuturing for cosmetic reasons, significant deep tear or puncture wounds, or hand wounds)
5. Lacerations associated with significant crush injury (where deep tissue necrosis may be ongoing)
6. All human bites, especially from closed-fist injury

46. Following a laceration or penetrating injury, how long before a tetanus infection usually begins?

Rarely, tetanus has been reported within a day of injury or > 60 days after injury. However, > 80% of tetanus cases occur from 3–14 days after the acute injury, and > 90% occur within 2–21 days. The average onset of symptoms is day 7. Following repeat immunization, protective concentrations of antibody appear in the vast majority of patients within 4–7 days after vaccination.

Wassilak SG: Timing of tetanus immunoprophylaxis in wound management. Pediatr Infect Dis J 9:67–68, 1990.

47. What are the recommendations for tetanus prophylaxis in a child with a laceration?

No. of Previous Immunizations	Most Recent Booster	Type of Wound	Recommendation for Children ≥ 7 Years of Age
Unclear or <3	—	Clean, minor	Adult-type tetanus vaccine
		Tetanus-prone	Adult-type tetanus vaccine and tetanus immunoglobulin
≥ 3	> 10 yrs	Clean, minor	Adult-type tetanus vaccine
		Tetanus-prone	Adult-type tetanus vaccine
≥ 3	5–10 yrs	Clean, minor	None
		Tetanus-prone	Adult-type tetanus vaccine
≥ 3	< 5 yrs	Clean, minor	None
		Tetanus-prone	None

In children < 7 years of age, other tetanus-containing vaccines (DTP, DTaP, DT) should be given rather than the adult-type tetanus vaccine (Td), depending on the immunization status and previous reactions. *Clean, minor wounds* generally are defined as wounds that are < 6 hours old; not infected or contaminated with feces, soil, or saliva; superficial enough to permit irrigation and debridement; and surrounded by viable tissues. Most are linear. *Tetanus-prone wounds* include all other wounds but especially those caused by puncture, crush injury, burns, or frostbite.

48. When is the use of lidocaine with epinephrine contraindicated as an anesthetic?

When there is question of tissue viability and in any instance in which vasoconstriction might produce ischemic injury to an "end organ" without an alternative blood supply (e.g., tip of nose, margin of ear, tip of finger or toe).

49. What makes TAC tick? What is it?

TAC is a method of needleless local anesthesia using a solution of **T**etracaine (1–2%), **A**drenaline (epinephrine, 1:1000), and **C**ocaine (4.0–11.8%). It is applied directly to the wound by dripping or brushing and is held in place for 10–15 minutes, until blanching occurs around the wound. Use near mucous membranes should be avoided because excessive absorption can lead to seizures. Care should also be taken not to use TAC near the eyes (because of the possibility of corneal abrasions) or on any end-artery site such as the fingertip or toe or ear margin (because of the risk of ischemia).

Of note, an alternative can be **LAT** (94% **L**idocaine, **A**drenaline [1:2000 epinephrine], 0.5% **T**etracaine). This solution can also be applied topically, and the elimination of the cocaine component reduces the potential for side effects as well as the cost.

Ernst AA, et al: Lidocaine-adrenaline-tetracaine gel versus tetracaine-adrenaline-cocaine gel for topical anesthesia in linear scalp and facial lacerations in children aged 5 to 17 years. Pediatrics 95:255–258, 1995.

50. In what situations is EMLA cream useful?

EMLA stands for **E**utectic **M**ixture of **L**ocal **A**nesthetics, which are lidocaine and prilocaine. EMLA is very useful in anesthetizing the skin prior to venipuncture, IV placement, injection, lumbar puncture, or circumcision. The cream is placed on the site and covered with an occlusive dressing for 1–2 hours. Obviously, its most practical use is for anticipated procedures.

51. Is the "DPT lytic cocktail" a thing of the past?

With the development of newer anesthetic and analgesic agents, it should be. **DPT** stands for **D**emerol (meperidine), **P**henergan (promethazine), and **T**horazine (chlorpromazine), and for many years, it has been a mainstay of pediatric sedation and analgesia. The combination of two phenothiazines and a long-acting narcotic runs counter to the ideal of rapid onset of action with reversibility that should characterize these types of medications. Problems with the DPT cocktail include its administration (IM), delayed onset of action , prolonged (up to 6 hours) sedation, hypotension, and respiratory depression.

Committee on Drugs: Reappraisal of lytic cocktail Demerol, Phenergan, and Thorazine (DPT) for the sedation of children. Pediatrics 95:598–602, 1995.

52. How is conscious sedation best managed in children?

There is no single best method for conscious sedation of pediatric patients for diagnostic, radiologic, or minor surgical procedures. Surveys indicate a wide variety of approaches are used in emergency rooms and radiology suites, including chloral hydrate, opioids (morphine, meperidine, fentanyl, butorphanol), benzodiazepines (diazepam, midazolam), barbiturates (pentobarbital, thiopental), and the DPT lytic cocktail.

Although conscious sedation by definition is a state of medically controlled depressed consciousness with a patent airway, maintained protective reflexes, and appropriate responses to stimulation on verbal command, the potential for rapidly developing problems should be anticipated. These can include hypoventilation, apnea, airway obstruction, or cardiorespiratory collapse. Consequently, keys to any pharmacologic method of conscious sedation are administration under supervised conditions (eliminating home treatment prior to office or hospital arrival), competent personnel capable of resuscitation, ongoing monitoring (especially the use of pulse oximetry), and sufficient equipment for resuscitation (e.g, positive pressure oxygen delivery system, suction apparatus).

Cote CJ: Sedation for the pediatric patient: A review. Pediatr Clin North Am 41:31–58, 1994.

Committee on Drugs: Guidelines for the monitoring and management of pediatric patients during and after sedation for diagnostic, dental and therapeutic procedures. Pediatrics 89:1110–1115, 1992.

RESUSCITATION

53. How does the CPR technique differ between an infant and a child?

In an infant, the heart is lower in relation to the external chest than in a child. Thus the proper position for chest compression is 1 finger-breadth below the intersection of the intermammary line. The rescuer should use 2 or 3 fingers to compress the sternum to a depth of 0.5–1.0 inches at a rate of at least 100 times/minute. The infant should be ventilated at a rate of 20 breaths/minute.

For older children (> 1 year old), the rescuer places the heel of the hand 2 finger-breadths above the sternal notch. Depth of compression is optimally 1.0–1.5 inches with a recommended rate of 80 times/minute. The older child should be ventilated at a rate of 16 breaths/minute.

54. What is the Thaler technique for infant CPR?

This is the technique of encirclement. The rescuer clasps the fingers together beneath the thoracic spine, encircles the chest with the hands and compresses with the thumbs. Care should be taken to minimize the limitation of chest movement during ventilation.

55. Can CPR cause rib fractures in infants?

Very unlikely. In one study of 91 infants who underwent autopsy and postmortem x-rays following CPR, none had rib fractures. Child abuse must always remain at the top of a list when rib fractures are identified.

Spevak MR, et al: Cardiopulmonary resuscitation and rib fractures in infants: A postmortem radiologic-pathologic study. JAMA 272:617–618, 1994.

56. Is there any use for the "precordial thump" in pediatric CPR?

Even in witnessed and documented ventricular fibrillation, the thump is felt *not* to be more effective than routine external compression in terms of converting the abnormal rhythm, and there is increased risk of internal organ damage.

57. If a child suddenly becomes asystolic and resuscitation is not initiated, what is the time course of pupillary changes?

15 seconds after arrest, pupillary dilatation begins and is complete at 1 minute 45 seconds.

58. Why is the airway of an infant or child more prone to obstruction than that of an adult?

1. An infant has less margin of safety because of the smaller airway diameter. Because airflow is inversely proportional to the airway radius raised to the fourth power (the oft-cited Poiseuille's law), small changes in the diameter of the trachea can result in very large drops in airflow.

2. The tracheal cartilage of an infant is softer and can result in collapse upon hyperextension. This is particularly important if CPR is performed with vigorous extension of the neck. Air exchange may then be obstructed.

3. In an infant, the lumen of the oropharynx is relatively smaller due to the larger size of the tongue and smaller size of the mandible.

4. In an infant, the larynx is funnel-shaped and more cephalad (opposite C2–3 vertebrae compared with opposite C4–6 vertebrae in an adult).

5. The narrowest portion of the airway in infants and children is at the cricoid ring, below the vocal cords.

6. Lower airways are smaller and less developed in children. The typical peanut and an infant's mainstem bronchus always seem to fit hand-in-glove.

59. What size endotracheal tube should be used for resuscitation?

A good rule of thumb:

$$ID\ (mm) = \frac{16 + age\ (yrs)}{4}$$

For example, a 2-year-old would warrant a 4.5-mm tube by this formula. Since this is an approximation, the next smaller or larger size tubes should be available. To convert internal diameter (ID) size to French catheter size, multiply by 4 (e.g., a 5.0 tube is 20 French).

60. What emergency drugs can be given via an endotracheal tube?

E-LAINE (Endotracheally—Lidocaine, Atropine, Isoproterenol, Naloxone, and Epinephrine).

61. Is there ever an indication for intracardiac epinephrine?

Outside of televised dramas, epinephrine is very rarely administered via the intracardiac route. Other methods of administration (peripheral or central IV, intraosseous or endotracheal tube) should be readily available. The use of intracardiac epinephrine interrupts CPR and can cause tamponade, coronary artery laceration, or pneumothorax. If epinephrine is accidentally given into the cardiac muscle rather than the ventricular chamber, intractable ventricular fibrillation or cardiac standstill may result.

62. What is the role of high-dose epinephrine in pediatric resuscitations?

Animal studies, anecdotal reports, and a small clinical trial in children showed that the use of epinephrine in higher doses (100–200 times normal) facilitated the return of spontaneous circulation better than the standard lower dose. Larger prospective studies in adults did not show an advantage. One retrospective study of pediatric out-of-hospital cardiopulmonary arrests also did not document any benefits. While the evidence accumulates, the American Heart Association recommends that after the first standard dose of IV or intraosseous epinephrine (0.01 mg/kg of a 1:10,000 solution), subsequent higher doses (0.1–0.2 mg/kg of a 1:1000 solution) might be effective. In the scenario of a witnessed cardiac arrest, the use of high-dose epinephrine should strongly be considered.

Brown CG, et al: A comparison of standard-dose and high-dose epinephrine in cardiac arrest outside the hospital. N Engl J Med 327:1051–1055, 1992.

Dieckmann RA, Vardis R: High-dose epinephrine in pediatric out-of-hospital cardiopulmonary arrest. Pediatrics 95:901–913, 1995.

63. How effective is intratracheal epinephrine?

Epinephrine is poorly absorbed from the lung, and if available, intraosseous or IV administration is preferable. If epinephrine is to be given via an endotracheal tube in an acute setting, it should be mixed with 1–3 ml of normal saline and instilled with a catheter or feeding tube beyond the end of the endotracheal tube to facilitate dispersal. The ideal endotracheal dose is unclear, but because of the poor absorption, initial higher doses (0.1–0.2 mg/kg of a 1:1000 solution) should be used.

64. When is atropine indicated during a resuscitation?

Atropine may be administered to the child with symptomatic bradycardia after other resuscitative measures (i.e., oxygenation and ventilation) have been initiated. It is useful in breaking the vagally mediated bradycardia associated with laryngoscopy and may have some benefit during the initial treatment of atrioventricular block. The deleterious effects of a slow heart rate are more likely to occur in a younger child, whose cardiac output is more dependent on rate changes than volume or contractility changes. Atropine is no longer routinely recommended in the treatment of asystole.

65. What risks are associated with administering an inappropriately low dose of atropine?

If the dose of atropine is too small, paradoxically worsening bradycardia may result. This is due to atropine's central stimulating effect on the medullary vagal nerve at lower doses, which slows atrioventricular conduction and heart rate. Standard dosing of atropine in a setting of bradycardia is 0.02 mg/kg IV. However, at least 0.1 mg should be used even in the youngest patient.

66. When is the use of calcium indicated during a resuscitation?
Routine use of calcium is no longer recommended during a resuscitation. There is evidence that calcium may increase postischemic injury in the intracranial reperfusion phase following resuscitation. Calcium use may be justified in three settings of resuscitation: (1) an overdose of a calcium channel blocker, (2) hyperkalemia resulting in cardiac dysrhythmia, and (3) infants and children with low serum calcium.

67. If electromechanical dissociation (EMD) is suspected, what should be done ASAP?
EMD exists when there is organized electrical activity on ECG without evidence of effective myocardial contraction (i.e., absent blood pressure or nonpalpable pulse). The electrical rate can be fast or slow, and the complexes narrow or wide. EMD is caused either by myocardial disease (hypoxic/ischemic myocardium due to respiratory arrest is most common in children) or by causes extrinsic to the heart. If prolonged myocardial ischemia is the cause of EMD, the prognosis is poor. However, rapid diagnosis of an extracardiac cause and its treatment may be life-saving. The extracardiac causes of EMD include hypovolemia, tension pneumothorax, cardiac tamponade, hypoxemia, acidosis, and pulmonary embolus. The treatment of EMD begins with the initiation of chest compressions and ventilation with 100% oxygen, followed by the administration of epinephrine and sodium bicarbonate. Extracardiac causes are treated with fluid administration, pericardiocentesis, or thoracentesis as indicated. Empiric administration of calcium is no longer felt to be of value.

68. Why should one bone up on the technique of intraosseous infusions?
Because of the difficulty and delays in establishing IV access in pediatric resuscitations, intraosseous infusions have become the first or very early second-line of therapy in emergency settings. An intraosseous line is a rapid means of vascular access and utilizes the marrow cavity of bone, which drains into the central venous system. Fluid, drug distribution, and rates are comparable to those in IV infusions. The technique is straightforward and involves placing a styleted needle, bone marrow needle, or intraosseous needle into the proximal tibia approximately 1–3 cm below and medial to the tibial tuberosity. Distal tibial and proximal femoral sites are less commonly used.

69. Is capillary refill still a useful clinical sign?
Capillary refill is the return to normal color of the pulp of the finger or fingernail after it has been compressed. In healthy children, a normal value is approximately 2 seconds. In theory, a normal refill time is a measure of adequate peripheral perfusion and thus normal cardiac output and peripheral vascular resistance. It has been used as a measure of perfusion in the settings of trauma and possible dehydration. However, it must be utilized in conjunction with other clinical features, because studies of its usefulness as a sole indicator of dehydration have shown it to have a low sensitivity and specificity. In one study of children with 5–10% dehydration, only 50% had prolonged capillary refill. In addition, lower ambient temperature has a significant effect on delaying capillary refill. Capillary refill should be measured in the upper extremity.
Baraff LJ: Capillary refill: Is it a useful clinical sign? Pediatrics 92:723–724, 1993.

70. Why are MAST trousers of potential value in pediatric resuscitation?
Pneumatic anti-shock garments (PASGs), or the MAST (military anti-shock trousers) suit, is a pneumatic device that inflates around the lower extremities, pelvis, and abdomen. It may be useful to augment blood pressure in hypotensive and hypovolemic patients, especially in the setting of pelvic and lower-extremity fractures. Potential negative effects include exacerbation of bleeding above the diaphragm, worsening of pulmonary edema, and the development of a compartment syndrome. The efficacy of MAST trousers has not been carefully studied in children.

71. Are steroids indicated in the treatment of shock in children?
No. The controversy has related primarily to the role of steroids in treating septic shock. There are data in animals that steroids given prior to, or concomitantly with, endotoxin can

improve survival. However, in multiple clinical trials in adults, early steroids have not been shown to decrease long-term mortality and actually may have contributed to increased mortality because of higher secondary infection rates in steroid-treated patients compared with controls. Data in children are lacking. However, by extrapolation, steroids at present are not indicated.

72. Is colloid or crystalloid better for the treatment of hypotension?

Colloid (blood, fresh frozen plasma or 5% or 25% salt-poor albumin) and crystalloid (Ringer lactate, normal saline) are equally effective for the treatment of hypovolemic hypotension. In the setting of hypovolemic shock, use whatever product is most readily available. Certain instances might warrant tailoring of the volume expander. Hypotension due to large recent blood loss is best treated with whole blood or packed red blood cells and plasma to correct the anemia. Ringer lactate would be less appropriate in the setting of hyperkalemia and hypotension because it contains 4 mEq K^+/L. One should always remember the risks of blood products as volume expanders and the cost of albumin, which is nearly 50–100 times that of normal saline.

73. What is the normal tidal volume of a child?

Approximately 7 ml/kg.

74. What is the proper treatment if a large bolus of air is accidentally injected into a 6-year-old child?

The main problem is that the air can block the right ventricular outflow tract or main pulmonary artery. This is similar to "vapor lock" in automobiles, in which air in the carburetor prevents fuel from flowing and a stall results. The patient should be placed in a steep head-down position with the right side up to trap air in the upper right ventricular chamber and prevent passage to the outflow tract. Therapeutic options include:

1. 100% oxygen
2. Careful monitoring, including ECG
3. Observation for symptoms or signs of dysrhythmia, hypotension, or cardiac arrest
4. If air is auscultated in the heart, a right ventricular tap should be considered.
5. If arrest occurs, standard CPR should be initiated, as manual compression may help to dislodge air emboli.

75. What is the effect of body temperature on arterial blood gases (ABGs)?

CO_2 and O_2 are more soluble and exert less partial pressure at lower temperatures. Therefore, blood sampled from a hypothermic patient and warmed to the standard 37° in the blood gas analyzer will have a higher partial pressure than exists in the patient. Similarly, blood sampled from the hyperthermic patient and cooled to 37° will have a lower partial pressure than exists in the patient. For each 1° C difference from 37°, the $PaCO_2$ changes by about 7% and the $PaCO_2$ by about 4.5%. Although much debate exists whether to use the "corrected" (patient body temperature) or "uncorrected" (37° C of blood gas analyzer) value, the difference in most clinical scenarios is not significant. In cases of extreme temperature differences (e.g,. hypothermia in cold-water near-drowning), the difference may be considerable.

76. How do pediatric and adult defibrillation differ?

1. Smaller dosing: 2 W-sec/kg and then doubled as needed
2. Smaller paddles: standard pediatric paddles are 4.5 cm in diameter compared with 8.0 cm in adults
3. Rarer use: ventricular fibrillation is uncommon in children

77. What is the difference between livor mortis and rigor mortis?

Livor mortis or dependent lividity is the gravitational pooling of blood that results in a line of mauve staining in the dependent half of a recently deceased body. It usually is noticeable 30 minutes after death and is very marked at 6 hours. **Rigor mortis** is the muscular stiffening and shortening that result from ongoing cellular activity and depletion of ATP after death, with increasing lactate and phosphate and salt precipitation. Neck and facial changes begin at 6 hours, shoulder and upper extremities at 9 hours, and trunk and lower extremities at 12 hours. Livor mortis and rigor mortis are absolute indications not to initiate a resuscitation. They should be looked for during the initial rapid assessment. In the confusion of the moment, they may be easily overlooked.

78. When should a failing resuscitation be stopped?

There is no precise answer. Some studies have suggested that when two rounds of medication (i.e., epinephrine and bicarbonate) have been given without clinical cardiovascular or neurologic improvement and/or > 15 minutes have elapsed since the initiation of resuscitation, the likelihood of death or survival with neurologic devastation greatly increases. Unwitnessed out-of-hospital arrests are nearly always associated with a poor outcome. In settings of hypothermia, asystolic patients should be rewarmed to 36° before resuscitation is discontinued.

79. How successful is pediatric emergency room resuscitation?

Unobserved cardiorespiratory arrest in children carries a grim prognosis, much worse than in adults. More than 90% do not survive. Of the survivors, nearly 100% are vegetative or have severe neurologic sequelae.

80. Why is resuscitation less successful in children than in adults?

Adults more commonly collapse and arrest from primary cardiac disease and associated dysrhythmias—ventricular tachycardia and fibrillation. These are more readily reversible and carry a better prognosis. Children, however, have cardiac arrest as a secondary phenomenon from other processes, such as respiratory obstruction or apnea, often associated with infection, hypoxia, acidosis, or hypovolemia. Primary cardiac arrest is rare. By the time a child has cardiac arrest, severe neurologic damage is almost always present.

81. What are the top ten errors in running a resuscitation?

One subjective list is as follows:
1. Leader of code not clearly designated
2. Failure to place nasogastric tube
3. Failure to give proper medications in response to situation
4. Failure to periodically assess breath sounds, pupils, pulses
5. Delay in access before attempting intraosseous line or other
6. Leader of code too involved with individual procedure
7. Failure to assign roles
8. Failure to assess patient initially
9. Failure to observe adequate cardiac compressions
10. Excessively lengthy resuscitation for out-of-hospital arrests

TOXICOLOGY

82. What are the most common poisonings in children under 6 years of age?

More than 1 million poisoning exposures for children under age 6 are reported to poison control centers annually. Approximately 60% are nonpharmaceuticals and 40% are pharmaceuticals. In descending order of frequency, the most common are

Nonpharmaceuticals	Pharmaceuticals
Cleaning products and polishes	Analgesics
Cosmetics and grooming products	Cough and cold preparations
Plants, including mushrooms and tobacco	Topical agents
Battery, toy, and other foreign bodies	Antimicrobials
Pesticides	Vitamins

Litovitz TL, et al: 1994 Annual Report of the American Association of Poison Control Centers Toxic Exposure Surveillance System. Am J Emerg Med 13:551–597, 1995.

83. How efficacious is ipecac?

Most studies have shown that < 25% of swallowed drug or marker substance is retrievable with ipecac-induced vomiting at > 30–60 minutes after ingestion. Thus, ipecac syrup has been deemphasized over the past several years and is generally no longer recommended in the emergency department in the management of the acutely poisoned patient. Activated charcoal is more commonly used as the first-line treatment. On the other hand, ipecac is still used and recommended as a first-aid agent in the home after consultation with a physician or poison control center. Syrup of ipecac (at a dose of 10 ml for infants 6–12 months old, 15 ml for children, and 30 ml for adolescents) will induce vomiting in nearly 100% of patients.

84. When is ipecac-induced vomiting contraindicated?

Coma, Convulsions, Caustics, and household hydroCarbons.

85. In what poisonings should whole bowel irrigation be considered?

This procedure involves the instillation of large volumes of iso-osmotic polyethylene glycol lavage solution (CoLyte, GoLytely) usually via a nasogastric tube. Its use is mainly in poisonings involving **iron** or **sustained-release pharmaceuticals** in which prolonged intestinal exposure is more likely to occur.

86. What is the value of activated charcoal in the treatment of poisonings?

Activated charcoal has a long history of safe and effective use. Its pores are designed to increase the surface area available for the adsorption of drugs, and thus it facilitates the trapping of toxins in the intestine for fecal removal. In addition, various drugs (e.g., carbamazepine, tricyclic antidepressants, meprobamate) exhibit a significant enterohepatic recirculation, and charcoal can disrupt this flow. Doses are 1 gm/kg, or about 20–30 gm in toddlers and 50–100 gm in adolescents, and can be repeated every 3–4 hours. The excretion of many drugs (e.g., benzodiazepines, carbamazepine, phenobarbital, phenothiazines, salicylates, theophylline, and tricyclic antidepressants) may be improved by multiple-dose activated charcoal.

87. In what settings is activated charcoal not advised?

Charcoal should not be given in poisonings involving:
1. Caustics (charcoal can interfere with possible endoscopy)
2. Drugs for which immediate oral antidotes are contemplated (e.g., late presentation of pure acetaminophen ingestion)
3. Clinical presentation of ileus, hematemesis, or severe vomiting
4. Household petroleum distillates (e.g., gasoline, kerosene) because of possible increased risk of aspiration
5. Compounds for which it is ineffective, including acids, alcohols, alkalis, cyanide, iron, heavy metals, and lithium

88. Should all children with ingestion be given a cathartic?

Cathartics may help to decrease absorption and lessen constipation caused by charcoal. Magnesium sulfate (250 mg/kg), magnesium citrate (4–8 ml/kg up to 300 ml), or sorbitol (70%, 1.5 gm/kg) are the usual choices. The contraindications are similar to those for activated charcoal. Care must be taken when cathartics are given to smaller children, as large volume loss may result. Repeated administration of magnesium-containing cathartics can cause hypermagnesemia, manifested by hypotonia, altered mental status, and in severe cases, respiratory failure.

Perry H, Shannon M: Emergency department gastrointestinal decontamination. Pediatr Ann 25:19–26, 1996.

89. How is the manipulation of urinary pH used in treating poisonings?

Acidification or alkalinization of the urine to enhance the excretion of weak acids and bases has been a traditional way to enhance the elimination of toxicologic agents. In recent years, its use has been limited because of the potential complications from fluid overload (e.g., pulmonary and cerebral edema), the risk of acidemia, and the use of other therapeutic advancements (e.g., hemodialysis). However, alkaline diuresis is still considered valuable in the management of acute overdoses of salicylates, barbiturates, or tricyclic antidepressants.

90. What ingestions and exposures have available antidotes?

Ingestion/Exposure	Antidote
Acetaminophen	N-acetylcysteine (Mucomyst)
Anticholinergics	Physostigmine
Benzodiazepines	Flumazenil
Beta-blockers	Glucagon
Carbon monoxide	Hyperbaric oxygen
Cyanide	Sodium nitrite, sodium thiosulfate
Digoxin	Digibind (anti-digoxin antibody)
Ethylene glycol	Ethanol
Iron	Deferoxamine
Isoniazid	Pyridoxine
Mercury	Dimercaprol, DMSA
Methanol	Ethanol
Methemoglobinemic agents	Methylene blue
Opiates	Naloxone
Organophosphates	Atropine, pralidoxime
Phenothiazines	Diphenhydramine
Warfarin	Vitamin K

From Fortenberry JD, Mariscalco MM: Poisonings. In Oski FA, et al (eds): Principles and Practice of Pediatrics, 2nd ed. Philadelphia, J.B. Lippincott, 1994, p 835; with permission.

91. Narcan is considered an antidote for which kinds of ingestions?

Narcan (naloxone) is an antidote for opioid drugs. In "low" doses (0.005–0.01 mg/kg), it effectively reverses the CNS and respiratory depression of morphine and heroin. It is also useful in reversing or improving the sensorium in overdoses due to many of the synthetic opioids, including propoxyphene, codeine, dextromethorphan, pentazocine, and meperidine. In these cases, a "high" dose is utilized, usually 0.01–0.1 mg/kg. In fact, there is no significant risk to using a high dose of Narcan in any pediatric overdose situation, although Narcan can produce withdrawal symptoms (i.e., GI upset, anxiety) in an addicted patient.

Many authorities now recommend the following regimen for all suspected opioid poisonings:
Coma without respiratory depression—1.0 mg
Coma with respiratory depression—2.0 mg
These doses may be repeated every 2–10 minutes up to a total dose of 8–10 mg before concluding that there is no effect.

92. Which ingestions are radiopaque on abdominal x-ray?

The mnemonic "CHIPS" indicates possible suspects.
C: Chloral hydrate
H: Heavy metals (arsenic, iron, lead)
I: Iodides
P: Phenothiazines, psychotropics (tricyclic antidepressants)
S: Slow-release capsules, enteric-coated tablets

The likelihood of radiopacity depends on numerous factors including weight of the patient, size of the ingestion, and composition of the pill matrix.

Barkin RM, et al: Poisoning and overdose. In Barkin RM, Rosen P (eds): Emergency Pediatrics, 4th ed. St. Louis, Mosby, 1994, p 335.

93. What is a toxidrome?

A *toxidrome* is a clinical constellation of signs and symptoms that is very suggestive of a particular poisoning or category of intoxication. For example, patients with salicylate overdose commonly present with fever, hyperpnea and tachypnea, abnormal mental status (ranging from lethargy to coma), tinnitus, vomiting, and sometimes oil of wintergreen odor from methylsalicylate.

94. What breath odors may be associated with specific ingestions?

Bitter almond	Cyanide
Fruity	Isopropanol, acetone, nail polish remover
Garlic	Arsenic, thallium, organophosphates
Minty	Mouthwash (often with high levels of ethanol), rubbing alcohol (often scented with oil of wintergreen or methylsalicylate)
Mothballs	Naphthalene, *p*-dichlorobenzene
Peanuts	Vacor rat poisons
Rotten eggs	Hydrogen sulfide
Shoe polish	Nitrobenzene

Woolf AD: Poisoning in children and adolescents. Pediatr Rev 14:411–422, 1993.

95. What are the limitations of the routine toxicology screen?

Most toxicology screens are intended to detect drugs encountered in substance abuse. Even in larger pediatric hospitals, comprehensive toxicology screens generally include only a fraction of the drugs available to children. Most blood screens analyze for common over-the-counter analgesics (e.g., acetaminophen, salicylates, ibuprofen) and various alcohols. Urine is often screened for substances of abuse and other common psychoactive drugs, including antidepressants, antipsychotics, benzodiazepines, sedative-hypnotics, and anticonvulsants. Other potential toxins which can cause mental status changes (e.g., carbon monoxide, chloral hydrate, cyanide, organophosphates) or circulatory depression (e.g., beta-blockers, calcium channel blockers, clonidine, digitalis) may not be included.

96. How do the types of alcohol ingestions vary?

All alcohols can cause CNS disturbances ranging from mild mentation and motor abnormalities to respiratory depression and coma. In addition, each type of alcohol can be associated with specific metabolic complications. **Ethanol** (present in adult beverages and as an additive in numerous over-the-counter products, especially mouthwash) can cause moderate metabolic acidosis and hypoglycemia. **Methanol** (present in Sterno and windshield wiper fluid) can cause severe, refractory acidosis and permanent retinal damage leading to blindness. **Isopropyl alcohol** (present in jewelry cleaners and rubbing alcohols) causes gastric irritation and mild ketosis but does not usually cause significant acidosis and/or hypoglycemia. **Ethylene glycol** (present in antifreeze) causes metabolic acidosis; in addition, it is metabolized to oxalic acid, which can cause renal damage by the precipitation of calcium oxalate crystals in the renal parenchyma. The calcium oxalate formation can also result in hypocalcemia.

97. Which alcohol is considered the most lethal?

Methanol. Small amounts of methanol (1 ml/kg) may be lethal. In addition, the early signs of methanol poisoning may be fairly subtle despite ingestion of a lethal or eye-damaging amount.

98. Why is ethanol used as an antidote in methanol ingestion?

Ethanol competitively inhibits the formation of methanol's toxic metabolites, formaldehyde and formic acid, by preferentially serving as a substrate for alcohol dehydrogenase.

99. How is the osmolar gap helpful in diagnosing ingestions?

The osmolar gap is the difference between the measured osmolarity (obtained from freezing point depression) and the calculated osmolarity (calculated = 2 [serum Na] + BUN/2.8 + glucose/18).

Normal osmolarity is about 290 mOsm/L. A significant osmolar gap suggests an alcohol poisoning, which typically produces exogenous osmoles.

100. If a child has ingested an acetaminophen-containing product, when should the first acetaminophen level be obtained?

A plasma level obtained four hours after ingestion is a good indicator of the potential for hepatic toxicity. Nomograms are available for determining risk. As a rule, doses under 150 mg/kg are unlikely to be harmful.

101. When should a NAC attack begin?

N-acetylcysteine (NAC) is a specific antidote for acetaminophen hepatotoxicity by serving as a glutathione-substitute in detoxifying the hepatotoxic metabolites. It should be used for any acetaminophen overdose with a toxic serum acetaminophen level within the first 24 hours after ingestion. It is especially effective if used in the first 8 hours after ingestion. If acetaminophen levels are not available on a rapid basis or the time since ingestion is not clear, it is preferable to initiate NAC (140 mg/kg orally and then 70 mg/kg orally every 4 hours for 17 doses) while awaiting consultation with a toxicologist or poison control center.

102. What quantity of ingested aspirin is cause for concern?

Generally, an acute salicylate overdose of 140 mg/kg will produce symptoms. In chronic salicylism, a dose that averages > 100 mg/kg/day for several days may also lead to toxic effects.

103. What features suggest the possibility of lead toxicity in a child?

Most children with elevated lead levels are asymptomatic. Plumbism, or lead intoxication, should be suspected if a child has **pica** and:

1. Vague abdominal complaints, such as anorexia, recurrent abdominal pain, constipation, and vomiting
2. Vague behavioral effects, such as hyperactivity, irritability, malaise, or lethargy
3. Progressive ataxia or seizure
4. A history of unexplained anemia
5. Basophilic stippling of peripheral RBCs
6. Any additional risk factors (see Question 105)

104. How do the signs and symptoms of acute and chronic lead intoxication differ?

Acute lead poisoning is rare in children and differs from chronic poisoning mainly in the occurrence of a reversible renal Fanconi-like syndrome. In **chronic** exposure, a glomerulonephritis with hypertension and renal failure may occur. The CNS effects are similar, however, and are the most feared consequences of pediatric plumbism. Lead encephalopathy may range from mild behavioral and cognitive dysfunction to severe, life-threatening coma, seizures, cerebral edema, and permanent neurologic sequelae in survivors.

105. Should all children be screened for elevated lead levels?

Because of substantial regional and local variations in the prevalence of elevated lead levels, the recommendation to screen all children is controversial. Some states have adopted universal screening because increased lead levels have been associated with slowed mental growth and behavior disorders. In general, it is advisable to screen high-risk children, including those:

1. Living in or visiting homes with peeling paint built before 1960 or undergoing renovation
2. Having a sibling or playmate with elevated lead
3. Living with an adult whose job or hobby involves lead
4. Living near an industry likely to release lead (e.g., smelting plant, battery-recycling plant)

106. Why is erythrocytic protoporphyrin (EP) no longer used as an initial screen for lead poisoning?

Elevated EP can be an indicator of abnormalities in heme biosynthesis, which can occur in lead poisoning. As the acceptable limit for blood lead has been progressively lowered (in 1991 to 10 mg/dl), the EP test is no longer considered sensitive. It identifies only a small percentage of children with blood levels of 10–25 mg/dl and misses > 50% of children with blood levels above 25 mg/dl. In addition, there is approximately a 2-week lag between significant lead accumulation and detectable rises in the EP level, therefore making it a poor indicator of recent lead exposure.

Weitzman M, Glotzer D: Lead poisoning. Pediatr Rev 12:461–468, 1992.

107. What are the environmental sources of lead other than lead-based paint?

Lead-contaminated water, lead dust carried into homes by clothing and shoes of lead-factory workers, improperly glazed "homemade" ceramics, moonshine liquor made with lead vats or tubes, and the burning of lead batteries as fuel are uncommon causes of lead poisoning. An organic-lead encephalopathy has also been reported in adolescents who willfully abuse leaded gasoline by chronically inhaling the fumes.

108. At what lead levels is chelation indicated?

< 25 µg/dl	Chelation not indicated
25–45 µg/dl	Chelation not routinely indicated, as no evidence exists that chelation avoids or reverses neurotoxicity.
	Some patients may benefit from (oral) chelation (e.g., succimer), especially if elevated levels persist despite aggressive environmental intervention and abatement.
45–70 µg/dl	Chelation indicated with either succimer or $CaNa_2EDTA$ (if no clinical symptoms suggestive of encephalopathy such as headache or persistent vomiting); if symptoms of encephalopathy, chelation with dimercaprol (BAL) and $CaNa_2EDTA$ indicated. Prior to chelation, an abdominal radiograph should be taken to evaluate for possible removable enteral lead.
> 70 µg/dl	Inpatient chelation therapy with dimercaprol and $CaNa_2EDTA$

Committee on Drugs: Treatment guidelines for lead exposure in children. Pediatrics 96:155–160, 1995.

109. What is the pathophysiologic basis for the toxicity in iron ingestions?

Iron is toxic in various ways. It has a direct caustic effect on the GI tract, and when absorbed in excess of the total iron-binding capacity, free iron causes shock due to vascular dilations. Hepatotoxicity results from accumulation of free iron in hepatocytes.

110. Which clinical and lab features correlate with an acutely elevated serum iron?

Iron levels in the toxic range (> 350 µg/dl) are associated with early (first 6 hours) symptoms such as nausea, vomiting, diarrhea, lethargy or coma, convulsions, and/or shock. Laboratory correlates of an elevated iron level include leukocytosis (> 15,000/mm³), hyperglycemia (> 150 mg/dl), and radiopaque tablets on abdominal x-ray.

111. How do the signs and symptoms of acute iron ingestion differ from those of other heavy metal poisonings?

Iron salt ingestion causes early GI symptoms and, in severe cases, hemorrhagic gastritis shock, and coma. After 24–48 hours, evidence of hepatic damage ensues.

Lead poisoning may cause mild GI symptoms; however, encephalopathy with cerebral vasculitis, increased intracranial pressure and coma, seizures, and severe neurologic damage are the most feared complications.

Acute **mercury salt** poisoning causes both a hemorrhagic gastroenteritis and renal damage. The liver is generally not injured.

Arsenic poisoning affects multiple organs with marked skin and hair changes, neurologic effects (encephalopathy, peripheral neuropathy, tremor, coma, convulsions), fatty infiltration of the liver, renal tubular and glomerular damage, and cardiac involvement with conduction delays and dysrhythmias.

112. What is the value of a deferoxamine challenge?

Deferoxamine challenge occasionally may be useful as an additional screening test for mild to moderate iron poisoning if "stat" iron levels are not available. In the asymptomatic or mildly symptomatic patient, a dose of 15 mg/kg (up to 1 gm maximum) may be given intramuscularly. A positive test (orange or "vin rose" tint to the urine) signifies the excretion of feroxamine (deferoxamine–iron chelate). All patients with a positive challenge test should be admitted for continuing chelation therapy. A negative challenge test in a patient with *significant* symptoms does not rule out iron toxicity and should not be relied upon.

113. Are acid or alkali ingestions more harmful?

Both acid and alkali ingestions may cause severe esophageal or gastric burns, but alkalis tend to be worse because they produce a relatively more penetrating liquefactive necrosis of the esophagus.

114. Are steroids helpful for caustic ingestion?

Steroids are controversial in the treatment of caustic ingestions. They are purported to reduce scar formation and strictures but may interfere with wound healing and predispose to perforation. Most authorities currently recommend steroids for all significant second-degree burns and advocate their omission for significant full-thickness burns (where their use might be hazardous as well as ineffectual) or first-degree burns (which are expected to heal without scarring regardless of treatment).

115. When does stricture formation occur in lye ingestion?

Although strictures may form as soon as 2–3 weeks after caustic ingestion, the development is somewhat variable and scarring may continue for ≥ 6 months after such an exposure. In general, in the followup of patients exposed to caustics, esophagoscopy and barium swallow are performed 3 weeks after ingestion if a significant burn was noted at the time of initial presentation. Clinical followup should occur for 6 months, at which time a repeat barium swallow should be considered. Occasionally, a mild stricture that has been relatively asymptomatic will become problematic after an interval of years, particularly following growth spurts (e.g., at adolescence). Long-term follow-up is also important because of the increased risk of carcinoma of the esophagus following ingestion of lye.

116. Which hydrocarbons pose the greatest risk for chemical pneumonitis?

The household hydrocarbons with **low viscosities** pose the greatest aspiration hazard. These include furniture polishes, gasoline and kerosene, turpentine and other paint-thinners, and lighter fuels.

117. Are there any indications for induced emesis in a hydrocarbon ingestion?

1. Those rare exposures due to inherently toxic compounds (e.g., carbon tetrachloride, toluene, benzene)
2. The occasional hydrocarbon–toxic compound combination, such as pesticides

118. Which patients with hydrocarbon ingestions should be admitted?

All patients with significant clinical findings or an abnormal chest x-ray 2–4 hours after ingestion should be admitted. Children with a history of exposure are safe to discharge if they have (1) no symptoms; (2) very transient coughing or gagging; (3) a normal physical exam after 4 hours; and (4) a normal chest x-ray after 4 hours.

119. What is the differential diagnosis in a 10-year-old boy who presents to the emergency department with delirium?

Delirium is defined as a transient and reversible dysfunction in cerebral metabolism manifest as decreased ability to maintain attention to external stimuli, disorganized thinking, reduced level of consciousness, perceptual disturbances, disorientation, and memory impairment. It can be the result of numerous causes, including toxins, as depicted by the foreboding mnemonic, "I WATCH DEATH":

I = Infectious	(encephalitis, meningitis, syphilis, AIDS)
W = Withdrawal	(alcohol, barbiturates, sedatives-hypnotics)
A = Acute metabolic	(acidosis, alkalosis, electrolyte disturbance, hepatic failure, renal failure)
T = Trauma	(heat stroke, postoperative, severe burns)
C = CNS pathology	(abscesses, hemorrhage, normal pressure hydrocephalus, seizures, stroke, tumors, vasculitis)
H = Hypoxia	(anemia, CO poisoning, hypotension, pulmonary/cardiac failure)
D = Deficiencies	(B_{12}, niacin, thiamine)
E = Endocrinopathies	(hyper-/hypoadrenalcorticism, hyper-/hypoglycemia)
A = Acute vascular	(hypertensive encephalopathy, shock, migraine)
T = Toxins/drugs	(medications, pesticides, solvents)
H = Heavy metals	(lead, manganese, mercury)

From Williams DT: Neuropsychiatric signs, symptoms, and syndromes. In Lewis M (ed): Child and Adolescent Psychiatry. Baltimore, Williams & Wilkins, 1991, p 343; with permission.

120. How are children with tricyclic antidepressant (TCA) overdose managed?

TCA overdose is one of the most serious and potentially lethal ingestions in children. These children usually need to be closely monitored in a hospital setting. Not all TCA ingestions result in life-threatening toxicity, but patients should be observed for at least 6 hours in an emergency department for any clinical symptoms including evidence of anticholinergic effects (sinus tachycardia, dilated pupils, and hot, flushed, dry skin), seizures, and ECG abnormalities (ventricular ectopy, QRS prolongation, or any evidence of frank dysrhythmias such as ventricular tachycardia). The later are the most feared complication TCA overdose in children.

The complete management of TCA overdose in children is complex but includes anticonvulsant therapy for seizures, sodium bicarbonate and occasionally magnesium sulfate to prevent and/or treat TCA-associated dysrhythmias, and fluids and vasopressors, including norepinephrine and dopamine, for hypotension.

121. What are the most feared complications of antihistamine overdose?

Antihistamine overdoses may cause a full-blown anticholinergic syndrome with agitation, hallucinations, and seizures; hot, dry, flushed skin; dilated pupils; tachycardia; hypertension; and dysrhythmias ("Mad as a hatter, hot as a hare, dry as a bone, red as a beet"). For severe agitation, hallucinations, or uncontrollable seizures, the use of physostigmine should be considered.

122. How are drug-induced dystonic reactions treated?

Dystonic reactions consist of twisting and writhing sustained movements of the neck, face, and proximal upper extremities that occur most commonly following ingestion of phenothiazines. Most children are treated with Benadryl (diphenhydramine, 1 mg/kg IV). In the adolescent or adult, Cogentin (benztropine, 1–2 mg IV or IM) can also be used.

123. What are the signs and symptoms of organophosphate poisoning?

Organophosphates inhibit cholinesterase and cause all the signs and symptoms of acetylcholine excess.

Muscarinic effects: increased oral and tracheal secretions, miosis, salivation, lacrimation, urination, vomiting, cramping, defecation, and bradycardia; may progress to frank pulmonary edema.

CNS effects: agitation, delirium, seizures, and/or coma.

Nicotinic effects: sweating, muscle fasciculation, and, ultimately, paralysis.

The mnemonic SLUDGE may be helpful in remembering these signs and symptoms: **S**alivation, **L**acrimation, **U**rination, **D**efecation, **GI** cramps, **E**mesis.

124. A child is brought to the ED with a temperature of 105°, hypertension, and involuntary muscle contraction. What kinds of poisoning should be considered?

The combination of severe hyperthermia and increased muscle activity is common for a number of acute drug overdoses as well as withdrawal from alcohol and sedative hypnotic agents. The common acute overdoses that may present this way include cocaine, amphetamines and other sympathomimetic agents, monoamine oxidase inhibitors, lithium, phencyclidine, and some anticholinergic agents (including TCAs). Occasionally, the syndrome is seen as part of the so-called neuroleptic-malignant syndrome, which occurs with therapeutic dosing of antipsychotic agents.

125. What metal intoxication can mimic Kawasaki syndrome?

Mercury. Acrodynia is the term applied to one form of mercury salt intoxication that results in a constellation of signs and symptoms very similar to that currently recognized as Kawasaki syndrome. The classic presentation of acrodynia was described in children exposed to calomel, a substance used in teething powders, which was essentially mercurous chloride. The symptom complex included swelling and redness of the hands and feet, skin rashes, diaphoresis, tachycardia, hypertension, photophobia, and an intense irritability with anorexia and insomnia. Infants were often very limp, lying in a frog-like position, with impressive weakness of the hip and shoulder girdle muscles. Similar symptoms have been described in children exposed to other forms of mercury, including broken fluorescent light bulbs or diapers rinsed in mercuric chloride.

126. What causes Minamata disease?

Methylmercury exposure. The term derivatives from Minamata, Japan, where in the 1950s the local population was exposed to methylmercury through the ingestion of fish caught in the heavily contaminated Minamata bay. Severe neurologic abnormalities developed in the older population, and 6% of children born from 1955–1959 had significant problems, including microencephaly and cerebral palsy.

Harada M: Minamata disease: Intrauterine and methylmercury poisoning. Teratology 18:285–288, 1978.

127. Where did the "mad hatter" get his name?

The encephalopathy of chronic elemental mercury poisoning was an occupational hazard of hat makers, who used mercury to produce felt.

128. How does the coma caused by barbiturates differ from that caused by psychotropic drugs?

Barbiturates are classic examples of the **sedative-hypnotic group** of drugs. Ingestions of these agents are manifested by a dose-dependent CNS depression with subsequent respiratory and cardiovascular depression. These patients usually have coma, occasionally with miotic pupils and depressed deep tendon reflexes; the coma is characterized by slowed vital signs and decreased muscle tone. This picture contrasts with that of the **psychotropic drugs** and **phenothiazines**, which often produce an anticholinergic effect, elevated vital signs, and increased muscle tone with progression to seizures.

129. Why is cyanide so toxic?

Cyanide ion binds to the heme-containing cytochrome a_3 enzyme in the electron transport chain of mitochondria, which is the final common pathway in oxidative metabolism. Thus, with a significant exposure, virtually every cell in the body becomes starved of oxygen at the mitochondrial level and is unable to function. The body does have minor routes of cyanide detoxification, including excretion by the lungs and liver via rhodanese, an hepatic enzyme that combines cyanide with thiosulfate to form the less toxic thiocyanate for renal excretion. However, these mechanisms are inadequate in the face of a significant cyanide exposure. As with carbon monoxide poisoning, symptoms tend to be most prominent among the metabolically active organ systems. In particular, the CNS is rapidly affected, causing headache and dizziness, which may progress to prostration, convulsions, coma, and death. Less severe ingestions may be noted initially by burning of the tongue and mucous membranes, with tachypnea and dyspnea due to cyanide stimulation of chemoreceptors.

130. Which kinds of plants account for the greatest percentage of deaths due to plant poisoning?

Mushrooms account for > 50% of all deaths due to plant poisoning. The most dreaded variety are the *Amanita* species, which initially cause intestinal symptoms by one toxin (phallotoxin) and then hepatic and renal failure by a separate toxin (amatoxin).

131. After an enjoyable takeout meal of moo goo gai pan, an 8-year-old presents with facial burning and headache. What is the likely diagnosis?

The **Chinese restaurant syndrome**. Several hours after ingestion of Chinese food, a patient may complain of burning and numbness of the face and neck, headache, and, occasionally, severe chest pain. Symptoms can persist up to 1–2 days. The pathophysiology remains unclear, but monosodium glutamate (MSG), a food additive, may be involved with glutamate acting as a neurotransmitter. Other studies suggest that the fermentation of typical ingredients in Chinese cooking (e.g., soy sauce, black beans, shrimp paste) may release histamines which account for the symptoms.

132. Is mistletoe toxic?

Mistletoe, the popular Christmas plant, is an evergreen with small white berries. Ingestions of small amounts of the berries, leaves, or stems may result in GI symptoms, including pain, nausea, vomiting, and diarrhea. Rarely, large ingestions have resulted in seizures, hypertension, and even cardiac arrest. In some countries, extracts of mistletoe have been used for illegal abortifacients, brewed in teas which are particularly toxic. In the United States, the typical call to a poison center concerns a child who eats one or two mistletoe berries, which in general, is unlikely to produce significant signs or symptoms. Kissing under the mistletoe may lead to greater hazards.

133. Should ingested disc batteries be removed?

Although the concern is that a disc battery may produce corrosive intestinal injury, most traverse the GI tract without incident. An initial x-ray for localization is indicated. If the disc battery is in the distal esophagus, removal is required. Otherwise, if the battery is in the stomach or beyond and the patient remains asymptomatic, watchful waiting is appropriate. If the battery is not seen in the stool by 5–7 days, a repeat x-ray should be obtained.

134. What is the best way to remove a foreign body from the esophagus?

Three methods are used:

1. *Esophagoscopy*, the most commonly used method, is done under general anesthesia.

2. A *Foley catheter* can be inserted beyond the foreign body, inflated, and then pulled back to remove the object. This extraction method is used by various centers, particularly for coins if the ingestion is < 24 hours old and no respiratory distress is present. Complications, such as airway obstruction by a displaced coin and esophageal perforation, are possible.

3. In *bougienage*, the object is forced into the stomach.

TRAUMA

135. In a child with head trauma, is a skull x-ray a good screening study?

Skull x-rays correlate very poorly with intracranial injury. As many as 90% of older patients with a skull fracture will not have intracranial pathology, and of those with documented intracranial pathology, as many as 50% will not have a fracture. Thus, a normal skull film may be falsely reassuring. Although it remains a controversial issue, the routine use of skull films in the setting of head trauma is declining. Specific indications may include assessment of possible treatable disruptions of the skull (e.g., penetrating trauma, foreign-body impaction, depressed skull fracture), trauma over the middle meningeal groove (where arterial bleeding caused by a fracture is more likely), or patients aged < 12 months with significant injury or suspected child abuse.

136. When is a CT scan indicated following head trauma?
1. Prolonged loss of consciousness (> 5 min) or amnesia
2. Penetrating trauma
3. Deteriorating or persistent altered level of consciousness
4. Focal neurologic abnormality
5. Seizure
6. Unremitting vomiting (> 6 hrs) or progressive headache
7. Depressed, compound, or suspected basilar skull fracture
8. Other significant injuries requiring general anesthesia

Adapted from Schutzman SA: Head injury. In Fleisher GR, Ludwig S (eds): Textbook of Pediatric Emergency Medicine, 3rd ed. Baltimore, Williams & Wilkins, 1993, p 272.

137. What types of localized anatomic pathology can develop after acute head trauma?

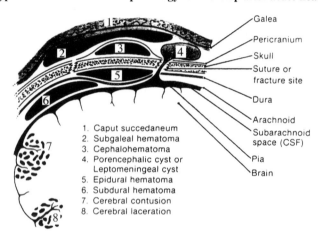

From Rosman NP, et al: Acute head trauma in infancy and childhood. Pediatr Clin North Am 26:708, 1979; with permission.

138. If a patient with head trauma has persistent hypotension and bradycardia despite resuscitative efforts, what should be considered?

Neurogenic shock. Trauma to the cervical or high thoracic spinal cord can often injure or ablate the descending sympathetic pathways, which results in the loss of vasomotor tone and sympathetic control of the heart. Treatment consists of cardiorespiratory support, atropine, fluid resuscitation, and sympathomimetics. The vast majority of patients respond to fluids alone.

139. Why is hyperventilation beneficial in head trauma with increased intracranial pressure (ICP)?

Following severe head trauma, cerebral blood flow and cerebral blood volume increase and can result in an elevated ICP. Severely increased ICP may compromise cerebral perfusion pressure (defined as the mean arterial pressure minus ICP) and contribute to ischemic injury. Cerebral blood flow is influenced by $PaCO_2$. The hyperventilation of a patient to reduce the $PaCO_2$ from

40 mmHg to 25–30 mmHg reduces cerebral blood volume by approximately 50%, lowering ICP and thus improving cerebral perfusion pressure.

140. When ICP is acutely elevated, how long before papilledema develops?

A minimum of 24–48 hours.

141. How do the signs of CNS herniation differ?

Unilateral herniation of temporal lobe (through rigid tentorium)—Ipsilateral fixed and dilated pupil and contralateral hemiparesis.

Cerebellar tonsils through foramen magnum—Abnormalities of tone and progressive respiratory distress.

Beware that these clinical findings tend to overlap, and an altered state of consciousness is often the initial symptom.

142. What are the components of the Glasgow Coma Scale?

Developed in 1974 by the neurosurgical department at the University of Glasgow, the scale was an attempt to standardize the assessment of the depth and duration of impaired consciousness and coma, particularly in the setting of trauma. The scale is based on eye opening, verbal responses, and motor responses, with a total ranging from 3–15.

Glasgow Coma Scale

Best verbal response*	5	Oriented, appropriate conversation
	4	Confused conservation
	3	Inappropriate words
	2	Incomprehensible sounds
	1	No response
Best motor response	6	Obeys a verbal command
(to command or pain,	5	Localizes
such as rubbing	4	Withdraws
knuckles on sternum)	3	Abnormal flexion (decorticate posturing)
	2	Abnormal extension (decerebrate posturing)
	1	No response
Eye opening	4	Spontaneous
	3	In response to verbal command
	2	In response to pain
	1	No response

* Children < 2 years should receive full verbal score for crying after stimulation.

143. How, when, and where are car seats to be used?

All 50 states require that children riding in cars always be restrained in an approved safety seat based on weight or height as follows:

< 20 lbs	Rear-facing infant seat
20–40 lbs	Forward-facing toddler seat
40–60 lbs	Booster seat with lap belt
> 60 lbs	Regular lap belt
> 48 in	Shoulder strap with belt

Schmitt BD, Headley RM: Ambulatory pediatrics. In Hay WW, et al (eds): Current Pediatric Diagnosis & Treatment, 12th ed. Norwalk, CT, Appleton & Lange, 1995, p 284.

144. What are the major signs of a blow-out fracture?

Traumatic force to the eye can result in a blow-out fracture affecting either the orbital floor or medial wall. The fracture may result from either a sudden increase in intraorbital pressure or from a direct concussive force to the bony walls. Symptoms and signs can include:

• Pain on upward gaze
• Diplopia on upward gaze
• Enophthalmos (i.e., posterior displacement of globe)
• Loss of sensation over upper lip and gums on injured side
• Inability to look upward on affected side due to entrapment of the inferior rectus muscle
• Crepitus over the inferior orbital ridge

145. How does the location of cervical spine fractures vary between younger children and older children/adults?

Younger children tend to have fractures of the upper cervical spine, whereas older children and adults have fractures more often involving the lower cervical spine, for the following reasons:

1. Changing fulcrum of spine: In an infant, the fulcrum of the cervical spine is at approximately C2–3; in a child aged 5–6 years, C3–4; by age 8 to adulthood, C5–6. These changes are in large part due to the relatively large head size of a child compared to an adult.
2. Younger children have relatively weak neck muscles.
3. Younger children have poorer protective reflexes.

Woodward GA: Neck trauma. In Fleisher GR, Ludwig S (eds): Textbook of Pediatric Emergency Medicine, 3rd ed. Baltimore, Williams & Wilkins, 1993, pp 1126–1127.

146. What is a hangman's fracture?

This fracture of the posterior elements of the C2 vertebra results from severe hyperextension of the neck. When the neck is placed in flexion, this may allow subluxation (spondylolisthesis) of C2 on C3, causing damage to the spinal cord.

147. Which patients have SCIWORA?

Up to two-thirds of children with spinal cord injuries have SCIWORA, which is Spinal Cord Injury Without Radiographic Abnormality. Most are < 8 years of age with symptoms and signs consistent with spinal cord injury, but x-ray and CT studies reveal no bony abnormalities. Various causes are suspected, including vascular trauma, ligamentous injury, or incomplete neuronal destruction. The more recent use of MRI in these children may help to clarify the cause(s).

Kriss VM, Kriss TC: SCIWORA (spinal cord injury without radiographic abnormality) in infants and children. Clin Pediatr 35:119–124, 1996.

148. How should the pupils be dilated?

Pupillary dilation is sometimes needed in the evaluation of eye trauma, in the search for retinal hemorrhages in suspected child abuse, in the ongoing examination of suspected increasing ICP (e.g., headaches, meningitis, head trauma), and in the ascertainment of papilledema prior to lumbar puncture. Pupillary control is dual—the pupillary dilator is sympathetically mediated; the pupillary sphincter is parasympathetically mediated (as is the ciliary muscle, which controls lens accommodation). Combinations of drops are often utilized involving sympathomimetics (e.g., phenylephrine 2.5%) and anticholinergics (e.g., tropicamide 0.5–1.0%, cyclopentolate 0.5%). All have rapid onsets (< 30 min) and short durations of action (e.g., phenylephrine, < 3 hrs; tropicamide, < 6 hrs). Local custom will prevail, but one simple method of dilation is 1 drop of tropicamide 0.5%, repeated if necessary. Darker eyes are more difficult to dilate and may require repeat dosing.

Chiaviello CT, Bond GR: Dilating the pupil in the pediatric emergency department. Pediatr Emerg Care 4:216–218, 1994.

149. When are drops for pupillary dilation contraindicated?

These drops should not be used in patients requiring sequential neurologic exams (e.g., after severe head trauma) where increasing ICP with herniation is possible. They are also contraindicated in the setting of acute-angle glaucoma. The risk of inducing glaucoma is very low in children, but if symptoms of glaucoma (e.g., moderate eye pain, decreased vision, cloudy cornea, asymmetric pupil size, poor pupillary reaction) are present, dilation should be deferred. Of note, all drops can have side effects, and these can be minimized by pressure over the medial canthus to avoid systemic absorption.

150. When should avulsed teeth be reimplanted?
Avulsion is the complete displacement of the tooth from its socket. Primary (i.e., baby) teeth should not be reimplanted as dental ankylosis may result. Secondary teeth should be repaired within 30 minutes to maximize the chance of tooth viability. A dislodged tooth should be gently rinsed, transported in milk or saliva or under a parent's tongue, and reimplanted temporarily until definitive dental care can be obtained.

151. What are the three most important considerations in evaluating nasal trauma?
1. *Bleeding.* If persistent, bleeding should be controlled with pressure, topical vasoconstrictors, topical thrombin, cauterization, and anterior or posterior nasal packing.
2. *Septal hematoma.* If the nasal septum is bulging into the nasal cavity, there is likely a hematoma which must be drained. If drainage is not done, abscess formation or pressure necrosis can result, leading to a saddle-nose deformity.
3. *Watery rhinorrhea.* This may be a sign of cribriform plate, suborbital ethmoid, sphenoid sinus, or frontal sinus fracture with CSF leak. Radioisotope scans or CT scan with metrizamide dye can confirm the fracture. Hospitalization is warranted if positive.

More extensive facial trauma requires evaluation for many items, especially midface fractures and eye damage. Determining if the nose is fractured is a lower priority item because fracture reduction is done only if there is distortion of the nose. Furthermore, such distortion cannot be properly assessed acutely due to swelling.

152. How long before a broken nose in a child must be reduced?
If a nasal bone fracture causes asymmetry, which is noted as the swelling from acute trauma subsides, the fracture should be reduced within 4–5 days. A longer delay may result in malunion.

153. How does one distinguish nasal mucosal drainage from CSF leakage?
This often becomes an issue when children have nasal rhinorrhea following trauma. The simplest test is to check the glucose concentration. The CSF glucose is normally 40–80 mg/dl, whereas the glucose concentration of nasal mucus is normally near 0.

154. Why is left shoulder pain after abdominal trauma a worrisome sign?
Whenever Kehr's sign is present, potential trouble lurks. Left shoulder pain can be a sign of splenic rupture. This sign can be elicited by LUQ palpation or by placing the patient in the Trendelenburg position.

155. In a 7-year-old boy with an x-ray-proven pelvic fracture, what urologic procedure is needed?
The urethra as it passes through the prostate is very close to the pubic bone and is thus susceptible to injury by a pelvic fracture. Urethral damage should be suspected in all patients with pelvic fractures, even those without hematuria. The recommended diagnostic procedure is a **retrograde urethrogram**. Of note, a boggy, high-riding prostate found on rectal exam and/or blood seen at the urethral meatus are clinical signs of possible urethral disruption.

156. How is zipper entrapment remedied?
This situation most commonly occurs in boys with intact foreskins. Following use of a local anesthetic (1% lidocaine without epinephrine), release is accomplished by simple manipulation of the zipper, cutting the median bar of the zipper with a wire cutter or dividing the zipper transversely.

6. ENDOCRINOLOGY

Lorraine E. Levitt Katz, M.D., and Daniel E. Hale, M.D.

ADRENAL DISORDERS

1. What is the differential diagnosis of primary adrenal insufficiency?

Inherited enzymatic defects: Congenital adrenal hyperplasia (multiple enzymatic defects)

Autoimmune: Isolated, autoimmune polyendocrine syndromes (APES I and II), Schmidt syndrome

Infectious: Tuberculosis, meningococcemia, disseminated fungal infections

Traumatic: Bilateral adrenal hemorrhage

2. What are the most common causes of secondary adrenal insufficiency?

Secondary causes can include failure of the hypothalamic and/or pituitary gland due to tumor, CNS trauma, irradiation, infection, or surgery. The most common cause, however, is prolonged glucocorticoid use for treatment of nonadrenal disease.

3. Can clinical clues suggest that adrenal insufficiency is a primary rather than secondary problem?

In primary adrenal insufficiency, ACTH levels rise due to disruption of the hormonal feedback loop. Hyperpigmentation can result from these elevated levels. In secondary adrenal insufficiency, ACTH levels are low, and no hyperpigmentation occurs. Furthermore, in secondary insufficiency, the zona glomerulosa of the adrenal gland (responsible for aldosterone secretion) remains intact. Therefore, hyperkalemia and/or volume depletion are distinctly uncommon, but hyponatremia may occur as a result of decreased capacity to excrete a water load. In contrast, primary deficiencies commonly lead to hyponatremia *and* hyperkalemia.

4. At what time should serum cortisol be tested?

The time depends on the question being addressed. If the question is whether the pituitary-adrenal axis is functioning normally, then cortisol should be measured at 8 AM and 11 PM. The response is also dependent on whether the patient is significantly stressed (e.g., serious illness) and has an established diurnal pattern. Morning values should be 8–19 µg/dl, and evening values should be 4–11 µg/dl. Hypofunction of the axis is likely to be demonstrated by a low AM cortisol, while hyperfunction is more likely to be shown by a high PM cortisol. More definitive evaluation of the axis can be obtained by using some combination of the cosyntropin stimulation test, corticotropin-releasing factor (CRF) test, and metyrapone test. If hyperfunction of the axis is suspected, 24-hour urinary free cortisol determination is more definitive, although multiple 24-hour urine collections may need to be obtained.

5. How does one choose between the cosyntropin stimulation test, metyrapone test, and CRF test as measures of adrenal function?

The choice of tests depends on the disease process suspected from the history and physical examination.

The **cosyntropin stimulation test** is solely a test of adrenal function and examines whether cortisol is present in the adrenal, which then can be released in response to a synthetic form of ACTH. It provides no information on whether the child produces normal amounts of ACTH or how long the cortisol took to accumulate. The test is used primarily in children with suspected intrinsic adrenal disease.

The **corticotropin-releasing factor** (CRF) **test** examines ACTH release by the pituitary in response to the normal hypothalamic releasing factor. It provides insight into the hypothalamic-pituitary axis, although it does not necessarily differentiate pituitary from hypothalamic disease. It only examines whether an acutely releasable pool of ACTH is available and provides no assurance that the hypothalamic regulation of this release is normal. The CRF test is of use in individuals with known or suspected pituitary or hypothalamic lesions.

The **metyrapone test**, although technically more difficult and prone to cause more symptoms, remains the best test of the integrity of the hypothalamic-pituitary-adrenal axis. This is because metyrapone blocks the synthesis of cortisol. The fall in cortisol serves as the physiologic stimulus to the hypothalamus-pituitary, which must, in turn, produce its respective hormones.

Riddick L, et al: Comparison of adrenocorticotropin and adrenal steroid responses to corticotropin-releasing hormone vs metyrapone testing in patients with hypopituitarism. Pediatr Res 36:215–220, 1994.

Grinspoon SK, Biller BMK: Laboratory assessment of adrenal insufficiency. J Clin Endocrinol Metab 79:923–931, 1994.

6. How is the cosyntropin stimulation test done?

Cosyntropin is a synthetic form of ACTH. It contains the first 25 amino acids in naturally occurring ACTH and exhibits all of the biologic functions of ACTH. Normally-functioning adrenal glands receive this exogenous signal and respond by increasing cortisol production.

The test: Prior to the study, blood is drawn for a baseline cortisol level. Cosyntropin (0.25 mg/m²) is then administered by IV push, and additional cortisol levels are drawn at 30 and 60 minutes. An incremental increase of plasma cortisol > 6 µg/dl to a maximum > 20 µg/dl is strong evidence of normal adrenal function. Levels of plasma cortisol less than expected indicate that the adrenal gland is not functioning normally and stress coverage is needed. Abnormal results provide no information on whether the problem is adrenal, pituitary, or both.

7. How is the metyrapone test done?

Metyrapone is an 11-hydroxylase inhibitor that blocks the conversion of 11-deoxycortisol to cortisol. As a consequence, cortisol levels fall. The decrease in serum cortisol levels is sensed by the pituitary gland, which responds by increasing ACTH production. This, in turn, increases adrenal activity and the production of 11-deoxycortisol. The protocol is detailed, but basically the increased levels of 11-deoxycortisol and ACTH can be measured in blood. Lack of an increase indicates pathology in the pituitary gland (e.g., secondary insufficiency), hypothalamus (e.g., tumor), or adrenal gland (e.g., suppression secondary to chronic steroid use).

8. In newborns with congenital adrenal hyperplasia (CAH), why are girls more likely to be diagnosed earlier than boys?

The most obvious clinical feature of CAH in the newborn period is ambiguous genitalia due to androgen excess. In boys, androgen excess does not cause any clearly abnormal appearance of the external genitalia. In girls, however, ambiguous genitalia are common. CAH should always be considered in the differential diagnosis of ambiguous genitalia, particularly in genetic females.

9. Describe the clinical features of the various forms of congenital adrenal hyperplasia (CAH).

CAH refers to a group of autosomal recessive disorders that result from various enzymatic defects in the biosynthesis of cortisol. Depending on the enzyme involved, the blockade can result in excesses or deficiencies in the other steroid pathways (i.e., mineralocorticoids and androgens). 21-Hydroxylase deficiency accounts for > 90% of cases; the complete (salt-losing) and partial (simple virilizing) forms occur in about 1/12,000 births and have an equal sex distribution. A late-onset or attenuated form (mild deficiency) manifests in adolescent females with hirsutism and menstrual irregularities.

Clinical Features of Disorders of Adrenal Steroidogenesis

ENZYME DEFECT	SEXUAL AMBIGUITY		POSTNATAL VIRILIZATION	SALT WASTING	HYPERTENSION
	FEMALE	MALE			
21-Hydroxylase					
Salt-wasting	+	0	+	+	0
Simple virilizing	+	0	+	0	0
Late-onset	0	0	+	0	0
11-Hydroxylase	+	0	+	0	+
17-Hydroxylase	0	+	0	0	+
18-Hydroxylase	0	0	0	+	0
3β-Hydroxysteroid dehydrogenase	+	+	+	+	0
Desmolase	0	+	0	+	0

10. How do the major steroid preparations vary in potency?

Relative Potencies of Glucocorticoids

NAME	RELATIVE GLUCOCORTICOID POTENCY	RELATIVE DOSING (mg)	RELATIVE MINERALO-CORTICOID POTENCY
Cortisone	1	100	++
Hydrocortisone	1.25	80	+
Prednisone	5	20	++
Prednisolone	5	20	++
Methylprednisolone	6	16	0
Fludrocortisone	20	*	+++++
Dexamethasone	50	1	0

* Not used for glucocorticoid therapy.
Adapted from Donohoue PA: The adrenal cortex. In Oski FA, et al (eds): Principles and Practice of Pediatrics, 2nd ed. Philadelphia, J.B. Lippincott, 1994, p 2003; with permission.

11. How do physiologic, stress, and pharmacologic doses of hydrocortisone differ?

Careful studies have shown that adrenal glucocorticoid production in the normal individual is about 7–8 mg/m^2/24 hr. Because 50–60% of oral hydrocortisone is absorbed, the recommended **physiologic replacement** orally is about 12–15 mg/m^2/24 hr.

Based on studies performed prior to the development of high-quality radioimmunoassays, a consensus developed that production of glucocorticoid increased about threefold when individuals were physiologically stressed. Hence, when the term **stress dose** is used, it generally means 50 mg of hydrocortisone/m^2/24 hr.

Glucocorticoids are extensively used in **pharmacologic doses** in the treatment of various inflammatory processes and in surgery or trauma to reduce or prevent swelling and inflammation. The doses are dependent on the underlying process and are often > 50 mg hydrocortisone/m^2/24 hr.

12. When does adrenal-pituitary axis suppression occur in prolonged glucocorticoid treatment?

As a general rule, the longer the duration of treatment and the higher the dose, the greater the risk of adrenal suppression. If pharmacologic doses of glucocorticoids are used for < 10 days, there is a relatively small risk of permanent adrenal insufficiency, while daily use > 30 days carries a high risk of transient or permanent adrenal suppression.

Probability of Adrenal Suppression

DURATION OF TREATMENT (DAYS)	DOSE	ADRENAL SUPPRESSION
< 3	< 3 ×	None
	> 3 ×	Unlikely
> 3 but < 10	> 1 ×	Unlikely
>10 but < 30	> 1 ×	Possible
> 30	> 1 ×	Possible
	Alternate day	
	> 1 ×	Probable
	Every day	

13. How rapidly should prescribed doses of steroids be reduced?

No single rule can cover all possible circumstances. The rapidity of tapering depends on the duration of treatment, the amount and type of glucocorticoid used, and the disease process under treatment.

1. The reduction from pharmacologic to physiologic doses is predicted on the underlying disease. For example, a child with lupus who has been maintained on pharmacologic doses for weeks may need to be tapered very slowly (10% increments every 2 weeks) in order to avoid a rebound of disease.

2. If there is no obvious reason to taper slowly, then the dose can be reduced by 50% every 2 days until the patient is on the equivalent of physiologic dosing (12–15 mg hydrocortisone/m^2/24 hr). The second phase, tapering from a physiologic dose, can then begin (see Question 14).

3. In cases of congenital adrenal hyperplasia or known hypopituitarism, reducing the dose below physiologic replacement amounts may be contraindicated.

14. A child has been on physiologic doses of prednisone (3–4 mg/m^2/day) for 4 months. What is the best way to discontinue the therapy safely?

1. Change to a hydrocortisone preparation with corresponding equivalency dose.

2. Reduce to ½ of physiologic dose for 2 weeks. If the child is stressed, the dose must be increased to an appropriate stress dose (50 mg/m^2/24 hr).

3. At the end of the second week, withhold the AM hydrocortisone dose and obtain an AM cortisol level.

    a. If AM cortisol is > 10 mg/dl, supplementation may be stopped. However, stress coverage is required until the adequacy of the adrenal-pituitary response to stress (ACTH stimulation test and/or metyrapone testing) can be determined.

    b. If AM cortisol is < 10 mg/dl, continue supplementation (6–8 mg/m^2/24 hr). Repeat AM cortisol in 1 month. Stress coverage must be maintained.

CALCIUM METABOLISM AND DISORDERS

15. Is it Chvostek's or Trousseau's sign that gets the tap?

Chvostek's. Both are clinical manifestations of hypocalcemia or hypomagnesemia that occur because of neuromuscular irritability.

Chvostek's sign: Tapping on the facial nerve in front of the ear results in movement of the upper lip.

Trousseau's sign: Inflating a blood pressure cuff at pressures greater than systolic for 2 minutes results in carpopedal spasm.

16. What are the causes of hypercalcemia?

Remember the "high fives" (**High 5-I's**) rule: **H** (hyperparathyroidism) plus the 5 **I's** (idiopathic, infantile, infection, infiltrations, and ingestions) and **S** (skeletal disorders).

Hyperparathyroidism
   Familial
   Isolated
   Syndromic
Idiopathic
   Williams syndrome
Infantile
   Subcutaneous fat necrosis
   Secondary to maternal
     hypoparathyroidism
Infections
   Tuberculosis

Ingestions
   Milk-alkali syndrome
   Thiazide diuretics
   Vitamin A intoxication
   Vitamin D intoxication
Infiltrations
   Malignancy
   Sarcoidosis
   Tuberculosis
Skeletal disorders
   Hypophosphatasia
   Immobilization
   Skeletal dysplasias

17. In what circumstances should hypoparathyroidism be suspected?

Historical

1. May occur as part of the autoimmune polyendocrine syndrome (see Question 27)
2. Associated with thymic aplasia and immunodeficiency (DiGeorge syndrome)
3. Damage may occur as a complication of neck surgery or irradiation

Clinical

1. Manifestations of hypocalcemia such as carpopedal spasm, bronchospasm, tetany, or seizures
2. Lenticular cataracts (which can occur in other causes of long-standing hypocalcemia)
3. Changing behaviors, ranging from depression to psychosis
4. Mucocutaneous candidiasis (seen in familial form)
5. Dry and scaly skin, psoriasis, and patchy alopecia
6. Brittle hair and fingernails
7. Enamel hypoplasia (if present during dental development)

Laboratory

1. Low serum calcium with elevated phosphate
2. Prolonged QT interval on ECG

18. An 8-year-old in a spica cast following hip surgery develops vomiting and a serum calcium of 15.3 mg/dl. What should be done?

A serum calcium concentration > 15 mg/dl or the presence of significant symptoms (vomiting, hypertension) constitutes a medical emergency and requires immediate intervention to lower the calcium level. The mainstay of treatment is isotonic saline at 2–4 times maintenance rates and furosemide (1 mg/kg IV, every 6 hrs). Furosemide is a potent diuretic and calciuric agent. Meticulous monitoring of input and output and of serum and urinary electrolytes (including serum magnesium) is vital. ECG monitoring is mandatory because hypercalcemia can be associated with conduction disturbances, including premature ventricular contractions, ventricular tachycardia, prolonged PR interval, prolonged QRS duration, and atrioventricular block.

19. If saline and furosemide fail as treatments for hypercalcemia, what other options are available?

The administration of glucocorticoids may decrease serum calcium levels by decreasing intestinal absorption of calcium. Bone antiresorptive agents, including mithramycin, calcitonin, and etidronate, have also been used successfully as therapies for hypercalcemia. Phosphate (1–2 mmol/kg/day given orally for 4–6 days, or 1 mmol/kg given over 6–8 hrs IV) has also been effective, but there is considerable risk of soft tissue calcification, especially with intravenous administration.

McKay C, Furman WL: Hypercalcemia complicating childhood malignancies. Cancer 72:256–260, 1993.

20. What are the main causes of hypocalcemia in children?

1. *Nutritional:* inadequate intake of vitamin D and/or calcium

2. *Renal insufficiency:* due to (a) increased serum phosphorus from decreased GFR with depressed serum calcium and secondary hyperparathyroidism or (b) decreased activity of renal α-hydroxylase, which is involved in converting the less-active 25-hydroxyvitamin D into the more active 1,25-$(OH)_2$ D.

3. *Nephrotic syndrome:* with lowered serum albumin, total calcium levels are reduced. Additionally, intestinal absorption of calcium is decreased, urinary losses of cholecalciferol-binding globulin are increased, and urinary losses of calcium are increased with prednisone therapy.

4. *Hypoparathyroidism:* (a) in infants, primary aplasia, hypoplasia, or DiGeorge syndrome or (b) in older children, autoimmune polyglandular disease or mitochondrial myopathy syndromes.

5. *Pseudohypoparathyroidism:* a peripheral resistance syndrome with elevated parathyroid hormone and normal renal function.

Fouser L: Disorders of calcium, phosphorus, and magnesium. Pediatr Ann 24:38–46, 1995.

CLINICAL SYNDROMES

21. How does the syndrome of inappropriate secretion of antidiuretic hormone (SIADH) develop?

Antidiuretic hormone (ADH) is released from the posterior pituitary gland and serves as a regulator of extracellular fluid volume. The secretion of ADH is regulated by changes in osmolality sensed by the hypothalamus and alterations in blood volume detected by carotid and left atrial stretch receptors. Intracranial pathology can increase the secretion of ADH directly by local CNS effects, and intrathoracic pathology can increase secretion by stimulating volume receptors. Medications (see Question 23) can directly promote ADH release as well as enhance its renal effects. SIADH is usually asymptomatic until symptoms of water intoxication and hyponatremia develop. Nausea, vomiting, irritability, personality changes, progressive obtundation, and seizures can result.

22. What are the 5 criteria for the diagnosis of SIADH?

1. Hyponatremia with reduced serum osmolality

2. Urine osmolality elevated compared with serum osmolality (a urine osmolality < 100 mOsm/dl usually excludes the diagnosis)

3. Urinary sodium concentration excessive for the extent of hyponatremia (usually > 20 mEq/L)

4. Normal renal, adrenal, and thyroid function

5. Absence of volume depletion

23. SIADH is associated with what conditions?

CNS abnormalities
- Infections (meningitis, encephalitis, abscess)
- Head trauma
- Postoperative (especially perinatal asphyxia)
- Hypoxic encephalopathy (especially pituitary manipulations)
- Tumor
- Hemorrhage (subarachnoid or intraventricular)
- Guillain-Barré syndrome

Intrathoracic disorders
- Infection (pneumonia, tuberculosis, empyema)
- Cystic fibrosis
- Positive-pressure ventilation
- Asthma
- Pneumothorax

Drug-related

Pituitary secretion enhanced
- Phenothiazines
- Vincristine
- Vinblastine
- Vidarabine
- Morphine

Renal effect enhanced
- Chlorpropamide
- Indomethacin

ADH analog
- Desmopressin (DDAVP)

24. What clinical features suggest diabetes insipidus?

Because diabetes insipidus is caused by insufficiency of ADH, or the inability to respond to ADH, the signs and symptoms tend to be directly related to excessive fluid loss. The clinical spectrum may vary depending on the child's age. The infant may present with failure to thrive secondary to chronic dehydration or with a history of repeated episodes of hospitalizations for dehydration. There may also be a history of intermittent low-grade fever. Other infants present with obesity, since the child's cry is interpreted as hunger rather than thirst and formula is given rather than water.

Often, caretakers report a large volume intake or an inability to keep a dry diaper on the infant. In the young child, diabetes insipidus may present as difficulty with toilet training. In the older child, the reappearance of enuresis, increasing frequency of urination, nocturia, or dramatic increases in fluid intake may herald the diagnosis. Frequent urination with large urinary volumes should lead to the suspicion of diabetes insipidus, and the absence of glucosuria is sufficient to rule out diabetes mellitus.

25. How is the diagnosis of diabetes insipidus (DI) made?

The child who sleeps for 8–12 hours without urinating or drinking fluids is unlikely to have DI. If the possibility of DI has been raised in such a child, measurement of the serum osmolality and urine osmolality shortly after awakening should be done. If the serum osmolality is normal (< 290 mOsm/L) and the urine is concentrated (> 800 mOsm/L), DI is unlikely.

In a child with a more compelling history (excessive thirst and urination, awakening at night to drink, water-craving behaviors), deprivation of water intake for a limited time accompanied by judicious monitoring of physical and biochemical parameters may be required. The diagnosis of DI rests on the demonstration of (a) an inappropriately dilute urine in the face of a rising or elevated serum osmolality; (b) urine output that remains high despite the lack of oral input; and (c) changes in physical parameters consistent with dehydration (weight loss, tachycardia, loss of skin turgor, dry mucous membranes). A child who, with water deprivation, appropriately concentrates urine and whose serum osmolality remains constant is unlikely to have DI.

If a child meets the criteria for the diagnosis of DI, the water-deprivation test is usually ended with the administration of some form of ADH, such as desmopressin (DDAVP) and the provision of fluids. If the urine subsequently becomes appropriately concentrated, this confirms the diagnosis of ADH deficiency (central DI). Failure to concentrate suggests renal resistance to ADH (nephrogenic DI).

Oberfield SE: Diabetes insipidus and other disorders of water balance. Pediatr Ann 9:384–389, 1980.

Blevins LS Jr, Wand GS: Diabetes insipidus. Crit Care Med 20:69–79, 1992.

26. Precocious puberty and café-au-lait spots are commonly seen in what syndrome?

McCune-Albright syndrome. This syndrome is the association of polyostotic fibrous dysplasia, precocious puberty, and café-au-lait pigmentation. These nevi classically have an irregular border ("coast of Maine"), while the lesions in neurofibromatosis have a more regular border ("coast of California"). McCune-Albright syndrome may occur in either an incomplete form (pigmented nevi and bony changes without precocious puberty) or expanded form (the hallmark features plus other findings such as gigantism, hyperthyroidism, Cushing syndrome, and ovarian cysts). It occurs most commonly in females. The syndrome is thought to be due to autonomous function of the involved gland (ovary, adrenal, thyroid).

27. What distinguishes MEN from APES?

Besides the occasional use of forks, the distinction involves the two groups of polyendocrine disorders. **MEN** (multiple endocrine neoplasia) involves the development of pluriglandular neoplasia. MEN type I (Werner syndrome) is characterized by adenomas of the pancreatic islet cells (with insulin and a gastrin production) and the pituitary gland (with prolactin secretion) and by hyperplasia or multiple adenomas of the parathyroids. MEN II (Sipple syndrome) is associated with medullary thyroid carcinoma, parathyroid adenomas, and, occasionally, pheochromocytomas. MEN III has features of MEN II plus multiple mucosal neuromas.

APES is autoimmune polyendocrine syndrome. APES I has its onset in childhood and is distinguished by hypoparathyroidism, adrenal insufficiency and mucocutaneous candidiasis. APES II occurs in adults and involves a variety of thyroid, adrenal, pancreatic, gonadal, and dermatologic abnormalities.

Caruso DR, et al: Multiple endocrine neoplasia. Curr Opin Oncol 3:103–108, 1991.
Riley WJ: Autoimmune polyglandular syndrome. Horm Res 38(suppl 2):9–15, 1992.

DIABETES MELLITUS

28. What are the risks of developing insulin-dependent diabetes mellitus (IDDM) if one sibling is affected?

Identical twins	> 50%
HLA identical	20%
HLA haploidentical	5%
HLA nonidentical	1%

Plotnick L: Insulin-dependent diabetes mellitus. Pediatr Rev 15:138, 1994.

29. Which markers are available to screen siblings for their likely risk of developing IDDM?

In addition to HLA testing, first-degree relatives of patients with IDDM can be screened by measuring islet cell antibodies, insulin autoantibodies, and the first-phase response to an intravenous glucose tolerance test. Efforts are under way to develop strategies to postpone or prevent the onset of overt diabetes mellitus. Two large clinical trials are under way: one using low-dose insulin treatment (Diabetes Prevention Trial 1) and the other using nicotinamide (European Nicotinamide Diabetes Intervention Trial). There are also some smaller trials with various immunosuppressive agents. The testing for risk is best done under the auspices of one of the research centers involved in these trials.

30. Is the use of cow's milk in infants linked to the later development of IDDM?

IDDM is believed most likely to result from an autoimmune destruction of pancreatic islet cells involving both a genetic predisposition and environmental insult. Multiple environmental factors, including viral infections and toxins, may serve as triggers. Some research suggests that antibodies to bovine serum albumin may be involved in the initiation of the autoimmune process.

Work Group on Cow's Milk Protein and Diabetes Mellitus: Infant feeding practices and their possible relationship to the etiology of diabetes mellitus. Pediatrics 94:752–754, 1994.

31. How long does the "honeymoon" period last in newly diagnosed insulin-dependent diabetics?

The "honeymoon" usually begins within 1–2 weeks after the initiation of insulin treatment. It is a period of falling or minimal exogenous insulin requirements that reflects continued residual endogenous insulin production. The duration of the honeymoon in a particular individual may last for a few weeks or months but is not predictable. However, evidence is accumulating that it may be prolonged by the maintenance of excellent control. Cessation of the honeymoon is often heralded by elevated fasting blood glucose levels prior to breakfast or by an increasing insulin requirement.

32. How do the types of insulin vary in their timing and duration of action?

Kinetics of Action of Insulins

	ONSET OF ACTION (HRS)	PEAK OF ACTION (HRS)	DURATION OF ACTION (HRS)
Regular	0.5–1	2–4	5–7
Insulin zinc (prompt, Semilente)	1–3	2–8	12–16
Isophane (NPH)	3–4	6–8	18–24
Insulin zinc (Lente)	1–3	9–12	24–28
Protamine zinc	4–6	14–24	36
Insulin zinc (extended, Ultralente)	4–6	18–24	24–36

For most children with juvenile-onset diabetes, the mainstays of treatment are regular and NPH insulin. The most widely used forms of insulin are those derived from recombinant DNA technology. The other forms (beef/pork, pure pork, modified pork) are becoming increasingly hard to obtain, although some patients and physicians feel that these have superior qualities compared to the recombinant forms. Children and adolescents treated with recombinant NPH seem to be somewhat more likely to have hypoglycemia prior to lunch and hyperglycemia prior to supper. If that pattern is noted, switching to an animal insulin or Lente may alleviate both problems.

33. What are the typical insulin dosages given after the "honeymoon" period?

Prepubertal children generally require about 0.5 U/kg/day, while postpubertal individuals require 0.75–1.0 U/kg/day. Athletes or those with a low caloric intake require less insulin.

34. When should the Somogyi phenomenon be suspected?

The Somogyi phenomenon is rebound hyperglycemia following an incident of hypoglycemia. This rebound is secondary to release of counter-regulatory hormones, which is the natural response to hypoglycemia. As tighter diabetic control is maintained, there is an increased likelihood of hypoglycemia and therefore the Somogyi phenomenon. If the hypoglycemia is recognized and treated promptly, rebound hyperglycemia is less likely to occur. Thus, the Somogyi is commonly reported more frequently at night because there is greater likelihood of unrecognized and untreated hypoglycemia when the child is asleep. The Somogyi phenomenon should be suspected when a child in excellent control begins to have intermittent high blood glucoses in the morning. If that pattern is noted, blood glucose should be checked at 2–3 AM on several nights to determine if hypoglycemia is occurring. If hypoglycemia can be documented, the dose of evening insulin should be decreased.

35. What causes the "dawn phenomenon"?

The term dawn phenomenon describes a rise in blood glucose that occurs in the early morning hours (5–8 AM), particularly in patients who have normal glucose levels throughout most of the night. The rise in glucose is thought to be due to several factors, including:

1. The normal increase in the AM cortisol
2. Cumulative effect of increased nocturnal growth hormone
3. Insulinopenia, due to the length of time since the pre-supper injection

In some instances, the dawn phenomenon can be satisfactorily managed by shifting the NPH dose to a later time (pre-bedtime snack) or by using Lente.

36. How rapidly can renal disease develop after the onset of diabetes mellitus?

Microscopic changes in the glomerular basement membrane are present by 2 years after the diagnosis of diabetes. Microalbuminuria is often present by 10–15 years, followed by a protein-uric period (> 0.5 gm/24 hrs). Beyond this point, there is a relentless decline in glomerular func-tion. An azotemic period begins on average by 17 years, and frank uremia occurs by 20 years. Retrospective studies suggest that as many as 50% of patients with IDDM diagnosed before age 30 will develop end-stage renal disease. Diabetic nephropathy accounts for 25% of patients re-ceiving long-term renal dialysis in the United States.

37. When does retinopathy develop following the onset of diabetes mellitus?

Retinal disease in patients with diabetes is characterized by either background (simple) or proliferative retinopathy. By 25–30 years after the diagnosis of diabetes, 90% of patients have demonstrable retinal lesions. The onset of the proliferative form of retinopathy carries a high risk of blindness. Vitreous hemorrhage, scarring, and retinal hemorrhage occur frequently. Approximately 10% of patients develop proliferative retinopathy within 14 years. The disease will proceed to blindness in about 45% of patients within 5 years of the onset of proliferative changes. Diabetes is the leading cause of adult blindness in the United States. It is important to remember that knowledge concerning dietary management has expanded, the quality of the in-sulin has improved, and the ability to maintain better diabetic control has changed dramatically in the past 20 years. Therefore, the prognosis for both renal and retinal injury may be signifi-cantly better than the statistics outlined above.

38. Describe the three forms of diabetic neuropathy.

1. *Mononeuropathy.* Involves a peripheral or cranial nerve. The usual presentation is the sudden appearance of foot drop, wrist drop, or paralysis of the III, IV, or VI cranial nerves. Generally, the abnormality subsides in several days.

2. *Symmetrical peripheral polyneuropathy.* A symmetrical sensory loss occurs in the distal lower extremities. Upper extremity involvement and motor deficits are uncommon. Numbness, tingling, and burning of the affected extremities are common and generally are worse at night. The pain may be severe on occasion. Due to the loss of sensory input, injuries may occur that are asymptomatic. Increased surveillance for these injuries in affected patients is required.

3. *Autonomic neuropathy.* This may result in orthostatic hypotension, sexual dysfunction, and motility disorders of the esophagus, stomach, gallbladder, small intestine, colon, and urinary bladder.

39. How is hemoglobin A₁C helpful in monitoring diabetic control?

Glycohemoglobin, also known as glycosolated hemoglobin or hemoglobin A_1C, is a hemo-globin-glucose combination formed nonenzymatically within the cell. Initially, an unstable bond is formed between glucose and the hemoglobin molecule. With time, this bond rearranges to form a more stable compound in which glucose is covalently bound to the hemoglobin molecule. The amount of the unstable form may rise rapidly in the presence of a high blood glucose level, while the stable form changes slowly and provides a time-average integral of the blood glucose concentration through the 120-day lifespan of the red blood cell. Thus, glycohemoglobin levels can provide an objective measurement of averaged diabetic control over time.

40. Is tight control of diabetes better than conventional control?

The Diabetes Control and Complications Trial (DCCT) followed over 1400 diabetics (nearly 200 of whom were adolescents). Study subjects were randomized to receive either standard diabetic therapy (e.g., twice daily insulin shots) or more intensive therapy (e.g., more frequent blood glucose monitoring and 3 or more shots daily). Intensive control reduced the risk of development of retinopathy by 53% and the occurrence of microalbuminuria by 55% compared with conventional control. The major adverse effect was a threefold increase in the rate of severe hypoglycemia. Whether the benefits of tighter control outweigh the potential risks of hypoglycemia in younger pediatric patients remains unknown.

DCCT Research Group: Effect of intensive diabetes treatment on the development and progression of long-term complications in adolescents with insulin-dependent diabetes mellitus: Diabetes Control and Complications Trial. J Pediatr 125:177–188, 1994.

Clark CM Jr, Lee DA: Prevention and treatment of the complications of diabetes mellitus. N Engl J Med 332:1210–1217, 1995.

41. Discuss general considerations regarding fluid management in diabetic ketoacidosis (DKA).

The most critical aspect of the management of diabetic ketoacidosis is the provision of adequate fluid. Rapid volume expansion with isotonic saline (20 ml/kg) should be undertaken in the first hour. Repeat boluses (10 ml/kg) may be necessary if the patient remains significantly hypotensive and/or tachycardic after the initial bolus. Subsequent fluid management must include:

1. Provision of maintenance fluids
2. Replacement of deficit, which is generally assumed to be 10–15% of body weight.
3. Replacement of ongoing urinary losses in excess of 3 ml/kg/hr.

As a general rule, approximately half of the deficit is replaced during the initial 16-hour period. Therapy must be individualized such that close attention is paid to the patient's input, output, vital signs, and perfusion status.

42. Why is a falling serum sodium concentration during the treatment of DKA of concern?

Most patients with DKA have a significant sodium deficit of 8–10 mEq/kg which needs to be replaced. Following initial fluid boluses, fluids containing 0.5 normal saline or greater may be required. As a general rule, the serum [Na] is low at the outset and rises throughout the course of treatment. An initial [Na] > 145 mEq/L suggests severe dehydration. An initial [Na] that is normal or low and begins to fall with treatment merits prompt attention since it indicates either inappropriate fluid management or the onset of inappropriate diuretic hormone secretion (SIADH) and can signal impending cerebral edema.

43. How should potassium deficits be replaced in children with DKA?

In almost all children, there is a potassium deficit of 6–10 mEq/kg, although the initial serum [K] value is often normal or high. if the initial [K] < 3.5 mEq/L, 60 mEq/L should be added to the infusion and close ECG monitoring should be instituted. If the initial [K] is 3.5–5.5, 40 mEq/L of potassium is used. When the initial [K] is > 5.5, only 20 mEq/L is recommended.

After the initial fluid bolus, the typical child in DKA will receive 0.5 normal saline containing 40 mEq/L of potassium. Half of the potassium may be given as potassium chloride and the other half as potassium phosphate. The initial rate will be about twice normal maintenance rates. It is strongly recommended that while the initial fluid bolus is being given, the physician carefully carefully calculate fluid and electrolyte replacement.

44. Why do potassium levels fall during management of DKA?

- Dilutional effects of rehydration
- Correction of acidosis (less K^+ exchanged out of cell for H^+ as pH rises)
- Insulin administration (increases cellular uptake of K^+)
- Ongoing urinary losses

Most patients are potassium-depleted, although the serum $[K^+]$ is usually normal or elevated. A low $[K^+]$ is particularly worrisome because it suggests severe potassium depletion.

45. Should bicarbonate be used in the treatment of children with DKA?

Pro	Con
Improved pH enhances myocardial contractility and response to catecholamines	Cardiac function problems are rare in children
Ventilatory response to acidosis blunted when pH < 7.0	Ventilatory response well maintained in children
No adverse effect of bicarbonate on oxygenation has been demonstrated clinically	May alter oxygen-binding of hemoglobin, potentially decreasing tissue oxygenation
Questionable relevance of CNS acidosis	Paradoxical CNS acidosis documented in humans
May be useful in the rare patient with hyperkalemia	Hypokalemia may result from uptake of K^+ as acidosis is corrected; low serum [K] is 6 times more common after bicarbonate treatment

The use of bicarbonate in the treatment of DKA in children has been both advocated and denounced. The establishment of an adequate intravascular volume and the provision of sufficient quantities of insulin are *far* more important in the treatment of DKA than bicarbonate. The decision to initiate bicarbonate therapy should be based on an arterial blood gas, *not* a venous blood gas. The three clear indications for bicarbonate therapy are:
1. Symptomatic hyperkalemia
2. Cardiac instability
3. Inadequate ventilatory compensation.

Each of these conditions requires admission to an intensive care unit where appropriate monitoring can be undertaken and ventilatory assistance provided if necessary.

46. When should glucose be added to the infusate in DKA?

When the glucose level approaches 300 mg/dl. It is usually wise to order the appropriate glucose-containing fluid in advance. This is easy to do because the rate of fall of glucose is predictable when a child is on continuous intravenous insulin. After the glucose-containing infusate is introduced, the glucose-free infusate can be kept at the bedside in case the blood glucose begins to rise excessively.

47. Is continuous or bolus insulin better in the treatment of DKA?

The choice of route of administration depends in part on the particular situation. For example, hourly IM injections are easier to manage while a child is being transported between institutions. Theoretically, continuous IV insulin is easier to titrate than IM injections. However, the differences are not clinically significant. More importantly, injection of insulin subcutaneously is inappropriate until adequate hydration is established and the acidosis is resolving ($[HCO_3^-] > 15$ mEq/L).

Continuous insulin is given initially at a rate of 0.1 U/kg/hr (after an initial bolus of 0.1 U/kg). This rate is adjusted to allow blood sugar to fall by about 100 mg/dl/hr. Alternatively, IM insulin can be used with an initial dose of 0.25 U/kg, followed by 0.1 U/kg/hr. Only regular insulin should be used. Intermediate or long-acting insulins are not appropriate in the treatment of DKA.

48. How is the transition made to intermittent insulin therapy as DKA is resolving?

The transition from insulin infusion to intermittent subcutaneous therapy is predicated on three factors:

1. *Normalization of biochemical parameters.* Insulin infusions should not be stopped until the blood sugar is < 300 mg/dl, pH is > 7.3, and HCO_3^- is > 15 mEq/L.

2. *Resumption of oral food intake.* As long as the patient is not eating and is receiving a constant supply of glucose by vein, it is easier to maintain a stable blood sugar using an insulin infusion rather than intermittent subcutaneous insulin. When oral intake is resumed, food is usually

provided on an intermittent (bolus) basis. It is then reasonable to provide insulin in an intermittent fashion as well.

3. *Convenience/normal schedule.* Patients with diabetes generally are placed on a four-times-daily insulin regimen for the initial 24–36 hour period after an episode of ketoacidosis. Regular insulin is given prior to meals and the bedtime snack. For the first dose of insulin after an episode of DKA, the child can be allowed to eat with the insulin drip running. If food is retained for 30 minutes without problems, a dose of subcutaneous insulin (0.25 U/kg) can be administered and the insulin infusion shut off. Subsequent doses of insulin should be given prior to meals.

49. What signs and symptoms suggest worsening cerebral edema during the treatment of DKA?

Cerebral edema accounts for the majority of the 1–2% of case fatalities that occur in DKA. It is unpredictable, occurring often as biochemical abnormalities are improving. It may be sudden in onset or occur gradually. Those most susceptible are children < 5 years of age and newly-diagnosed diabetics. Signs and symptoms include:

- Decreasing sensorium
- Sudden and severe headache
- Incontinence
- Vomiting
- Change in vital signs
- Combativeness, disorientation, agitation
- Ophthalmoplegia
- Pupillary asymmetry or sluggish responses
- Papilledema
- Seizure

Early recognition is vital because intervention (e.g., IV mannitol, intubation, hyperventilation) can improve outcome in 50% of patients.

Rosenbloom AL, Schatz DA: Diabetic ketoacidosis in childhood. Pediatr Ann 23:284–288, 1994.

GROWTH DISTURBANCES

50. Do children grow in a steady fashion or in spurts?

While it is commonly believed that children grow in steady small increments, multiple studies using very frequent precise measurements (e.g., the knemometer which measures leg length with great precision) have shown that growth in children (and even the fetus) is more likely saltatory. As grandmothers claimed correctly, growth seems to occur in spurts in periods up to 24 hours with variable inactive intervals.

Lampl M: Evidence of saltatory growth in infancy. Am J Hum Biol 5:641–652, 1993.

51. How do the growth rates of boys and girls differ?

In both both boys and girls, the rate or velocity of linear growth begins to decelerate at about 2 years of age. In girls, this deceleration continues until approximately age 11 years, at which time the adolescent growth spurt begins. For boys, the deceleration continues until about 13 years. The peak rate of increase in males occurs at age 14 years.

52. What is the best predictor of a child's eventual adult height?

Mid-parental height. This is an estimate of a child's expected genetic growth potential based on parental heights (preferably measured rather than by history).

For girls ([father's height – 13 cm] + [mother's height])/2.

For boys: ([mother's height + 13 cm] + [father's height])/2.

This gives a rough range (± 5 cm) of expected adult height. The predicted height can be compared with the present height percentile and any significant deviation can be a clue of an abnormal growth pattern in a child.

53. When have most children achieved the height percentiles consistent with parental height?

By age two. Rough estimates of ultimate adult height can be obtained by taking a boy's length at age 2 and a girl's length at 18 months and doubling them.

54. Name the seven major categories of causes of short stature.
   1. Familial
   2. Constitutional delay ("late bloomer")
   3. Chronic disease (e.g., inflammatory bowel disease, chronic renal failure, renal tubular acidosis, cyanotic congenital heart disease)
   4. Chromosomal/genetic (e.g., Turner's [45 XO], 18q–, Down, achondroplasia)
   5. Endocrine (e.g., hypothyroidism, growth hormone deficiency, hypopituitarism, hypercortisolism [endogenous and exogenous])
   6. Psychosocial (e.g., chaotic social situation, orphanage)
   7. Intrauterine (e.g., small for gestational age)
   Familial patterns and constitutional delay account for the largest percentage of determined causes.

55. In a child with short stature, what rate of growth makes an endocrinologic cause unlikely?
   Rates of growth are age-dependent. In general, a growth rate of ≥ 6 cm/yr between ages 2–5 years or ≥ 5 cm/yr in children between age 5 and the adolescent growth spurt makes an endocrinologic cause of short stature less likely. The importance of sequential measurements using standard growth charts cannot be underestimated. Growth rates below the 3rd percentile or crossing percentiles downward warrant further investigation.

56 In evaluating a short child, why should you ask about the time the parents reached puberty?
   The age at which puberty occurred in other family members may help identify children with constitutional delay, since this entity tends to run in families. Most women will remember their age at menarche, and this age can be used as a reference for the age at which other pubertal events occurred. The strongest association for pubertal delay is between father and son. The most useful reference point for adult males is the age at which they reached adult height, since almost all normal males will have reached their adult height by 18 years of age (around high school graduation). Significant growth beyond this age suggests a history of pubertal delay.

57. What other historical information is helpful in the diagnosis of short stature?
   The gestational and birth history are often revealing. About one-third of small-for-date infants, while growing at normal rates, remain small throughout childhood and are unlikely to achieve a height consistent with their genetic potential. Girls with Turner syndrome are often short at birth, and many are noted to have edema of the hands and feet in the newborn period.
   A **review of systems** should be undertaken with particular emphasis on systemic disease, intracranial pathology, and medication usage. Growth failure in inflammatory bowel disease may precede the onset of clinical disease by more than a year. Chronic headaches or visual difficulties may presage pituitary or hypothalamic pathology. Frequent use of steroidal hormones may suppress linear growth. Changes in the level of activity, sleeping patterns, or bowel habits can be an early indication of thyroid disease, while failure to change shoe size and excess abdominal obesity suggest a deficiency of growth hormone. An examination of photographs taken of the child and the child's siblings at various ages can be helpful in separating familial changes from clinical problems.
   Access to **previous growth records** is absolutely essential since endocrine diseases affect the rate of linear growth. These records can often by obtained from the school, family physician, child's "baby book," or the door jam in the family home. If records are not available, it is useful to obtain heights every 3 months over a 6–12-month period prior to the initiation of extensive testing. Linear growth rate can be determined from accurate sequential height measurements. It is essential that this process be standardized and that the same observer obtain the measurement.

58. Are upper to lower body ratios helpful in the diagnosis of growth problems?
   Disproportionate short stature generally refers to an inappropriate ratio between truncal length and limb length (upper to lower segment ratio). It is important that the ratio be compared to individuals of similar age and race, because there are both age-related and racial differences in

the ratio. In the infant, the head and trunk are quite long relative to the limbs, so that the ratio of truncal length to limb length is about 1.7.

Throughout childhood this ratio declines, so that by 7–10 years of age this ratio is about 1.0. Variance from the normal ratio may occur in bony dysplasias (e.g., achondroplasia and hypochondroplasia), in certain syndromes (e.g., Marfan syndrome), and after specific types of therapy (e.g., spinal irradiation).

59. What laboratory studies should be obtained when evaluating short stature?

Extensive laboratory tests are generally not indicated unless the growth rate is abnormally low. Laboratory testing may include any or all of the following: complete blood count, urinalysis, chemistry panel, sedimentation rate, thyroxine, TSH, insulin-like growth factor-I (IGF-I), and IGF-binding protein-3 (IGFBP-3).

Random growth hormone levels are of little value because they are generally low in the day-time, even in children of average height. IGF-I (or somatomedin C) mediates the anabolic effects of growth hormone, and levels correlate well with growth hormone status. However, IGF-I can also be low in nonendocrine conditions, such as malnutrition and liver disease.

IGFBP-3, the major binding protein for IGF-I in serum, is also regulated by growth hormone. IGFBP-3 levels generally indicate growth hormone status and are less affected by nutritional factors than IGF-I. Many endocrinologists now use IGF-I and IGFBP-3 as their initial screening tests for GH deficiency.

Rosenfeld RG, et al: Diagnostic controversy: The diagnosis of childhood growth hormone deficiency revisited. J Clin Endocrinol Metab 80:1532–1540, 1995.

Evans AJ: Screening tests for growth hormone deficiency. J R Soc Med 88:161P–165P, 1995.

60. In a very obese child, how does height measurement help to determine whether an endocrinopathy might be the cause?

In children with simple obesity (e.g., familial), linear growth is enhanced, whereas in endocrinopathies it is impaired. If the height of a child is at or greater than mid-parental height percentile, an endocrine cause of the obesity is unlikely.

61. How does a growth chart help in the diagnosis of failure to thrive?

If an infant is demonstrating deceleration of a previously established growth pattern or growth consistently less than the 5th percentile, the pattern of growth of head circumference, height, and weight can help establish the likely cause. There are three main types of impaired growth: Type I (retardation of weight with near-normal or slowly decelerating height and head circumference), Type II (near-proportional retardation of weight and height with normal head circumference), and Type III (concomitant retardation of weight, height, and head circumference). See charts on next page.

From Roy CC, Silverman A, Alagille DA: Pediatric Clinical Gastroenterology, 4th ed. St. Louis, Mosby-Year Book, 1995, pp 4–8; with permission.

62. Why is a bone age determination so helpful in evaluating short stature?

The rate of bony maturation corresponds better with physical development than with chronologic age. Standards of normal skeletal radiographic maturation are available, and all children with possible pathologic short stature should have radiographs obtained for comparison. Generally, a radiograph of the left hand and wrist is obtained, but occasionally a more complete bone age using the knees, elbows, and ankles is required. A single bone age is of value in differentiating familial short stature and genetic diseases, in which bone age is normal, from other causes of short stature. A delayed bone age (> 2 SD below the mean) which correlates with the child's height age (age on growth chart at which child's height would be on the 50th percentile) is suggestive of constitutional delay, while a markedly delayed bone age is suggestive of endocrinologic disease. Serial bone ages each 6–12 months are often helpful, since in both the normal child and the child with constitutional delay, the bone age will advance in parallel with chronologic age. In endocrinologic disease, the bone age falls progressively further behind chronologic age.

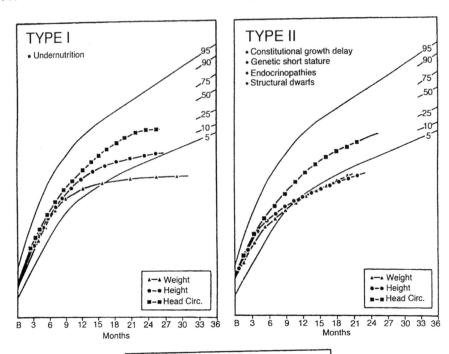

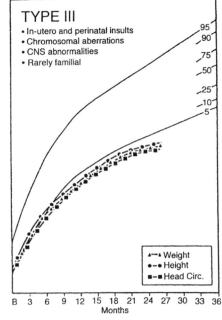

Bone age may be normal or delayed in chronic disease, dependent on the severity of disease, its duration, and type of treatment used.

63. What features suggest constitutional delay as a cause of short stature?
1. No symptoms or signs of systemic disease
2. Bone age delayed up to 2–4 years but consistent with height age
3. Period of poorest growth occurring often from ages 18–30 months, with steady linear growth thereafter (normal rate of growth for bone age)
4. Parental or sibling history of delayed development
5. Height predictions consistent with family characteristics

64. How is constitutional delay managed?
If the results of history, physical examination, and clinical laboratory evaluation are unremarkable, the child is seen once every 3–6 months for accurate height measurements and determination of growth rate. A bone age is done yearly to assess progression of bony maturation. In constitutional delay, the rate of bone maturation should keep pace with chronologic age. In children who are of mid-to-late pubertal ages (girls > 13, boys > 14 yrs) but showing minimal or no signs of puberty, selective use may be made of estrogen or testosterone supplementation to initiate puberty.

65. What are the causes of growth hormone (GH) deficiency?
Growth hormone deficiency can result from isolated defects of GH biosynthesis and release or from a malignancy or structural abnormalities involving the pituitary and hypothalamus. In recent years, it has been increasingly recognized that both chemotherapy and craniospinal irradiation affect GH production. Trauma or disease involving the base of the skull (e.g., Wegener's granulomatosis) may also affect its production.

66. How is growth hormone production tested?
GH production is extremely variable from day to day, even in normal children. Production by the pituitary is affected by a host of factors, including sleep and psychologic state, medications, and nutrition, as well as input from the hypothalamus and higher brain centers. These factors make testing for GH difficult. Furthermore, there is good evidence that specific subsets of children (e.g., those with Turner syndrome) make insufficient GH on a daily basis while they respond normally to pharmacologic stimuli.

Testing for GH can be divided into **pharmacologic stimulation** and **physiologic evaluation**. Stimulation tests rely on specific agents known to cause the normal pituitary to release GH. Extensive protocols are available for this type of testing; the general protocol is to obtain a baseline blood level GH quantitation, followed by administration of the pharmacologic agent, and then repetitive blood specimens are drawn at various times afterward. The limitations of these tests are that (1) they only measure the acutely releasable pool and provide no information on how long the pool took to accumulate; (2) 5–10% of normal children will fail to respond to any single provocative agent; and (3) some children will give a normal response although they do not produce normal amounts of GH on a daily basis.

Physiologic testing potentially provides a more reliable indicator of how the hypothalamic-pituitary axis performs under the "usual" conditions. This testing requires either serial 24-hour urine collections for GH or the collection of blood every 20 minutes for a 12–24-hour period. These studies are problematic because of methodologic issues. For example, the act of withdrawing blood every 20 minutes may be stressful and painful or alter the normal sleep cycle, and these stimuli that may affect pituitary GH production or its regulation.

67. When did growth hormone become available by recombinant DNA technology?
Since 1983, all GH given in the U.S. has been made by recombinant techniques. Before that, U.S. GH was still extracted from collections of human pituitary glands. There were case reports of patients receiving the human-derived hormone who developed Creutzfeldt-Jakob disease, a

neurodegenerative disorder caused by a slow virus or prion (proteinaceous infectious particle) with a long latency period. Many patients may still be at risk. Recombinant therapy has allowed more widespread use of GH in trials for short-stature syndromes (e.g., Turner, Noonan, Prader-Willi, Down syndrome) and children with short stature due to chronic illness.

68. Does the use of growth hormone in patients with short stature unassociated with GH deficiency result in increasing the predicted final adult height?

An ongoing area of study and controversy. In children with idiopathic or familial short stature, the outcome of treatment remains unclear. In these patients, while height velocity increases with the initial use of GH, increased rates of bone maturation may result in height changes less than predicted. It should be noted that the use of an expensive therapy for short patients without GH deficiency remains heavily debated.

Furlanetto RW, et al: Guidelines for the use of growth hormone in children with short stature. J Pediatrics 127:857–867, 1995.

69. What are the clinical manifestations of growth hormone excess?

Prior to puberty, the cardinal manifestations are an increase in growth velocity with minimal bone deformity and soft tissue swelling—a condition called **pituitary gigantism**. Hypogonadotropic hypogonadism and delayed puberty often coexist with GH excess, and affected children exhibit eunuchoid body proportions. If the GH excess occurs after puberty (after epiphyseal closure), the more typical features of **acromegaly** occur, including coarsening of the facial features and soft tissue swelling of the feet and hands. GH excess is rare in children.

70. List the causes of tall stature.

Constitutional (familial)

Endocrine causes
    Somatotropin excess (pituitary gigantism)
    Androgen excess (tall as children,
        short as adults)
        True sexual precocity
        Pseudosexual precocity
    Androgen deficiency (normal height
        as children, tall as adults)
        Klinefelter syndrome
        Anorchia (infection, trauma, idiopathic)
    Hyperthyroidism

Genetic causes
    Klinefelter syndrome
    Syndromes of XYY, XXYY
        (tall as adults)

Miscellaneous syndromes and entities
    Marfan syndrome
    Cerebral gigantism (Soto syndrome)
    Total lipodystrophy
    Diencephalic syndrome
    Homocystinuria

From Gotlin RW, et al: Endocrine disorders. In Hay WW, et al (eds): Current Pediatric Diagnosis and Treatment, 12th ed. Norwalk, CT, Appleton & Lange, 1995, p 885; with permission.

HYPOGLYCEMIA

71. How is hypoglycemia defined?

A serum glucose of < 50 mg/100 ml is defined as hypoglycemia in childhood. Some argue for lower levels being used for term and preterm infants; however, these arguments are based on population sampling data rather than on physiology. Hypoglycemia is a laboratory finding, and its presence should lead to a diligent search for the underlying pathology.

72. Describe the clinical findings associated with hypoglycemia.

Neuroglycopenic symptoms include irritability, headache, confusion, unconsciousness, and seizure. Adrenergic signs include tachycardia, tremulousness, diaphoresis, and hunger. Any combination of the above signs and symptoms should lead to the measurement of the blood glucose level.

73. What are the causes of childhood hypoglycemia?

No single cause predominates in any age group. Therefore, the entire differential diagnosis must be considered in any child who presents with hypoglycemia.

Differential Diagnosis of Childhood Hypoglycemia

Increased glucose utilization
    Hyperinsulinism—islet-cell adenoma or hyperplasia (nesidioblastosis), oral hypoglycemic agents, exogenous insulin

Decreased glucose production
    Inadequate glycogen reserves—enzymatic defects in glycogen synthesis and glycogenolysis
    Ineffective gluconeogenesis—inadequate substrate, (e.g., ketotic hypoglycemia), enzymatic defects

Diminished availability of fats
    Depleted fat stores
    Failure to mobilize fats (e.g., hyperinsulinism)
    Defective utilization of fats—enzymatic defects in fatty acid oxidation (e.g., medium-chain acyl CoA dehydrogenase deficiency)

Decreased fuels and fuel stores
    Fasting, malnutrition, prolonged illness, malabsorption

Increased fuel demand
    Fever, exercise

Inadequate counter-regulatory hormones
    Growth hormone or cortisol deficiency, hypopituitarism

---

74. An unconscious 3-year-old is brought to the emergency department with a serum glucose concentration of 26 mg/dl. What other laboratory tests should be done?

The principal laboratory evaluations should include the measurement of (1) the metabolic compounds associated with fasting adaptation, (2) the hormones that regulate these processes, and (3) drugs that can interfere with glucose regulation.

A 3-ml red-top tube of blood can be sent for measurement of:
- Markers of principal regulatory hormones: insulin, growth hormone, cortisol
- Markers of fatty acid metabolism: ketones (β-hydroxybutyrate and acetoacetate), free fatty acids, total and free carnitine
- Markers of gluconeogenic pathways: lactate, pyruvate, alanine

Urine can be tested for:
- Ketones
- Metabolic byproducts associated with known causes of hypoglycemia (e.g., organic acids, amino acids)
- Toxicology screen, especially for alcohol, salicylates

Taken together, these tests provide valuable clues as to the cause. For example, low levels of ketones and free fatty acids suggest that fat was not appropriately mobilized. As a consequence, ketones were not formed by the liver. Those biochemical abnormalities are seen in hyperinsulinemic states and can be confirmed by documenting a high level of circulating insulin. Low urinary ketones also suggest an enzymatic defect in fatty acid oxidation.

If appropriate studies are not obtained at the time of presentation and the cause remains unknown, a careful fasting study must be undertaken to evaluate fasting adaptation, since repeated profound hypoglycemic episodes are associated with significant morbidity and mortality.

75. In patients with acute hypoglycemia, what are the treatment options?

The principal acute treatment is provision of **glucose** orally or intravenously. If the patient is alert, orange juice or cola (4–8 oz) may be given. If the patient is obtunded, intravenous glucose (2–3 ml/kg of $D_{10}W$ or 1 ml/kg of $D_{25}W$) should be administered rapidly. If venous access cannot be achieved promptly, glucose can be provided via a nasogastric tube, as glucose is rapidly absorbed from the gut. The risk of prolonged hypoglycemia far outweighs the risk associated with passage of a nasogastric tube in an obtunded patient. Subsequently, the blood sugar should be monitored closely and, if necessary, maintained by the constant infusion of glucose (6–8 mg/kg/min). $D_{10}W$ given at about 1.5 times maintenance dose approximates that glucose rate. Larger quantities may be necessary, and the blood sugar should be closely followed.

Glucagon promotes glycogen breakdown. In settings where glycogen stores have not been depleted (e.g., insulin overdose), 1 mg of glucagon intramuscularly or subcutaneously will raise blood glucose levels.

Glucocorticoids should not be used routinely. Their only clear indication is in known primary or secondary adrenal insufficiency. In other settings, they have little acute value and may cloud the diagnostic process.

HYPOTHALAMIC/PITUITARY DISORDERS

76. What clinical signs or symptoms suggest hypothalamic dysfunction?

The signs and symptoms of hypothalamic dysfunction are as variable as the processes controlled by the hypothalamus, ranging from disorders of hormonal production to disturbances of thermoregulation. Precocious or delayed sexual maturation represent the most common presentations of hypothalamic endocrine abnormality in childhood. Diabetes insipidus, psychic disturbances, and excessive sleepiness are found in about one-third of all patients with hypothalamic dysfunction and may be the first manifestation of disease. Eating disorders (obesity, anorexia, bulimia) and convulsions are also reported. Dyshidrosis and disturbances of sphincteric control are occasionally seen.

77. List the intracranial or systemic processes that can interfere with hypothalamic-pituitary function.

Intracranial
- Congenital
  Inherited deficiencies of gonadotropin-releasing factor (GnRF), growth-hormone-releasing hormone (GHRH)
  Syndromic—Laurence-Moon-Biedl, Prader-Labhart-Willi syndromes
  Structural—craniopharyngioma, Rathke pouch cyst, hemangioma, hamartoma
- Infectious—meningitis, encephalitis
- Tumors—glioma, dysgerminoma, ependymoma
- Trauma—subarachnoid or intraventricular hemorrhage, surgical stalk section
- Idiopathic

Systemic
- CNS abnormality demonstrable by scan or biopsy
  Kernicterus, congenital infection, sarcoidosis, Langerhans cell histiocytosis (eosinophilic granuloma), tuberculosis, neurofibromatosis, leukemia
- CNS involvement is functional
  Anorexia nervosa, psychosocial dwarfism, chronic illness

78. What is the significance of an enlarged sella turcica on a skull film?

The sella turcica derives its name from the Latin words for *Turkish saddle*. The name reflects the anatomic shape of the saddle-like prominence on the upper surface of the sphenoid bone in the middle cranial fossa above which sits the pituitary gland. A variety of conditions can lead to sellar enlargement, including tumors of the pituitary or functional hypertrophy of the pituitary, which may occur in primary hypothyroidism or primary hypogonadism. Modern imaging techniques have supplanted the skull series as a tool for searching for pituitary or hypothalamic disease; however, an enlarged sella may be noted on children in whom skull series are obtained for other reasons (i.e., head trauma).

79. Which tests are useful in studying suspected hypothalamic and pituitary malfunction?

The choice of tests depends on the spectrum of historical features and clinical findings, but it is essential to rule out structural pathology prior to searching for functional abnormalities. Skull films are not adequate for this purpose; therefore, either an **MRI** or **CT scan** is required.

Studies of the pituitary-hypothalamus may include any or all of the following:

1. **Prolactin.** Random levels tend to be elevated in the presence of hypothalamic lesions. A normal level does not rule out structural abnormalities.

2. **Thyrotropin-releasing hormone provocative test (TRH test).** TRH normally promotes the rapid release of thyroid-stimulating hormone (TSH) by the pituitary. In the presence of pituitary or hypothalamic dysfunction, the release of TSH is often blunted and delayed. TRH also promotes release of prolactin. In hypothalamic dysfunction, the prolactin response is often altered as well.

3. **Growth hormone production tests** (see Question 65). These tests are generally indicated only if the child's growth rate is subnormal. Growth hormone releasing factor is now available for testing the pituitary responsiveness. It has proven useful, in some instances, in delineating pituitary causes of growth hormone underproduction from primary hypothalamic disease.

4. **Gonadotropin-releasing hormone (GnRH) provocative test.** Random levels of leuteinizing hormone and follicle-stimulating hormone are not generally helpful if one is searching for pituitary hypofunction. The results of the GnRH test must be correlated with the age of the child, since there are developmental changes in the response to GnRH.

5. **Metyrapone test** (see Question 7).

6. Simultaneous **urine and serum osmolalities.** A normal serum osmolality and a concentrated urine osmolality tend to rule out diabetes insipidus. If these results are equivocal, a water deprivation test may be required.

SEXUAL DIFFERENTIATION AND DEVELOPMENT

80. An infant is born with suspected ambiguous genitalia. What features of history and physical examination are key in the evaluation?

History: One should search for evidence of maternal androgen ingestion (rare now, but common in the 1960s with certain progestational agents), other hormonal use (e.g., for infertility or endometriosis), alcohol use, parental consanguinity, previous neonatal deaths, or a family history of previously affected children.

Physical examination: The presence of a gonadal structure in the labioscrotal fold strongly implies the presence of some Y chromosomal material. Gonads containing both ovarian and testicular components (ovotestes) have been found in the inguinal canal. However, it is rare to find an ovary in the inguinal canal. In the absence of a palpable gonad, no conclusions can be drawn regarding probable chromosomal sex. The size of the phallic structure and the location of the urethral meatus provide no information regarding genetic or chromosomal make-up. However, phallic size and function are important considerations when determining gender-of-rearing.

The presence of midline abnormalities (e.g., cleft palate) suggests hypothalamic or pituitary dysfunction, while congenital anomalies such as imperforate anus suggest structural derangements. Digital rectal exam will confirm the patency of the anus and may allow palpation of the uterus. Other anomalies should be noted since ambiguous genitalia can be a feature of numerous syndromes.

81. What is the most common cause of ambiguous genitalia?

There are numerous causes of ambiguous genitalia, and no particular cause appears to predominate. Nature is capable of endless variety; therefore, great caution must be exercised in assigning a diagnosis and gender to an affected child.

Undervirilized male (XY karyotype)

- Androgen resistance
    - Complete—testicular feminization
    - Partial
- Defects in androgen synthesis
    - 3β-Hydroxysteroid dehydrogenase deficiency
    - 5α-Reductase deficiency

Virilized female (XX karyotype)
• Excess androgen
  Congenital adrenal hyperplasia
    21-Hydroxylase deficiency
    3β-Hydroxysteroid dehydrogenase deficiency
  Maternal androgen exposure
    Medication
    Virilizing adrenal tumor
Intersex (mosaic karyotypes; e.g., XO/XY)
Structural abnormalities

82. Which studies are essential in the evaluation of ambiguous genitalia?

1. *Ultrasonography:* This test is the most helpful in identifying internal structures, particularly the uterus and occasionally the ovaries. The absence of a uterus suggests that testes were present early in gestation and produced müllerian-inhibiting factor, causing regression of the müllerian-derived ducts (and thus the uterus). The injection of contrast medium into the urethrovaginal opening(s) will often demonstrate a pouch posterior to the fused labioscrotal folds. Occasionally, the cervix and cervical canal will be highlighted by this study as well.

2. *Chromosomal analysis:* Obviously useful in predicting gonadal content. Of note, buccal smears searching for clumps of nuclear membrane chromatin (Barr bodies), representing the inactive X chromosome in girls, should not be used (even preliminarily) because of their high rates of inaccuracy.

3. *Measurement of adrenal steroids* (17-hydroxyprogesterone, 11-deoxycortisol, 17-hydroxypregnenolone). 17-Hydroxyprogesterone is the precursor elevated in the most common variety of congenital adrenal hyperplasia associated with ambiguous genitalia (21-hydroxylase deficiency).

4. *Measurement of testosterone and dihydrotestosterone* (DHT).

As important and useful as the testing is, it is also useful to have input from staff with expertise in this area, including a geneticist, pediatric endocrinologist, and pediatric urologist. It is also essential that information be synthesized by this group after all data are available and that it be communicated to the family by a single spokesperson.

83. What major criteria are used to define a micropenis?

To be classified as a micropenis, the phallus must meet two major criteria:

1. The phallus must be normally formed, with the urethral meatus located on the head of the penis and the penis positioned in an appropriate relationship to the scrotum and other pelvic structures. If these features are not present, then the term micropenis should be avoided.

2. The phallus must be > 2.5 SD below the appropriate mean for age. For a term newborn, this means that a penis < 2 cm in stretched length is classified as a micropenis.

It is essential that the phallus be measured appropriately. This entails the use of a rigid ruler pressed firmly against the pubic symphysis, depressing the suprapubic fat pad as much as possible. The phallus is grasped gently by its lateral margins and stretched. The measurement is taken along the dorsum of the penis. Note should also be made of the breadth of the phallic shaft. Micropenis must be recognized early in life so that appropriate diagnostic testing can be done.

   Lee PA, et al: Micropenis. I. Criteria, etiologies and classification. Johns Hopkins Med J 146:156–163, 1980.

84. What causes a micropenis?

Regression of the müllerian system, fusion of the labioscrotal folds, and migration of the urethral meatus occur during the first trimester of gestation. Further growth of the phallus during the second and third trimester is dependent on the production of testosterone by the fetal testis in response to fetal pituitary luteinizing hormone (LH). Growth hormone also enhances penile growth in utero. Thus, the following disorders can result in micropenis:

• Hypothalamic/pituitary dysfunction—isolated, Kallmann syndrome, Prader-Willi syndrome, septo-optic dysplasia

- Testicular dysfunction or failure—intrauterine testicular torsion (vanishing testes syndrome), testicular dysplasia
- Complex (testicular and/or pituitary) or idiopathic—Robinow, Klinefelter, other X polysomies
- Partial androgen resistance

85. Outline the three main concerns in the initial evaluation of a 1-month-old with micropenis.

1. *Is there a defect in the hypothalamic-pituitary-gonadal axis?* Specific tests include measurement of testosterone, dihydrotestosterone, LH, and follicle-stimulating hormone (FSH). Because circulating levels of these hormones are normally quite high in the neonatal period, measurement of random levels during the first 2 months of life may be useful in identifying diseases of the testes and pituitary. Beyond 3 months of age, the tests are generally not useful because the entire axis becomes quiescent and remains so until late childhood. Depending on the patient's age, provocative tests may be necessary including: (a) repetitive testosterone injection to evaluate the ability of the penis to respond to hormonal stimulation, (b) use of human chorionic gonadotropin (hCG) as a stimulus for testosterone production by the testes, and (c) GnRH administration to examine the responsiveness of the pituitary to stimulation. The trial of testosterone therapy is especially important because it indicates whether phallic growth is possible, and if not, gender reassignment becomes a consideration.

2. *Does a possible pituitary deficiency involve other hormones?* Isolated growth hormone deficiency, gonadotropin deficiency, and panhypopituitarism have been associated with micropenis. The presence of hypoglycemia, hypothermia, or hyperbilirubinemia (e.g., associated with hypothyroidism) in a child with micropenis should lead one to search for other pituitary hormone deficits and structural abnormalities of the CNS (e.g., septo-optic dysplasia).

3. *Is there a renal abnormality?* Because of the association of genital and renal abnormalities and nature's endless variations, it may be important in some cases to obtain an abdominal and pelvic ultrasound to better define the internal anatomy.

86. Review the spectrum of androgen resistance syndromes.

In males, the testis-determining factor (TDF, formerly "HY antigen") is encoded on the short arm of the Y chromosome. TDF induces the gonads to develop into testes. In the testes, Sertoli cells secrete müllerian inhibiting factor (MIF), and the müllerian ducts (responsible for the proximal vagina, uterus, and fallopian tubes) regress. Leydig cells secrete testosterone, which maintains the wolffian ducts (responsible for seminiferous tubules). Testosterone is converted by 5α-reductase to dihydrotestosterone (DHT), which virilizes the urogenital sinus and external genitalia. If there is no TDF, the cascade does not begin and the internal and external development is female.

Androgen resistance syndromes usually refer to peripheral defects, which can vary from a lack of receptors (androgen insensitivity) to a deficiency in 5α-reductase. In complete androgen insensitivity (testicular feminization), an XY male appears externally to be completely female. Because MIF production has also occurred, no internal female organs are present. Affected individuals often present at adolescence with primary amenorrhea. In 5α-reductase deficiency, external virilization of the genitalia is incomplete, and these children usually present at birth with ambiguous genitalia.

Griffin JE: Androgen resistance—The clinical and molecular spectrum. N Engl J Med 326:611, 1992.

87. If a third grade girl, age 9, develops breast buds and pubic hair, is this normal or precocious?

Precocious puberty is the appearance of physical changes associated with sexual development earlier than normal. In practical terms, this means the appearance of breast buds (Tanner stage II) and pubic hair (Tanner stage II) before 8 years of age in the female. Any vaginal bleeding occurring before age 10 years is suspicious, especially if it is not preceded by significant breast and pubic hair development. In the male, the appearance of pubic hair or genital development before 9 years is considered precocious.

88. Breast buds are noted on a 2-year-old girl. Is this worrisome?

Premature thelarche, or the development of breast buds, is the most common variation of normal pubertal development. A form of mild estrogenization, it typically occurs between ages 1 and 4. It is usually benign and should not be associated with the onset of other pubertal events. Precocious puberty, rather than simple premature thelarche, should be suspected if:
- Breast, nipple, and areolar development reach Tanner III stage
- Androgenization with pubic and/or axillary hair begins
- Linear growth accelerates

Ongoing parental observation and periodic re-examination are all that are required if there are no signs of progression.

89. How should a 6-year-old with axillary hair be evaluated?

The growth of axillary hair is stimulated by androgen. Therefore, a **history** should be taken, searching for possible androgen exposure or other evidence of androgenization, such as increased oiliness of skin, adult-type body odor or acne. Information should be gathered about the progression of these changes and any accompanying factors such as mood swings and accelerated growth rates. The **family history** should be reviewed for individuals who were early maturers or who are excessively hirsute, since many partial forms of adrenal hyperplasia are familial. **Physical examination** should search for other evidence of androgenization, such as facial or pubic hair, enlargement of the phallus, or acne. In girls, the stage of breast development and vaginal estrogenization should be noted. In boys, testicular volume and scrotal development should be determined. If axillary hair is the only finding on physical examination, no further investigation is warranted, and the child should return in 3–4 months for re-evaluation of progression and height velocity.

90. On re-evaluation of this 6-year-old, there are now signs of progression. How should you proceed?

Girl: If there is additional evidence of both androgenization and estrogenization, then the approach is essentially that for precocious puberty. If only androgenization is seen, then the most likely source is the adrenal (although the ovary does contribute to androgen production). The differential diagnosis in this case is simple premature adrenarche, a partial defect in adrenal steroid production, or androgen-producing tumor of the adrenal or ovary. Premature adrenarche is by far the most common of these problems and is characterized by gradual progression of pubertal changes, usually accompanied by a slightly accelerated rate of growth and bone maturation. The evaluation of this girl would include an adrenal androgen panel (17-OH progesterone, 17-OH pregnenolone, dehydroepiandrosterone sulfate [DHEA-S], androstenedione) and bone age. Mild elevations of DHEA-S are the typical finding in premature adrenarche, while more marked elevation of one or more of the precursors is anticipated in the partial defects in adrenal steroid biosynthesis.

Boy: The evaluation depends on whether there is testicular enlargement. If testicular enlargement is bilateral, then the evaluation is that for central precocious puberty. If only one testes is enlarged, this raises concerns about testicular pathology. Testosterone is likely to be elevated above the prepubertal range. If there is no testicular enlargement, then the most probable source of androgen is the adrenal. In this case, an adrenal androgen panel and bone age should be obtained.

Winter JS: Hyperandrogenism in female adolescents. Curr Opin Pediatr 5:488–493, 1993.

Kletter GB, Kelch RP: Disorders of puberty in boys. Endocrinol Metab Clin North Am 22:425–477, 1993.

91. Which aspects of the physical exam are particularly important in evaluating a patient with precocious puberty?

1. *Evidence of CNS mass:* examination of optic fundus for possible increased intracranial pressure; visual fields testing for evidence of optic nerve compression by a hypothalamic or pituitary mass

2. *Evidence of androgenic influence:* presence of acne, facial and axillary hair; increased muscle bulk and definition; extent of other body/pubic hair; in boys, increased scrotal rugation accompanied by thinning and pigmentation, penile elongation

3. *Evidence of estrogenic influence:* size of breast tissue and nipple/areolar contouring; vaginal mucosa color (increased estrogen causes cornification of vaginal epithelium with a color change from prepubertal shiny red to a more opalescent pink); labia minor (become more prominent and visible between the labia majora as puberty progresses)

4. *Evidence of gonadotropic stimulation:* testicular enlargement > 2.5 cm in length or > 4 ml in volume (preferably measured using a Prader orchidometer of labeled volumetric beads). Of note, pubertal development without testicular enlargement usually suggests adrenal pathology.

5. *Evidence of other mass:* asymmetric testicular enlargement; hepatomegaly; abdominal mass

92. Which radiologic and laboratory tests are indicated for evaluation of precocious puberty?

The evaluation may often be costly and complex, and in most cases, a specific cause will not be identified. As a general rule, the younger the child and the more rapid the onset of the condition, the greater the likelihood of detecting pathology. While precocious puberty occurs 80% of the time in girls, boys are more likely to have identifiable pathology.

Radiologic evaluation

1. *Bone age:* This study helps to determine the duration of exposure to the elevated sex hormone. A significantly advanced bone age compared with chronologic age suggests long-term exposure.

2. *Abdominal and pelvic ultrasound:* In boys, this test identifies possible adrenal masses, and in girls, adrenal masses, ovarian masses, or cysts. Increased uterine size and echogenicity suggest endometrial proliferation in response to circulating estrogen.

Laboratory

1. LH, FSH, estradiol, testosterone

2. Adrenal steroid levels (17-hydroxyprogesterone, androstenedione, cortisol). More extensive testing may be needed in a virilized child if the initial studies are normal.

3. Provocative testing of the hypothalamic-pituitary axis (using a synthetic GnRH) or of the adrenal gland (using an ACTH agonist [cosyntropin]) may be needed, especially in the child presenting with slight but progressive pubertal changes.

Rosenfield RL: Puberty and its disorders in girls. Endocrinol Metab Clin North Am 20:15–42, 1991.

Kappy MS, Ganong CS: Advances in the treatment of precocious puberty. Adv Pediatr 41:223–261, 1994.

93. Discuss the terms denoting aspects of precocious sexual development.

The terms used to describe precocious puberty reflect the fact that normal puberty is an orderly process by which female children are feminized and male children masculinized. The development of breast tissue without pubic hair is called *premature thelarche.* If pubic hair subsequently develops, the term *precocious puberty* is used. If pubic hair develops without breast tissue, it is *premature pubarche.* Since pubic hair development in the female is thought to be due to adrenal androgens, the term *premature adrenarche* is commonly used. If the pubertal changes are early and appear to proceed in the orderly fashion of breast budding, pubic hair development, growth spurt, and finally menstruation, the term *true precocious puberty* is used. When some of the changes of puberty are present but their appearance is isolated or out of normal sequence (e.g., menses without breast development), the term *pseudo-precocious puberty* is used. When the changes of puberty are consistent with the child's gender, they are called *isosexual;* when they are discordant with gender, they are *heterosexual.*

To illuminate, the child with 3-cm breast buds bilaterally and no pubic hair could be labeled using any of the following terms: premature thelarche, "early" precocious puberty, isosexual precocious puberty, and some others.

THYROID DISORDERS

94. Which thyroid function tests are standard?

Diseases of the thyroid represent a heterogeneous group of disorders. As such, there are no "standard" thyroid function studies appropriate for all children with suspected thyroid disease. The choice of laboratory tests is based on the results of a careful history and physical examination.

Clinical findings suggesting **hyperthyroidism:** A thyroid-stimulating hormone (TSH) and thyroxine (T_4) level should be obtained. TSH suppression is probably the most sensitive indictor of hyperthyroid status. If the patient is symptomatic and has a suppressed TSH with a normal T_4, it will be necessary to obtain a triiodothyronine (T_3) radioimmunoassay, since cases of T_3-thyrotoxicosis do occur. If the patient is asymptomatic but has an elevated T_4, then some measure of binding capacity should be obtained, such as a T_3 uptake.

Clinical findings consistent with **hypothyroidism:** The laboratory evaluation consists of the quantitation of T_4 and TSH. A low T_4 and elevated TSH are diagnostic of hypothyroidism.

95. What is the significance of anti-thyroid antibodies in children?

In the pediatric population, **chronic lymphocytic thyroiditis** is the most common cause of **hypothyroidism**. The antibodies that are generally available as markers for this condition include antimicrosomial, antithyroglobulin, and antithyroidal peroxidase antibodies. Most laboratories will run at least 2 of these assays. A titer > 1:2000 on any assay provides strong evidence in favor of the diagnosis, but the absence of antibodies does not rule out chronic lymphocytic thyroiditis. High titers may be seen in Graves disease. Low titers may be present with a wide range of systemic diseases, particularly autoimmune processes.

Nordyke RA, et al: The superiority of antimicrosomal over antithyroglobulin antibodies for detecting Hashimoto's thyroiditis. Arch Intern Med 153:862–865, 1993.

96. Of what value is the T_3 resin uptake (T_3RU) test?

The T_3RU test is a measure of serum thyroid-binding capacity. Because T_4 is primarily protein-bound, only a small amount exists in the unbound (free) state. Physiologically, the free T_4 is the metabolically active compound, but it is technically complex to assay directly. In most cases, it has proved simpler to measure T_3RU and total T_4 and to calculate the amount of T_4 that is unbound. In primary thyroidal disease, the T_3RU and the T_4 should go in the same direction (i.e., both increased or both decreased). If they go in opposite directions, it is probably a binding problem.

97. Which signs and symptoms in an infant suggest congenital hypothyroidism?

Symptoms	Signs
Lethargy	Hypotonia, slow reflexes
Poor feeding	Poor weight gain
Prolonged jaundice	Jaundice
Constipation	Distended abdomen
Mottling	Acrocyanosis
Cold extremities	Coarse features
	Large fontanels/wide sutures
	Hoarse cry
	Goiter

98. What causes congenital hypothyroidism?

- Primary—agenesis/dysgenesis, ectopic, dyshormonogenesis
- Secondary—hypopituitarism, hypothalamic abnormality

- Other
  Transient
  Maternal factors—goitrogen ingestion, iodide deficiency
  Autoimmune thyroiditis
  Pseudo-hypothyroidism—thyroid-binding globulin (TBG) deficiency, prematurity,
  euthyroid sick syndrome

99. How common is goiter in newborns with congenital hypothyroidism?

Congenital goiter is seen in only 20% of newborns with congenital hypothyroidism. Maternal ingestion of antithyroid medications, iodides, and goitrogens, congenital thyroid dyshormonogenic defects, and congenital hyperthyroidism are associated with palpable thyromegaly. Goiter in the newborn is difficult to recognize because of the infant's relatively short neck and increased subcutaneous fat. Palpation of the neck is often overlooked in newborn exams.

100. How effective are screening programs for congenital hypothyroidism?

Screening programs correctly identify 90–95% of children affected with congenital hypothyroidism. Screening programs are most likely to miss infants with large ectopic glands, those with partial defects in thyroidal hormone biosynthesis, and individuals with secondary (pituitary or hypothalamic) disease. If an infant presents with a clinical picture of hypothyroidism and has had a normal newborn screen, it is important to realize that the false-negative rate of the screening is up to 10%.

101. What drug preparations are recommended for thyroid replacement therapy in children with congenital or acquired hypothyroidism?

L-Thyroxine is the medication of choice for treatment of hypothyroidism. Infants generally need higher doses relative to body weight than do older children. The smallest available tablets are 25 μg, which are scored. There is no oral suspension. L-Thyroxine is readily soluble in liquid and can be crushed and dissolved immediately prior to administration.

Initial Dosages for Thyroid Replacement in Infants

WEIGHT (kg)	L-THYROXINE (μg)
< 3.5	25
3.5–5.0	37.5
5.0–7.5	50
7.5–10.0	62.5
10.0–20.0	75
> 20.0	2–3 μg/kg

After therapy is started, thyroid tests (T_4, TSH) should be repeated in 4–6 weeks, and the dosage adjusted according to test results and clinical findings. Optimally, the TSH should be normalized. In infants with congenital hypothyroidism, this goal is not always achievable without making the child clinically hyperthyroid. In that circumstance, the T_4 value should be maintained in the upper half of the normal range for age, and trends in the TSH can be followed.

102. Discuss the risks in delaying treatment for congenital hypothyroidism.

Therapy should begin as early as possible because outcome is related to the time treatment is started. Because < 20% of patients will have distinctive clinical signs at 3–4 weeks of age, screening is now performed on all newborns in the United States at 2–3 days of age, and most affected children are started on therapy prior to 1 months of age. The prognosis for intellectual development is directly related to the amount of time from birth to the initiation of therapy. Children begun on hormone replacement at < 30 days of age have a mean IQ of 106, but those whose treatment started at 3–6 months have a mean IQ of 70.

103. If a goiter is noted during a routine exam of an asymptomatic 7-year-old boy, what should be the next course of action?

The evaluation of a child with goiter is generally simple. In the absence of signs of thyroidal disease, history should be obtained regarding recent exposure to iodine or other halogens. A family history should be obtained regarding thyroidal disease since thyroiditis tends to run in families. The initial laboratory evaluation is typically T_4, TSH, and anti-thyroidal antibodies. If there is discrete nodularity within the thyroid or the gland is rock hard or tender, then further diagnostic evaluation (ultrasound, CT scan) may be indicated. Parathyroid enlargement or lymphoma may be misdiagnosed as a goiter.

104. What are the causes of acquired hypothyroidism in childhood?

The most common cause is chronic lymphocytic thyroiditis.

Common Causes of Acquired Thyroid Disease in Childhood and Adolescence

Chronic lymphocytic thyroiditis (autoimmune thyroiditis, Hashimoto thyroiditis)

Associated with chromosomal abnormalities (e.g., trisomy 21, Turner syndrome)

Associated with other endocrine diseases
  Diabetes mellitus, hypoadrenalism (Schmidt syndrome)
  Autoimmune polyendocrine syndromes

Associated with congenital infection (e.g., rubella, toxoplasmosis)

Subacute thyroiditis (DeQuervain), postviral

Goitrogen ingestion (e.g., iodides, expectorants, thioureas)

Thyroid removal or I^{131} ablation

Infiltrative disease (e.g., cystinosis, Langerhans cell histiocytosis)

Hypothalamic or pituitary disease

"Late onset" congenital (e.g., large ectopic)

Pseudohypothyroidism (e.g., TBG deficiency, peripheral resistance to thyroid hormone, euthyroid sick syndrome)

Lafranci S: Thyroiditis and acquired hypothyroidism. Pediatr Ann 21:29, 32–39, 1992.
Rapoport B: Pathophysiology of Hashimoto's thyroiditis and hypothyroidism. Annu Rev Med 42:91–96, 1991.

105. What is the most common clinical presentation of Hashimoto thyroiditis?

Chronic lymphocytic thyroiditis (CLT), also called Hashimoto disease or autoimmune thyroiditis, is the most common thyroid problem in children and is thought to be caused by an autoimmune organ-specific process. Although symptoms of hypo- or hyperthyroidism may be present, the preponderance of pediatric patients are asymptomatic, and the condition is detected by the presence of a goiter.

106. Are the antibodies in chronic lymphocytic thyroiditis a cause or effect?

The diagnosis of CLT is primarily based on the demonstration of antithyroglobulin and/or antimicrosomal antibody in high titers (> 1:2000). These antibodies are not the cause of the thyroiditis, but instead they simply reflect the immunologic response to release of intracellular and intrafollicular elements into the bloodstream. Low titers of anti-thyroidal antibodies may be observed in other thyroid diseases (e.g., Graves) and in children with systemic autoimmune processes (e.g., systemic lupus erythematosus). Antibodies may not be detectable in 10–20% of individuals with CLT.

Weetman AP: Autoimmune thyroiditis: Predisposition and pathogenesis. Clin Endocrinol 36:307–323, 1992.
McLachlan SM, Rapoport B: The molecular biology of thyroid peroxidase; Cloning, expression and role of autoantigen in autoimmune thyroid disease. Endocr Rev 13:192–206, 1992.

107. What should a parent be told about the prognosis of a child who has euthyroid goiter caused by chronic lymphocytic thyroiditis?

About half of all children who present with euthyroid goiter will have resolution of the goiter over several years regardless of whether or not thyroxine replacement is given. However, it is not possible to predict which children will recover completely, which will remain euthyroid with goiter, and which will become hypothyroid. Any child identified with thyroid disease should have T_4 and TSH values monitored yearly.

108. What other autoimmune endocrine diseases are associated with chronic lymphocytic thyroiditis?

Adrenal insufficiency (Schmidt syndrome), diabetes mellitus, and autoimmune polyendocrine syndrome (Type II).

109. What does a normal T_4 and an elevated TSH suggest?

The diagnosis of hypothyroidism is based on finding both a low T_4 and an elevated TSH. However, on occasion, the T_4 can be maintained in a normal range by increased stimulation of the thyroid gland by TSH. This combination of laboratory values is suggestive of a failing thyroid and is referred to as **compensated hypothyroidism**. Since TSH is the most useful physiologic marker for the adequacy of a circulating level of thyroid hormone, an elevated TSH is an indication for thyroid replacement therapy. If the TSH is only minimally elevated and the child is asymptomatic, it is worthwhile to wait 4–6 weeks and repeat the T_4 and TSH levels before instituting therapy.

110. What is the most common cause of hyperthyroidism in children?

Graves disease is a multisystem disease characterized by hyperthyroidism, infiltrative ophthalmopathy, and, occasionally, an infiltrative dermopathy. The features of this disease may occur singly or in any combination. In the pediatric population, the ophthalmopathy seems to be less severe, and the dermopathy is rare. The full syndrome may never develop. There has been a tendency to use the terms Graves disease, thyrotoxicosis, and hyperthyroidism interchangeably, but there are many other causes of hyperthyroidism in childhood.

Non-Graves Causes of Hyperthyroidism in Children

Excess TSH	Thyroid inflammation
TSH producing tumor	Subacute thyroiditis
Abnormal thyroid stimulation	Hashimoto thyroiditis
TSH receptor antibody	Exogenous hormone
Thyroid autonomy	Hormone ingestion
Adenoma	Ectopic thyroid tissue
Multinodular goiter	

111. Describe the typical features of hyperthyroidism due to Graves disease.

History: The onset of symptoms is usually gradual, with increasing emotional lability and deteriorating school performance. Since the onset of Graves disease and puberty may coincide, many parents initially attribute the psychologic changes to adolescence. The younger child may simply be thought to be "hyperactive." Sleep disturbances, nervousness, and weight loss may be noted as well as easy fatigability and heat intolerance. Observation of the child's behavior while the history is being obtained from the parent is often instructive.

Physical examination: The oral temperature may be slightly increased (100°F). Weight may be low for height, and many children will be tall for age and genetic potential. Some children will have experienced an acceleration in growth rate at the same time that their behavior began to deteriorate. However, the onset of puberty may be delayed or accelerated. The pulse rate is usually inappropriately high for age. A widened pulse pressure or elevated blood pressure is often noted, although this is a more variable finding in children than in adults. A hyperactive pre-cordium may accompany the changes in blood pressure, and a functional systolic murmur may be heard. Two- to fourfold thyroid enlargement is a consistent finding. The thyroid is usually firm, symmetrical, smooth, and nontender. The presence of a discrete node or area of tenderness warrants further investigation.

Sills IN: Hyperthyroidism. Pediatr Rev 15:417–421, 1994.

112. What causes Graves disease?

Graves disease is an autoimmune disorder in which TSH receptor antibodies bind to the TSH receptor, resulting in stimulation of thyroid hormone production and subsequent hyperthy-roidism. Most thyroid receptor antibodies belong to the IgG class. The general name used for these antibodies is **human thyroid-stimulating immunoglobulins**, formerly called long-acting thyroid stimulator.

113. How is the hyperthyroidism of Graves disease distinguished from that occasionally found in chronic lymphocytic thyroiditis?

Patients with hyperthyroidism due to CLT may be indistinguishable from those with Graves disease. The presence of ophthalmologic findings points toward the latter entity, but the absence of exophthalmos does not rule out Graves disease. The demonstration of human thyroid-stimulat-ing antibodies is confirmatory of the Graves diagnosis, but these tests may not be readily avail-able. The best way to distinguish between these two entities is by determining the uptake of radioactive iodine 6 and 24 hours after the administration of the isotope. Low or normal uptake supports the diagnosis of CLT, whereas elevated uptakes at 6 and 24 hours are more indicative of Graves disease.

114. In the child or adolescent with Graves disease, what other endocrine abnormalities can be observed?

A great number of endocrinologic functions are altered in Graves disease, but only a few of these changes are clinically relevant to children and adolescents.

1. Hyperthyroidism may be associated with either delayed or early *puberty*. The mecha-nisms for these alterations are not well understood.

2. Postpubertal females often have *menstrual irregularity* prior to treatment. The inter-menstrual interval may be either prolonged or shortened, and menstrual flow may be diminished. In rare circumstances, frank amenorrhea may occur.

3. *Hypercalcemia* has been noted in patients with hyperthyroidism, and the serum *alkaline phosphatase* may also be elevated in affected children. These changes are similar to those found in hyperparathyroidism. However, parathyroid hormone levels are low or undetectable. True hy-perparathyroidism and Graves disease may coexist and should be suspected if the hypercalcemia does not improve as the hyperthyroidism is controlled.

4. The manifestation of *thyroid hormone excess*—flushing, sweating, tachycardia, GI hy-permotility—are similar to those seen in carcinoid syndrome. However, the plasma serotonin concentration, urinary 5-hydroxyindoleacetic acid excretion, and platelet monoamine oxidase ac-tivity are normal.

115. Why does exophthalmos occur in Graves disease?

The reason is unknown, but several facts suggest an autoimmune process:

1. Histologic studies reveal lymphocytic infiltration of the retrobulbar muscles.
2. Circulating lymphocytes are sensitized to an antigen unique to the retrobulbar tissues.
3. The thyroglobulin—antithyroglobulin antibody complexes found in patients with Graves disease bind specifically to the extraorbital muscles.

116. What treatment options are available for children with Graves disease?

The three types of therapy are antithyroid medication, radioactive (^{131}I) ablation, and subtotal thyroidectomy.

Treatment Modalities for Graves Disease in Children

	MEDICAL	[131]I	SURGICAL
Contraindications	Noncompliance Previous drug reaction	Pregnancy Prepubertal (?)	Inadequate presurgical preparation
Effectiveness	65–95%	90–100%	80–100%
Pretreatment	None	Antithyroidal medications stopped 3–5 days prior prior to [131]I	Preferably euthyroid with thionamides, then iodine treatment for 7–14 days to involute thyroid
Treatment	Dosage based on body weight	Dosage based on estimated gland size and I uptake	Removal of all thyroidal tissue except that near vital structures
Acute complications	Drug reaction GI upset Arthralgias	Hyperthyroidism Tenderness	Vocal cord paralysis Bleeding at surgical site Hypocalcemia
Long-term complications	Essentially none; complications due to drug resolve when drug is discontinued	Hypothyroidism Genetic or radiation damage	Hypothyroidism Hypoparathyroidism Vocal cord paralysis

Klein I, et al: Treatment of hyperthyroid disease. Ann Intern Med 121:281–288, 1994.
Caruso DR, Mazzaferri EL: Intervention in Graves' disease: Choosing among imperfect but effective treatment options. Postgrad Med 92(8):128–129, 133–134, 1992.

117. Describe the principal modes of actions and side effects of medications used to treat Graves disease.

The thionamide derivatives, propylthiouracil, and methimazole are the keystones of long-term management. However, their effective onset of action is slow since they block synthesis but not release of thyroid hormone. Propranolol is useful in treating many of the β-adrenergic effects of hyperthyroidism. It is used during the acute management of Graves disease but should be discontinued when the thyroid disease is controlled. Iodide, which can transiently block thyroid hormone release, and glucocorticoids are useful "stopgap" medications while awaiting the inhibitory effects of the thionamides. They are generally used only when the patient is acutely symptomatic (thyroid storm).

Drug	*Effects*	*Adverse Reactions*
Propylthiouracil (PTU)	Blocks organification of iodide and peripheral conversion of T_4 to T_3	Agranulocytosis (1%) All reactions (5%), including arthralgias, neuritis, hepatitis, rash, urticaria, lupus-like syndrome, loss of taste
Methimazole	Blocks organification of iodide	Agranulocytosis (0.2%) All reactions (10%) (same as for PTU)
Propranolol	Decreases adrenergic component of thyrotoxicosis May impair peripheral T_4 conversion	Bradycardia, hypotension, hypoglycemia
Iodine-saturated solution (SSKI)	Blocks T_4 release by thyroid gland Useful for acute management	Acneiform skin rash, drug fevers, conjunctivitis, vasculitis, eosinophilic granulocytosis

118. Has radioactive iodide fallen into disfavor as a treatment option for Graves disease?

On the contrary, radioactive iodide (^{131}I) is increasing in popularity. Concern had been voiced about the possible risk of thyroid carcinoma, leukemia, thyroid nodules, or genetic mutations, but as the individuals treated with ^{131}I during childhood have been followed for prolonged periods, experience suggests that children are *not* at a significantly increased risk.

Farrar JJ, Toft AD: Iodine-131 treatment of hyperthyroidism: Current issues. Clin Endocrinol (Oxf) 35:207–212, 1991.

119. During a routine physical exam, a solitary thyroid nodule is palpated on a asymptomatic 10-year-old. Can a "wait and see" approach be taken?

Absolutely not. In children with a solitary nodule, about 30–40% have a carcinoma, 20–30% have an adenoma, and the remainder will have thyroid abscess, thyroid cyst, multinodular goiter, Hashimoto thyroiditis, subacute thyroiditis, or nonthyroidal neck mass. Given the relatively high incidence of carcinoma, a thyroidal mass demands prompt evaluation. Previous irradiation to the head or neck is associated with a significantly increased incidence of thyroid carcinoma. A family history of thyroid disease increases the likelihood of chronic lymphocytic thyroiditis or Graves disease. The presence of tenderness or palpation or high titers of anti-thyroid antibodies points away from a malignant process. However, in all cases, radiologic studies should be undertaken, and in many cases, surgical exploration is required.

120. How should this solitary thyroid nodule be investigated?

The principal tools used in the investigation of a thyroid mass are ^{123}I scanning and ultrasound. **Ultrasound** is useful in delineating the size of the mass, its anatomic relationship to the rest of the thyroid, and the presence of cystic structures. **^{123}I imaging** that reveals a single nonfunctioning mass ("cold" nodule) suggests a carcinoma or adenoma and is a clear indication for surgery. Patchy uptake is more characteristic of chronic lymphocytic thyroiditis, while a poorly functioning lobe may be found in a subacute thyroiditis.

121. How is the euthyroid sick syndrome diagnosed?

This syndrome is an adaptive response to slow body metabolism. It is also called the low T_3 syndrome because the most consistent finding is a depression of serum T_3. Reverse T_3 (rT_3), a metabolically inactive metabolite, is increased, although this is rarely measured. T_4 and TBG levels may be low or normal. Free T_4 levels and TSH levels are normal. In sick preterm infants, the clinical picture is often confusing because levels of T_4, free T_4, and T_3 are naturally low. Infants and children with the euthyroid sick syndrome generally revert to normal as the primary illness resolves.

7. GASTROENTEROLOGY

David A. Piccoli, M.D., and Chris A. Liacouras, M.D.

CLINICAL ISSUES

1. How is ascites diagnoses by physical examination?

Severe ascites is commonly diagnosed by observation of the child in a supine and then upright position. Bulging flanks, umbilical protrusion, and scrotal edema (in males) are generally evident. Three main techniques are used when the diagnosis is not obvious:

1. **Fluid wave:** This sign can be elicited in a cooperative patient by tapping sharply on one flank while receiving the wave with the other hand. The transmission of the wave through fatty tissue should be blocked by a hand placed on the center of the abdomen.

2. **Shifting dullness:** With the patient supine, percussion of the abdomen will demonstrate a central area of tympany at the top surrounded by flank percussion dullness. This dullness shifts when the patient moves laterally or stands up.

3. **"Puddle sign":** A cooperative and mobile patient may be examined in the knee-chest position. The pool of ascites is tapped while you listen for a sloshing sound or change in sound transmission with the stethoscope.

Small amounts of ascites can be extremely difficult to detect on physical exam in children. Although ascites can be demonstrated on radiographs, the most sensitive and specific test is an abdominal-pelvic ultrasound, which an detect as little as 150 ml of ascitic fluid.

2. How does the major cause of ascites in neonates differ from that in older children?

Older children: portal hypertension due to hepatic (e.g., chronic liver disease of multiple etiologies), prehepatic (e.g., portal vein thrombosis), or posthepatic (e.g., congestive heart failure, constrictive pericarditis) conditions.

Infants: urinary ascites due most commonly to obstructive renal disease (e.g., posterior urethral values)

3. Which features on plain radiographs are suspicious for ascites?
- Separation of bowel loops
- Abdominal haziness
- Indistinct psoas muscle shadow
- Increased pelvic density in the upright position
- McCort sign: increased distance (> 2 mm) between the properitoneal fat stripe and the right colon
- Hellmen sign: appearance of a radiolucent shadow between the lateral wall of the liver and the abdominal wall
- Dog ear sign: radiodensity superior and lateral to the bladder
- Obliteration of the lower lateral hepatic angle

Cochran WJ: Ascites. In Oski FA (ed): Principles and Practice of Pediatrics, 2nd ed. Philadelphia, J.B. Lippincott, 1994, p 1904.

4. In addition to serum amylase, what other tests are useful in the diagnosis of pancreatitis?

Multiple laboratory abnormalities can exist in pancreatitis, and although serum amylase is the most widely used test for diagnosis, it may not be the most sensitive or specific. It is usually elevated in the first 12 hours but then may return to normal within 24–72 hours. The serum lipase remains elevated for longer periods of time. Other tests have been advocated as being more useful for pancreatic injury than a simple serum amylase:

- Cationic trypsinogen
- Amylase:creatinine clearance ratio (> 5% suggests pancreatitis)
- Elevated hepatic transaminases, hyperglycemia, and hypocalcemia
- Abdominal x-rays showing pancreatic calcifications or abdominal ileus
- Abdominal ultrasonography revealing increased density, pancreatic enlargement, or pseudo-cyst formation.

Of note, falsely elevated serum amylase can occur if amylase is released from other injured areas (e.g., salivary gland in mumps, intestine in Crohn disease, ovary and fallopian tube in salpingitis). Isoenzyme determinations can help to identify the source if the clinical picture is confusing.

5. What are the most frequent causes of pancreatitis in children?

Acute pancreatitis in children is relatively rare. Most cases are due to drugs, infections (primarily viral), systemic illness, or trauma. In up to 25% of cases, an etiology is not identified.

- Drugs/toxins: Alcohol, L-asparaginase, high-dose corticosteroids, sulfasalazine, thiazides, valproic acid
- Infections: Viral (mumps, coxsackie virus, Epstein-Barr virus, rubella, influenza A), *Mycoplasma pneumoniae*, salmonella, ascariasis
- Systemic disease: Cystic fibrosis, diabetes mellitus, Henoch-Schönlein purpura, Kawasaki syndrome, renal failure, sarcoidosis, systemic lupus erythematosus
- Trauma
- Anatomic abnormalities: Biliary obstruction (stones, tumors), duodenal ulcer
- Congenital abnormalities: Annular pancreas, choledochal cyst, pancreatic divisum
- Metabolic: Hypercalcemia, hypertriglyceridemia, Reye syndrome
- Miscellaneous: Familial, refeeding syndrome (following malnutrition)
- Idiopathic

Lerner A, et al: Pancreatic diseases in children. Pediatr Clin North Am 43:125–156, 1996.

6. In what clinical settings is rectal prolapse most commonly seen?

- Constipation
- Malnutrition
- Cystic fibrosis
- Myelomeningocele
- Ehlers-Danlos syndrome
- Celiac disease
- Severe coughing (e.g., pertussis)
- *Enterobius vermicularis* (pinworm) infestation
- Abnormalities of sacrum or coccyx

7. Which agents are known to cause food poisoning in children?

Food poisoning is best defined as a gastrointestinal upset resulting in nausea, vomiting, and diarrhea, with or without fever, and appearing within 72 hours of ingestion of food contaminated by microorganisms or toxins. The likely offending agents vary according to the nature and time of onset of symptoms after the ingestion.

Onset within 1–6 hrs, nausea and vomiting, no fever
  Staphylococcus aureus toxin
  Bacillus cereus
Abdominal cramps and diarrhea within 8–16 hrs
  Clostridium perfringens
  Bacillus cereus
Fever, abdominal cramps, diarrhea within 16–48 hrs
  Salmonella
  Shigella
  Vibrio parahaemolyticus
  Invasive *Escherichia coli*
  Campylobacter jejuni
Abdominal cramps, watery diarrhea within 16–72 hrs
  Enterotoxigenic *E. coli*
  V. parahaemolyticus

V. cholerae, non-O1
V. cholerae, O1 (endemic area)
Fever, abdominal cramps within 16–48 hrs
   Yersinia enterocolitica
Nausea, vomiting, paralysis within 18–36 hrs
   Clostridium botulinum

Tauxe RV, Hughes JM: Food-borne disease. In Mandell GL, Bennett JE, Dolin R (eds): Principles and Practice of Infectious Diseases, 4th ed. New York, Churchill Livingstone, 1995, pp 1012–1024.

8. How should the bowel be prepared prior to colonoscopy?

Children < 1 year of age
  Clear liquids for 24 hours
  Pediatric Fleet enemas the night before and the morning of the exam
Children > 1 year of age
  Clear liquids for 48 hours
  X-prep (senna extract) or magnesium citrate orally on 2 successive nights prior to exam
  Adult Fleet enema the night before and the morning of the exam

GoLytely or CoLyte (2–4 liters over 3–4 hours) administered orally or via nasogastric tube the night before the procedure may be substituted in children over 5 years of age. It must be used with caution in younger children.

9. List the indications for lower GI colonoscopy or endoscopy in children.

- Hematochezia in absence of anal source
- Chronic diarrhea of unclear etiology
- Colitis of unclear etiology
- Diagnosis and management of inflammatory bowel disease
- Abnormality on barium enema
- History of familial polyposis
- Persistent severe unexplained lower abdominal pain
- Removal of foreign body
- Ureterosigmoidostomy, surveillance
- Dilation of a colonic stricture

10. When is colonoscopy contraindicated?

- Suspected perforation
- Recent abdominal surgery
- Inadequate bowel preparation
- Massive lower GI bleeding
- Toxic megacolon
- Unstable medical illness
- Coagulopathy

Fox VL: Colonoscopy. In Walker WA, et al (eds): Pediatric Gastrointestinal Disease, 2nd ed. St. Louis, Mosby, 1996, pp 1533–1541.

11. In children with recurrent abdominal pain, what historical features suggest a possible serious cause?

Recurrent abdominal pain is the most common chronic pain syndrome encountered in pediatrics. The vast majority have no identifiable organic basis. Features that may suggest an identifiable cause include:

- Pain localizing away from the umbilicus
- Abnormalities in bowel function (constipation, diarrhea, incontinence)
- Vomiting
- Pain that awakens a child at night
- Pain with radiation to the back, shoulder, or lower extremities
- Dysuria
- Rectal bleeding
- Constitutional symptoms (fever, weight loss, altered rate of growth, rash, arthralgia)
- Presentation at age < 4 or > 15
- Family history of GI or systemic illness (peptic ulcer disease, inflammatory bowel disease, lactose intolerance)

Oberlander TF, Rappaport LA: Recurrent abdominal pain. Pediatr Rev 14:313–319, 1993.

12. How does the average volume of a swallow in a child compare with that of an adult?
Child (age 1¼–3½ yrs):   4.5 ml   Adult male: 21 ml
Adult female: 14 ml   Average: 0.27 ml/kg
Jones DV, Work CE: Volume of a swallow. Am J Dis Child 102:427, 1961.

13. What is intractable singultus?
Persistent hiccups.

CONSTIPATION

14. When is the first stool normally passed?
Ninety-nine percent of infants will pass a stool within the first 24 hours, and 100% by 48 hours. Failure to pass a stool can be an indication of intestinal obstruction or anatomic abnormality. Approximately 95% of patients with Hirschsprung disease and 25% of patients with cystic fibrosis do not pass their first stool in the first 24 hours. The rule of early passage does not apply to premature babies, in whom delayed evacuation (> 24 hrs) is common, particularly with extreme prematurity.

15. What constitutes constipation in childhood?
Strictly speaking, constipation is defined as infrequent stooling, difficulty passing feces, or chronic fecal retention. Normal stool frequency varies from several times a day to 1 stool every 3 days. In children, constipation should be considered when the normal stooling pattern becomes more infrequent, when stools become hard or are difficult to expel, or when the child exhibits withholding patterns or behavioral changes toward moving his or her bowels. Soiling, or encopresis, can be a sign of constipation.

16. How should children with constipation be evaluated?
Any child suspected of having constipation should undergo a full history and physical examination. Common clinical features include a history of difficulty passing stools, withholding behavior, intermittent passage of extremely large stools, soiling, abdominal pain, rectal pain, or the development of anal fissures. An examination of the abdomen may reveal hard mobile masses which represent palpable stool. A rectal examination is extremely important. The presence of large amounts of stool in the rectal vault almost always indicates functional constipation. If no stool is present, Hirschsprung disease and abnormal anorectal anatomy should be considered. Abdominal radiographs can be used to show the degree of fecal retention and can be used to monitor treatment in children who have severe functional constipation.

17. Which clinical features differentiate chronic retentive constipation from Hirschsprung disease?

Functional Constipation	Hirschsprung Disease
Meconium passes within 24 hrs	Meconium passes after 24 hrs
Vomiting unusual	Vomiting common
Begins during toilet training	Begins shortly after birth
Soiling (encopresis) occurs	Soiling very rare
No enterocolitis	Enterocolitis
Palpable stool in rectal vault	No stool in rectal vault
Dilated anal canal	Narrow anal canal
Normal growth	Failure to thrive

18. How is Hirschsprung disease diagnosed?
Hirschsprung disease results from the failure of normal migration of ganglion cell precursors to their location in the GI tract during gestation. The loss of ganglion cells always begins distally

in the rectum, involves a contiguous portion of the colon, and can extend to variable lengths in the large and small intestine. Involvement can vary from total aganglionosis to short-segment disease. In Hirschsprung disease, a prone abdominal x-ray typically reveals a lack of air in the rectal vault. The diagnosis can be made by obtaining an unprepped *barium enema*, which will demonstrate a change in the caliber of the large intestine at the site where normal bowel meets aganglionic bowel (transition zone). An unprepped barium enema is required, since the use of cleansing enemas can dilate the abnormal portion of the colon and remove some of the distal impaction, thereby resulting in a false-negative result. Following the study, retention of barium for 24 or more hours is suggestive of Hirschsprung disease or a significant motility disorder. *Rectal suction biopsies or full-thickness surgical biopsies* will confirm the absence of ganglion cells. Anal manometry is less reliable in children and in small infants requires specialized equipment.

19. How is encopresis defined?

Encopresis, or fecal soiling, may be defined as the involuntary passage of fecal material in an otherwise healthy and normal child. Children with encopresis typically sense no urge to defecate. Fecal soiling is almost always associated with severe functional constipation.

20. How should children with chronic constipation and encopresis be managed?

Therapy for constipation and encopresis requires a multimodal approach.

1. The rectosigmoid colon should be aggressively cleansed of fecal material. Commonly, multiple enemas over 2 or 3 days are needed. Adult enemas should be used in children over the age of 2.

2. An oral lubricant, such as mineral oil or Kondremul, is necessary to promote continued passage of stool. In difficult cases, stimulant medications, such as milk of magnesia or Haley's MO, can be substituted. While fecal soiling typically improves rapidly, a maintenance dose of mineral oil may be required for a prolonged period of time.

3. It is extremely important to educate patients and parents about the mechanics of the disorder. A high-fiber diet, defined periods of toilet-sitting, and a behavior modification system rewarding normal bowel movements are essential for eventual success.

Loening-Baucke V: Encopresis and soiling. Pediatr Clin North Am 43:279–298, 1996.

21. How does the use of mineral oil affect the absorption of fat-soluble vitamins?

Mineral oil is extensively used for treatment of functional constipation. While several case reports have shown that the long-term use of mineral oil can potentially alter the absorption of fat-soluble vitamins (A, D, E, K), vitamin deficiencies rarely occur. However, when mineral oil is prescribed, a multivitamin supplement (given at a different time than the mineral oil) is commonly added to the child's diet.

DIARRHEA

22. Which is a better predictor of bacteria as a cause of diarrhea: blood in the stool or neutrophils (PMNs) in the stool?

Stool PMNs are more reliable as indicators of a bacterial etiology than a positive stool guaiac test for blood. While about 30–50% of patients with blood in the stool will have a bacterial etiology, up to 70% will not. Thus, the presence of blood has a fair specificity but poor sensitivity. Stool PMNs, on the other hand, have a specificity and sensitivity of around 85% with a positive predictive value of around 60%.

DeWitt T, et al: Clinical predictors of acute bacterial diarrhea in young children. Pediatrics 76:551–556, 1985.

23. How is the stool examined for white blood cells?

Unlike dipstick testing for urine white blood cells, you must find stool PMNs the old-fashioned way. A thin smear of fresh stool is placed on a slide and air-dried. The sample is covered with methylene blue for about 5 seconds, gently rinsed with tapwater, and air-dried again. The quantity of PMNs seen per high-power microscopic field can be classified as occasional, scattered, or diffuse.

24. Which historical questions are key in seeking the cause of diarrhea?

1. Recent medications, especially antibiotics
2. History of immunosuppression (e.g., recurrent major infections, history of malnutrition, AIDS, recent measles)
3. Illnesses in other family members or close contacts
4. Travel outside the United States
5. Travel to rural or seacoast areas (e.g., with consumption of untreated water, raw milk, raw shellfish)
6. Attendance in day care
7. Recent foods
8. Presence of family pets

25. How do patterns of acute diarrhea vary by the pathogen involved?

Secretory/Enterotoxigenic	Inflammatory
Characterized by watery diarrhea and absence of fecal leukocytes	Characterized by dysentery (i.e., symptoms and bloody stools), fecal leukocytes, and erythrocytes
Food poisoning (toxigenic)	
Staphylococcus aureus	*Shigella*
Bacillus cereus	Invasive *E. coli*
Clostridium perfringens	*Salmonella*
Enterotoxigenic *Escherichia coli*	*Campylobacter*
Vibrio cholerae	*Clostridium difficile*
Giardia lamblia	*Entamoeba histolytica*
Cryptosporidium	
Rotavirus	
Norwalk-like virus	

From Northrup RS, Flanigan TP: Gastroenteritis. Pediatr Rev 15:463, 1994; with permission.

26. How quickly can the mucosa of the gut repair itself after a bout of viral gastroenteritis?

Acute viral gastroenteritis is usually a self-limited disease. Histologic recovery of the intestinal epithelium can be expected 7–10 days after virus excretion has ceased. Functional recovery of the bowel occurs shortly thereafter. Occasionally, in infants < 12 months of age, a severe postviral enteritis may occur for up to 6–12 weeks. Normally, the differentiated enteric epithelium replenishes itself every 3–5 days.

27. What is the best way to feed an outpatient infant who has an acute bout of diarrhea complicated by mild dehydration?

The AAP's Committee on Nutrition in 1985 recommended rapid rehydration over 4–6 hours with an oral glucose-electrolyte rehydration solution, followed by diluted formula or milk. Use of a lactose-free formula was not routinely recommended. For older infants or children, dietary supplementation with nonlactose, complex carbohydrate-rich foods, such as rice, cereal, bananas, or potatoes, was suggested within 24 hours after successful rehydration. This contrasted with the traditional approach of rehydration with clear fluids for 24–48 hours followed by a slowly advancing concentration of diluted milk or formula and the BRAT diet (bananas, rice, apples, toast and tea) or a regular diet for older children as the diarrhea resolved. Recent data indicate that earlier initiation of full-strength formula does not worsen and may decrease the duration of diarrhea, although data are conflicting regarding the use of full-strength lactose-free vs. lactose-containing formula. By one survey, two-thirds of practicing pediatricians recommend a lactose-free formula.

Bezerra JA, et al: Treatment of infants with acute diarrhea: What's recommended and what's practiced. Pediatrics 90:1–4, 1992.

Provisional Committee on Quality Improvement: Practice parameter: The management of acute gastroenteritis in young children. Pediatrics 97:424–436, 1996.

28. How do the various oral electrolyte replacement solutions differ in composition from other liquids commonly used in rehydration?

Oral Replacement Solutions (ORS)

SOLUTION	CARBOHYDRATE* (g/L)	SODIUM (mEq/L)	POTASSIUM (mEq/L)	BASE (mEq/L)	OSMOLALITY (mOsm/L)	CALORIES (cal/100 ml)
Diarrhea	—	50–100	25–35	25–40	250–300	—
WHO (recommended)	G: 20	60–90	20–30	25–35	< 300	8
WHO ORS	G: 20	90	20	30	300	8
Pedialyte	G: 25	45	20	30	260	10
Ricelyte	R: 30	50	25	34	210	12
Cereal-based ORS	St: 50	60–90	20	30	315	42
Gatorade	G: 50	20	3	3	330	10
Chicken broth	0	250	5	0	450	0
Cola	F/G: 50–150	2	0.1	13	550	12–16
Apple juice	F/G/S: 100–150	3	30	0	700	15–18
Tea	0	0–1	0–1	0	0–5	0

* G, glucose; F, fructose; R, rice syrup solids; S, sucrose; St, starch.

Each solution has some advantages and disadvantages. Many home remedies are either very deficient or very excessive in electrolytes or sugar. A main problem with recommended ORS solutions is their low caloric content, but development of cereal-based and polymer-based solutions, which increase calories without increasing osmolality, is in progress.

29. How can the WHO oral electrolyte (rehydration) solution be duplicated?
The WHO solution is 2% glucose, 20 mEq K^+/L, 90 mEq Na^+/L, 80 mEq Cl^-/L, and 30 mEq bicarbonate/L. This solution is approximated by adding ¾ tsp of salt, 1 tsp of baking soda, 1 cup of orange juice (for KCl), and 8 tsp of sugar to a liter of water.

30. When is antidiarrheal pharmacologic treatment indicated in children?
Antidiarrheal agents include (1) anti-infective/antibiotic agents, (2) antimotility agents (e.g., opiates, diphenoxylate), (3) antisecretory agents (e.g., loperamide, somatostatin), and (4) binding agents (e.g., pectin, cholestyramine, charcoal, attapulgite). Antidiarrheal medications are seldom indicated in pediatrics. In most cases, treatment of diarrhea consists of fluid and electrolyte replacement by oral rehydration solutions. Antibiotics are useful in only a number of bacterial and parasitic diseases. Rarely, antidiarrheal agents are indicated in those children who have chronic diseases, such as cholestatic liver disease (cholestyramine), inflammatory bowel disease, short-gut syndrome, or other secretory diarrheas (loperamide). Opiates are almost never indicated.
Provisional Committee on Quality Improvement: Practice parameter: The management of acute gastroenteritis in young children. Pediatrics 97:424–436, 1996.

31. Why is true diarrhea in the first few days of life especially concerning?
In addition to the greater potential for dehydration in a newborn, diarrhea in this age group more commonly is associated with major congenital intestinal defects involving electrolyte transport (e.g., congenital sodium- or chloride-losing diarrhea) or carbohydrate absorption (e.g., congenital lactase deficiency). While viral enteritis can occur in the nursery, any newborn with true diarrhea warrants thorough evaluation and possible referral to a tertiary center.

32. Why is salmonella enteritis so concerning if present in a child less than 12 months of age?
In older children with salmonella gastroenteritis, secondary bacteremia and dissemination of disease rarely occur. In infants, however, 5–40% may have positive blood cultures for salmonella,

and in 10% of these cases, salmonella can cause meningitis, osteomyelitis, pericarditis, and pyelonephritis. Thus, in infants < 1 year old, outpatient management of diarrhea assumes even greater significance, particularly if salmonella is suspected.

Management of Salmonella Enteritis in the First Year of Life

	MANAGEMENT
First Evaluation	
Colitis (dysentery, heme positive stool, fecal WBCs)	Stool culture Blood culture if < 3 mos of age or temperature > 39.5°C
Diarrhea (no colitis)	Consider viral or other causes first Stool culture if diarrhea prolonged (≥ 5 days) Stool and blood culture if < 3 mos and exposure to salmonella
Follow-up	
Persistent diarrhea	Stool culture
Positive stool culture (blood culture +)	Admit, repeat cultures (including CSF) Systemic parenteral antibiotics (e.g., ceftriaxone, cefotaxime) regardless of appearance on repeat examination
Positive stool culture (blood culture −)	
Toxic, ill, or immunocompromised	As if blood culture-positive
Febrile, nontoxic	Admit, blood culture, systemic parenteral antibiotics if < 3 mos
Afebrile, improving	Home observation, periodic reexamination

Adapted from St. Geme JW III, et al: Consensus management of Salmonella infection in the first year of life. Pediatr Infect Dis J 7:615–618, 1988; with permission.

33. What are the etiologies of traveler's diarrhea?

The etiologies vary by location, but toxigenic *Escherichia coli* is clearly the most commonly identified cause.

Microorganism	*Average Frequency (%)*	*Range (%)*
Toxigenic *E. coli*	40–60	0–72
Invasive *E. coli*	< 5	0–5
Shigella	10	0–30
Salmonella	< 5	0–15
Campylobacter jejuni	< 5	0–15
Vibrio parahaemolyticus	< 5	0–30
Aeromonas	< 5	0–30
Giardia lamblia	<5	0–6
Entamoeba histolytica	< 5	0–6
Rotavirus	5	0–36
No pathogen identified	40	20–85

From Gorbach SL, et al: Infectious diarrhea and bacterial food poisoning. In Sleisinger MH, Fordtran JS (eds): Gastrointestinal Disease, 5th ed. Philadelphia, W.B. Saunders, 1993, p 1153; with permission.

34. How can traveler's diarrhea be prevented?

Four strategies can be used to prevent traveler's diarrhea: (1) anticipatory guidance regarding food and beverage intake, (2) bismuth subsalicylate (3) anti-infective drugs, and (4) symptomatic control and medications with direct action on the GI tract.

In high-risk areas in developing countries, avoid previously peeled raw fruits and vegetables and any foods or beverages prepared with tap water. Prophylactic bismuth subsalicylate (Pepto-Bismol) has been shown to minimize diarrheal illness in up to 75% of adults. While some authorities recommend its use in children, others argue against it because of the risk of salicylate intoxication. Prophylactic use of antimicrobial agents such as trimethoprim-sulfamethoxazole, neomycin, doxycycline, and ciprofloxacin can decrease the frequency of traveler's diarrhea in children and adults. However, routine use of antibiotics is not recommended because of potential risks of allergic drug reactions, antibiotic-associated colitis, and development of resistant organisms. If symptoms develop, empiric therapy is indicated, and the regimen of trimethoprim-sulfamethoxazole and imodium (for children age > 2 years) is very effective. Immunization, while potentially an ideal solution, at present is not an alternative.

35. Which bacterial gastroenteritides may benefit from antimicrobial therapy?

Enteropathogen	Indication or Effect
Shigella	Shortens duration of diarrhea Eliminates organisms from feces
Campylobacter jejuni	Shortens duration Prevents relapse
Salmonella	Indicated for Infants < 12 mos Bacteremia Metastatic foci (e.g., osteomyelitis) Enteric fever
Escherichia coli	
EPEC (enteropathogenic)	Use primarily in infants Intravenous use if invasive disease
ETEC (enterotoxigenic) EIEC (enteroinvasive)	Most illnesses brief and self-limited
EHEC (enterohemorrhagic)	Antibiotic therapy does not appear to prevent progression to hemolytic-uremic syndrome
Yersinia enterocolitica	None for gastroenteritis alone, but indicated if suspected septicemia or other localized infection
Clostridium difficile	10–20% relapse rate
Aeromonas hydrophila	Efficacy not clearly established

36. List the differential diagnosis of chronic diarrhea by age group.

Newborns	Infants	Toddlers	Older Children
Congenital short gut	Protein sensitization	Postgastroenteritis diarrhea	Lactose intolerance
Congenital lactose intolerance	Infection	Dietary (allergy, excess fruit juice ingestion)	Infection
Malrotation with intermittent volvulus	Parenteral diarrhea (urinary or upper respiratory infection)	Toddler's diarrhea	Inflammatory bowel disease
Ischemia	Immunoglobulin deficiency	Hyperthyroidism	Irritable bowel
Defective Na+/H+ exchange	Postgastroenteritis diarrhea	Sucrase-isomaltase deficiency	Laxative abuse
Congenital chloride diarrhea	Cystic fibrosis	Constipation/impaction with overflow	
Microvillus disease	Celiac disease	Teething (?)	
	Clostridium difficile		

From Gryboski J: The child with chronic diarrhea. Contemp Pediatr 10:73, 1993; with permission.

37. How does secretory diarrhea differ from osmotic diarrhea?

Stools	Osmotic Diarrhea	Secretory Diarrhea
Electrolytes	Na$^+$ < 70 mmol/L	Na$^+$ > 70 mmol/L
Osmotic gap*	> 100 mOsm	< 50 mOsm
pH	< 5	> 6
Reducing substance	Present	Absent
Volume	< 20 ml/kg/day	> 20 ml/kg/day
After fasting	< 10 ml/kg/day	> 20 ml/kg/day
Blood/pus/fat	Present or absent	Absent

* Osmotic gap = osmolality of the fecal fluid minus the sum of the concentrations of the fecal electrolytes
From Mehta DI, Lebenthal E: New developments in acute diarrhea. Curr Probl Pediatr 24:99, 1994; with permission.

38. How should children with secretory diarrhea be managed?

It is important to identify an etiology for secretory diarrhea. After the child is taken off feeds, a vigorous attempt must be initiated to maintain fluid and electrolyte balance. If this is successful, the child should be evaluated for proximal small bowel damage, enteric pathogens, and a baseline malabsorptive workup. If abnormalities of the mucosal integrity are suspected, a small bowel biopsy is performed, and if the findings are significantly abnormal, the patient may be given parenteral alimentation and gradual refeeding. Electron microscopy may reveal congenital abnormalities of the microvillus membrane and brush border.

If the evaluation is negative, hormonal causes of secretory diarrhea (such as a VIPoma, hypergastrinoma, or carcinoid syndrome) must be considered. The list of active GI hormones is rapidly expanding, and unusual tumors stimulating diarrhea have been identified. Bacterial overgrowth may cause a secretory process, although usually this diarrhea will abate somewhat with fasting. A number of congenital abnormalities have been identified and are classified under the diagnosis of intractable diarrhea of infancy. if no etiology is identified, severe protracted disease may occur, and central parenteral alimentation is initiated. Careful monitoring and maintenance of intravenous access are critical because of marked fluid shifts.

39. How common is asymptomatic *Clostridium difficile* carriage?

C. difficile is the agent most often implicated in antibiotic-associated colitis. Fever, abdominal pain, and bloody diarrhea begin as early as a few days after starting antibiotics (especially clindamycin, ampicillin, cephalosporins). The diagnosis in infancy is more difficult because the carriage rate for *C. difficile* is relatively high. Neonates have a colonization rate of about 20%, infants 30–40%, older children 10%, and adolescents 5%. Toxin assays are more indicative of *C. difficile*-associated disease than culture. However, the toxin may be present without any symptoms, especially in infants.

Kelley CP, et al: *Clostridium difficile* colitis. N Engl J Med 330:257–262, 1994.

40. Which antibiotics most commonly cause pseudomembranous colitis?

Pseudomembranous colitis is a severe condition seen in patients undergoing intensive antibiotic therapy. It is associated with profuse diarrhea, which may be watery or mucoid, and is usually green, foul-smelling, and often bloody, and is accompanied by abdominal cramps. Fever and leukocytosis are common, and stool smears frequently show leukocytes. Diagnosis is made by sigmoidoscopy, which reveals pseudomembranous plaques or nodules. The causative agent is toxin-producing *Clostridium difficile*. Pseudomembranous colitis has been reported most commonly with ampicillin, clindamycin, and cephalosporins, but most antibiotics may cause this condition.

41. What are the therapeutic alternatives for treatment of pseudomembranous colitis?

If the disease is not severe, children may be treated with withdrawal of antibiotics and good supportive care. More severely ill children should be treated with oral vancomycin or metronidazole. Some clinicians have advocated cholestyramine to bind *C. difficile* toxin.

42. How helpful is eosinophilia as a diagnostic sign of parasitic disease?

Normally, the total eosinophil count does not exceed $500/mm^3$. As a screening tool for suspected parasitic disease (e.g., in symptomatic patients returning from foreign travel), it has a very poor positive-predictive value (15–55%). Its negative-predictive value is better (73–96%), particularly if sequential eosinophil counts remain normal.

Mawhorter SD: Eosinophilia caused by parasites. Pediatr Ann 23:405–413, 1994.

43. Name the three most common presentations of giardiasis.
- Asymptomatic carrier state
- Chronic malabsorption with steatorrhea and failure to thrive
- Acute gastroenteritis with diarrhea, weight loss, abdominal cramps, abdominal distention, nausea, and vomiting

44. How reliable are the various diagnostic methods for detecting giardia?

Single stool exam for trophozoites or cysts—50–75%
Three stool exams (ideally 48 hours apart) for same—95%
Single stool exam and stool ELISA test for giardia antigen—> 95%
Duodenal aspirate or string test—> 95%
Duodenal biopsy (gold standard)—closest to 100%

45. Which patients are particularly susceptible to giardiasis?

Those with cystic fibrosis, chronic pancreatitis, achlorhydria, agammaglobulinemia, and hypogammaglobulinemia.

46. What are the clinical features of cryptosporidial enteritis?

Most reported cases occur in immunocompromised patients, although limited outbreaks have occurred in normal hosts. Children infected with HIV are particularly susceptible. Acute infection typically has an incubation period of 1–7 days. The clinical features include fever, abdominal pain, nausea, vomiting, high-output diarrhea, and failure to thrive. The illness may resolve within a few days, or it may be prolonged for several weeks. Asymptomatic carriage has been reported.

47. What is the triad of findings in acrodermatitis enteropathica?

Diarrhea, hair loss, and dermatitis are the presenting signs of this rare autosomal recessive disorder. The name nicely describes the disorder. There is a classic **acral** distribution of the rash. It is usually eczematous, often with a vesiculobullous or pustular component, and involves skin around body orifices as well. As for **enteropathica**, serum zinc levels are extremely low, secondary to impaired GI absorption. Dietary insufficiency of zinc may give an identical clinical picture. This has been found in children on long-term total parenteral nutrition without sufficient zinc and in very premature infants due to decreased stores and increased requirement.

48. What features characterize "toddler's diarrhea"?

Toddler's diarrhea, also known as chronic nonspecific diarrhea and even irritable bowel syndrome, is a clinical entity of unclear etiology that occurs in infants between 6 and 40 months, often following a distinct identifiable enteritis and treatment with an antibiotic. Loose, nonbloody stools (at least two per day but usually more) occur without associated symptoms of fever, pain, or growth failure. Malabsorption is not a key feature.

Multiple causes may be present: overconsumption of fruit juices, relative intestinal hypermotility, increased secretion of bile acids and sodium, intestinal prostaglandin abnormalities. The diagnosis is one of exclusion, and toddlers should be evaluated for disaccharide intolerance, protein hypersensitivity, parasitic infestation, and inflammatory bowel disease. Treatment consists of re-assurance, careful growth assessment, and psyllium bulking agents (as initial therapy). Other agents used with success have been cholestyramine and metronidazole.

49. In what settings can diarrhea be a severe life-threatening illness?

Severe diarrhea of any cause can lead to dehydration, which can cause significant morbidity and mortality. However, diarrhea can be a sign of a serious associated illness which in itself can be life-threatening:

Intussusception	Salmonella gastroenteritis (neonatal)
Hemolytic-uremic syndrome	Hirschsprung disease (with toxic megacolon)
Pseudomembranous colitis	Inflammatory bowel disease (with toxic megacolon)

Fleisher GR: Diarrhea. In Fleisher GR, Ludwig S (eds): Textbook of Pediatric Emergency Medicine, 3rd ed. Baltimore, Williams & Wilkins, 1993, p 153.

50. How is the degree of dehydration estimated in a child?

Clinical Findings to Estimate the Degree of Dehydration

SIGNS AND SYMPTOMS	MILD	MODERATE	SEVERE
Body fluid lost (ml/kg)	< 50	50–100	> 100
Weight loss	< 5%	5–10%	> 10%
State of shock	Impending	Compensated	Uncompensated
General appearance	Thirsty, alert, restless	Thirsty, restless or lethargic, irritable to touch, younger children more likely drowsy	Drowsy; limp, cold, sweaty; older may be apprehensive; infants may be comatose
Vital Signs			
Systolic BP	Normal	Normal (orthostatic)	Very low or absent
Heart rate	Normal	Slight elevation (orthostatic)	Very elevated
Respiration	Normal	Deep, may be rapid	Deep and rapid (hyperpnea)
Other Exam			
Radial pulse	Normal rate and strength	Rapid and weak	Feeble, rapid, may be impalpable
Capillary refill	< 2 sec	2–3 sec	> 3 sec
Skin elasticity	Retracts immediately	Retracts slowly	Retracts very slowly (> 3 sec)
Anterior fontanel	Flat	Depressed	Sunken
Mucous membranes	Normal/dry	Very dry	Very dry/cracked
Tears	Present	Absent	Absent
Skin color	Pale	Gray	Mottled
Lab Tests			
Urine			
Volume	Decreased (< 2–3 ml/kg/hr)	Oliguric (1 ml/kg/hr) (< 1 ml/kg/hr)	Anuric
Osmolarity (mOsm/L)	600	800	Maximal
Specific gravity	1.010	1.025	Maximal
Blood			
pH	7.40–7.22	7.30–6.92	7.10–6.80
BUN	Upper normal	Elevated	High
HCO_3^-	Lower normal	Decreased (16–19 mEq/L)	Very decreased (< 16 mEq/L)

Adapted from Shaw KN: Dehydration. In Fleisher GR, Ludwig S (eds): Textbook of Pediatric Emergency Medicine, 3rd ed. Baltimore, Williams & Wilkins, 1993, p 148.

51. How accurate is blood urea nitrogen (BUN) as a means of assessing dehydration in children?

Notoriously unreliable. The BUN does not begin to rise until the glomerular filtration rate falls to approximately one-half of normal. It then rises about 1% each hour. It may rise even less in a fasting child with disease. In a prospective study, Bonadio et al. found that 80% of patients judged to be 5–10% dehydrated by common physical findings may have a normal BUN.

Bonadio WA, et al: Efficacy of measuring BUN in assessing children with dehydration due to gastroenteritis. Ann Emerg Med 18:755–757, 1989.

FOOD ALLERGIES

52. What are the most common food allergies in children?

Egg, cow's milk, and peanut account for 75% of abnormal food challenges. Soy, wheat, fish, and chicken are also common allergens.

53. Are food allergies in infants more or less common than generally perceived?

As the saying goes, "it depends on where your bread is buttered." Nearly a third of parents report that their infant has an adverse food reaction, most equating this with allergy. In pediatric circles, the general perception is that true food allergies are relatively rare. The answer, as custom, lies somewhere between. A prospective study in Colorado of 489 infants followed from birth to age 3 showed 8% had allergies confirmed by food challenge. In Denmark, a prospective study of nearly 1800 infants showed a prevalence of cow's milk allergy of 2.2%. Of note, the natural history of food allergies in infants is disappearance in nearly 90% of cases by age 3.

Bock SA: Prospective appraisal of complaints of adverse reactions to foods in children during the first three years of life. Pediatrics 79:683–688, 1987.

Host A, Halken S: A prospective study of cow's milk allergy in Danish infants during the first three years of life. Allergy 45:587–596, 1990.

54. How are adverse food reactions characterized?

Food allergy: Ingestion of food results in hypersensitivity reactions mediated most commonly by IgE.

Food intolerance: Ingestion of food results in symptoms not immunologically mediated, and causes may include toxic contaminants (e.g., histamine in scromboid fish poisoning), pharmacologic properties of food (e.g., tyramine in aged cheeses), digestive and absorptive limitations of host (e.g., lactase deficiency), or idiosyncratic reactions.

55. What are the manifestations of milk protein allergy in childhood?

Milk protein allergy and milk intolerance have been blamed for nearly every symptom in infancy. It is important to distinguish between a milk protein allergy, a lactose intolerance, and the common side effects of significant milk ingestion.

Acute manifestations	Subacute symptoms
Angioedema	Chronic vomiting
Urticaria	Intestinal obstruction
Acute vomiting and diarrhea	Persistent diarrhea
Anaphylactic shock	Malabsorption
GI bleeding	Protein-losing enteropathy
	Hypoproteinemia with or without edema
	Upper GI bleeding
	Lower GI bleeding
	Hemoptysis
	Abdominal distention
	Failure to thrive
	Colic

Diarrhea of variable severity is the most common manifestation of a milk protein allergy. Histologic abnormalities of the small intestinal mucosa have been documented, with the most severe form seen as a flat villous lesion. Protein-losing enteropathy may result from disruption of the surface epithelium. The stools of children with primary milk protein intolerance often contain blood. At sigmoidoscopy there is an erythematous and friable mucosa, and biopsies demonstrate a cellular infiltration, often with eosinophils, and changes in the surface and glandular epithelium. **Heiner syndrome** is hematemesis and hemoptysis with failure to thrive associated with milk allergy.

56. Can laboratory tests confirm a diagnosis of milk allergy?

The laboratory tests available are *not* sensitive or specific enough to confirm the diagnosis fully. Tests of humoral or cellular immune function, RAST tests, intradermal skin testing, and IgE levels have not been diagnostic. Specific assays for serum immunoglobulins directed against individual proteins in milk formulas may be useful. The peroral small bowel biopsy may show signs of superficial damage, but postenteritis syndrome, celiac disease, and other diseases also present with this finding. The accurate diagnosis of milk protein allergy still relies on the clinical challenge test.

57. Why is the DBPCFC a must in diagnosing food allergy?

The double-blind placebo-controlled food challenge (DBPCFC), while in need of a catchier acronym, is the gold standard for evaluating food allergies. The initial choice of food to be tested is usually based on history, skin tests, or RAST testing. In a fasted patient without recent antihistamine use, small quantities of the chosen food (or placebo) are given in lypholized form (food rapidly frozen and dehydrated under high vacuum), capsules or liquid. The quantities are doubled every 30–60 minutes as the patient is observed for up to 8 hours, depending on the anticipated reaction. Observers must be capable of responding to possible anaphylaxis, which usually occurs in the first 2 hours. If no reaction has occurred, the observer should knowingly give the food being tested to ensure that a false-negative test has not occurred.

58. Why can children who are allergic to nuts usually eat peanuts without any problem?

Tree nuts (e.g., almonds, Brazil nuts, cashews, pecans, pistachios, and walnuts) are a relatively common cause of food allergy in adults and less commonly in children. Peanuts are a legume (like soy) and have no cross-reactivity with members of the nut family.

59. Does delaying the introduction of solid foods until 4–6 months reduce the risk of food allergies?

This remains unclear and relatively unstudied, but usually recommended. The theoretical reason for the delay is to allow intestinal mucosal maturation with less "leakiness" so that fewer antigens can penetrate and initiate an immunologic response. One setting in which delay appears to have proven benefit is in children with a strong family history of atopic dermatitis. Limiting solid foods in the first 4–6 months and also minimizing exposure to major allergenic foods (e.g., cow's milk, egg, peanut) diminish the prevalence and extent of atopic dermatitis.

Kajosaari M, Saarinen UM: Prophylaxis of atopic disease by six month's total solid food elimination. Arch Paediatr Scand 72:411–414, 1983.

GASTROESOPHAGEAL REFLUX

60. How rapidly do infants outgrow gastroesophageal reflux (GER)?

As a rule, in infants who have significant primary GER, 50% resolve by 6 months, 75% by 12 months, and 95% by 18 months.

Boyle JT: Gastroesophageal reflux in the pediatric patient. Gastroenterol Clin North Am 18:315–337, 1989.

61. What factors can contribute to the process of gastroesophageal reflux?

GER is defined as the egress of gastric contents proximal to the stomach. There are a variety of factors that contribute to GER in children. Anatomic abnormalities such as a hiatal hernia or defective diaphragmatic or crural musculature can cause GER. Anatomic abnormalities distal to the stomach, such as malrotation or duodenal webs may cause intermittent partial obstruction or mechanical delayed gastric emptying. Functional abnormalities such as a decreased resting lower esophageal sphincter (LES) pressure, an increase in transient LES relaxations, delayed gastric emptying, increased intra-abdominal pressure, esophageal dysmotility, or abnormal esophageal acid clearance have also been implicated. The process can be exacerbated by medications that alter gastric acid production or diminish LES competence or by constant horizontal positioning, as occurs in some children with psychomotor disorders.

Holloway RH, Dent J: Pathophysiology of gastroesophageal reflux. Gastroenterol Clin North Am 19:517–535, 1990.

62. Which test is most reliable for the diagnosis of GER?

The diagnosis can be made either clinically or by diagnostic testing. Clinically, reflux should be suspected in any child who demonstrates frequent, effortless vomiting or regurgitation without evidence of GI obstruction. With regard to diagnostic testing, the upper GI barium study is not sensitive for identifying reflux, as it is seen in only 50% of affected patients. The "milk scan" is a more physiologic test, but it detects only postprandial reflux. Unfortunately, significant damage occurs during nocturnal reflux, which cannot be modeled by a "milk scan." Endoscopically, the presence of histologic esophagitis is suggestive but not diagnostic of reflux. Scintigraphy, a non-invasive test utilizing radiolabeled meal, is very specific but only moderately sensitive in predicting reflux. The **24-hour pH probe** continues to be the most reliable test for the diagnosis of GER.

63. How are the complications of GER treated?

Simple GER	**Failure to thrive**
Counseling	Nutritional rehabilitation
Thickened feeding	Nasogastric feeding
Positional therapy	**Apnea**
Prokinetic agents (bethanecol,	Monitoring
metoclopramide, cisapride)	Fundoplication, if severe
Esophagitis	**Recurrent aspiration**
Antacids	Fundoplication
Cimetidine, ranitidine, or	Jejunal feeding
famotidine	**Failure of medical and nutritional therapy**
Sucralfate	Fundoplication

64. What are the endoscopic and pathologic findings in GER?

Simple reflux has no pathologic correlate. If reflux is complicated by esophagitis, there may be erythema, edema, friability, or frank ulceration of the distal esophagus. Histologically, the diseased portion of the esophagus may demonstrate neutrophilic or eosinophilic infiltration into the epithelium and occasionally ulceration.

65. An infant with known GER who periodically arches his or her back likely has what syndrome?

Sandifer syndrome is paroxysmal dystonic posturing with opisthotonus and unusual twisting of the head and neck (resembling torticollis) in association with GER. Typically, an esophageal hiatal hernia is also present.

66. How effective are milk-thickening agents as a treatment for GER?

While not as effective as once thought, thickened feedings do alleviate GER in 40–50% of infants, especially when the child is placed in the prone position with the head elevated approximately 30°.

67. Should antacids used in the treatment of GER be given before, during, or after feedings?

Antacids should be given 60–90 minutes following a meal and/or before bedtime. Antacids are used to buffer gastric acid, and the buffering capacity lasts up to 1 hour. Meals also buffer gastric acid, and thus antacids have minimal effect when given with meals.

68. What are common side effects of antacids?

Diarrhea, eructation, flatulence, nausea, vomiting, rash, and constipation. Rarely, antacids can cause hypophosphatemia, hypocalcemia, hypermagnesemia, gastric bezoars, abnormal gastric emptying, and fecaliths.

69. Does the use of theophylline worsen GER?

The effect of theophylline on the development of GER is controversial. While theophylline has been reported to inhibit lower esophageal sphincter tone, several studies have shown that the use of theophylline and/or bronchodilators causes no significant increase in the frequency or severity of GER.

70. What is the Nissen fundoplication?

The Nissen fundoplication is the most commonly performed anti-reflux surgical procedure. It involves wrapping a portion of the gastric fundus 360° around the distal esophagus in an effort to tighten the gastroesophageal junction.

71. Which infants are candidates for fundoplication?

The vast majority of infants with developmental reflux do not require fundoplication. It is indicated in patients with recurrent aspiration, refractory or Barrett's esophagitis, reflux-associated apnea, and reflux-associated failure to thrive which is refractory to medical therapy. Patients with severe reflux and psychomotor retardation should be evaluated for a fundoplication if a feeding gastrostomy is contemplated.

72. What are the infectious causes of esophagitis?

Fungal	Bacterial
Candida albicans	*Helicobacter pylori*
Aspergillus	Protozoan
Torulopsis glabrata	*Trypanosoma cruzi*
Viral	*Cryptosporidium*
Cytomegalovirus	
Varicella-zoster	
Herpes	

GASTROINTESTINAL BLEEDING

73. What features on physical exam can help identify an unknown cause of GI bleeding?

Skin	Signs of chronic liver disease (e.g., spider angiomas, venous distension, caput medusae, jaundice)
	Signs of coagulopathy (e.g., petechiae, purpura)
	Signs of vascular dysplasias (e.g., telangiectasia, hemangiomas)
	Signs of vasculitis (e.g., palpable purpura on legs and buttocks suggests Henoch-Schönlein purpura)
Head and neck	Signs of epistaxis (especially before placing nasogastric (NG) tube, which can induce bleeding)
	Hyperpigmented spots on lips and gums (suggests Peutz-Jeghers syndrome, which is associated with multiple intestinal polyps)
	Webbed neck (suggests Turner syndrome, which is associated with GI vascular malformations and inflammatory bowel disease)

Cardiac	Murmur of aortic stenosis (in adults, associated with vascular malformations of the ascending colon, although this association not certain in children)
Abdomen	Splenomegaly or hepatomegaly (suggests portal hypertension and possible esophageal varices)
	Ascites (suggests chronic liver disease and possible varices)
Rectal	Perianal ulcerations and skin tags (suggest inflammatory bowel disease)
	Presence of polyps, melena or hematochezia

Mezoff AG, Preud'homme DL: How serious is that GI bleed? Contemp Pediatr 11:60–92, 1994.

74. In acute GI bleeding, how may vital signs indicate the extent of volume depletion?

It is important to remember that in acute bleeding in children, it may take from 12–72 hours for full equilibration of a patient's hemoglobin to occur. Vital signs are much more useful in patient management in the acute setting.

Vital Signs	Blood Volume Loss
Tachycardia without orthostasis	5–10% loss
Orthostatic changes: 　Pulse increases by 20 bpm 　BP decreases by 10 mmHg	> 10% loss
Hypotension and resting tachycardia	30% loss
Nonpalpable pulses	> 40% loss

From Mezoff AG, Preud'homme DL: How serious is that GI bleed? Contemp Pediatr 11:62, 1994; with permission.

75. What is the simplest way of differentiating upper GI from lower GI bleeding?

Nasogastric lavage. After insertion of a soft NG tube (12 Fr in small children, 14–16 Fr in older children), 3–5 ml/kg of room-temperature normal saline is instilled, and if bright red blood or coffee-ground material is aspirated, the test is positive. A pink-tinged effluent is not a positive test because it can simply denote dissolution of a clot and not active intestinal bleeding. By definition, upper GI bleeding occurs proximal to the ligament of Treitz. If the lavage is negative, it is unlikely that the bleeding is above this ligament and rules out gastric, esophageal, or nasal sources. However, bleeding from duodenal ulcers and duodenal duplications may sometimes be missed by these aspirates.

76. How does the type of bloody stool help pinpoint the location of a GI bleed?

1. **Hematochezia** (bright red blood):
   Normal stool spotting on toilet tissue likely suggests distal bleeding, such as anal fissure, juvenile colonic polyp.
   Mucous or diarrheal stools (especially if painful) indicates left-sided or diffuse colitis
2. **Melena** (black, tarry stools) indicates blood denatured by acid and usually implies a lesion likely before the ligament of Treitz. However, melena can be seen in Meckel's diverticulum (due to denaturation by anomalous gastric mucosa).
3. **Currant jelly** (dark maroon) **stools** usually come from the distal ileum or colon and often are associated with ischemia, as with intussusception.

Since blood is a cathartic, intestinal transit time can be greatly accelerated and makes defining the site of bleeding by the magnitude and color of the blood difficult. This difficulty underscores the importance of the initial NG tube insertion.

77. What can cause false-negatives and false-positives in stool testing for blood?

Hemoglobin and its various derivatives (e.g., oxyhemoglobin, reduced hemoglobin, methemoglobin, carboxyhemoglobin) can serve as catalysts for the oxidation of guaiac (HemOccult) or benzidine (Hematest) when a hydrogen peroxide developer is added, producing a color change.

False negatives	Ingestion of large doses of ascorbic acid
	Delayed transit time or bacterial overgrowth allowing bacteria to degrade the hemoglobin to porphyrin
False positives	Recent ingestion of red meat or peroxidase-containing fruits and vegetables (e.g., broccoli, radishes, cauliflower, cantaloupes, turnips)

78. How do the causes of lower GI bleeding vary by age group?

Newborns	Infants	Children
Anal fissure	Anal fissure	Anal fissure
Allergic proctocolitis	Infectious diarrhea	Polyp
Infectious diarrhea	Allergic proctocolitis	Infectious diarrhea
Hirschsprung disease	Meckel's diverticulum	Lymphonodular hyperplasia
Necrotizing enterocolitis	Intussusception	Inflammatory bowel disease
Volvulus	GI duplication	Henoch-Schönlein purpura
Stress ulcer	Peptic ulcer	Meckel's diverticulum
Vascular malformation	Foreign body	Peptic ulcer
GI duplication		Hemolytic uremic syndrome
		Vascular malformations

* In order of frequency.
From Mezoff AG, Preud'homme DL: How serious is that GI bleed? Contemp Pediatr 11:82, 1994; with permission.

79. A previously asymptomatic 18-month-old presents with large amounts of painless rectal bleeding (red but mixed with darker clots). What is the likely diagnosis?

Meckel's diverticulum. This outpouching occurs from the failure of the intestinal end of the omphalomesenteric duct to obliterate. Up to 2% of the population may have a Meckel's diverticulum, and about half contain gastric mucosa. Most are usually silent throughout life. Meckel's is twice as common in males and usually presents in the first 2 years of life as massive painless bleeding, red or maroon in color. Tarry stools are observed in about 10% of cases. A history of previous minor episodes may be obtained. The presentation can range from shock to intussusception with obstruction, volvulus, or torsion. Meckel's diverticulitis, which occurs in 10–20% of cases, may be indistinguishable from appendicitis.

80. What percentage of patients with Meckel's diverticulum will have a falsely negative technetium-99m scintiscan?

Up to 45%. If clinical suspicion remains high, a nuclear medicine study with tagged RBCs or surgical or laparoscopic exploration is indicated.

Teitelbaum DH, et al: Laparoscopic diagnosis and excision of Meckel's diverticulum. J Pediatr Surg 29:495–497, 1994.

81. How can the reliability of the Meckel's scintiscan be improved?

This radionuclide study employs ^{99m}Tc pertechnetate, which is taken up by the heterotopic gastric muscosa. Both pentagastrin (an HCl-stimulating hormone) or H_2 antagonists (e.g., cimetidine) may improve sensitivity. False-positives can occur in other anomalies containing ectopic gastric mucosa (e.g., duplication cysts) or inflammatory bowel disease. False-negative studies also occur, and angiography may be needed (especially with brisk bleeding). In rare instances, the diagnosis is made only at the time of laparotomy.

82. Describe the management for massive upper GI bleeding.

Massive upper GI hemorrhage is a life-threatening emergency, and initial therapy precedes the specific diagnostic evaluation. Management includes:

- Brief history and character of bleeding, previous episodes, bleeding disorders
- Vital signs
- Intravascular access and serologic studies (CBC, LFTs, coagulation profile, crossmatch)
- Nasogastric tube insertion
- Full history and physical examination
- Transfusion and intravascular support
- Determination of probable etiology

    1. Peptic disease
        Diagnostic endoscopy
        Therapeutic endoscopy
        H2-blockers, antacids,
           sucralfate
        If no resolution,
           Surgical repair of ulcer
           Partial resection

    2. Variceal bleeding
        Diagnostic endoscopy
        Therapeutic endoscopy
        Vasopressin
        Sengstaken-Blakemore tube
        If no resolution,
           Emergency portosystemic shunt
           Esophageal devascularization

    3. Mallory-Weiss tear
    4. Superficial vascular anomaly
        Endoscopic ablation

83. How do the causes of upper GI bleeding vary by age group?

Newborns	Infants	Children
Swallowed maternal blood	Epistaxis	Epistaxis
Hemorrhagic gastritis	Gastritis	Tonsillitis/sinusitis
Stress ulcer	Esophagitis	Gastritis
Idiopathic	Stress ulcer	Gastric/duodenal ulcer
Coagulopathy	Gastric/duodenal ulcer	Medications
Gastric outlet obstruction	Foreign bodies	Mallory-Weiss tears
Gastric volvulus	Gastric volvulus	Tumors
Pyloric stenosis	Esophageal varices	Hematologic disorders
Antral or pyloric webs		Esophageal varices
		Münchausen/Münchausen-by-proxy syndrome

* In order of frequency.
From Mezoff AG, Preud'homme DL: How serious is that GI bleed? Contemp Pediatr 11:82, 1994; with permission.

84. Why is the buffering of gastric acid important in controlling upper GI bleeding?

1. Acid is ulcerogenic and can cause and propagate erosions.
2. Coagulation is better in a neutral or alkaline environment than in an acidic one.
3. Platelet plugs are disrupted by gastric pepsins, but these pepsins function less well in a neutral or alkaline environment

Mezoff AG, Preud'Homme DL: How serious is that GI bleed? Contemp Pediatr 11:79, 1994.

85. Name the six most common causes of massive GI bleeding in children.

- Esophageal varices
- Hemorrhagic gastritis
- Peptic ulcer (mainly duodenal)
- Meckel's diverticulum
- Crohn disease with ileal ulcer
- Arteriovenous malformation

Treem WR: Gastrointestinal bleeding in children. Gastrointest Endosc Clin North Am 5;78, 1994.

HEPATIC/BILIARY DISEASE

86. What are the most sensitive indicators of hepatic function?

The most sensitive indicator of hepatic disease is the fasting serum bile salt assay. Bile salts are synthesized and excreted by the liver to promote fat absorption and conserved by ileal reabsorption into the enterohepatic circulation. While highly sensitive, this assay is of no use in hepatic failure. Since hepatic failure denotes the impairment of hepatic function, the most clinically useful assays monitor the processes of synthesis, detoxification, excretion, and metabolic regulation. Synthesis of serum proteins, such as albumin, and clotting factors are important indicators of hepatic function, but interpretation can be complicated by infection., disseminated intravascular coagulation, and third-space fluid shifts. Other measures of true hepatic function include transamination and urea synthesis and drug detoxification and elimination. Tests of aminopyrine, methacetin, caffeine, and galactose metabolism have all been recently used in an attempt to quantify hepatic function in a meaningful way.

87. How should a normal child with isolated hepatomegaly be evaluated?

All children with isolated hepatomegaly should have a careful history and physical examination. Family history of liver disease, previous exposure to hepatitis, foreign travel, blood transfusions, and drugs or toxins should be determined. One should verify that the liver is indeed large and not displaced by adjacent structures or hyperinflation. The consistency, character, and tenderness of the liver will provide information about possible etiologies. The spleen should be carefully palpated. Cutaneous signs of chronic liver disease and portal hypertension, lymphadenopathy, retinal pathology, cardiac lesions, and abdominal venous hums may indicate a particular etiology. Isolated hepatomegaly without splenomegaly or CNS involvement should be evaluated systematically to conserve resources.

88. What is the differential diagnosis for hepatomegaly?

Hepatocytic inflammation
    Infectious (bacterial, viral, mycobacterial, fungal, abscess, parasitic)
    Noninfectious (toxic, drug-induced, autoimmune, postobstructive)
Kupffer cell (septicemia/systemic infection, malignancy, granulomatous hepatitis, vitamin A
    toxicity)
Congestion (congestive heart failure, Budd-Chiari, sickle cell, vascular tumors)
Infiltration
    Nonneoplastic (extramedullary hematopoiesis, cysts, benign tumors)
    Neoplastic (Langerhans cell histiocytosis, leukemia, lymphoma, metastatic tumors,
        hepatoblastoma, hepatocellular carcinoma)
Storage (glycogen storage disease, mucopolysaccharidoses, lipidoses, gangliosidoses)
Metabolic (α1-antitrypsin disease, galactosemia, hereditary fructose intolerance, hereditary
    tyrosinemia, Wilson disease, hemochromatosis, Reye syndrome, fatty-acyl-CoA dehy-
    drogenase deficiency)
Steatosis (malnutrition, hyperalimentation, acute refeeding, steroids)
Portal tract (congenital hepatic fibrosis, idiopathic cirrhosis)
Bile duct abnormalities (arteriohepatic dysplasia, obstruction, biliary atresia, sclerosing
    cholangitis)
Miscellaneous (juvenile rheumatoid arthritis, systemic lupus erythematosus, cerebrohepatorenal
    syndrome, cystic fibrosis, endocrine [hypopituitarism, hypothyroidism, hypocorticolism])

89. A 3-year-old who experiences mild fluctuating jaundice in times of illness "just like his Uncle Kevin" is likely to have what condition?

Gilbert syndrome is due primarily to a decrease in hepatic glucuronyl transferase activity. Normally, bilirubin is diconjugated to glucuronic acid. In Gilbert's, the defective total conjugation results in increased production of monoglucuronides in bile and mild elevation in serum unconjugated (indirect) bilirubin. The syndrome is inherited in an autosomal dominant fashion with incomplete penetrance (boys outnumber girls by 4:1). Frequency of this gene in the population is estimated at 2–6%. Elevations of bilirubin are noted during times of medical and physical stress, particularly fasting.

90. List the most common causes of direct hyperbilirubinemia in an infant.
Biliary atresia, α_1-antitrypsin deficiency, arteriohepatic dysplasia, and cholestasis secondary to total parenteral nutrition or sepsis in the premature infant.

91. What types of liver injury are associated with various drugs?

Type of Liver Injury	Drug
Zonal liver necrosis	Acetaminophen
	Phenytoin
	Isoniazid
	Ketaconazole
Cholestasis	
Canalicular	Sex hormones
	Cyclosporine
Hepatocanalicular	Erythromycin
	Chlorpromazine
	Azathioprine
	Cimetidine
Microvesicular steatosis	Valproic acid
	Tetracycline
Granulomatous hepatitis	Sulfonamides
	Carbamazepine
Biliary cirrhosis	Methotrexate

From Mews C, Sinatra F: Chronic liver disease in children. Pediatr Rev 14:429, 1993; with permission.

92. What are the causes of chronic hepatitis in children?

Viral Hepatitis
Hepatitis B
Hepatitis C
Delta hepatitis
Cytomegalovirus

Autoimmune hepatitis
Anti-smooth muscle antibody-positive
Anti-liver-kidney microsomal
  antibody-positive

Metabolic/genetic disorders
Wilson disease
α_1-antitrypsin deficiency
Cystic fibrosis
Steatohepatitis

Toxic hepatitis
Drugs
Hepatotoxins
Radiation

From Mews C, Sinatra F: Chronic liver disease in children. Pediatr Rev 14:427, 1993; with permission.

93. In children with α_1-antitrypsin deficiency, which organ system is initially involved, lung or liver?
α_1-Antitrypsin is a major inhibitor of several proteolytic enzymes, primarily leukocyte elastase. It was first described in adults with chronic obstructive pulmonary disease. Since leukocyte elastase functions relatively unchecked, elastic fibers in the lung are digested with resultant destruction of alveolar walls and eventual panacinar emphysema. However, since the pulmonary effects take years to evolve, this condition rarely presents with pulmonary disease in children. More common presentations are neonatal cholestasis, hepatomegaly, chronic hepatitis, or, rarely, cirrhosis with liver failure. The pathophysiology of the liver disease is less clear. α_1-antitrypsin is synthesized in the liver, and in affected children, variants of the protein may be blocked from

release from the hepatocyte. Some studies suggest that the buildup of these variants may be toxic and lead to chronic liver injury.

94. How is Pi typing useful in the evaluation of α₁-antitrypsin deficiency?

Pi typing (short for protease inhibitor typing) takes advantage of the fact that there are over 70 variants of the α_1-antitrypsin protein, each with a different electrophoretic mobility. Alleles are inherited in a codominant fashion, and thus a gene from each parent is expressed in one individual. MM is the normal phenotype and has the highest activity. ZZ has the lowest activity and most common association with liver disease. PiMM is the most common Pi type, with a distribution of about 87%, PiMS represents 8% and PiMZ 2%. The incidence of PiZZ ranges between 1:2000–5000.

95. An infant with cholestasis, triangular facies, and a pulmonic stenosis murmur is likely to have what syndrome?

One of the most common etiologies of neonatal cholestasis and hepatitis is arteriohepatic dysplasia, or **Alagille syndrome**. Now called **syndromic bile duct paucity**, it consists of a constellation of conjugated hyperbilirubinemia and cholestasis, typical triangular facies, cardiac lesions of pulmonic stenosis, peripheral pulmonic stenosis, or occasionally more significant lesions, butterfly vertebrae, and eye findings of posterior embryotoxon and Axenfeld anomaly, or iris processes. The patient may have extreme cholestasis, with pruritus and marked hypercholesterolemia. Although some patients have mental deficiency, most are normal. The usual mode of inheritance of Alagille syndrome is autosomal dominant.

96. Describe the clinical findings in portal hypertension.

Obstruction to portal flow is manifest by two physical signs: **splenomegaly** and **increased collateral venous circulations**. Collaterals are evident on physical examination in the anus and abdominal wall and by special studies in the esophagus. Hemorrhoids may suggest collaterals, but in older patients these are present in high frequency without liver disease, and thus their presence has no predictive value. Dilation of the paraumbilical veins produces a rosette around the umbilicus (the caput medusae), and the dilated superficial veins of the abdominal wall are visible. A venous hum may be present in the subxiphoid region, from varices in the falciform ligament.

97. How do the clinical presentations of acute and chronic liver failure vary?

Hepatic failure may be acute and fulminant or it may follow a prolonged chronic course. In **fulminant hepatic failure**, there is a worsening of the hyperbilirubinemia and a decreased synthetic capacity which is evidenced by a worsening coagulation profile (vitamin-K resistant) and decreasing concentrations of fibrinogen, urea, and serum albumin. Encephalopathy, with concomitant increases in serum ammonia, may develop. As the liver mass shrinks, hepatic transaminases (a marker of liver damage) may paradoxically fall toward normal. These patients are at high risk for hypoglycemia.

Chronic hepatic failure, caused by a wide variety of infectious, toxic, and metabolic abnormalities, is characterized by jaundice and cutaneous manifestations (spider angiomas, caput medusae, palmar erythema). Fluid retention, development of ascites, renal hypoperfusion, and metabolic acidosis may occur. Mental status alterations and tremulous asterixis are chronic neurologic features. Ominous signs are GI bleeding, renal failure, cerebral edema, and coma.

98. A patient with liver failure develops confusion. Why worry?

Hepatic encephalopathy can present as either a rapid progression to coma or as mild fluctuations in mental status over extended times. A single underlying cause has not been established, but suspected toxins include ammonia, other neurotoxins, and a relatively increased GABA activity. **Management** is as follows:

1. Treat any precipitating factors (e.g., infection, hemorrhage)
2. Limit protein to 0.5–2.0 gm/kg/day

3. Use modified amino acid preparations
4. Administer lactulose, 1 ml/kg every 6 hrs, until diarrhea begins and then titrate to achieve mild diarrhea
5. Peritoneal dialysis may be indicated in severe coma and prior to liver transplantation
6. Intracranial pressure monitoring in advanced cases

99. In children with liver failure, how should GI hemorrhage be managed?
1. Pass an NG tube to monitor upper GI hemorrhage in patients with portal hypertension
2. Daily vitamin K IV (0.2 mg/kg) for 3 days, and continue if response is seen
3. Judicious administration of fresh frozen plasma for clinical bleeding
4. Have blood cross-matched at all times; for children with variceal bleeding, have 40 ml/kg whole blood and 0.2 U/kg platelets available
5. For gastritis or peptic ulceration, treat with cimetidine (30 mg/kg/day) and maintain gastric pH > 5

100. Liver transplantation in children: what is the long-term outcome?
In the past two decades, since the introduction of cyclosporine, the long-term outcome for patients with liver transplantation has improved markedly. Initially, the one-year survival rate was less than 50% for children. Current one-year survival rates for infants are > 80% with very little mortality from the first to the fifth year after transplant. The greatest improvement in the mortality rate has occurred in the pretransplantation waiting period. Initially, > 50% of infants died while on the transplantation list because of inadequate organ supply. Although regional centers for allotment and fair priority scoring systems have helped in part, the most significant advancement has been the development of technology allowing reduced size "split-livers" from adults to be used in infants. The use of living-related donors in the future may also help the organ supply for livers.

101. Which patients are at risk for cholelithiasis?

	Pigment Stone	*Cholesterol Stone*
Demography		
Race	—	Native American
Sex	—	Females
Age	—	Adolescence
Diet	—	Obesity
Total parenteral nutrition	+++	—
Hemolytic disease (esp. sickle cell disease, thalassemia, hereditary spherocytosis)	+++	—
Cystic fibrosis	—	+++
Ileal disease	—	+++
Defects in bile salt synthesis	—	+++
Hypertriglyceridemia	—	+++
Diabetes mellitus	—	+++

Adapted from Shaffer EA: Gallbladder disease. In Walker WA, Watkins JB (eds): Pediatric Gastrointestinal Disease. Philadelphia, B.C. Decker, 1991, p 1154; with permission.

102. Are there predisposing factors for cholecystitis in children and adolescents?
Most are conditions that predispose to the formation of gallstones. Acalculous cholecystitis occurs in only about 15% of cases. In addition to the risk factors for gallstones (see Question 101), other predisposing factors include pregnancy, obesity, and family history of biliary disease.

INFLAMMATORY BOWEL DISEASE

103. How do ulcerative colitis and Crohn disease vary in the intestinal distribution?
   Ulcerative colitis is limited to the superficial mucosa of the colon. It always involves the rectum and extends proximally to a variable extent. Limited distal ulcerative colitis has been termed ulcerative proctitis and in children may have a better prognosis. Regional enteritis, or **Crohn disease**, is a transmural inflammation of the bowel that may affect the entire tract from the mouth to the anus. The syndrome of limited Crohn colitis may be difficult to differentiate from ulcerative colitis.

104. What features differentiate ulcerative colitis from Crohn disease?

	Ulcerative Colitis	*Crohn Disease*
Incidence (10–19-year olds)	2/100,000	3.5/100,000
Onset during childhood	15–20%	20–25%
Clinical presentation	Diarrhea—50%	Diarrhea—80%
	Rectal bleeding— > 90%	Rectal bleeding—50%
	Weight loss—65%	Weight loss—85%
	Growth failure—10%	Growth failure—35%
	Pain with defecation	Anorexia, postprandial pain; extraintestinal signs may predominate
Site of disease at presentation	Rectal involvement—100%	Ileum ± colon—50–70%
	Left-sided colitis—50–60%	Colon alone—10–20%
	Severe pancolitis—10%	Proximal small bowel—10–15%
		Gastroduodenal— < 5%
Endoscopic findings	Continuous inflammation	Focal or segmental inflammation
	100% rectal involvement	Rectal sparing
	Erythema, edema, friability, ulceration on abnormal mucosa	Aphthous or linear ulcerations on normal-appearing mucosa
		Cobblestoning
		Abnormal terminal ileum— > 50%
Histologic findings	Mucin depletion	Epithelioid granulomas
	Villous mucosal surface pattern	Histiocytic infiltrates
	Crypt abscesses	Pericryptitis
	Epithelial atypia	Submucosal extension of inflammation
	Continuous disease	Discontinuous disease

From Hofley PM, Piccoli DA: Inflammatory bowel disease in children. Med Clin North Am 78:1283, 1994; with permission.

105. As the severity of ulcerative colitis increases, how does the treatment vary?
   Treatment varies according to the age of the patient and the duration and severity of disease. Sulfasalazine is the usual first therapy in all cases of ulcerative colitis, except if the patient is G6PD-deficient or highly sulfa-allergic. Folate supplementation should be given concomitantly. Steroid or 5-aminosalicylic acid enemas may control distal-limited disease. In more severe cases, prednisone (or any of the steroid group) is used to induce remission. When outpatient therapy is unsuccessful, elemental diets or parenteral alimentation are instituted. Long courses of intake restriction and aggressive intravenous nutritional therapy are likely to be efficacious. Immunosuppressive therapy (azathioprine) may have a role in the maintenance of remission. When medical therapy fails or when toxic megacolon is present, surgical therapy is necessary.
   Hanaver SB: Drug therapy: Inflammatory bowel disease. N Engl J Med 334:841–848, 1996.

106. In a child diagnosed with inflammatory bowel disease (IBD), what are the potential long-term complications?

The complications and presentations of IBD have considerable overlap.

1. *Severe perianal disease* can be a debilitating complication. More prevalent in Crohn disease, it may range from simple skin tags to total devastation of the perineum. Deep perianal abscesses can interfere with the ability to sit and walk, and open drainage is often necessary. More extensive surgical removal may result in damage to the sphincter and subsequent incontinence. Fistulization to the vagina, bladder, or skin may occur.

2. In Crohn disease, *enteroenteral fistulae* may occur and "short-circuit" the absorptive process. The thickened bowel may obstruct or perforate, requiring operation. The recurrence rate is high after surgery, repeated operations are often necessary, and short bowel syndrome may result. In many cases a permanent ostomy is placed, although pouch construction and continent ileostomies have become more common.

3. In ulcerative colitis, the patient may require *surgery* because of the severity or duration of disease. In the past, most patients had total colectomy and ileostomy, but the current recommended procedure is a subtotal colectomy and an endorectal pullthrough with rectal mucosal stripping. This procedure maintains intestinal continuity, and the patient develops normal rectal continence, although with increased stool frequency.

4. *Toxic megacolon* may occur with either form of IBD but is much more common with ulcerative colitis. After a progressive course, fever and a decrease in diarrhea usually herald a distended, tender, and tympanitic abdomen. The profound dilation of the bowel may be segmental or total, and massive hemorrhage or perforation may ensue. Mortality is high if toxic megacolon is not identified and treated aggressively.

5. *Growth retardation and delayed puberty* are seen in both diseases but are more common in Crohn disease. The insidious onset may result in several years of linear growth failure before the correct diagnosis is made. With epiphyseal closure, linear growth is terminated, and short adult stature will be permanent.

6. *Hepatic complications* of IBD include chronic active hepatitis and sclerosing cholangitis, which may require liver transplantation.

7. *Nephrolithiasis* may occur in patients with resections or steatorrhea due to increased intestinal absorption of oxalate.

8. Chronic reactive and restrictive *pulmonary disease* has been noted.

9. Arthralgias are common, but destructive *joint disease* is uncommon.

107. Are children with IBD at increased risk for malignancy?

The risk of malignancy has not been studied systematically in pediatric populations with IBD. The risk in adults depends both on the disease and its duration. After 10 years of ulcerative colitis, the risk rises dramatically (1–2% increased incidence of malignancy per year). The risk is felt to be higher in patients with pancolitis compared to those with limited left-sided disease. The carcinomas associated with ulcerative colitis are often poorly differentiated and metastasize early. They have a poorer prognosis and are more difficult to identify by radiographic and colonoscopic examinations. Most authors indicate that carcinoma of the bowel is much less common in Crohn disease, although this has been disputed. The risk of lymphoma is increased in patients with Crohn disease. Immunosuppressive therapy such as azathioprine may also increase the risk of neoplasia.

108. When is surgery indicated in IBD in children?

Crohn disease	Ulcerative colitis	
Perforation with abscess formation	Urgent:	Hemorrhage
Obstruction with or without stenosis		Perforation
Uncontrolled massive bleeding		Toxic megacolon
		Acute fulminant colitis unresponsive to maximal medical therapy

Crohn disease	Ulcerative colitis	
Draining fistulas and sinuses	Elective:	Chronic disease with recurrent severe exacerbations
Toxic megacolon		
Growth failure in patients with localized areas of resectable disease		Continuous incapacitating disease despite adequate medical treatment
		Growth retardation with pubertal delay
		Disease of > 10 years' duration with evidence of epithelial dysplasia

From Hofley PM, Piccoli DA: Inflammatory bowel disease in children. Med Clin North Am 78:1293–1295, 1994; with permission.

109. Which has a better prognosis, Crohn disease or ulcerative colitis?

The outcome for patients with ulcerative colitis is better unless toxic megacolon or carcinoma develops. In these patients, surgery is curative, and the chronic morbidity depends on the type of surgery employed. Patients with Crohn disease can be expected to lead a functional and productive life. However, as many as three-fourths require surgery within 5 years, and only half of those with growth failure achieve significant catch-up growth.

MALDIGESTION/MALABSORPTION

110. What bedside tests on a stool specimen are helpful in establishing carbohydrate malabsorption as a contributing factor to diarrhea?

- Stool pH: The pH is tested on litmus paper and acidic pH (< 5.5) is suggestive of carbohydrate malabsorption.
- Clinitest: This tests for reducing substances (e.g., lactose). If positive, it is suggestive of carbohydrate malabsorption. When testing for sucrose, the specimen must first be hydrolyzed with acid, because sucrose is a nonreducing substance.

111. How is the lactose breath hydrogen test done?

Actually, this test may be done for any carbohydrate. It measures the end-products of bacterial fermentation (i.e., hydrogen) which are exhaled by a patient following ingestion of a substrate. The test uses the presence of hydrogen-producing bacteria in the colon to determine the degree of malabsorption of a specific sugar. Lactose is most commonly tested. After a preingestion measurement of breath hydrogen, 2 gm/kg (up to 50 gm) of lactose in a 20% solution of water is consumed by the patient. Lactose, which is not digested and/or absorbed, reaches the large intestine where it is catabolized by bacteria, producing hydrogen gas. The hydrogen is subsequently excreted in the lungs. Samples of air are collected at 30-minute intervals, and excretion curves calculated using gas chromatography and compared with normals. False-negatives can occur if antibiotics have recently been given or in approximately 1% of the population who are colonized with bacteria that are non-hydrogen-producers.

112. Which other tests can be used to evaluate suspected carbohydrate malabsorption?

Carbohydrate malabsorption is characterized by abdominal pain, typanitic abdominal distension, watery and frothy stools, increased flatulence, nausea, and occasional vomiting. As noted, stool can be tested for an acidic pH and the presence of reducing substances. Disaccharide absorption (and rarely monosaccharide disorders) can be assayed by breath tests which evaluate specific sugar absorption. Other tests include:

1. D-Xylose absorption test evaluates the absorption of a monosaccharide (from the jejunum) which requires neither pancreatic digestion nor surface hydrolysis. D-Xylose (14.5 gm/m^2 up to 25 gm) is administered orally, and blood and urine levels are determined at set intervals. At 1 hour, blood levels should be 20 mg/dl, and by 5 hours, more than half of the ingested dose should have been excreted in urine. An abnormal result occurs with diminished surface area (e.g., celiac disease), bacterial overgrowth, and altered transit.

2. **Biopsy** directly assays multiple enzymes in the small intestine.

3. **Pancreatic exocrine function:** Although fat and protein malabsorption commonly predominate in pancreatic insufficiency, polysaccharide digestion can also be abnormal. Pancreatic function can be assayed directly by obtaining duodenal secretions or indirectly by the bentiromide absorption test.

113. Name the four varieties of lactose intolerance in childhood.

1. **Primary** or **congenital alactasia** is a rare disorder caused by absent or markedly decreased lactase in small intestinal biopsies specimens. The levels of other surface enzymes are normal. This rare autosomal recessive disorder presents at birth in infants fed a lactose-containing formula with severe watery diarrhea which resolves when lactose intake is eliminated.

2. **Acquired** or **postenteritis** lactose intolerance is due to the destruction of the superficial mucosa of the small intestine and its resident lactase. Resolution of this syndrome occurs following repair of the microvillus environment.

3. **Term** and **preterm newborns** have a limited capacity to hydrolyze lactose in the first few weeks of life. In certain situations this may be clinically important, but in normal breastfed infants, it does not justify formula changes. Stool-reducing substances are commonly present in breastfed infants' stools.

4. **Late-onset** lactose intolerance is due to the progressive decrease in small intestinal lactase activity seen in many ethnic groups during childhood. Some 15–80% of adults are lactose malabsorbers and, in many, this defect is uniform and severe. These patients have distension, bloating, discomfort, nausea, or diarrhea following ingestion of lactose-containing foods.

114. How does late-onset lactase deficiency vary by ethnicity?

After high levels in infancy, lactase levels decline progressively; after age 5 years, most people have lactase levels of about 10% of infancy. Since it is statistically more common to have these lower levels, the term *deficiency* may be a misnomer. Lactose intolerance may develop if excessive lactose loads are ingested.

Approximate Percentage of Low Lactase Activity by Ethnic Group

United States		Worldwide	
White	20%	Dutch	0%
Hispanic	50%	French	32%
Black	75%	Filipino	55%
Native American	90%	Vietnamese	100%

115. What conditions produce secondary lactose deficiency?

Any disorder that alters the mucosa of the proximal small intestine may result in secondary lactose intolerance. For this reason, the lactose tolerance test is commonly used as a screening test for intestinal integrity, although this has the disadvantage of concomitantly identifying all primary lactose malabsorbers. Although a combination of factors is present in many disease processes, secondary lactose intolerance can be organized into lesions of the microsurface, total surface, transit time, and site of bacterial colonization in the small bowel.

At microvillus/brush border	Bulk intestinal surface area
Postenteritis	Short bowel syndrome
Bacterial overgrowth	Bacterial overgrowth in proximal small bowel
Inflammatory lesions (Crohn disease)	Altered transit with early lactose entry
At level of the villus	into colon
Celiac disease	Hyperthyroidism
Allergic enteropathy	Dumping syndromes
Eosinophilic gastroenteropathy	Enteroenteral fistulas

116. Which disorders of carbohydrate absorption are inherited?

Monosaccharides	Polysaccharides
Glucose-galactose malabsorption	Congenital amylase deficiency
Disaccharides	Pancreatic insufficiency syndromes
Congenital alactasia (lactase deficiency)	Shwachman syndrome
Congenital sucrase-isomaltase deficiency	Cystic fibrosis
Trehalose deficiency	

Glucose-galactose malabsorption is an autosomal recessive disorder of carrier-mediated transport; patients have a normal ability to absorb fructose. Sucrase-isomaltase deficiency is the most common of the congenital abnormalities of carbohydrate absorption; the combined defect always coexists, and incidence is as high as 10% in some populations. By contrast, congenital lactase deficiency is extremely rare. Trehalose is a brush border enzyme whose only function is to digest trehalose. The source of trehalose is mushrooms, and occasionally gas and diarrhea attributed to rich or spicy foods may be due to this deficiency. Obviously, this disease is of little clinical importance (except to mushroom farmers). Additionally, all humans lack enzymes to digest stachyose and raffinose, two sugars in high concentration in beans. This explains the "beans syndrome," which for most people is clinically similar to lactose intolerance.

117. What is gluten?

After starch has been extracted from wheat flour, gluten is the residue that is left. This residue is made up of multiple proteins that are distinguished by their solubility and extraction properties. For example, the alcohol-soluble fraction of wheat gluten is wheat gliadin. It is this protein component that is primarily responsible for the mucosal injury that occurs in the small bowel in patients with sprue.

118. Why does the flat villous lesion in the small intestine develop in celiac disease?

The relationship of the small intestinal flat villous lesion to celiac disease is well established, but the pathogenesis is still unclear. One theory is that an intestinal enzyme that normally digests gluten is absent, resulting in a toxic reaction that produces changes in the intestinal epithelium. This enzyme has been actively sought but never conclusively proven. A number of immunologic abnormalities have been suggested in celiac patients. Children with celiac disease have circulating antigliadin antibodies, and there is an increase in IgA- and IgM-containing plasma cells in the lamina propria. The number of intraepithelial lymphocytes is also increased. Each of these phenomena may disappear on a prolonged gluten-free diet. Celiac disease is associated with HLA B8, DR3, and DR7. The lectin hypothesis is based on the theory that a cell surface membrane defect may allow gluten to act as a lectin, and the subsequent reaction cause cell toxicity. Other hypotheses have focused on an increased permeability of the mucosal barrier or precipitation by viral infections.

119. What clinical features suggest celiac disease?

Gluten-sensitive enteropathy (celiac disease) is a relatively common cause of severe diarrhea and malabsorption in infants and children. Children with celiac disease commonly present between ages 9 and 24 months with failure to thrive, diarrhea, abdominal distention, muscle wasting, and hypotonia. After several months of diarrhea, growth slows. Weight typically decreases before height. Often, these children become irritable and depressed and display poor intake and symptoms of carbohydrate malabsorption. Vomiting is less common. On examination, the growth defect and distention are commonly striking. There may be a generalized lack of subcutaneous fat, with wasting of the buttocks, shoulder girdle, and thighs. Edema, rickets, and clubbing may also be seen.

120. How is the diagnosis of celiac disease confirmed?

To diagnose celiac disease, **multiple small bowel biopsies** must be obtained. In a typical sequence, the first biopsy on gluten should show villous atrophy, with increased crypt mitoses and disorganization and flattening of the columnar epithelium. This should resolve fully on the second biopsy after a strict gluten-free diet. To confirm the diagnosis and eliminate the possibility of a coincidental recovery after an infectious enteritis, a third biopsy must be obtained after the patient has again been challenged with gluten. This biopsy again must show the manifestations of the disease. The increasing utility of commercial antigliadin antibodies may shorten the expense and invasiveness of this sequence. In many patients, the titer falls dramatically with treatment and increases again with challenge. Unfortunately, the currently available tests are not sensitive or specific enough to be used alone for diagnosis.

121. In addition to celiac disease, what disorders are associated with a flat villous lesion?

Acute enteritis
    Bacterial disease
    Viral disease
    Protozoal (*Giardia*)
    Radiation enteritis
Allergic enteropathy
    Milk-soy protein allergy
    Celiac disease
    Eosinophilic gastroenteritis
Immunoregulatory abnormalities
    Immunodeficiency
    Graft vs. host disease

Chronic enteritis
    Tropical sprue, Whipple disease
    Intractable enterocolitis
    Lymphoma
Malnutrition
    Protein calorie
    Folate deficiency
    Iron deficiency
Congenital
    Congenital villous atrophy

122. How is the steatocrit measured?

Excessive fat in the stool is a measure of malabsorption, and usually a 24-hour collection and analysis is done. However, the steatocrit is a rapid measurement of the percentage of fat in a spot sample of stool. It is done by taking 0.5 gm of stool and homogenizing it with 0.05 gm of sand and 2 ml of water. From this slurry, a microhematocrit tube is filled, spun, and the percentage of fat layer calculated (much like a spun hematocrit). Newborns normally excrete up to 15% fat, and this percentage falls with age. A value above 5% is abnormal for any child over age 3.

Phuapradit P: The steatocrit: A simple method for estimating stool fat content in newborn infants. Arch Dis Child 56:725–727, 1981.

NUTRITION

123. In the world of ideal pediatric nutrition, what are the various requirements for protein, fat, and carbohydrates?

Protein should account for 7–15% of caloric intake and should include a balance of the 11 essential amino acids. Protein requirements range from 0.7–2.5 gm/kg/day. Fats should provide 30–50% of caloric intake. While most of these calories are derived from long-chain triglycerides, sterols, medium-chain triglycerides, and fatty acids may be important in certain diets. Linoleic acid and arachidonic acid are essential for tissue membrane synthesis, and approximately 3% of intake must be composed of these triglycerides. The remaining 50–60% of calories should come from carbohydrates. About half of these are contributed by mono- and disaccharides, such as sucrose and lactose, and the remainder as starch.

124. Which fatty acid is the most essential?

Linoleic acid. It is converted to longer chain fatty acids with multiple double bonds, which are essential components of membranes. Arachidonic acid is also a component of membranes, but it can be synthesized from linoleic acid. A dietary intake of linoleic acid at a level of 1–2% of dietary calories will prevent both the biochemical and clinical manifestations of essential fatty acid deficiency. Oral fats high in linoleic acid include safflower oil (72%), sunflower oil (61%), and corn oil (54%).

125. If recommended caloric intakes are maintained, what is normal daily weight gain in young children?

Age	Weight Gain (grams)	Recommended Caloric Intake (kcal/kg/day)
0–3 mos	26–31	100–120
3–6 mos	17–18	105–115
6–9 mos	12–13	100–105
9–12 mos	9	100–105
1–3 yrs	7–9	100
4–6 yrs	6	90

It should be noted that when babies are primarily breastfed, growth during months 3–18 is less than that indicated in the table. On average, breastfed babies gain 0.65 kg less than formula-fed infants in the first year of life.

Dewey KG, et al: Growth of breast-fed and formula-fed infants from 0 to 18 months: The DARLING Study. Pediatrics 89:1035–1041, 1992.

National Research Council, Food and Nutrition Board: Recommended Daily Allowances. Washington, D.C., National Academy of Sciences, 1989.

126. What is the calorie-nitrogen ratio?

The relationship between energy and protein intake. Usually a ratio of 150:1 or more is required, but this ratio is modified in states of increased protein utilization or decreased protein metabolism.

127. What are the recommended bottle feedings by age?

Age	No. of Feedings	Oz per Feeding
Birth–1 wk	6–10	1–3
1 wk–1 mo	7–8	2–4
1 mo–3 mos	5–7	4–6
3 mos–6 mos	4–5	6–7
6 mos–9 mos	3–4	7–8
10 mos–12 mos	3	7–8

128. Why is honey not recommended for infants in the first year of life?

Honey, as well as some commercial corn syrups, has been associated with infantile botulism. *Clostridium botulinum* spores contaminate the honey and are ingested. In infants, intestinal colonization and multiplication of the organism may result in toxin production and lead to symptoms of constipation, listlessness, and weakness.

129. How is nutritional status objectively assessed in children?

1. The most easily obtainable information comes from a carefully plotted *growth chart*. Anthropometric data give an estimate of the height, weight, and head circumference of a child, compared to a population standard. Growth curves also provide a plot of weight for height (or stature). At any single point in time, this is a more accurate representation of the current nutritional status of the child. A change in the child's percentile after the first 6–12 months may signify the presence of a nutritional problem or systemic disease.

2. *Compare actual with ideal body weight* (average weight for height age). The ideal body weight is determined by plotting the child's height on the 50th percentile and recording the corresponding age. The 50th percentile weight for that age is obtained, and this ideal body

weight is divided by the actual weight. The result is expressed as a percentage, the percent ideal body weight, which gives a better stratification of patients with significant malnutrition. A %IBW of > 120 is obese, 110–120 is overweight, 90–110 normal, 80–90 mild wasting, 70–80 moderate wasting, and < 70 severe wasting.

3. *Measurement of midarm circumference* provides information about the subcutaneous fat stores, and the midarm-muscle circumference (calculated from the triceps skinfold thickness) estimates the somatic protein or muscle mass. Subscapular skinfold thickness measurements may be preferable in infants. These values can be used to calculate the percent body fat in children. Potential errors in calculation arise when there is overhydration or underhydration, extreme obesity, musculoskeletal disorders, and profound mental-motor retardation.

4. *Laboratory assessment* of nutritional status can provide objective data about the patient. Vitamin and mineral status can be directly assayed. Measurements of albumin (half-life 14–20 days), transferrin (half-life 8–10 days), and prealbumin (half-life 2–3 days) can provide information about protein synthesis, but each may be affected by certain diseases. The ratio of albumin to globulin may decrease in protein malnutrition. The creatinine height index is a measure of lean body mass, which decreases as muscle protein is used as an energy source. Specific measurements of nitrogen balance may be obtained to determine the degree of protein anabolism or catabolism.

130. What are the medical consequences of obesity in children and adolescents?

1. Increased height
2. Early menarche
3. Advanced bone age
4. Increased blood pressure
5. Increased incidence of sleep apnea
6. Increased incidence of cholelithiasis
7. Increased long-term cardiovascular risks

131. How can examination of the head alone suggest problems of malnutrition?

Clinical Sign	*Nutrient Deficiency*
Epithelial	
Skin	
Xerosis, dry scaling	Essential fatty acids
Hyperkeratosis, plaques around hair follicles	Vitamin A
Ecchymoses, petechiae	Vitamin K
Hair	
Easily plucked, dyspigmented, lackluster	Protein-calorie
Nails	
Thin, spoon-shaped	Iron
Mucosal	
Mouth, lips, and tongue	B vitamins
Angular stomatitis (inflammation at corners of mouth)	B_2 (riboflavin)
Cheilosis (reddened lips with fissures at angles)	B_2, B_6 (pyridoxine)
Glossitis (inflammation of tongue)	B_6, B_3 (niacin), B_2
Magenta tongue	B_2
Edema of tongue, tongue fissures	B_3
Spongy, bleeding gums	Vitamin C
Ocular	
Conjunctival pallor due to anemia	Vitamin E (premature infants), iron, folic acid, vitamin B_{12}, copper
Bitot's spots (grayish, yellow, or white foamy spots on the whites of the eye)	Vitamin A
Conjunctival or corneal xerosis, keratomalacia	Vitamin A
Periorbital edema	Protein

132. What causes Harrison grooves?

Harrison grooves are horizontal depressions extending from the lower end of the sternum to the midaxillary line along the 6th and 7th costal cartilages. This corresponds to the sites of attachment of the anterior portion of the diaphragm. The grooves can be congenital, a sign of rickets, or rarely, associated with atrial septal defects.

133. How do marasmus and kwashiorkor differ clinically?

Although both disorders are due to a deficiency in energy intake, the syndromes differ dramatically because of the available protein sources. **Kwashiorkor** is edematous malnutrition due to low serum oncotic pressure. The low serum proteins result from a disproportionately low protein intake compared to the overall caloric intake. These children appear replete or fat, but have dependent edema, hyperkeratosis, and atrophic hair and skin. They generally have severe anorexia, diarrhea, and frequent infections and may have cardiac failure. **Marasmus** is severe nonedematous malnutrition caused by a mixed deficiency of both protein and calories. Serum protein and albumin levels are usually normal, but there is a marked decrease in muscle mass and adipose tissue. Signs are similar to those noted in hypothyroid children, with cold intolerance, listlessness, thin sparse hair, dry skin with decreased turgor, and hypotonia. Diarrhea, anorexia, vomiting, and recurrent infections may be noted.

134. With what laboratory tests should a patient on hyperalimentation be monitored?

* Daily until stable, then twice per week
     Serum glucose, sodium, potassium, chloride, bicarbonate
     BUN and creatinine
     Calcium, phosphate, magnesium
* Weekly
     Complete blood count with platelets
     Bilirubin and LFTs
     Cholesterol and triglycerides
     Albumin, total protein, total iron-binding capacity
* As indicated by disease state
     Serum B_{12}, iron, trace elements, serum amino acids

135. What are the major complications of intravenous hyperalimentation?

Mechanical, infectious, and metabolic.

1. **Mechanical complications** vary with the type of infusion and the delivery system, and include local or distant site thrombosis, perforation of the vasculature or heart, and accidental breakage or infiltration of the infusate into the subcutaneous, pleural, or pericardial space. Unfortunately, accidental dislodgment or disconnection is all too common in pediatric patients, and an emergency clamp should always be accessible.

2. Line-associated **sepsis** is a life-threatening complication that is associated with poor line aseptic technique. Any patient with fever and a central line should have an immediate set of peripheral and "line" cultures obtained and be started on antibiotics pending the results. Because sepsis can be seeded by contaminated IV solutions, all equipment should be cultured in suspected line sepsis.

3. The **metabolic complications** of hyperalimentation may be limited by close monitoring but potentially span an enormous range including:

     * Congestive heart failure and pulmonary edema from excessive infusate
     * Hyper- and hypoglycemia
     * Electrolyte, mineral, and vitamin disorders
     * Hyperlipidemia
     * Metabolic acidosis
     * Hyperammonemia
     * Anemia

• Demineralization of bone (i.e., rickets)
• Hepatic disorders (e.g., cholestasis, cholelithiasis, hepatitis)
• Eosinophilia (of unknown cause)

PEPTIC ULCER DISEASE

136. What are the signs and symptoms of primary peptic ulcer (PUD) in childhood?:
Abdominal pain is the most common symptom of primary PUD. It is present in 90% of patients. While the quality and character of the pain can be variable, it is usually localized to the epigastric region. Classically, ulcer pain is temporally related to meals, but in children, this association occurs only about half the time. **Nocturnal pain** occurs in about 60% of patients and is a key feature in distinguishing organic from nonorganic pain. **Melena** is a feature in about a third of cases. Vomiting, hematemesis, and perforation are uncommon features.

137. How does the presentation of secondary ulcer disease differ from primary PUD?
Secondary ulcers, in association with other conditions, are often silent until very acute symptomatology develops. **Pain** occurs only in about 25% of patients, but 80% develop **melena**, 60% have **hematemesis**, and 30% have **perforation**, often with severe bleeding and shock. The secondary ulcers have much higher mortality, morbidity, and need for surgical intervention. In primary PUD, symptoms are often recurrent and protracted. Delays in diagnosis can last for up to 2–4 years.

138. What conditions are associated with secondary ulcers in children?
• *Systemic diseases:* sepsis, acidosis, sickle cell anemia, cystic fibrosis, systemic lupus erythematosus, renal failure, severe hypoglycemia
• *Traumatic injury:* head trauma, burns, major surgery
• *Drugs/toxins:* corticosteroids, nonsteroidal anti-inflammatory drugs, theophylline, tolazoline, aspirin

139. What treatments are available for PUD in children?
Acid-neutralizing antacids
    Effective in promoting ulcer healing
    Used more commonly for symptomatic pain relief because of poor compliance due to large volumes (0.5 ml/kg/dose) required for therapy and potential side effects (e.g., diarrhea and constipation)
    Side effects (e.g., diarrhea and constipation)
H_2-receptor antagonists
    Include cimetidine, ranitidine, famotidine
    Well-tolerated in children with few side effects
    Also effective as prophylaxis in setting of systemic illness, head trauma, or surgery
"Proton pump" inhibitors
    Prototype is omeprazole, a substituted benzimidazole, which irreversibly binds to the gastric parietal cell, inhibiting H^+–K^+ exchange
    Limited data on use in children
Sucralfate
    Chemical complex of sucrose actasulfate and aluminum hydroxide which binds to the ulcer base and acts as a barrier; adsorbs pepsin and neutralizes hydrogen ions
Anticholinergics
    Decrease acid secretion
    At effective doses, side effects (e.g., dry mouth and blurred vision) may be significant
Antibiotics
    As treatment for *Helicobacter pylori* infection
    Most effective treatment remains unclear, but combination therapy with amoxicillin, bismuth subsalicylate (Pepto-Bismol), and metronidazole has an eradication rate of 60–90%

140. What is the relationship of *Helicobacter pylori* infection with antral gastritis, peptic ulcer disease, and recurrent abdominal pain in children?

An area of considerable interest, debate, and research. In adults, *H. pylori* has been associated with duodenal ulceration in over 90% of patients and with gastric ulceration in 70% of patients. However, asymptomatic colonization complicates the picture. In asymptomatic adult volunteers, 20–25% of patients have *H. pylori* colonization, as contrasted with only 4% of asymptomatic children. Studies seem to indicate that in children, there is a strong relationship between *H. pylori* and antral gastritis and primary duodenal ulcer disease, but a weak relationship between *H. pylori* and gastric ulcers and recurrent abdominal pain.

Bourke B, et al: *Helicobacter pylori* infection and peptic ulcer disease in children. Pediatr Infect Dis J 15:1–12, 1996.

Macarthur C, et al: *Helicobacter pylori*, gastroduodenal disease, and recurrent abdominal pain in children. JAMA 273:729–734, 1995.

141. What methods are available for detecting the presence of *Helicobacter pylori* in the stomach or duodenum?

Non-invasive tests
    Stable isotope ^{14}C-urea breath test
    Serum ELISA IgG and IgA titers
Invasive tests
    Culture of biopsy specimen
    Identification of histologic gastritis
    Special stains for *H. pylori*

H. pylori produces urease, which can metabolize urea and produce CO_2, which is then exhaled by the patient. ^{14}C-labeled urea, given orally to the patient, exploits this peculiar metabolic step. If *H. pylori* is present in the proximal GI tract, labeled CO_2 is released. This is a reliable test, but requires (nonradioactive) labeled substrate and a mass-spectroscopy center for the assay. The ELISA assay detects the presence of antibody but is not as reliable for differentiating active disease from asymptomatic colonization. Levels of antibody titer may have some future role in monitoring therapeutic response.

The definitive diagnosis of *H. pylori*-associated gastritis requires endoscopic mucosal biopsies of the gastric antrum. The biopsy is cultured for *H. pylori* by direct inoculation of fresh minced tissue onto special media in the endoscopy lab. Multiple specimens are also sent for histologic evaluation. Convincing evidence of *H. pylori* disease occurs when there is gastritis, and special stains (silver stain or acridine orange) identify the organism in the overlying mucus. When *H. pylori* occurs in the absence of gastritis or ulcer disease, as commonly happens in adults, the bacterial presence may indicate colonization rather than infection.

142. Which patients should be evaluated for Zollinger-Ellison syndrome (ZES)?

ZES, a rare diagnosis in children, is ulcer disease caused by a gastrin-secreting tumor (gastrinoma). Patients usually present with symptoms secondary to peptic ulcer disease, and nearly all patients with ZES develop ulcers at some time in the course of the disease. In general, these ulcers are more persistent and progressive and commonly less responsive to treatment. Although the duodenal bulb is the most common location for both ZES and non-ZES associated ulcers, atypical ulcers in the distal duodenum or jejunum are more common in ZES. In children, any ulcer that does not heal after the first course of therapy should be investigated, as should patients with gastric acid hypersecretion and prominent gastric rugae.

143. How is the diagnosis of Zollinger-Ellison syndrome confirmed?

A simple screening test is the **fasting serum gastrin level**, which should be obtained when the patient is not receiving acid blockade (H_2 blockers) or antacids. An elevated level requires prompt further investigation. Usually, the gastrin level is at least threefold elevated in patients with ZES. Unfortunately, many patients with an elevated gastrin level do not have ZES. Furthermore, some patients with a normal gastrin level may have a hormone-secreting tumor.

When the diagnosis is strongly suspected but the serum gastrin concentration is low, a **gastric acid secretion test** is useful. Arteriography and CT scanning may be useful in locating a tumor, but in a large number of cases, even exploratory laparotomy may not identify the lesion.

SURGICAL ISSUES

144. What is the natural history of an umbilical hernia?

Most umbilical hernias < 0.5 cm spontaneously close before a patient is 2 years old. Those between 0.5 cm and 1.5 cm take up to 4 years to close. If the umbilical hernia is > 2 cm, it may still close spontaneously but may take up to 6 years or more. Unlike an inguinal hernia, incarceration and strangulation are very rare in an umbilical hernia.

Yazbeck S: Abdominal wall developmental defects and omphalomesenteric remnants. In Roy CC, et al (eds): Pediatric Clinical Gastroenterology, 4th ed. St. Louis, Mosby-Year Book, 1995, pp 134–135.

145. Which umbilical hernias warrant surgical repair?

Because of the high probability of self-resolution, indications for surgery are controversial. Some authorities argue that a hernia > 1.5 cm at age 2 years warrants closure due to its likely persistence for years. Others argue that since the likelihood of incarceration is small for umbilical hernias, surgical closure is warranted prior to puberty only for persistent pain, history of incarceration, or associated psychologic disturbances.

146. When should an infant with inguinal hernia have it electively repaired?

Once the diagnosis of inguinal hernia is made, it should be repaired as soon as possible. In a large study of children with incarcerated hernia, 40% of patients had a known inguinal hernia prior to incarceration and 80% were awaiting elective repair. Eighty percent of the children with incarceration of a hernia were infants under age 1 year, and especially in this age group, delay of repair should be minimized.

Stylianos S, et al: Incarceration of inguinal hernia in infants prior to elective repair. J Pediatr Surg 18:582–583, 1993.

147. How are incarcerated inguinal hernias reduced?

Incarceration occurs most commonly in the first year of life. Because the infant will likely need to be admitted, nothing should be given to eat or drink. Reduction is most easily accomplished if the infant is calm (preferably asleep), warm, and, if possible, in a slightly reverse Trendelenburg position. Analgesia, such as 0.1 mg/kg/IV of morphine, may facilitate the relaxed state. With one hand, the examiner stabilizes the base of the hernia by the internal inguinal ring and, with the other hand, milks the sac distally to progressively force fluids and/or gas through the ring to eventually allow complete reduction. If unsuccessful, immediate surgery is indicated.

148. Under what clinical settings should manual reduction of an inguinal hernia not be attempted?

When the patient has clinical findings of shock, perforation, peritonitis, GI bleeding or obstruction, or evidence of gangrenous bowel (bluish discoloration of the abdominal wall).

149. How do causes of intestinal obstruction vary by age?

Infant/young child

Pyloric stenosis	Intussusception
Inguinal hernia	Appendicitis
Malrotation	Intestinal duplication
Intestinal atresia or stenosis	Omphalomesenteric remnants
Intraluminal web	Hirschsprung disease
Adhesions	

Older child

Appendicitis (perforated)	Intussusception (lead-point)
Adhesions	Malrotation
Inguinal hernia	Omphalomesenteric remnants
Inflammatory bowel disease	

From Caty MG, Azizhan RG: Acute surgical conditions of the abdomen. Pediatr Ann 23:194, 1994; with permission.

150. What is the significance of green vomiting in the first 72 hours of life?

In the neonatal period, green vomiting should always be interpreted as a sign of potential intestinal obstruction requiring surgical intervention. In one study of 45 infants with green vomiting, 20% had surgical conditions (e.g., malrotation, jejunal atresia, jejunal stenosis), 10% had nonsurgical obstruction (e.g., meconium plug and microcolon), and 70% had idiopathic vomiting which self-resolved. If plain radiographs are equivocal or abnormal, upper or lower GI contrast studies should be done.

Lilien LD, et al: Green vomiting in the first 72 hours in normal infants. Am J Dis Child 140:662–664, 1986.

151. What are the clinical findings of malrotation of the intestine?

Malrotation of the intestine is due to the abnormal rotation of the intestine around the superior mesenteric artery during embryologic development. Arrest of this counterclockwise rotation may occur at any degree of rotation. The lesion may present with in utero volvulus or may be asymptomatic throughout life. Infants may present with intermittent vomiting or complete obstruction. Any infant with bilious vomiting should be considered emergent and requires careful evaluation for volvulus and other high-grade surgical obstructions. Recurrent abdominal pain, distention, or lower GI bleeding may result from intermittent volvulus. Full volvulus with arterial compromise results in intestinal necrosis, peritonitis, perforation, and an extremely high incidence of mortality. Because of the extensive nature of the lesion, postoperative short gut syndrome is present in many patients who require resection.

152. Describe the x-ray findings associated with malrotation.

The upper GI series will show malposition and malfixation of the ligament of Treitz. The proximal small bowel may be located in the right upper quadrant, but this is not always true. The cecum viewed from either the upper GI series or barium enema may be unfixed or malpositioned. In both malrotation and volvulus, the plain films may be entirely normal. There may be proximal obstruction with gastroduodenal distention. In volvulus, the barium studies may show an obstruction near the gastroduodenal junction, often with a twisted appearance.

153. In an asymptomatic child with an incidental finding of malrotation, is surgery indicated?

Because of the persistent possibility of acute volvulus and intestinal obstruction, surgery is *always* indicated when intestinal malrotation is diagnosed.

154. In what settings should intussusception be suspected?

Ileocolic intussusception is twice as common in boys and usually occurs before the second year of life. Half of all cases occur between 3 and 9 months. Most cases do not have any identifiable etiology, but there is a seasonal clustering in the spring and fall which may be related to the increase in respiratory and enteric infections during those times, with resultant reactive intestinal lymphoid tissue. Colicky pain is seen in over 80% of cases but may be absent. It typically lasts 15–30 minutes, and the baby usually sleeps between attacks. In about two-thirds of cases, there is blood in the stool (currant jelly stools). Other presentations include massive lower GI bleeding or blood streaking on the stools. The infant may appear quite toxic, dehydrated, or in shock. Fever and tachycardia are common. A right lower quadrant mass may be palpable, or the area may feel surprisingly empty. Distention may accompany decreased bowel sounds. Radiographs typically demonstrate a small bowel obstruction pattern, but the diagnostic study of choice is a barium enema, which should be performed in all children with symptoms < 48 hours in duration. In 80% of cases, the barium enema under fixed hydrostatic pressure will reduce the intussusception. If this is unsuccessful, surgical reduction is necessary.

155. How commonly does intussusception present with the classic findings?

The classic triad of symptoms of intussusception consists of **colicky pain, vomiting,** and passage of **bloody mucous** stool. Unfortunately, this classic presentation is the exception. In one study of 583 patients, 80% of patients did not have this triad of symptoms, about 30% had blood in the stool, and this percentage dropped to about 15% if the abdominal pain was present for < 12 hours. Palpation of a mass can suggest the diagnosis, but a high degree of suspicion is key.

Bruce J, et al: Intussusception: Evolution of current management. J Pediatr Gastroenterol Nutr 6:663, 1987.

156. What causes intussusception?

Intussusception is caused by one proximal segment of the bowel being invaginated and progressively drawn caudad and encased by the lumen of distal bowel. This causes obstruction and may occlude the vascular supply of the bowel segment. There is commonly a lead point on the proximal bowel which initiates the process. Lead points have included lymphoid hyperplasia, hypertrophied Peyer's patches, eosinophilic granuloma of the ileum, lymphoma, lymphosarcoma, leiomyosarcoma, leukemic infiltrate, polyps, duplication cysts, ectopic pancreas, Meckel's diverticulum, hematoma, Henoch-Schönlein syndrome, worms, foreign bodies, and appendicitis.

157. What is the most common type of intussusception?

Ileocolic intussusception. It is also the most common cause of intestinal obstruction in infancy). Cecocecal and colocolic intussusceptions are less common. Gastroduodenal intussusception is rare and is usually associated with a gastric mass lesion such as a polyp or a leiomyoma. Enteroenteral intussusception is seen after surgery and in patients with Henoch-Schönlein syndrome.

158. How frequently does intussusception recur?

Idiopathic ileocolic intussusception recurs in about 3% of all cases. Intussusceptions in older children tend to recur at a higher frequency if the causative lesion is not removed. It is important to investigate cases of recurrent intussusception for an underlying lesion.

159. Duodenal or jejunoileal atresia—which is associated with other embryonic abnormalities?

Duodenal atresia is caused by a persistence of the proliferative stage of gut development and a lack of secondary vacuolization and recanalization. It is associated with a high incidence of other early embryonic abnormalities. Extraintestinal anomalies occur in two-thirds of patients. In jejunoileal atresia, the lesion occurs after the establishment of continuity and patency, as evidenced by distal meconium seen in these patients. The etiology is postulated to be a vascular accident, volvulus, or mechanical perforation. Jejunoileal atresias are usually not associated with any other systemic abnormality.

160. How does the infant with biliary atresia classically present?

In classic cases, a term infant develops a recognizable jaundice by the third week of life, with increasingly dark urine and acholic stools. Usually the child appears well, with acceptable growth. The skin color sometimes appears somewhat greenish yellow. The spleen becomes palpable after the third or fourth week, at which time the liver is usually hard and enlarged. In other cases, the jaundice is clearly present in the conjugated form during the first week of life. There is also a strong association between the polysplenia syndrome and biliary atresia.

161. What are the complications of the Kasai procedure?

The Kasai procedure is a hepatic portoenterostomy. The remnants of the extrahepatic biliary tree are identified, and a cholangiogram is performed to verify the diagnosis. Dissection and resection of the remaining extrahepatic ducts and the fibrous plate present at the porta are then performed. A Roux-en-Y jejunal limb is constructed to drain bile from the porta, and in some cases, this limb is temporarily exteriorized at a double-barrel ostomy. Postoperative complications include intestinal obstruction, early and late ascending cholangitis, peristomal breakdown, and stomal varices. In nearly half the cases, the procedure does not establish bile flow, and in most patients, there is ongoing inflammation and the development of portal hypertension.

162. When should a Kasai procedure be performed?

As soon as possible. Earlier operation results in a dramatically improved outcome. Patients operated before 70 days of age have increased likelihood of a successful procedure, although exceptions at both ends of this spectrum are common. Some surgeons now suggest that infants diagnosed late in the course should have a primary liver transplant rather than a hepatic portoenterostomy.

163. Why is distinguishing between a high and low imperforate anus so important?

The distinction is based on whether the blind end of the terminal bowel or rectum ends above (high-type) or below (low-type) the level of the pelvic levator musculature. The patients with high-type imperforations will have ectopic fistulae (rectourinary, rectovaginal), urologic anomalies (hydronephrosis or double collecting system), and lumbosacral spine defects (sacral agenesis, hemivertebrae). The surgical repair in these patients is much more extensive, and future problems of incontinence, fecal impaction, and strictures are much more likely.

164. What is the classic presentation of pyloric stenosis?

An infant 3–6 weeks of age presents with progressive nonbilious projectile vomiting leading to dehydration with hypochloremic, hypokalemic, metabolic alkalosis. On physical exam, a pyloric "olive" is palpable and peristaltic waves are visible.

165. How is pyloric stenosis diagnosed?

If the classic signs and symptoms are present in association with the typical blood chemistry findings (hypochloremia, hypokalemia, metabolic alkalosis), the diagnosis can be made on clinical grounds. If the diagnosis is in doubt, ultrasound can be used to visualize the hypertrophic pyloric musculature. Upper GI contrast studies demonstrate pyloric obstruction with the characteristic "string sign" and enlarged "shoulders" bordering the elongated and obstructed pyloric channel.

166. What is the mechanism of hyperbilirubinemia in babies with pyloric stenosis?

Unconjugated hyperbilirubinemia has been noted in 10–25% of babies with pyloric stenosis. While an enhanced enterohepatic circulation for bilirubin probably plays a role in the pathogenesis of the hyperbilirubinemia, hepatic glucoronyl transferase activity is markedly depressed in these jaundiced infants. The mechanism of diminished glucoronyl transferase activity is not known, although inhibition of the enzyme by intestinal hormones has been suggested.

167. In a patient with suspected pyloric stenosis, why is an acidic urine very worrisome?

As vomiting progresses in infants with pyloric stenosis, a worsening hypochloremic metabolic alkalosis develops. Multiple factors (e.g., volume depletion, elevated aldosterone levels) result in maximal renal efforts to reabsorb sodium. In the distal tubule, this is typically achieved by exchanging sodium for potassium and hydrogen. When total body potassium levels are very low, hydrogen is preferentially exchanged, and a paradoxic aciduria develops (in the setting of an alkaline plasma). This acidic urine is an indication that intravascular volume expansion and electrolyte replenishment (especially chloride and potassium) are urgently needed.

168. What syndromes are associated with pyloric stenosis?

- Trisomy 18
- Long-arm depletion 21
- Turner syndrome
- Smith-Lemli-Opitz syndrome
- Cornelia de Lange syndrome

169. What is the short bowel syndrome?

The short bowel syndrome results from extensive resection of the small intestine. Normally, the majority of carbohydrates, proteins, fats, and vitamins are absorbed in the jejunum and proximal ileum. The terminal ileum is responsible for the uptake of bile acids and vitamin B_{12}. Short bowel syndrome results in failure to thrive, malabsorption, diarrhea, vitamin deficiency, bacterial contamination, and gastric hypersecretion.

170. Why are infants with short bowel syndrome prone to renal calculi?

Chronic intestinal malabsorption results in an increase of intraluminal fatty acids, which saponify with dietary calcium. Thus, nonabsorbable calcium oxalate does not form, excessive oxalate is absorbed, and hyperoxaluria with crystal formation results.

171. In extensive small bowel resection, how much is "too much"?

Infants who retain 20 cm of small bowel as measured from the ligament of Treitz can survive if the ileocecal valve is intact. If the ileocecal valve has been removed, the infant usually requires a minimum of 40 cm of bowel to survive. The importance of the ileocecal valve appears to relate to its ability to retard transit time and minimize bacterial contamination of the small intestine.

172. What conditions may mimic appendicitis?

- Gastroenteritis
- Mesenteric adenitis
- Constipation
- Pelvic inflammatory disease
- Pyelonephritis
- Right lower lobe pneumonia
- Ruptured ovarian follicle/ovarian torsion
- Inflammatory bowel disease
- Henoch-Schönlein purpura
- Primary peritonitis
- Perforated peptic ulcer
- Pancreatitis

From Caty MG, Azizhan RG: Acute surgical conditions of the abdomen. Pediatr Ann 23:193, 1994; with permission.

173. How helpful are ancillary studies in the diagnosis of appendicitis?

The diagnosis of appendicitis remains a clinical one. The classic picture in children is a period of **anorexia** followed by **pain, nausea**, and **vomiting**. Abdominal pain begins periumbilically and then shifts after 4–6 hours to the right lower quadrant. Fever is low grade. Peritoneal signs are detected on exam.

However, ancillary studies may have value in equivocal cases. *WBC count* > 18,000/mm³ or a marked left shift is unusual in uncomplicated cases and suggests perforation or another diagnosis. A *urinalysis* with many WBCs suggests a urinary tract infection as the primary pathology. On a plain *radiograph*, a calcified fecalith may be seen in 5–10% of cases. A fecalith commonly precedes inflammation, and surgery is usually indicated. *Barium enema*, with only partial filling of the appendix or with evidence of a mass effect, is highly suggestive of appendicitis. An *ultrasound* revealing an enlarged noncompressible appendix is also highly suggestive and may tip the scales toward surgical exploration.

174. In children taken to surgery for appendicitis, how often is perforation of the appendix present?

It depends to a large extent on the age of the child (and, of course, on the skill of the clinician). Unfortunately, due to the variable location of the appendix, the clinical presentation of pain in appendicitis is often very different from the classical case. The younger the child, the more difficult the diagnosis. In infants < 1 year of age, nearly 100% of patients who come to surgery have a perforation. Fortunately, appendicitis is rare in this age group because the appendiceal opening at the cecum is much larger than the tip and obstruction is unusual. In children < 2 years, 70–80% are perforated, and in those up to 5 years, 50% are perforated. Particularly in younger children, a high index of suspicion is necessary and rapid diagnosis is critical. If the onset of symptoms can be pinpointed (usually anorexia related to a meal), 10% of patients will have perforation in the first 24 hours, but over 50% will perforate by 48 hours.

8. GENETICS

Elaine H. Zackai, M.D., JoAnn Bergoffen, M.D.,
Alan E. Donnenfeld, M.D., and Jeffrey E. Ming, M.D., Ph.D.

AUTOSOMAL TRISOMIES

1. Excluding chromosomal analysis, what laboratory tests suggest that a woman is carrying a fetus with trisomy 21?

The combination of low levels of **maternal serum alpha-fetoprotein** and **unconjugated estriol** and elevated levels of **human chorionic gonadotropin** (the so-called triple screen) can identify 60% of fetuses with Down syndrome with a false-positive rate of 5–7%. Abnormal screening tests can prompt definitive studies of chromosomal analysis.

2. What are the main advantages of chorionic villus sampling (CVS) over amniocentesis?

CVS is the aspiration of chorionic villi via a transcervical catheter or transabdominal needle using ultrasound guidance. The main advantage of CVS is that it can be done between 10–12 weeks of gestation compared with the usual 16-week timing of amniocentesis.

3. Describe the features of the three most common autosomal trisomies.

Common Autosomal Trisomies

FEATURE	TRISOMY 21	TRISOMY 18	TRISOMY 13
Eponym	Down syndrome	Edward syndrome	Patau syndrome
Liveborn incidence	1/800	1/8000	1/15,000
Tone	Hypotonia	Hypertonia	Hypo- or hypertonia
Cranium/brain	Mild microcephaly, flat occiput, 3 fontanels	Microcephaly, prominent occiput	Microcephaly, sloping forehead, occipital scalp defects, holoprosencephaly
Eyes	Upslanting, epicanthal folds, speckled iris (Brushfield spots)	Small palpebral fissures, corneal opacity	Micro-ophthalmia, hypotelorism, iris coloboma, retinal dysplasia
Ears	Small, low-set, over-folded upper helix	Low-set, malformed	Low-set, malformed
Facial features	Protruding tongue, large cheeks, low flat nasal bridge	Small mouth, micrognathia	Cleft lip and palate
Skeletal	Clinodactyly 5th digit, gap between toes 1 and 2, excess nuchal skin, short stature	Clenched hand, absent 5th finger distal crease, hypoplastic nails, short stature, thin ribs	Postaxial polydactyly, hypoconvex fingernails, clenched hand
Cardiac defect	40%	60%	80%
Survival	Long-term	90% die within first year	80% die within first year
Other features	(see below)	Rocker bottom feet, polycystic kidneys, dermatoglyphic arch pattern	Genital anomalies, polycystic kidneys, increased nuclear projections in neutrophils

4. Are Brushfield spots pathognomonic for Down syndrome?

No. Brushfield spots are speckled areas that occur in the periphery of the iris. They are seen in about 75% of patients with Down syndrome but also in up to 10% of normal newborns.

5. What clinical findings occur most frequently in Down syndrome infants?

Frequency of Positive Phenotypic Findings in Infants with Down Syndrome

Sagittal suture separated	98%	Muscle weakness	81%
Oblique palpebral fissure	98	Hypotonia	77
Wide space between first and second toes	96	Brushfield spots	75
False fontanel	95	Mouth kept open	65
Plantar crease between first and second toes	94	Protruding tongue	58
Hyperflexibility	91	Epicanthal folds	57
Increased neck tissue	87	Single palmar crease	50–55
Abnormally shaped palate	85	Brachyclinodactyly	50–51
Hypoplastic nose	83		

Modified from Pueschel SM: The child with Down syndrome. In Levine et al: Developmental-Behavioral Pediatrics. Philadelphia, W.B. Saunders, 1983, p. 356; with permission.

6. What is the chance that a newborn with a simian crease has Down syndrome?

A single transverse palmar crease is present in 4% of normal newborns. Bilateral palmar creases are found in 1%. These features occur twice as commonly in males than females. However, 50–55% of newborn infants with Down syndrome have a single transverse crease. Since Down syndrome occurs in 1/800 live births, the chance that a newborn with a simian crease has Down syndrome is only **1 in 60**.

7. What is the expected intelligence and personality of a child with Down syndrome?

The IQ range is generally 35–65, with a mean reported IQ Of 54. Occasionally, the IQ may be higher. Intelligence deteriorates in adulthood, with clinical and pathologic findings consistent with advanced Alzheimer disease. Autopsy results from brains of deceased adults with Down syndrome reveal both neurofibrillary tangles and senile plaques, as found in Alzheimer disease. By age 40, the mean IQ is 24. Children with Down syndrome are generally affectionate and docile. They tend toward mimicry and are noted usually to enjoy music, having a good sense of rhythm. However, 13% have serious emotional problems, and coordination is usually poor.

8. What causes the dementia of Down syndrome?

Pathologic evidence of senile dementia or Alzheimer disease (i.e., senile plaques, neurofibrillary tangles, and granulovascuolar degeneration) was reported in individuals with Down syndrome for the first time in 1929. Currently, it is believed that overexpression of a gene for the amyloid precursor (PreA4) located on the long arm of chromosome 21 may lead to amyloid deposition in Down syndrome patients.

Rumble B, et al: Amyloid A4 protein and its precursors in Down syndrome and Alzheimer's disease. N Engl J Med 320:1446–1452, 1989.

9. Why do older individuals with Down syndrome rarely develop atherosclerotic heart disease?

The enzyme cystathionine β-synthase (CBS) is needed to form cystathione from homocysteine and serine. Deficiency of this enzyme results in homocystinuria, which is characterized by precocious atherosclerosis and plasma accumulation of methionine and homocysteine. The gene for CBS is found on chromosome 21, and its activity is increased in cultured fibroblasts of Down syndrome patients. The plasma level of homocysteine has also been shown to be lower in Down syndrome patients after an overnight fast and a methionine load. It has been suggested that the higher enzymatic activity could be related to the lower incidence of atherosclerosis in individuals with Down syndrome.

10. Why is maternal age of 35 at delivery chosen as the cutoff for recommending amniocentesis for chromosome analysis?

There is a well-known association between advanced maternal age and trisomies (including XXY, XXX, trisomy 13, 18, and 21).

Maternal Age	Approximate Risk of Down Syndrome
30	1:1000
35	1:365
40	1:100
45	1:50

Most cases of Down syndrome involve nondisjunction at meiosis I in the mother. This may be related to the lengthy stage of meiotic arrest between oocyte development in the fetus until ovulation, which may occur as much as 40 years later.

11. What percentage of all babies with Down syndrome are born to women over the age of 35?

Only 20%. While their individual risk is higher, women in this age bracket account for only 5% of all pregnancies in the United States.

Haddow JE, et al: Prenatal screening for Down syndrome with use of maternal serum markers. N Engl J Med 327:588–593, 1992.

12. What percentage of cases of Down syndrome are due to translocations?

3.3% of all cases of Down syndrome are due to unbalanced Robertsonian translocations in which a third copy of chromosome 21 is present, attached to an acrocentric chromosome. The chance of translocation Down syndrome is two to three times greater in children of younger mothers (6–8% of mothers under 30). One of three infants with translocation Down syndrome will have a parent with a Robertsonian translocation. Two-thirds of the time, translocation Down syndrome occurs as a de novo event in the infant.

13. What is the overall recurrence risk of Down syndrome?

In chromosomally normal women under age 40, the recurrence risk for Down syndrome is 1% (assuming the father's chromosomes are also normal). Above age 40, the risk of having a child with Down syndrome increases, primarily as a function of maternal age. If the mother carries a translocation, the recurrence risk is 10%. If the father carries a translocation, the recurrence risk is 3–5%. One theory for this observed discrepancy between maternal and paternal rates of translocation Down syndrome is hindered motility of chromosomally abnormal sperm.

14. Does advanced paternal age increase the risk of having a child with trisomy 21?

There does not appear to be an increased risk of Down syndrome associated with paternal age until after age 55. Some studies have noted an increased risk of Down syndrome after this age, although others have not. The reports are controversial, and the statistical analysis needed to perform such a study is cumbersome. It is known that approximately 10% of all trisomy 21 cases derive the extra chromosome 21 from the father.

15. Why has the incidence of Down syndrome decreased from 1.6/1000 live births to 1.0–1.2/1000 live births over the past 25 years?

The decrease in incidence is a result of the reduction of births in older women and prenatal diagnosis. The risk for older women has not changed, but at the present time only 20% of children with Down syndrome are born to mothers over 35 years of age, whereas 25 years ago 50% of the children with Down syndrome were born to older mothers.

16. Which is technically correct: Down's syndrome or Down syndrome?

In 1866, John Langdon Down, physician at the Earlswood Asylum in Surrey, England, described the phenotype of a syndrome which now bears his name. However, it was not until 1959 that it was determined that this disorder is caused by an extra chromosome 21. The correct designation is Down syndrome.

CLINICAL ISSUES

17. What genetically inherited disease has the highest known mutation rate per gamete per generation?

Neurofibromatosis. The estimated mutation rate for this disorder is 1×10^{-4} per haploid genome. The clinical features are café-au-lait spots and axillary freckling in childhood followed by development of neurofibromas in later years. There is approximately a 10% risk of malignancy with this condition, and mental deficiency is common.

18. Which disorders with ethnic and racial predilections most commonly warrant maternal screening for carrier status?

Disorder	Ethnic or Racial Group	Screening Marker
Tay-Sachs disease	Ashkenazi Jewish, French French Canadian	Decreased serum hexosaminidase A concentration
Sickle cell anemia	Black African, Mediterranean, Arab, Indian Pakistani	Presence of sickling in hemolysate followed by confirmatory hemoglobin electrophoresis
Alpha- and beta-thalassemia	Mediterranean, Southern and Southeast Asian, Chinese	Mean corpuscular volume $< 80 \ \mu m^3$, followed by confirmatory hemoglobin electrophoresis

From D'Alton ME, DeCherney AH: Prenatal diagnosis. N Engl J Med 328:115, 1993; with permission.

19. Why are mitochondrial disorders transmitted from generation to generation by the mother and not the father?

Mitochondrial DNA abnormalities (e.g., many cases of ragged red fiber myopathies) are passed on from the mother because mitochondria are present in the cytoplasm of the egg and not the sperm. Transmission to males or females is equally likely; however, expression is variable because mosaicism with normal and abnormal mitochondria in varying proportions is very common.

Johns DR: Mitochondrial DNA and disease. N Engl J Med 333:638–644, 1995.

20. Which syndromes are associated with advanced paternal age?

Advanced paternal age is well documented to be associated with new dominant mutations. The assumption is that the increased mutation rate is due to accumulation of new mutations from many cell divisions. The more cell divisions, the more likely an error (mutation) will occur. The mutation rate in fathers > 50 is five times higher than the mutation rate in fathers < 20 years of age. Common autosomal dominant new mutations that have been recently mapped and identified are **achondroplasia** (Shiang et al., 1994), **Apert syndrome** (Wilkie et al., 1995), and **Marfan syndrome** (Dietz et al., 1991).

Dietz HC, Cutting GR, Pyeritz RE, et al: Marfan syndrome caused by a recurrent de novo missense mutation in the fibrillin gene. Nature 352:337–339, 1991.

Shiang R, Thompson LM, Zhu YZ, et al: Mutations in the transmembrane domain of FGFR3 cause the most common genetic form of dwarfism, achondroplasia. Cell 78:335–342, 1994.

Wilkie AO, Slaney SF, Oldridge M, et al: Apert syndrome results from localized mutations of FGFR2 and is allelic with Crouzon syndrome. Nature Genetics 9:165–172, 1995.

21. What is the most common genetic-lethal disease?

Cystic fibrosis (CF). A genetic-lethal disease is one that interferes with a person's ability to reproduce due to early death (before childbearing age) or impaired sexual function. CF is the most common autosomal recessive disorder in whites, occurring in 1/1600 (1 of every 20 individuals is a carrier for this condition). CF is characterized by widespread dysfunction of exocrine glands, chronic pulmonary disease, pancreatic insufficiency, and intestinal obstructions. Males are azospermic. The median survival is approximately 29 years.

22. Assuming that the husband is healthy and that no one in the wife's family has cystic fibrosis, what is the risk that a couple will have a child with cystic fibrosis if the husband's brother has the disease?

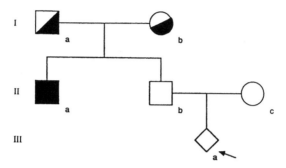

1. Since IIa is affected with CF, both his parents must be carriers.
2. The chance of IIb being a carrier is 2/3, since we know he is not affected by CF.
3. The risk of IIc being a carrier is 1/20 (the population risk).
4. The chance of IIIa being affected is: father's carrier risk × mother's carrier risk × the chance that both will pass on their recessive CF gene to their child; $\frac{2}{3} \times \frac{1}{20} \times \frac{1}{4} = \mathbf{1/120}$.

23. What are the "fat baby" syndromes?
 • Prader-Willi (obesity, hypotonia, small hands and feet)
 • Beckwith-Wiedemann (macrosomia, omphalocele, macroglossia, ear creases)
 • Sotos (macrosomia, macrocephaly, large hands and feet)
 • Weaver (macrosomia, accelerated skeletal maturation, camptodactyly)
 • Laurence-Moon-Biedl (obesity, retinal pigmentation, polydactyly)
 • Infants of diabetic mothers

24. What is the H₃O of Prader-Willi syndrome?
 Hyperphagia, hypotonia, hypopigmentation, and **obesity.** Up to 50% of patients, most with mental retardation, have a deletion on the long arm of chromosome 15. The gene(s) responsible for Prader-Willi syndrome are subject to parental imprinting. Imprinting refers to the process by which expression of a gene depends on whether it has been inherited from the mother or the father (reviewed by Deal, 1995). The gene(s) associated with Prader-Willi syndrome are paternally imprinted, meaning that loss of the paternal copy will result in the phenotype of Prader-Willi (Knoll et al., 1989; Robinson et al., 1991). A closely related area of the long arm of chromosome 15 is maternally imprinted, and loss of the maternal copy leads to Angelman syndrome (Chan et al., 1993). Angelman syndrome is characterized by severe developmental delay, abnormal gait, inappropriate laughter, and excessive movements, especially of the arms.

Chan C-TJ, Clayton-Smith J, Cheng X-J, et al: Molecular mechanisms in Angelman syndrome: A survey of 93 patients. J Med Genet 30:895–902, 1993.

Deal CL: Parental genomic imprinting. Curr Opin Pediatr 7:445–458, 1995.

Knoll JHM, Nicholls RD, Magenis RE, et al: Angelman and Prader-Willi syndromes have a chromosome 15 deletion but differ in parental origin of the deletion. Am J Med Genet 32:285–290, 1989.

Robinson WP, Bottani A, Xie YG, et al: Molecular, cytogenetic, and clinical investigations of Prader-Willi syndrome patients. Am J Hum Genet 49:1219–1234, 1991.

25. Name the two most common forms of dwarfism recognizable at birth.
 There are 21 different skeletal dysplasia syndromes that were classified at the International Nomenclature of Constitutional Diseases of Bone meeting as "recognizable at birth." The most common is **thanatophoric dwarfism**, a lethal chondrodysplasia characterized by flattened,

U-shaped vertebral bodies, telephone-receiver-shaped femurs, macrocephaly, and redundant skinfolds causing a pug-like appearance. Thanatophoric means death-loving (an apt description). The incidence is 1 in 6400 births. **Achondroplasia** is the most common viable skeletal dysplasia, occurring 1 in 26,000 live births. Its features are small stature (mean adult height 4'2"), macrocephaly, depressed nasal bridge, lordosis, and a trident hand. Some patients develop hydrocephalus due to a small foramen magnum. X-ray findings include narrowing of the interpedicular distance as one proceeds caudally. Both achondroplasia and thanatophoric dysplasia are due to mutations in fibroblast growth factor receptor 3 (Tavormina et al., 1995). In achondroplasia the mutation is in the transmembrance domain, while the mutation in thanatophoric dysplasia is either in the intracellular domain (type II) or the extracellular domain (type I).

Tavormina PL, Shiang R, Thompson LM, et al: Thanatophoric dysplasia (types I and II) caused by mutations in fibroblast growth factor receptor 3. Nature Genetics 9:321–328, 1995.

26. What are the risks of having a second child with autism?

The prevalence of autism in the siblings of autistic children has been estimated to be about 2–3%, which is 50–100 times greater than the expected rate of autism in the population (4–5/10,000). However, many families choose to limit further child bearing, and therefore, this estimate may be low. The genetics of autism are still unclear.

Folstein SE, Piven J: Etiology of autism: Genetic influences. Pediatrics 87(suppl):767–773, 1991.

27. What chromosomal abnormality is found in cri du chat syndrome?

Cri du chat syndrome is due to a deletion of material from the short arm of chromosome 5 (i.e., 5p–) which causes many problems including growth retardation, microcephaly, and severe mental retardation. Patients have a characteristic *cat-like cry* in infancy from which the syndrome derives its name. In 85% of cases, the deletion is a de novo event. In 15%, it is due to malsegregation from a balanced parental translocation.

28. Which syndromes are characterized by a senile-like appearance?
• Progeria (alopecia, atrophy of subcutaneous fat, skeletal dysplasia, early death)
• Werner syndrome (cataract, thick skin, sparse, gray hair)
• Cockayne syndrome (growth deficiency, retinal degeneration, impaired hearing, thick skin)
• Rothmund-Thomson syndrome (poikiloderma, cataract, ectodermal dysplasia)

29. List the syndromes and malformations associated with congenital limb hemihypertrophy.
• Russell-Silver syndrome
• Conradi-Hünermann syndrome
• Klippel-Trenaunay-Weber syndrome
• Beckwith-Wiedemann syndrome
• Wilms tumor
• Hypomelanosis of Ito
• CHILD syndrome (**C**ongenital **H**emidysplasia, **I**chtyosiform erythroderma, **L**imb **D**efects)
• Neurofibromatosis

One of every 32 patients with isolated hemihypertrophy is at risk for developing Wilms tumor. For this reason, renal and abdominal ultrasound should be offered periodically in childhood as a screening device for patients with hemihypertrophy.

30. Which genetic disorders are associated with hypoplastic left heart syndrome?

While most newborns with hypoplastic left heart syndrome have this defect as an isolated abnormality, several syndromes in which this congenital heart malformation is a component have been identified: Down syndrome, Turner syndrome, Smith-Lemli-Opitz syndrome, trisomy 13, trisomy 18, and Ivemark syndrome. Before extensive reconstructive surgery is attempted, it may be prudent to obtain a chromosomal analysis in cases where malformations are noted.

31. In the evaluation of a stillborn infant, how does the general appearance of the fetus suggest a likely etiology?

A *fresh embryo* or fetus implies a rapid expulsion after intrauterine or intrapartum death. These fetuses are usually without major anomalies and have normal karyotypes. Causes of death commonly are placental abruption, cord accidents, and ascending infection. A *macerated embryo* or fetus indicates prolonged retention in utero. In this circumstance, structural anomalies or chromosomal abnormalities are more frequent.

32. In which fetal and infant deaths are autopsies strongly advised?
1. Infants with external or suspected internal structural abnormalities
2. Infants with intrauterine growth retardation
3. Infants with nonimmune hydrops
4. Families with a previous unexplained loss
5. Infants with no obvious cause of death
6. Macerated fetuses

In addition to an autopsy, other studies that should be considered include chromosomal analysis, skeletal radiographs, placental and cord histologic studies, titers for congenital infection, and, if hydropic, evaluation for a hemoglobinopathy (e.g., alpha thalassemia), or possible metabolic storage disease.

Curry CJR: Pregnancy loss, stillbirth, and neonatal death. Pediatr Clin North Am 39:157–192, 1992.

33. How should women with recurrent pregnancy loss be evaluated?
Couples with recurrent pregnancy loss, variably defined as either two or three losses, should be considered for the following evaluations:

1. Cytogenetic analysis of both parents to rule out mosaicism or a balanced translocation.
2. Hysterosalpingogram to rule out malformations of the uterine cavity (congenital, DES-induced, myomas, and intrauterine synechiae)
3. Infectious workup for *Mycoplasma, Chlamydia,* and other pathogens
4. Immunologic evaluation for antiphospholipid antibody, anticardiolipin antibody, and antinuclear antibody (e.g., systemic lupus erythematosus)
5. Hormonal—endometrial biopsy or progesterone level analysis to rule out a luteal phase defect
6. Thyroid function tests
7. Evaluation of any suspected systemic illnesses

34. Give 8 reasons why a disease might be genetically determined but the family history be negative.
1. Autosomal recessive inheritance
2. X-linked recessive inheritance
3. Genetic heterogeneity (e.g., retinitis pigmentosa may be transmitted as AR, AD, or X-linked recessive)
4. Spontaneous mutation
5. Nonpenetrance
6. Expressivity (i.e., variable expression)
7. Extramarital paternity
8. Phenocopy (i.e., an environmentally determined copy of a genetic disorder)

Juberg RC: . . . but the family history was negative. J Pediatr 91:693–694, 1977.

DYSMORPHOLOGY

35. How are structural dysmorphisms categorized?
1. *Malformation:* a problem of poor formation (likely genetically based) in which the abnormality is present at the onset of development (e.g., hypoplastic thumbs of Fanconi syndrome)
2. *Disruption:* an extrinsic destructive process interferes with previously normal development (e.g., thalidomide causing limb abnormalities)
3. *Deformation:* an extrinsic mechanical force causes abnormalities, which are usually asymmetrical (e.g,. breech position causing tibial bowing and positional club feet)
4. *Dysplasia:* an abnormal cellular organization or function that generally affects only a single tissue type (e.g., cartilage abnormalities that result in achondroplasia)

36. What are the principal kinds of morphologic defects in infants with multiple anomalies?
1. *Developmental or polytopic field defect:* a pattern of anomalies derived from the distur-bance of a single region or part of an embryo which responds as a coordinated unit to extrinsic or intrinsic influences. Field defects are believed to be derivatives of a single malformative or disruptive process. For example, if the rostral mesoderm is disturbed early in development, mul-tiple anomalies of the head and face can occur.
2. *Sequence:* a pattern of multiple anomalies derived from a single known (or presumed) prior anomaly or mechanical factor. For example, the entity of micrognathia, glossoptosis, and cleft soft palate is more properly called the Pierre Robin sequence (rather than syndrome) be-cause the small mandible likely causes the developing tongue to be pushed posteriorly, which does not allow the posterior palatal shelves to close properly.
3. *Syndrome:* the nonrandom occurrence of multiple anomalies, with such an increased fre-quency that a pathogenetically causal relationship (often of unknown cause) is felt to be involved. For example, chromosomal syndromes (e.g., Down) have characteristic clinical features.
4. *Association:* the nonrandom occurrence of multiple anomalies without a known field defect, sequence initiator, or causal relationship, but with such a frequency that the malforma-tions have a statistical connection.

37. What is the difference between a major and a minor malformation?
Major malformations are unusual morphologic features that cause medical, cosmetic, or de-velopmental consequences to the patient. Minor anomalies are features that do not cause medical or cosmetic problems. Approximately 14% of newborn babies will have a minor malformation, whereas only 2–3% of newborns will have a major anomaly.

38. Identify the most common major congenital anomalies in the U.S.
Anencephaly and **spina bifida**. The combined prevalence is 0.5–2.0/1000 live births.

39. What is the clinical significance of a minor malformation?
Recognition of minor malformations in a newborn may serve as an indicator of altered mor-phogenesis or as a valuable clue to the diagnosis of a specific disorder. The presence of several minor malformations is unusual and often indicates a serious problem in morphogenesis. For exam-ple, when three or more minor malformations are discovered in a child, there is a > 90% risk of a major malformation also being present. The most common minor malformations involve the face, ears, hands, and feet. Almost any minor defect may occasionally be found as an unusual familial trait.

40. How common are minor anomalies in newborns?

Common Minor Anomalies

PHYSICAL FEATURE	BLACK INFANTS (%)	WHITE INFANTS (%)
Palpable metopic suture	42	64
Third sagittal fontanel	10	3
Double hair whorl	6	7
Overfolded ear helix	51	38
Preauricular sinus	5	0.8
Preauricular tag	0.7	0.3
Epicanthal folds, bilateral	1	1.4
Brushfield spots, bilateral	0.2	7
Anteverted nostrils	2	2.6
Supernumerary nipple	2.2	0.2
Umbilical hernia	6	0.7
Sacral dimple	0.6	4.8
Clinodactyly of both 5th fingers	4.5	5.2
Syndactyly, 2nd–3rd toes	0.5	0.6

Adapted from Holmes LB: Congenital malformations. In Behrman BE (ed): Nelson Textbook of Pediatrics, 14th ed. Philadelphia, W.B. Saunders, 1992, p 295, with permission

41. What are the 3 principal types of sequences?

1. *Malformation* sequences (resulting from poor formation of tissues)
2. *Deformation* sequences (resulting from mechanical factors)
3. *Disruptive* sequences (initiated by a disruptive process)

Examples include:

- DiGeorge sequence
- Early urethral obstruction sequence
- Extrophy of cloaca sequence
- Oligohydramnios sequence
- Caudal dysplasia sequence
- Pierre Robin sequence
- Extrophy of bladder sequence
- Rokitansky sequence
- Sirenomelia sequence
- Early amnion rupture sequence
- Jugular lymphatic obstruction sequence

42. Describe the most common associations.

CHARGE—**C**oloboma of the eye, **H**eart defects, **A**tresia of the choanae, **R**etardation (mental and growth), **G**enital anomalies (in males), **E**ar anomalies

MURCS—**M**üllerian duct aplasia, **R**enal aplasia, **C**ervicothoracic **S**omite dysplasia

VATER—**V**ertebral, **A**nal, **T**racheo-**E**sophageal, **R**enal or **R**adial anomalies

VACTERL—VATER anomalies plus **C**ardiac and **L**imb anomalies

43. What are the major vascular disruption sequences?

1. *Poland anomaly*—unilateral defect of the pectoralis muscle and syndactyly of the hand. This is thought to be due to an early deficit of blood flow through the subclavian artery to the distal limb and pectoral region.

2. *Hydranencephaly*—congenital absence of the cerebral hemispheres. Although the cause of this devastating defect can be varied, bilateral internal carotid artery occlusion has been commonly postulated.

3. *Proximal focal femoral hypoplasia*—unilateral dysgenesis of the proximal femur. Etiologies for this defect include familial genetic disorders, teratogenic influences, viral agents, maternal diabetes, trauma, and ischemia caused by vascular disruption.

4. *Oromandibular-limb hypogenesis spectrum*—craniofacial, limb, and often brain defects. This spectrum of anomalies suggests a diffuse disruptive vascular occlusion or hemorrhagic etiology.

44. What malformations are associated with oligohydramnios and polyhydramnios?

In early pregnancy (< 4 mos), the majority of amniotic fluid is produced by transudation through the placental membranes and fetal skin. Later in pregnancy, the bulk of amniotic fluid arises as a product of fetal urination. At term, the fetus swallows approximately 500 ml of amniotic fluid per day and urinates an equivalent amount. Fetal urine production increases rapidly from 3.5 ml/hr at 25 weeks to 25 ml/hr at term. Any malformation that leads to impaired urine production will cause oligohydramnios, including renal dysplasia, renal agenesis, and bladder outlet obstruction. When uteroplacental insufficiency occurs, the fetus is often faced with poor nutritive and volume support. The fetus becomes intravascularly depleted, leading to increased fluid conservation and decreased urine output, causing oligohydramnios. Oligohydramnios is often associated with intrauterine growth retardation.

The etiology of polyhydramnios may be broken down into maternal causes (30%), fetal causes (30%), and idiopathic causes (40%). Maternal disorders, such as diabetes, erythroblastosis fetalis, and preeclampsia, are often associated with excess amniotic fluid. Fetal disorders that commonly predispose to polyhydramnios are CNS anomalies (anencephaly, hydrocephaly, neurologic disorders, etc.), GI disorders (tracheoesophageal fistula, duodenal atresia), fetal circulatory disorders, and multiple gestation. The etiology for polyhydramnios in fetuses with CNS and upper GI anomalies is presumed to be impaired fetal swallowing ability.

45. What causes Potter syndrome?

Potter syndrome has come to be synonymous with fetal malformations caused by extreme oligohydramnios. Lack of amniotic fluid leads to fetal compression, a squashed, flat face, clubbing of the feet, pulmonary hypoplasia, and, commonly, breech presentation. Normal fetal lung development is dependent on in utero "breathing" and inhalation of amniotic fluid. In the absence of amniotic fluid, pulmonary hypoplasia occurs and is the cause of death for most fetuses with Potter syndrome. The underlying mechanism in Potter syndrome was initially reported to be renal agenesis or renal dysplasia. However, bladder outlet obstruction and prolonged premature rupture of the membranes may also cause this sequence. Some prefer that Potter syndrome be defined solely as renal agenesis.

46. If an infant is born with Potter syndrome, why should the parents undergo a renal ultrasound?

Renal agenesis is thought to be a sporadic or multifactorial condition, although autosomal dominant inheritance with variable expression (i.e., unilateral renal agenesis in a parent) has also been postulated. For this reason, obtaining a renal ultrasound on parents of a child with renal agenesis is advised. If the parents have normal renal evaluations, the empirically determined recurrence risk is approximately 3%. If one of the parents has unilateral renal agenesis, the recurrence risk may be as high as 50% due to a presumed autosomal dominant gene.

47. How do clinodactyly, syndactyly, and camptodactyly differ?

- *Clinodactyly:* curvature of a toe or finger (usually the fifth) due to hypoplasia of the middle phalanx, which is the last fetal bone to develop in the hands and feet. Normal curvature can consist of up to 8° of in-turning. Curvature beyond this is considered a minor anomaly.
- *Syndactyly:* an incomplete separation of fingers (usually 3rd and 4th) or toes (usually 2nd or 3rd)
- *Camptodactyly:* abnormal persistent flexion of fingers or toes

48. Name the three major types of dermal ridge patterns.

Dermal ridge patterns are formed early in embryogenesis. Their pattern is influenced by genetic inheritance, the influence of teratogens, congenital infections, and chromosomal abnormalities. The distal phalanges have a variety of dermal ridge patterns that can be classified in three major types: **arches, whorls,** and **loops.** Infants with trisomy 18 commonly have a high frequency of arches, an unusual finding in chromosomally normal individuals. In the foot, there is a pattern at the base of the great toe. In 50% of patients with trisomy 21, a simple arch pattern (called an open field) will be found. This occurs in < 1% of controls.

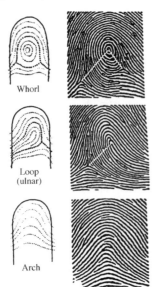

Whorl

Loop
(ulnar)

Arch

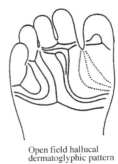

Open field hallucal
dermatoglyphic pattern

From Holt S: The genetics of dermal ridges. Br Med Bull 17:247, 1961; with permission.

49. Are preauricular ear tags a significant finding?
Preauricular pits and tags are minor anomalies that occur in about 0.3–1.0% of individuals, with a wide variance in frequency among racial groups. They are twice as common in females as in males and can be inherited as an autosomal dominant trait. They are believed to represent remnants of early embryonic branchial cleft or arch structures. As isolated findings, they do not warrant additional evaluations.

50. What is the proper way to test for low-set ears?
This designation is made when the upper portion of the ear (helix) meets the head at a level below a horizontal line drawn from the lateral aspect of the palpebral fissure. The best way to measure is to align a straight edge between the two inner canthi and determine whether the ears lie completely below this plane. In normal individuals, approximately 10% of the ear is above this plane.

From Feingold M, Bossert WH: Normal values for selected physical parameters: An aid to syndrome delineation. In Bergsma D (ed): The National Foundation-March of Dimes Birth Defects Series 10:9, 1974.

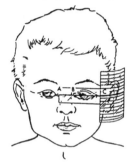
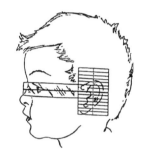

51. Where is the Darwinian tubercle located?
Also called the auricular tubercle, this is a cartilaginous bump on the upper part of the outer ear below and posterior to the helix. It is a minor variant that should not be considered an anomaly.

52. Why do the sclerae of patients with osteogenesis imperfecta appear blue?
Phylogenetically, the sclerae are closely related to the skeleton. In many animals, the sclera contains cartilage and osseous material. The primary component of sclera in humans is collagen. It is not surprising that in osteogenesis imperfecta and many other connective tissue diseases, the sclerae are abnormally thin and transparent, since abnormal collagen formation is the underlying defect in many of these disorders. The bluish color of the sclera in patients with connective tissue (especially collagen) diseases is thought to be due to visualization of the bluish-colored uvea (the eye layer behind the retina) as seen through a more transparent sclera. Uvea literally means grape, the name being derived from the similarity in their colors.

53. What is the significance of lip pits?
Lip pits derive from small, accessory salivary glands that fistulize on either side of the midline lower lip. This finding is most characteristic of Van der Woude syndrome, whose other features are cleft lip and/or palate and missing second premolars. Inheritance is autosomal dominant, yet variable expression often occurs, and in some cases only the lip pits will be present without the associated cleft lip and/or palate. Lip pits are seen less commonly in the rare popliteal pterygium syndrome.

54. What is the inheritance pattern of cleft lip and palate?
Most cases of cleft lip and palate are inherited in a polygenic or multifactorial pattern. The male to female ratio is 3:2, and the incidence in the general population is approximately 1/1000. Recurrence risk after one affected child is 3–4%; after two affected children, 8–9%.

55. How can hypertelorism be rapidly assessed?
If an imaginary third eye would fit between the eyes, hypertelorism is possible. Precise measurement involves measuring the distance between the center of each eye's pupil. This is a difficult measurement in newborns and uncooperative patients because of eye movement. In practice, the

best way to determine hypotelorism or hypertelorism is to measure the inner and outer canthal distances, then plot these measurements on standardized tables of norms.

56. Which syndromes are associated with iris colobomas?

Colobomas of the iris are due to abnormal ocular development and embryogenesis. They are frequently associated with chromosomal syndromes, most commonly trisomy 13, 4p−, 13q−, and triploidy. In addition, they may be commonly found in the CHARGE association, Goltz syndrome, and Rieger syndrome. Whenever iris colobomas are noted, chromosome analysis is recommended. The special case of complete absence of the iris (aniridia) is associated with the development of Wilms tumor and may be caused by an interstitial deletion of the short arm of chromosome 11.

57. How large is the posterior fontanel in the healthy term infant?

In 97% of full-term infants, the posterior fontanel is normally fingertip size or smaller. Large posterior fontanels can be seen in infants with congenital hypothyroidism, skeletal dysplasias, or increased intracranial pressure.

58. On which side does the newborn "crown" usually sit?

In the fetus, hair follicles on the skin surface grow downward during weeks 10–16. During this time, the brain and scalp expand outward in a dome-like fashion, pulling the follicles in different directions, and at 18 weeks, when the hair erupts, patterns are set. The "crown," or parietal hair whorl, is the focal point of this outgrowth. At birth, it is usually a few centimeters anterior to the posterior fontanel. 55% of single parietal scalp whorls are left of midline (presumably secondary to the larger size of the left brain), 30% are right-sided, and 15% are midline. 5% of normal individuals have bilateral hair whorls. Abnormal positioning of the hair whorl (particularly a posterior location) can be seen in microcephaly.

GENETIC PRINCIPLES

59. Why is chromosomal banding such a valuable asset?

Chromosome banding was introduced in the early 1970s and has revolutionized cytogenetics. Prior to banding, all chromosomes appeared as solid, dark figures and could not be individually identified. Stains such as Giemsa and quinacrine can now be used to differentially stain certain chromosome regions, producing a characteristic striped pattern that can accurately identify each chromosome. Even small chromosome fragments can often be identified on the basis of their banding patterns. Contiguous gene disorders are syndromes due to a microdeletion of specific chromosomal regions. Examples of microdeletion syndromes include Prader-Willi syndrome, Angelman syndrome, Miller-Dieker syndrome, and DiGeorge/velocardiofacial syndrome. While the deletions are sometimes detectable on a karyotype, submicroscopic deletions cannot be visualized even on high-resolution chromosome banding. These deletions can be detected by fluorescent in situ hybridization (FISH). In this technique, a DNA probe specific for the chromosomal region of interest is hybridized to the chromosomes. A fluorescent signal is attached to the probe so that the number of copies of the DNA corresponding to the probe can be determined for each cell. Normally, two copies of each region, one on each chromosome, should be present. If a deletion has occurred, only one of the copies will be seen. This technique has aided in the diagnosis of microdeletion syndromes that were formerly difficult to detect because of their small size (Gopal Rao et al., 1995).

Gopal Rao VVN, Roop H, Carpenter NJ: Diagnosis of microdeletion syndromes: high-resolution chromosome analysis versus fluorescence in situ hybridization. Am J Med Sci 309:208–212, 1995.

60. Why has the polymerase chain reaction (PCR) revolutionized molecular genetics?

Most DNA techniques require a microgram of DNA, and this amount is often difficult to obtain. PCR is a technique that allows a millionfold amplification of a specific DNA fragment from a sample as small as a billionth of a microgram. The DNA to be amplified is denatured by heating the sample. In the presence of DNA polymerase and excess deoxynucleotide triphosphates, oligonucleotides that hybridize specifically to the target sequence prime new DNA synthesis.

The first cycle is characterized by a product of indeterminate length. However, the second cycle produces the discrete short product which accumulates exponentially with each successive round of amplification. This leads to the millionfold amplification of the discrete fragment over the course of 20–30 cycles. PCR and other recently developed molecular techniques have led to a boom in the identification of genes associated with clinical disorders (Muenke, 1995).

Muenke M: Finding genes involved in human developmental disorders. Curr Opin Genet Dev 5:354–361, 1995.

61. How are restriction enzymes used in the diagnosis of genetic disorders?

Restriction enzymes (restriction endonucleases) are enzymes purified from bacteria which cut double-stranded DNA at precise nucleotide sequences. Each enzyme is named for the organism from which it was obtained (e.g., *Eco*RI from *Escherichia coli*), and each has its own specific recognition sequence of 4–8 bases (e.g., GAATTC). If there is an alteration at this recognition site, the sequence becomes unrecognizable to the restriction enzyme, and the DNA will not be cut. Restriction enzyme analysis is one approach for direct detection of some mutant genes. For example, the sickle cell mutation (adenine changes to thymine at codon 6) alters the recognition site for the restriction enzyme *Mst*II. Cleavage at the normal location does not occur in the DNA molecules that contain the mutation, and a longer fragment is created. Techniques are available to size the resulting enzyme fragments to see if a normal or variant fragment (i.e., gene) exists.

62. Why is RFLP an MVP in genetic analysis?

The lengths of DNA digested by restriction enzymes result in fragments of various sizes. If a patient has a mutation, the size of the fragments may vary because the DNA sequence at the restriction site has been altered. These restriction fragment length polymorphisms (RFLP) may be inherited with certain diseases and differ from the general population when certain restriction enzymes and identifying DNA probes are used. Comparative analysis can identify carriers.

63. What is a linkage map?

Linkage is the coinheritance of two or more nonallelic genes because their loci are in close proximity on the same chromosome. A linkage map is a chromosome map showing the relative positions of genetic markers of a given species, as determined by linkage analysis.

64. How does mosaicism develop?

Mosaicism is the possession of multiple chromosomally different cell lines in a single individual. Most mosaicism involves the sex chromosomes and occurs because of defects in mitosis in an early embryo. Normally, chromosomes duplicate and separate equally in mitotic division. Mosaicism occurs when the chromosomes fail to separate (mitotic nondisjunction) or fail to migrate (anaphase lag). In general, the greater the proportion of abnormal cell lines, the more abnormal the phenotype. The earlier in embryonic development an abnormal cell line is established, the higher the percentage of abnormal cells in that individual.

65. What causes chimerism in infants?

The term *chimera* is derived from the Greek mythological monster which, according to Homer, had the head of a lion, body of a goat, and tail of a dragon. In cytogenetic parlance, chimerism is the presence of two or more cell lines in an individual which are derived from two separate zygotes. The most common cause of chimerism is the mixing of blood from unlike-sexed twins, resulting in a karyotype of 46,XX/46,XY. Chimerism can also result from the admixture of cells from a nonviable twin into a surviving fetus or, most rarely, from incorporation of two zygotes into a single embryo.

66. What is the risk of having a child with a recessive disorder when the parents are first or second cousins?

First cousins may share more than one deleterious recessive gene. They have $\frac{1}{8}$ of their genes in common, and their progeny are homozygous at $\frac{1}{16}$ of their gene loci. Second cousins have only $\frac{1}{32}$ genes in common. The risk that consanguineous parents will produce a child with a severe or lethal abnormality is 6% for first-cousin marriages and 1% for second-cousin marriages.

67. Identify the common symbols used in the construction of a pedigree chart.

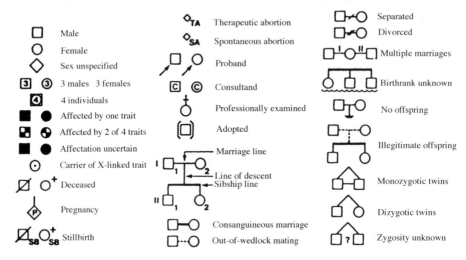

68. How does a reciprocal translocation differ from a robertsonian translocation?

A chromosome translocation is a transfer of chromosomal material between two (or more) nonhomologous chromosomes. The exchange is usually **reciprocal** (the two segments trading places). The genetic content of the individual is therefore complete but rearranged. **Robertsonian** translocation represents a special variety of chromosome translocation in which the long arms of two acrocentric chromosomes (#13, 14, 15, 21, or 22) fuse at their centromeres. The breaks may occur within, above, or below the centromeres. The short arms are usually lost, but this does not produce an abnormality since the genetic material on the short arms of acrocentric chromosomes occurs in multiple copies throughout the genome. A phenotypically normal individual with a robertsonian translocation has only 45 chromosomes inasmuch as the long arms of two acrocentric chromosomes are fused into one.

69. Why is a parent with a 14;21 robertsonian translocation at risk for having multiple miscarriages and/or children with birth defects?

When a parent with a translocation undergoes gametogenesis, six chromosomally different types of gametes can be formed due to unequal segregation of chromosomes during meiosis. The possible outcomes are trisomy 14 (which will abort), monosomy 14 (which will abort), monosomy 21 (which will abort), normal, trisomy 21 (Down syndrome), and a balanced robertsonian translocation (just like the parent).

70. How can an autosomal recessive disease occur when only one parent is a carrier?

Uniparental disomy is an inheritance pattern in which a child receives two identical chromosomes from one parent and none from the other. The most likely explanation is an abnormality in meiosis whereby one gamete receives an extra copy of a homologous chromosome due to an error in separation. This gamete with two copies from one parent then unites with the gamete of the other parent. If the second gamete lacks that particular chromosome (i.e., nullisomic gamete), a normal karyotype results. If the second gamete contains that particular chromosome, a trisomic zygote results. During embryonic development, this trisomy may be lost, resulting in a normal karyotype. Uniparental disomy has been reported in some patients with Prader-Willi, Angelman, and Beckwith-Weidemann syndromes as well as cystic fibrosis and hemophilia A.

71. How can the same genotype lead to different phenotypes?

In parental imprinting (an area of the regulation of gene expression that is incompletely understood), the expression of an identical gene is dependent on whether the gene is inherited from the mother or father. For example, in Huntington disease, the clinical manifestations occur much earlier if the gene is inherited from the father rather than the mother. Modification of the genes by methylation of the DNA during development has been hypothesized as one explanation of the variability.

72. 46,XY,t(4:8)(p21;q22)—what does it all mean?

46	Normal number of chromosomes
XY	Genetic male
t(4:8)	The first set of parentheses refers to the chromosomes. The symbol in front indicates the change: **t** stands for reciprocal translocation, **del** for deletion, **dup** for duplication, and **inv** for inversion.
(p21;q22)	The second set of parentheses refers to the bands on the chromosomes. The short arm symbol is **p**; the long arm symbol is **q**.

In this case, a genetic male with a normal number of chromosomes has a reciprocal translocation between the short arm of chromosome 4 at band 21 and the long arm of chromosome 8 at band 22.

SEX CHROMOSOME ABNORMALITIES

73. What are the features of the four most common sex chromosome abnormalities?

Most Common Sex Chromosome Disorders

	47,XXY (KLINEFELTER)	47,XYY	47,XXX	45,X (TURNER)
Frequency of live births	1/2000	1/2000	1/2000	1/8000
Maternal age association	+	–	+	–
Phenotype	Tall, eunuchoid habitus, underdeveloped secondary sexual characteristics, gynecomastia	Tall, severe acne, indistinguishable from normal males	Tall, indistinguishable from normal females	Short stature, web neck, shield chest, pedal edema at birth, coarctation of the aorta
IQ and behavior	80–100; behavioral problems	90–110; behavioral problems; aggressive behavior	90–110; behavioral problems	Mildly deficient to normal intelligence; spatial-perceptual difficulties
Reproductive function	Extremely rare	Common	Common	Extremely rare
Gonad	Hypoplastic testes, Ledig cell hyperplasia, Sertoli cell hypoplasia, seminiferous tubule dysgenesis, few spermatogenic precursors	Normal size testes, normal testicular histology	Normal size ovaries, normal ovarian histology	Streak ovaries with deficient follicles

From Donnenfeld AE, Dunn LK: Common chromosome disorders detected prenatally. Postgrad Obstet Gynecol 6:5, 1986; with permission.

74. What did Lyon hypothesize?

The Lyon hypothesis is that in any cell, only one X chromosome will be functional. Any other X chromosomes present in that cell will be condensed, late replicating, and inactive (called the Barr body). The inactive X may be either paternal or maternal in origin, but all descendants of a particular cell will have the same parentally derived chromosome inactive. Inactivation is initially random, occurring at the 16-day (blastocyst) stage of embryonic development. For example, in normal females (46,XX), one X chromosome is inactive. In normal males (46,XY), the X is always active, since it is the only one present. In 48,XXXY individuals, there will be two inactive X chromosomes per cell. The process of X inactivation allows for gene dosage compensation in females and poly-X males.

75. Is it possible to get identical twins of different sexes?

Yes. If anaphase lag (loss) of a Y chromosome occurs at the time of cell separation into twin embryos, a female fetus with karyotype 45,X (Turner syndrome) and a normal male fetus (46,XY) results.

76. How commonly does mosaicism occur in Turner syndrome?

At least 35% of chromosome abnormalities in individuals with Turner syndrome are mosaics. The most common are 45,X/46,XX, and 45,X/46,XX/47,XXX, and 45,X/46,XY. Whenever a cell line with a Y chromosome is identified in a phenotypic female, gonadectomy is recommended due to a high risk of malignancy in the gonads of these individuals.

77. Of the four most common types of sex chromosomal abnormalities, which is identifiable at birth?

Only infants with **Turner syndrome** have physical features easily identifiable at birth. Features include:

- Dorsal hand and pedal edema
- Web neck (pterygium colli)
- Broad chest with wide-spaced nipples
- Prominent ears
- Low posterior hairline
- Congenital elbow flexion (cubitus valgus)
- Narrow, hyperconvex nails
- Short fourth metacarpal and/or metatarsal

78. What causes the webbing of the neck in Turner syndrome?

Failure of canalization between the cervical and jugular lymphatic vessels causes trapped lymphatic fluid to accumulate progressively and to form large posterior nuchal cysts called cystic hygromas. Occasionally, resolution of fluid accumulation may occur during gestation with regression of the cystic hygroma, formation of nuchal webbing (called pterygium colli), nuchal skin redundancy, alteration in the zone of hair growth, protrusion of the lower auricles, and morphologic alterations of the fetal face. This is known as the **jugular lymphatic obstruction sequence.** It is hypothesized that if only a partial or temporary obstruction occurs, egress of lymphatic fluid may be possible, and the cystic hygroma will resolve with only redundant nuchal skinfolds remaining. Therefore, the entire obstruction sequence will not develop. However, others believe that the pathogenesis of the web neck is not related to lymphatic obstruction but occurs as a primary developmental defect due to the chromosomal abnormality.

79. Describe the similarities and differences between Noonan syndrome and Turner syndrome.

Similarities: short stature, web neck, cardiac defects, low posterior hairline, broad chest, wide-spaced nipples, edema of the dorsum of the hands and feet, cubitus valgus

Differences:	**Turner syndrome**	**Noonan syndrome**
	Affects females only	Affects both males and females
	Chromosome disorder (45,X)	Normal chromosomes, autosomal dominant disorder
	Near-normal intelligence	Mental deficiency
	Coarctation of aorta is most common cardiac defect	Pulmonary stenosis is most common cardiac defect
	Amenorrhea and sterility due to ovarian dysgenesis	Normal menstrual cycle in females

80. What is the most common inherited form of mental retardation?

Fragile X syndrome.

81. What is the nature of the mutation in fragile X syndrome?

When the lymphocytes of an affected male are grown in a folate-deficient medium and the chromosomes examined, a substantial fraction of X chromosomes demonstrate a break near the distal end of the long arm. This site, the fragile X mental retardation-1 gene (FMR-1), was identified and sequenced in 1991. At the center of the gene is a repeating trinucleotide sequence (CGG) which, in normal individuals, repeats 6–45 times. However, in carriers, the sequence expands to 50–200 times (called a premutation), and in fully affected individuals, it expands to

200–600 copies. These longer sequences cause malfunctioning of the gene (Fu et al., 1991). Expansion of trinucleotide repeat sequences are responsible for several other diseases (Carpenter, 1994), including the neurodegenerative disorders myotonic dystrophy (Brook et al., 1992), spinocerebellar ataxia type 1 (Orr et al., 1993), Kennedy disease (La Spada et al., 1991), and Huntington disease (Huntington's Disease Collaborative Research Group, 1993).

Brook JD, McCurrach ME, Harley HG, et al: Molecular basis of myotonic dystrophy: Expansion of a trinucleotide (CTG) repeat at the 3' end of a transcript encoding a protein kinase family member. Cell 68:799–808, 1992.

Carpenter NJ: Genetic anticipation. Expanding tandem repeats. Neurol Clin North Am 12:683–697, 1994.

Fu YH, Kuhl DP, Pizzuti A, et al: Variation of the CGG repeat at the fragile X site results in genetic instability: Resolution of the Sherman paradox. Cell 67:1047–1058, 1991.

Huntington's Disease Collaborative Research Group: A novel gene containing a trinucleotide repeat that is expanded and unstable on Hungtington's disease chromosomes. Cell 72:971–983, 1993.

La Spada AR, Wilson EM, Lubahn DB, et al: Androgen receptor gene mutations in X-linked spinal and bulbar muscular atrophy. Nature 352:77–79, 1991.

Orr HT, Chung MY, Banfi S, et al: Expansion of an unstable trinucleotide CAG repeat in spinocerebellar ataxia type 1. Nature Genetics 4:211–226, 1993.

82. What are the associated medical problems in fragile X syndrome in males?

Flat feet (80%), macro-orchidism (80% after puberty), mitral valve prolapse (50–80% in adulthood), recurrent otitis media (60%), strabismus (30%), refractive errors (20%), seizures (15%), scoliosis (< 20%).

Hagerman RJ: Fragile X syndrome. In Parker S, Zuckerman B (eds): Behavioral and Developmental Pediatrics. Boston, Little, Brown, & Co., 1995, pp 153–156.

83. What is the outcome for girls with fragile X?

Heterozygous females who carry the fragile X chromosome have more behavioral and developmental problems (including attention deficit hyperactivity disorder), cognitive difficulties (50% with an IQ in the mentally retarded or borderline range), and physical differences (prominent ears, long and narrow face). Cytogenetic testing is recommended for all sisters of fragile X males.

Hagerman RJ, et al: Girls with fragile X syndrome: Physical and neurocognitive status and outcome. Pediatrics 89:395–400, 1992.

TERATOLOGY

84. Which drugs are known to be teratogenic?

Most teratogenic drugs exert a deleterious effect in a minority of exposed fetuses. Exact malformation rates are unavailable due to the inability to perform a statistical evaluation on a randomized, controlled population. Known teratogens include:

Drug	Major Teratogenic Effect	Drug	Major Teratogenic Effect
Thalidomide	Limb defects	Androgens	Virilization
Lithium	Ebstein tricuspid valve anomaly	Tetracyline	Teeth and bone maldevelopment
Aminopterin	Craniofacial and limb anomalies	Streptomycin	Ototoxicity
Methotrexate	Craniofacial and limb anomalies	Warfarin	Nasal hypoplasia, bone maldevelopment
Phenytoin	Facial dysmorphism, dysplastic nails	Penicillamine	Cutis laxa
Trimethadione	Craniofacial dysmorphism, growth retardation	Accutane retinoic acid)	Craniofacial and cardiac
Valproic acid	Neural tube defects	Propylthiouracil	Goiter
Diethylstilbestrol (DES)	Müllerian anomalies, clear cell adenocarcinoma	Radioactive iodine	Hypothyroidism

85. Describe the characteristic features of the fetal hydantoin syndrome.

Craniofacial: Broad nasal bridge, wide fontanel, low-set hairline, broad alveolar ridge, metopic ridging, short neck, ocular hypertelorism, microcephaly, cleft lip/palate, abnormal or low-set ears, epicanthal folds, ptosis of eyelids, coloboma, and coarse scalp hair

Limbs: Small or absent nails, hypoplasia of distal phalanges, altered palmar crease, digital thumb, and dislocated hip

Approximately 10% of infants whose mothers took phenytoin (Dilantin) during pregnancy have a major malformation; 30% have minor abnormalities.

From Briggs GC, Freeman RK, Yaffe SJ: Drugs in Pregnancy and Lactation, 3rd ed. Baltimore, Williams & Wilkins, 1990; with permission.

86. Does cocaine cause fetal malformations?

Yes. Several malformations are associated with maternal cocaine use. All are believed to be due to a disruption in normal organ growth and development as a result of vascular insufficiency. Intestinal atresias due to mesenteric artery vasoconstriction or thrombosis and urinary tract anomalies, including urethral obstruction, hydronephrosis, and hypospadias, are most commonly reported. Limb reduction defects, often described as transverse terminal defects of the forearm or amputation of the digits of the hands and feet, have also been identified. The type of disruption will depend on the timing of cocaine exposure during pregnancy, the dosage and frequency of cocaine administration, and susceptibility of the embryo or fetus. The teratogenic influences of cocaine are not limited to the first trimester. Vasoconstriction may lead to infarction in a wide variety of organs; however, it is most common in the fetal brain. Additionally, uteroplacental insufficiency due to vasculopathy, chronic abruption, thrombosis, or a combination of these problems is a well-known cause of intrauterine growth retardation in cocaine-exposed fetuses.

87. What amount of alcohol is safe to ingest during pregnancy?

This is unknown. The full dysmorphologic manifestations of fetal alcohol syndrome are associated with heavy intake. However, most infants will not display the full syndrome. For infants born to women with lesser degrees of alcohol intake during pregnancy who demonstrate more subtle abnormalities (e.g., cognitive and behavioral problems), it is more difficult to ascribe risk because of confounding variables (e.g., maternal illness, pregnancy weight gain, other drug use, especially marijuana). Furthermore, it appears that infants prenatally exposed to similar amounts of alcohol are likely to have different consequences for reasons that are unclear. Because current data do not support the concept that any amount of alcohol is safe during pregnancy, the AAP recommends abstinence from alcohol for women who are pregnant or planning to become pregnant.

Committee on Substance Abuse and Committee on Children with Disabilities: Fetal alcohol syndrome and fetal alcohol effects. Pediatrics 91:1004–1006, 1993.

88. What are the frequent features of the fetal alcohol syndrome?

Skull	Microcephaly, mid-face hypoplasia
Eyes	Short palpebral fissures, epicanthal folds, ptosis, strabismus
Mouth	Hypoplastic philtrum, thin upper lip, prominent lateral palatine ridges, retrognathia in infancy, micrognathia or relative prognathia in adolescence
Nose	Flat nasal bridge, short and upturned nose
Cardiac	Ventricular septal and atrial septal defects
Skeletal	Pectus excavatum, altered palmar crease patterns, small fifth fingernails
Skin	Hemangiomas
CNS	Mild to moderate mental retardation, poor coordination, fine motor impairment, hypotonia, irritability in infancy, hyperactivity in childhood
Growth	Prenatal: small for gestational age Postnatal: < 2 SD for length and weight, disproportionately diminished adipose tissue

89. What happens to children with fetal alcohol syndrome when they grow up?

A follow-up study of 61 adolescents and adults revealed that relative short stature and microcephaly persisted, but facial anomalies became more subtle. Academic functioning, particularly in arithmetic, was delayed to the early grade-school level. Intermediate or significant maladaptive behavior was present in 100% of patients. Severely unstable family environments were common.

Streissguth AP, et al: Fetal alcohol syndrome in adolescents and adults. JAMA 265:1961–1967, 1991.

9. HEMATOLOGY AND IMMUNOLOGY

Bruce P. Himelstein, M.D., Steven D. Douglas, M.D., and Alan R. Cohen, M.D.

APLASTIC ANEMIA

1. What are the causes of acquired aplastic anemia?

Although most cases are idiopathic, a variety of associated conditions include:

Radiation	*Immune diseases*
Drugs and *chemicals*	Eosinophilic fasciitis
Regular: cytotoxic, benzene	Hypoimmunoglobulinemia
Idiosyncratic: chloramphenicol, anti-	*Thymoma*
inflammatory drugs, antiepileptics, gold	*Pregnancy*
Viruses	*Paroxysmal nocturnal hemoglobinuria*
Epstein-Barr virus	*Preleukemia*
Hepatitis	
Parvovirus	
HIV	

From Alter BP, Young NS: The bone marrow failure syndromes. In Nathan DG, Oski FA (eds): Hematology of Infancy and Childhood, 4th ed. Philadelphia, W.B. Saunders, 1993, p 217; with permission.

2. What distinguishes severe from mild or moderate aplastic anemia?

Severe disease implies a hypocellular bone marrow biopsy and marked abnormalities in at least two of three cell lines, demonstrated in peripheral blood by: neutrophil count < 500 cells/mm^3, platelet count < 20,000 mm^3, or reticulocyte count < 1% after correction for the hematocrit. Categorization has important prognostic and therapeutic implications.

3. What is the outcome for treated and untreated aplastic anemia?

In the absence of treatment, approximately 25% of children with severe acquired aplastic anemia survive for > 2 years. With anti-thymocyte globulin therapy, survival is 50–80% at 2 years. When bone marrow transplantation is performed using a histocompatible sibling donor, the 2-year survival rate exceeds 80%. In light of these statistics, the usual approach to the newly diagnosed child with severe acquired aplastic anemia is to perform bone marrow transplantation if there is a histocompatible sibling to serve as the donor.

4. Discuss the therapeutic alternatives to bone marrow transplantation in children with aplastic anemia.

Approximately 75–80% of children with severe aplastic anemia do not have an identical sibling as a donor for bone marrow transplantation. Without this preferred treatment, alternative therapies include:

1. *Anti-thymocyte* or *anti-lymphocyte globulin* (ATG or ALG) derived from horses immunized with human lymphocyte subclasses or thymocytes

2. *Immunosuppressive agents*, such as cyclosporine

3. *Growth factors*, such as granulocyte–macrophage colony-stimulating factor (GM-CSF) and granulocyte colony-stimulating factor (G-CSF).

GM-CSF raises the neutrophil count in many patients with aplastic anemia, but unfortunately it is least effective in those with the most severe neutropenia. Furthermore, GM-CSF does not consistently raise the hemoglobin level or platelet count. A tri-lineage response awaits the development of new growth factors or combinations of growth factors.

D'Andrea AD: Cytokine receptors in congenital hematopoietic disease. N Engl J Med 330:839–846, 1994.

Guinan EC, et al: Evaluation of granulocyte-macrophage colony-stimulating factor for treatment of pancytopenia in children with Fanconi anemia. J Pediatr 124:144–150, 1994.

5. Is aplastic anemia a preleukemic condition?

Some patients who ultimately turn out to have leukemia may initially present with low peripheral blood counts, a hypoplastic bone marrow, and some blasts but not enough to make a conclusive diagnosis of leukemia. However, it is usually obvious from the beginning that these patients do not have the typical marrow findings of acquired aplastic anemia (i.e., not associated with an increased number of blasts). Patients with Fanconi anemia have a propensity to develop leukemia, but the malignancy is probably a result of underlying chromosomal defects in this disorder rather than the aplastic anemia. Patients with the usual form of acquired aplastic anemia may have a lifetime risk of leukemia or other clonal disorders as high as 25%.

6. What is the probable diagnosis in a 6-year-old with pancytopenia, short stature, abnormal thumbs, and areas of hyperpigmentation?

Fanconi anemia, or constitutional aplastic anemia, is a disorder in which numerous physical abnormalities are often present at birth, and aplastic anemia occurs around age 5 years. The more common physical abnormalities include hyperpigmentation, anomalies of the thumb and radius, small size, microcephaly, and renal anomalies, such as absent, duplicated, or horseshoe kidneys. Mental retardation is found in fewer than one-fourth of affected patients. When patients are recognized early in life on the basis of the physical abnormalities, the early signs of bone marrow failure may be detected before clinical problems related to pancytopenia occur. Increased fetal hemoglobin may be present in the first year of life. Mild thrombocytopenia may occur in infancy or early childhood, but the platelet count may remain only slightly depressed for 4 or 5 years until the usual picture of bone marrow failure occurs.

7. Which test is most diagnostic of Fanconi anemia?

Chromosomal breakage analysis. On studies of peripheral blood lymphocytes, a high percentage of patients with Fanconi anemia will have chromosomal breaks, gaps, or rearrangements. Treatment with clastogenic agents (e.g., diepoxybutane) results in greater breakage than occurs in normal individuals.

8. How is transient erythroblastopenia of childhood (TEC) distinguished from Diamond-Blackfan syndrome?

Both are disorders of red cell production that occur in early childhood. It is extremely important to distinguish TEC from Diamond-Blackfan syndrome—TEC is a self-limited disorder, whereas Diamond-Blackfan syndrome usually requires life-long treatment. While there is an overlap in the age of presentation, Diamond-Blackfan syndrome commonly causes anemia in the first 6 months of life, whereas TEC occurs more frequently after age 1 year. Both disorders are characterized by a low hemoglobin level and an inappropriately low reticulocyte count. The bone marrows may be indistinguishable, showing reduced or absent erythroid activity in both cases. The red cells in patients with Diamond-Blackfan syndrome have fetal characteristics that are useful in distinguishing this disorder from TEC, including increased mean cell volume, elevated level of hemoglobin F, and presence of i antigen. The level of adenine deaminase may be elevated in patients with Diamond-Blackfan syndrome but normal in children with TEC.

CLINICAL ISSUES

9. What is the hemoglobin value (lower limit of normal) below which children are considered to be anemic?

Newborn infant (full term)	13.0 gm/dl	4–8 yrs	11.5
3 mos	9.5	8–12 yrs	11.5
1–3 yrs	11.0	12–16 yrs	12.0

Dallman P, Siimes MA: Percentile curves for hemoglobin and red cell volume in infancy and childhood. J Pediatr 94:27, 1979.

10. Who gets "statistical anemia"?

By definition, 2.5% of healthy children (i.e., 2 SD below the mean) will have an anemia un-related to iron deficiency, infection, or hemoglobinopathy. As the prevalence of iron deficiency declines (primarily from the use of iron-fortified formulas and cereals), the likelihood of anemia being a variation of normal rather than a pathologic condition increases.

11. Why is there a racial difference in hemoglobin concentrations?

Multiple nutritional surveys in the United States have shown that black children of all ages have lower mean hemoglobin levels (0.5–1.1 gm/dl) and lower mean hematocrit values (1–3%) than whites, Hispanics, and Asians. Socioeconomic status, environmental factors, and iron defi-ciency do not appear to explain the difference. Mild hereditary conditions more common in blacks (e.g., thalassemias, hemoglobin S trait, hemoglobin C trait) may explain a significant por-tion of the difference.

Rana SR, et al: Hemoglobin S and C traits: Contributing causes for decreased mean hematocrit in African-American children. Pediatrics 91:800–802, 1993.

12. In patients with severe chronic anemia, how rapidly should transfusions be given?

The main concern is that excessively rapid transfusions could lead to congestive heart fail-ure. A safe regimen for patients with a hemoglobin < 5 gm/dl is to transfuse packed red blood cells at a rate of 1–2 ml/kg/hr by continuous infusion until the desired target is reached. One ml/kg will raise the hematocrit by 1%.

Jayabose S, et al: Transfusion therapy for severe anemia. Am J Pediatr Hematol Oncol 15:324–327, 1993.

13. When does the physiologic anemia of infancy occur?

Physiologic anemia occurs at 8–12 weeks in full-term infants and 6–8 weeks in premature infants. Full-term infants may exhibit hemoglobin levels as low as 9 gm/dl at this time and very premature infants as low as 7 gm/dl.

14. Why does the physiologic anemia of infancy occur?

The mechanism(s) responsible for physiologic anemia is not completely understood. Red blood cell (RBC) survival time is decreased in both premature and full-term infants. Furthermore, the ability to increase erythropoietin production in response to ongoing tissue hy-poxia is somewhat blunted, even though the response to exogenous erythropoietin is normal. The precise signals that tell infants to increase RBC production are not clear. However, factors that control the infant's ability to deliver oxygen to tissues (e.g., oxygen saturation, hemoglo-bin-oxygen dissociation curve, cardiac output, red cell mass) as well as the metabolic demands of these tissues appear to be important. Some of the postnatal fall in hemoglobin concentration is undoubtedly dilutional due to an increasing plasma volume and stable or falling hemoglobin concentration.

15. In what settings of shortened RBC survival can the reticulocyte count be normal or decreased?

As a rule, the reticulocyte count is elevated in conditions of shortened RBC survival (e.g., hemoglobinopathies, membrane disorders) and decreased in anemias characterized by impaired RBC production (e.g., iron deficiency, thalassemias). The reticulocyte count may be abnormally low in the former category if a coexistent aplastic or hypoplastic crisis is occurring. The bone marrow suppression can be precipitated suddenly by acute infection (such as parvovirus) or drugs. Chronically, the marrow may become unresponsive secondary to micronutrient deficiency (e.g., iron, folate) or a reduction in erythropoietin production as seen in chronic renal failure.

16. How does the pathophysiology of anemia differ in acute and chronic infection?

Chronic infection and other inflammatory states impair the release of iron from reticuloen-dothelial cells, thereby decreasing the amount of this necessary ingredient available for RBC pro-duction. Giving additional iron under these circumstances further increases reticuloendothelial iron stores and does little to help the anemia. *Acute infection* may cause anemia through a variety of mechanisms, including bone marrow suppression, shortened RBC lifespan, red cell fragmentation, and immune-mediated RBC destruction.

17. What causes "ringed sideroblasts" in sideroblastic anemias?

Sideroblastic anemias comprise a rare group of disorders in which iron incorporation into the porphyrin ring to form heme is impaired. The result is an accumulation of excessive iron in the mitochondria of the nucleated red cells. These cells, when stained for iron, are known as **ringed sideroblasts** because of the presence of stainable iron in the mitochondria which encircle the nucleus. Congenital sideroblastic anemia may be inherited in a sex-linked (i.e., male) pattern. Acquired sideroblastic anemia can be associated with drugs or toxins that affect heme synthesis (e.g., lead, isoniazid), malignancy (e.g., early myelogenous or myelomonocytic leukemia), or chronic inflammatory disease (e.g., juvenile rheumatoid arthritis).

18. Describe the differential diagnosis for children presenting with splenomegaly and anemia.

The main question is whether the anemia is the cause of the splenomegaly or the splenomegaly is the cause of the anemia. Examples of anemia causing splenomegaly include hemolytic anemias in which the spleen plays an active role, such as membrane disorders, sickling disorders, and thalassemia syndromes. The major example of splenomegaly causing anemia is hypersplenism due to chronic liver disease and portal hypertension. In this instance, the anemia results from sequestration of RBCs in the enlarged spleen. Accompanying features usually include mild leukopenia and thrombocytopenia.

Anemia causing splenomegaly	Splenomegaly causing anemia
• Membrane disorders	• Cirrhotic liver disease
• Hemoglobinopathies	• Cavernous transformation of portal vessels
• Enzyme abnormalities	• Storage diseases
• Immune hemolytic anemia	• Persistent viral infections

19. How common are significant hematologic manifestations of lead toxicity?

The importance and frequency of hematologic manifestations of lead toxicity have been overstated. Although lead poisoning is generally listed as a cause of microcytic anemia, this is a rare event in severe lead intoxication. In children with significantly increased lead burden (≥ 50 $\mu g/100$ ml) and without iron deficiency, about 10–15% are anemic, but only about 2–4% have a microcytic anemia.

Cohen AR, et al: Reassessment of the microcytic anemia of lead poisoning. Pediatrics 67:904–906, 1981.

20. A 14-month-old presents with marked cyanosis, lethargy, and normal oxygen saturation by pulse oximetry after drinking from a neighbor's well. What is the likely diagnosis?

Methemoglobinemia should always be considered when a patient presents with cyanosis without demonstrable respiratory or cardiac disease. The most common causes are oxidant toxins, such as antimalarial drugs or nitrates in food or well water, inherited abnormalities of the enzymes that maintain hemoglobin iron in the reduced state, and the abnormal M hemoglobins that seem to stabilize hemoglobin in the ferric form.

Symptoms can range from simple cyanosis (methemoglobin < 30%) to headache, lethargy, and altered consciousness (30–70%). Levels above 70% can be fatal. In an acute situation when levels are > 30%, 1–2 mg/kg of **1% methylene blue** solution should be administered intravenously over 5 minutes and repeated in 1 hour if symptoms are still present. Failure to respond to therapy should raise the possibility of G6PD deficiency, which prevents the conversion of methylene blue to the metabolite that is active in the treatment of methemoglobinemia. In these cases, hyperbaric oxygen therapy or exchange transfusion may be necessary. Chronic methemoglobinemia, as observed with inherited enzyme abnormalities or M hemoglobinopathies, may result in chronic cyanosis without symptoms. In these patients, oral ascorbic acid may occasionally be useful. Of note, patients with cyanosis due to methemoglobinemia can have normal oxygen saturation as measured by pulse oximetry since the oximeter operates by measuring only hemoglobin that is available for saturation.

21. How can the diagnosis of methemoglobinemia be made at the bedside?

In methemoglobinemia, the inability of the red cell to maintain hemoglobin iron in the ferrous (Fe^{2+}) state leads to a loss of oxygen-carrying capacity. When a drop of blood from a patient with methemoglobinemia is placed on a piece of filter paper, it generally has a brownish color. When the filter paper is waved in the air, the color of the blood remains brown because the hemoglobin is unable to bind oxygen. In contrast, blood from a normal individual turns from brown to red when the filter paper is waved in the air.

22. Why are infants at greater risk for the development of methemoglobinemia?

1. *Anti-oxidant defense mechanisms* (e.g., soluble cytochrome b_5 and NADH-dependent cytochrome b_5 reductase) are 40% lower in infants than teenagers.

2. Infants' *intestinal pH* is relatively alkaline compared with older children's. If nitrates are ingested (as in fertilizer-contaminated well water), this higher pH more readily allows bacterial conversion of nitrate to nitrite, which is a potent oxidant.

3. More susceptible to various *oxidant exposures:* nitrate reductase from undercooked spinach, menadione (vitamin K_3) for prevention of neonatal hemorrhage, over-the-counter teething preparations with benzocaine, or metoclopramide for gastroesophageal reflux.

Bunn HF: Human hemoglobins: Normal and abnormal. In Nathan DG, Oski FA (eds): Hematology of Infancy and Childhood, 4th ed. Philadelphia, W.B. Saunders, 1993, pp 720–727.

23. Which organs produce erythropoietin?

The **kidney** is the primary manufacturing site, but the cell of origin is unclear. The fetal **liver** and, to a lesser extent, adult liver are also capable of production. The role of macrophages in synthesis is disputed.

Jelkmann W: Erythropoietin: Structure, control of production, and function. Physiol Rev 72:449–489, 1992.

24. What are indications for erythropoietin (EPO) therapy in the pediatric population?

The most clearly proven indication is therapy for the anemia associated with end-stage renal disease. Other indications include anemia induced by chemotherapy, anemia for HIV-positive patients on antiretroviral therapy, and anemia of chronic disease. The use of EPO in the neonatal setting as a treatment for various types of anemia (e.g., anemia associated with prematurity, fetal isoimmune hemolytic anemia) remains under study. EPO has no proven benefit in sickle cell anemia.

25. What are the adverse effects of erythropoietin?

The most common general side effects include an influenza-like syndrome, development of iron deficiency in the absence of iron supplementation, and neutropenia (rarely). Side effects such as hypertension, clotting of vascular access devices, and seizures are much more prevalent in adults being treated for end-stage renal disease.

Bennett WM: Side effects of erythropoietin therapy. Am J Kidney Dis 18(suppl):84–86, 1991.

26. In what circumstances is it best to transfuse filtered rbcs?

When packed red cells are prepared from whole blood and then filtered, most of the remaining white cells are removed from the product. Since febrile transfusion reactions are usually due to leukocytes, filtered red cells are an ideal product for patients who have experienced such reactions to previous blood transfusions. Filtered red cells may also be effective in reducing the transmission of cytomegalovirus because of the removal of the white cells that normally carry this virus. In addition, filtered red cells reduce the risk of HLA sensitization in patients with diseases that may later be treated by bone marrow transplantation.

COAGULATION DISORDERS

27. What features on history or physical exam help pinpoint the cause of a bleeding problem?
While there can be considerable overlap, in general, qualitative or quantitative *platelet* problems result in petechiae, especially on dependent parts of the body and mucosal surfaces. Additional manifestations of platelet disorders include epistaxis, hematuria, menorrhagia, and gastrointestinal hemorrhages. Ecchymoses are suspicious for *coagulation factor deficiencies* or *platelet* problems when they occur in unusual areas, are out of proportion to the extent of described trauma (also seen in child abuse), or are present in different stages of healing. Delayed bleeding from old wounds and extensive hemorrhaging (particularly into joint spaces) are also suggestive of coagulation protein disorders. Bleeding from multiple sites in an ill patient is worrisome for *disseminated intravascular coagulation*. Of note, if a patient has tolerated tonsillectomy and/or adenoidectomy or multiple wisdom teeth extraction (all major stresses on the overall system of hemostasis), a significant inherited bleeding disorder is unlikely.

28. What are the inheritance patterns of the common bleeding disorders?
Factor VIII and factor IX deficiency are inherited in a sex-linked pattern so that females are carriers and males are affected. The inheritance of von Willebrand disease, the most common coagulopathy, is autosomal dominant, as are the other clotting factor deficiencies. In general, heterozygotes for clotting factor deficiencies are not clinically affected. However, evidence indicates that some heterozygotes for deficiencies or dysfunction of anticoagulant proteins, such as protein C and antithrombin III, may have problems related to hypercoagulation such as venous thrombosis.

29. Why is the lack of a family history of bleeding problems only moderate evidence against the likelihood of hemophilia A in a patient?
The abnormal factor VIII gene responsible for hemophilia A exhibits marked heterogeneity, and up to a third of cases (either the immediate carrier mother or the son himself) may have developed a spontaneous mutation. In addition, if an affected family member has mild hemophilia but has not had a substantial hemostatic challenge (e.g., tonsillectomy), the manifestations of the disease might not have surfaced.

30. Do females have any manifestations of hemophilia?
Although factor VIII and factor IX deficiencies usually occur in males (because of their X-linked recessive inheritance), female carriers can have reduced factor levels (30–50%) due to extreme lyonization (i.e., random inactivation of one X chromosome). Because some female carriers can be at significant risk of hemorrhage during surgery, screening for an underlying factor VIII or IX deficiency is recommended by many authorities.
Lusher J, et al: Severe factor VIII and factor IX deficiency in females. Am J Med 65:637, 1978.

31. Which is more common, factor VIII or factor IX deficiency?
Factor VIII deficiency (hemophilia A) is more common, affecting 80–85% of all patients with factor deficiency.

32. How are the doses of replacement factor calculated for a hemophiliac with or without life-threatening hemorrhage?
For moderate (1–5% of normal factor levels) to severe (< 1% of normal) hemophilia, factor VIII or factor IX concentrates are the treatments of choice. For minor hemorrhages, such as knee and elbow bleeds, factor levels should be increased to 20–30% of normal. For major bleeding episodes, such as hip bleeds, intracranial hemorrhage, or bleeding around the airway, factor levels should be raised to 70–100%. Each unit of factor VIII or factor IX is equivalent to the activity in 1 ml of normal plasma. One unit/kg should increase the factor VIII level by 2% and the factor IX level by 1%.
Cohen AJ, et al: Treatment of inherited coagulation disorders. Am J Med 99:675–682, 1995.

33. What can cause an elevation of the prothrombin time (PT) with other coagulation testing being normal?

Factor VII deficiency. PT measures the function of the common pathway factors (including X, V, II, fibrinogen) as well as the extrinsic pathway (tissue factor and factor VII). The activated partial thromboplastin time (aPTT) measures the common pathway plus the function of the intrinsic pathway (including factors XII, XI, IX, VIII).

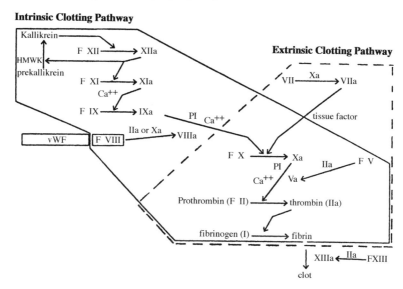

Adapted from Montgomery RR, et al: Newborn haemostasis. Clin Haematol 14:443, 1985; with permission.

34. What are the half-lives of exogenously administered factors VIII and IX?

The half-lives for the *first* doses of factors VIII and IX are 6–8 hours and 4–6 hours, respectively. With *subsequent* doses, factor VIII has a half-life of 8–12 hours, while factor IX has a half-life of 18–24 hours. Thus, for serious bleeding, the second dose of factor VIII should be given 6–8 hours after the first, while the second dose of factor IX should be given 4–6 hours after the first. Subsequent doses are usually given every 12 hours for factor VIII replacement and every 24 hours for factor IX, but measurement of actual factor levels may be necessary to guide therapy in life-threatening situations.

35. In hemophiliacs who develop inhibitors to factor infusions, what differentiates "low responders" from "high responders"?

About 15–40% of patients with hemophilia A (but < 5% with hemophilia B) develop IgG antibodies to factor VIII following infusion. Depending on the extent of response, the development of inhibitors can greatly complicate management. **Low responders** do not exhibit significant increases in titers with repeated transfusions and can be treated with increased amounts of factor VIII. **High responders** have an anamnestic response to factor replacement, and repeated treatments can result in substantial elevations in inhibitor titers. A variety of approaches may be tried including:

1. Activated and nonactivated prothrombin complex concentrates (to bypass the block)
2. Activated factor VII concentrates (to utilize the extrinsic pathway)
3. Porcine factor VIII (which has little cross-reactivity with human factor VIII)
4. In emergent situations, administration of large quantities of factor VIII, sometimes after plasmapheresis to lower inhibitor levels. This treatment, however, will lead to even higher inhibitor titers in a matter of days.

36. What is the role of desmopressin (DDAVP) in the treatment of hemophilia?

DDAVP, a synthetic analog of vasopressin, increases levels of factor VIII and von Willebrand factor perhaps by allowing release from storage sites. It can be used for patients with mild hemophilia or von Willebrand disease. A dose of 0.3 μg/kg given intravenously will raise baseline levels by 300–400% in many individuals.

37. Who gets "hemophilia C"?

More commonly called factor XI deficiency, this is an uncommon cause of hemophilia (< 5% of total patients). Unlike the X-linked nature of hemophilia A and B, it is an autosomal recessive disease that occurs most frequently in Ashkenazi Jews.

Asadai R, et al: Factor XI deficiency in Ashkenazi Jews in Israel. N Engl J Med 325:153–158, 1991.

38. Why is factor IX deficiency also called "Christmas disease"?

In 1952, investigators in England noted that when blood from one group of hemophiliacs was added to the blood of another group of hemophiliacs, the clotting time was shortened. This provided the basis for the discovery of plasma substances in addition to what was then called antihemophilic globulin (and now called factor VIII) responsible for normal clotting. Although it would be the stuff of Hollywood if the revelation had occurred while St. Nicholas was handing out departmental gifts, the truth is that the name was derived because the first patient examined in detail with the unusual clotting deficiency (later designated as factor IX) was a boy named Christmas. As Frank Capra might have scripted it, the publication of the landmark article did occur in the last week in December 1952.

Biggs R, et al: Christmas disease: A condition previously mistaken for haemophilia. BMJ 262:1378–1382, 1952.

39. What causes the coagulation abnormalities in von Willebrand disease?

von Willebrand disease is actually a group of disorders that involves the von Willebrand factor (vWF), which is a multimeric glycoprotein complexed to factor VIII in the plasma. It serves as a bridge between damaged endothelium and adhering platelets and facilitates platelet attachment. von Willebrand disease is a heterogenous disorder caused by qualitative or quantitative abnormalities in vWF. Either variety of abnormality can result in improper formation of a platelet plug and reduction in factor VIII quantities (due to the importance of vWF in minimizing the clearance of factor VIII from plasma and in accelerating its cellular synthesis). Coagulation abnormalities in children with severe disease can include a prolonged bleeding time, prolonged PTT, decreased factor VIII coagulant activity, decreased factor VIII antigen, and decreased ability of patient plasma to induce aggregation of normal platelets in the presence of ristocetin.

40. What are the best screening diagnostic tests for suspected von Willebrand disease?

The diagnosis can be difficult because test results can vary widely among patients. Stress, pregnancy, or medications (e.g., oral contraceptives) can cause variation even in an individual patient. Although the bleeding time and PTT are often abnormal, in milder disease, they are frequently normal. Thus, they are insensitive alone as screening tests. However, if in addition to the bleeding time and PTT, the vWF activity (i.e., ristocetin cofactor activity) is measured, over 90% of patients with von Willebrand disease will demonstrate at least one abnormality. More extensive (and expensive) testing, including vWF antigen, factor VIII clotting activity, ristocetin-induced platelet aggregation, and multimer analysis, can be done to determine subtype or to eliminate false-negatives if clinical suspicion remains high.

Werner EJ: Relative value of diagnostic studies for von Willebrand disease. J Pediatr 121:34–38, 1992.

41. Name the three most common variants of von Willebrand disease.

The diagnosis of von Willebrand disease is complicated by the multiple variations of the condition. The three most common variants include:

Common Variants of von Willebrand Disease

	TYPE I	TYPE IIA	TYPE IIB
Frequency	70–80%	10–12%	3–5%
Genetic transmission	Autosomal dominant	Autosomal dominant	Autosomal dominant
Ristocetin cofactor activity	↓	↓↓↓	±↓
Low-dose ristocetin-induced platelet aggregation	Normal	Normal	Increased
Multimeric electrophoretic pattern	Normal mixture (various sizes)	Large and intermediate forms absent	Large multimers absent

Adapted from Montgomery RR, Scott JP: Hemostasis: Diseases of the fluid phase. In Nathan DG, Oski FA (eds): Hematology of Infancy and Childhood, 4th ed. Philadelphia, W.B. Saunders, 1993, p 1622; with permission.

42. In what settings outside the newborn period can vitamin K abnormalities contribute to a bleeding diathesis?

Vitamin K is essential for gamma-carboxylation of both procoagulants (including factors II, VII, IX, X) and anticoagulants (proteins C and S). Gamma-carboxylation occurs in the liver and converts the proteins to their functional forms. Vitamin K is obtained in three ways: (1) as dietary fat-soluble K_1 (phytonadione) from leafy vegetables and fruits, (2) as K_2 (menaquinone) from synthesis by intestinal bacteria, and (3) as water-soluble K_3 (menadione) from commercial synthesis. *Malabsorptive intestinal disorders* (e.g., cystic fibrosis, Crohn disease, short bowel syndrome), *prolonged antibiotic therapy* (which diminishes intestinal bacteria), *prolonged hyperalimentation without supplementation*, and *malnutrition* can result in diminished stores. *Chronic hepatic disorders* (e.g., hepatitis, α_1-antitrypsin deficiency) can diminish both absorption of fat-soluble vitamin K (secondary to diminished bile salt production) and utilization of vitamin K in factor conversion. *Drugs* that can disrupt vitamin K include phenobarbital, phenytoin, rifampin, and warfarin.

43. What is the best test for distinguishing between coagulation disturbances secondary to hepatic disease, DIC, and vitamin K deficiency?

Factors II, V, VII, IX, and X are made in the liver, and all of these factors except factor V are vitamin K-dependent. Therefore, measurement of **factor V** is a useful test to distinguish liver disease from vitamin K deficiency, since this factor is reduced in the former and normal in the latter disorder. Factor VIII is reduced in patients with DIC because of the consumptive process, but this factor is normal or increased in liver disease and vitamin K deficiency. Therefore, the **factor VIII** level is a good test to distinguish DIC from the other two disorders.

Coagulation Abnormalities in Liver Disease, Vitamin K Deficiency, and DIC

	FACTOR V	FACTOR VII	FACTOR VIII
Liver disease	Low	Low	Normal or increased
Vitamin K deficiency	Normal	Low	Normal
DIC	Low	Low	Low

44. What is treatment of choice for DIC?

DIC occurs most commonly in the context of bacterial sepsis and hypotension. The best treatment is reversal of the hypotension through treatment of the infection and appropriate fluid management. If bleeding is severe or if hemorrhage is occurring in a life-threatening location, platelets and fresh frozen plasma should be given to make up for the loss of these elements which are occurring from consumption. The idea that the administration of these products "fuels the fire," thereby accelerating the thrombotic process, is interesting but clinically of little or no value.

If DIC fails to respond to these measures, heparin may be administered in an attempt to interrupt the consumptive process. However, heparin has not been proved to be effective in increasing survival in patients with sepsis and DIC. The replenishment of depleted antithrombin III levels with antithrombin III concentrate may decrease the risk of new thromboses.

45. How is anticoagulant therapy monitored in children?
The goal of standard *heparin* therapy is to raise the **PTT** to 1.5–2 times the normal level. However, the relationship between heparin level and prolongation of the PTT depends on the particular reagents that are used in the coagulation laboratory. Therefore, it is useful to check with the coagulation laboratory to see if they have established a range for the PTT at therapeutic heparin levels. Low molecular weight heparin, which is gaining usage at a rapid rate, does not require monitoring of the PTT under normal circumstances because the dose-response with this form of heparin is much more predictable. The reduction in laboratory costs partially offsets the higher cost of the drug itself.

Changes in the **PT** are used to monitor *warfarin* therapy. In the past, the prolongation of the PT by 1.5 times normal was the usual therapeutic goal. However, differences in reagents used in different laboratories made it difficult to monitor individual patients tested in different laboratories or to compare patients enrolled in multicenter clinical trials. The INR provides a measure of prolongation of the PT that is standardized against a common reagent. Thus, a therapeutic INR of 2–4 means the same thing no matter where the test is performed.

46. What are the four most common hereditary deficiencies that predispose a child to thrombosis?
1. *Factor V Leiden:* An abnormal factor V protein that is resistant to the normal antithrombotic effect of protein C.
2. *Protein C deficiency:* Protein C inactivates factors V and VIII and stimulates fibrinolysis. Homozygous individuals can present in the newborn period with purpura fulminans.
3. *Protein S deficiency:* Protein S serves as a cofactor for the expression of activated protein C.
4. *Antithrombin III deficiency:* Antithrombin III is involved in the inhibition of thrombin, factor X, and to a lesser extent, factor IX.

GRANULOCYTE DISORDERS

47. Describe the life cycle of a polymorphonuclear (PMN) leukocyte.
It takes about 14 days for an immature myeloblast to develop into a mature PMN. After departing the bone marrow, the PMN circulates in the blood for up to 20 hours and then migrates to tissue where it resides for 1–2 days.

48. Define neutropenia.
Neutropenia is arbitrarily defined as an absolute neutrophil count (ANC) of < 1500/mm³. The ANC is determined by multiplying the percentage of bands and neutrophils by the total white blood cell count. An ANC of < 500/mm³ is severe neutropenia. As a rule, the lower the ANC, the greater the risk of infectious complications. In the first 2 years of life (outside the neonatal period) when normal white blood counts are generally lower, an ANC < 1000/mm³ is considered neutropenic.

49. What is the most common cause of transient neutropenia in children?
Viral infections, including influenza, adenovirus, coxsackie virus, respiratory syncytial virus (RSV), hepatitis A and B, measles, rubella, Epstein-Barr virus, cytomegalovirus, and varicella. The neutropenia usually develops in the first 2 days of illness and may persist for up to a week. Multiple factors likely contribute to the neutropenia, including a redistribution of neutrophils (increased margination rather than circulation), sequestration in reticuloendothelial

tissue, increased utilization in injured tissues, and marrow suppression. In general, otherwise healthy children with transient neutropenia due to viral infections are at low risk for serious infectious complications.

50. Excluding intrinsic defects in myeloid stem cells, what conditions are associated with neutropenia in children?

1. *Bone marrow replacement:* tumor infiltration, myelofibrosis
2. *Drug:* sulfonamides, penicillin, antithyroid drugs, phenothiazines, benzodiazepines, aspirin, gold salts, acetaminophen
3. *Immunologic:* neonatal isoimmune (secondary to maternal IgG directed against fetal neutrophils), autoimmune (e.g., antineutrophil antibodies in systemic lupus erythematosus)
4. *Metabolic:* hyperglycinemia, isovaleric acidemia, propionic acidemia, methylmalonic acidemia, glycogen storage disease type IB
5. *Nutritional:* anorexia nervosa, marasmus, B$_{12}$/folate deficiency, copper deficiency
6. *Sequestration:* splenic enlargement

Curnutte JT: Disorders of granulocyte function and granulopoiesis. In Nathan DG, Oski FA (eds): Hematology of Infancy and Childhood, 4th ed. Philadelphia, W.B. Saunders, 1993, pp 945–949.

51. How should an infant or child with neutropenia be evaluated?

The evaluation of the patient with neutropenia should begin with a good history, focusing on prior illness or infection, toxin or drug exposure, growth and development, and family history. If the data are available, prior blood counts should be reviewed to determine if the neutropenia is newly acquired, longstanding, or congenital. Physical examination should focus on a search for mucosal or skin infection and phenotypic abnormalities, which may suggest another primary disorder such as Fanconi anemia, cartilage-hair hypoplasia, or Shwachman-Diamond syndrome. Delayed growth may be a clue to repeated infections or accompanying abnormalities such as malabsorption in Shwachman-Diamond syndrome.

If other cytopenias are present, a bone marrow examination is indicated immediately to rule out infiltrative disease or one of the bone marrow failure syndromes. If the neutropenia is isolated, any drugs which may be causative should be discontinued and all underlying infections or systemic illnesses treated. If the neutropenia persists, one should obtain serial blood counts to determine whether the low neutrophil count reoccurs in a predictable sequence, which would suggest the diagnosis of cyclic neutropenia.

Other diagnostic tests depend upon historical elements and available laboratory findings which might suggest an etiology. Relevant diagnostic tests might include viral serology, pancreatic function testing for babies with a history of diarrhea or growth failure to rule out Shwachman-Diamond syndrome, folate and vitamin B$_{12}$ levels if dietary history or blood cell morphology suggests a megaloblastic anemia, blood counts on family members if the family history is positive for repeated infections or early death, and evaluation for autoimmune or metabolic causes in the patient with multi-system disease.

52. What should top your diagnostic list in a 5-year-old with short stature, steatorrhea, neutropenia, and metaphyseal dysostosis on x-ray?

Shwachman-Diamond syndrome comprises a constellation of findings, including pancreatic insufficiency (resulting in malabsorption and failure to thrive), bone marrow failure, short stature, and characteristic bony changes. A unifying cause has not been identified.

53. What is the significance of a leukemoid reaction?

A leukemoid reaction usually refers to a white cell count > 50,000/mm^3 and an accompanying shift to the left. Causes include bacterial sepsis, tuberculosis, congenital syphilis, congenital or acquired toxoplasmosis, and erythroblastosis fetalis. Infants with Down syndrome may also have a leukemoid reaction that is often confused with acute leukemia during the first year of life.

54. Name the three most common causes of eosinophilia in children in the U.S.

Eosinophilia, usually defined as > 10% eosinophils or an absolute eosinophil count of $\geq 1000/mm^3$, is most commonly seen in three atopic conditions: **atopic dermatitis, allergic rhinitis**, and **asthma**.

55. Which conditions can be associated with extreme elevations of eosinophils in children?

• Visceral larval migrans (toxocariasis)
• Other parasitic disease (trichinosis, hookworm, ascariasis, strongyloidiasis)
• Eosinophilic leukemia
• Hodgkin disease
• Drug hypersensitivity
• Idiopathic hypereosinophilic syndrome

Lukens JN: Eosinophilia in children. Pediatr Clin North Am 19:969–981, 1972.

56. When is the best time to draw blood for evaluation of eosinophilia?

Midnight. Circulating blood eosinophils have a diurnal variation, with the highest values occurring near midnight and the lowest around noontime. This pattern may be a reflection of the diurnal nature of cortisol secretion, which is lower in the evening. Exogenous steroid administration is known to lower peripheral eosinophil counts. However, the small clinical significance (and large family repercussions) do not warrant midnight phlebotomy.

57. Which disorders are associated with basophilia?

1. *Hypersensitivity reactions:* drug or food hypersensitivity, urticaria
2. *Inflammation/infection:* ulcerative colitis, rheumatoid arthritis, influenza, chickenpox, tuberculosis
3. *Myeloproliferative diseases:* chronic myelogenous leukemia, myeloid metaplasia

Curnutte JT: Disorders of granulocyte function and granulopoiesis. In Nathan DG, Oski FA (eds): Hematology of Infancy and Childhood, 4th ed. Philadelphia, W.B. Saunders, 1993, p 957.

58. How do children with neutrophil disorders present?

Neutrophil disorders include those affecting quantity (e.g., various neutropenias) and function (e.g., chemotaxis, phagocytosis, bactericidal activity). These defects should be considered part of the differential diagnosis in patients with *delayed separation of the umbilical cord, recurrent infections with bacteria or fungi* of low virulence (but minimal problems with recurrent viral or protozoal infections), *poor wound healing*, and *specific locales of infection* (e.g., recurrent furunculosis, perirectal abscesses, gingivitis).

59. How is white cell function evaluated in children with suspected disorders?

Neutrophils and monocyte/macrophages are enumerated and examined morphologically after histochemical staining. Monoclonal antibodies directed against CD14 (a surface antigen on monocytes) are used in conjunction with flow cytometry to quantify the number of monocyte/macrophages. Suspected abnormalities in hexose monophosphate activity (as seen in children with chronic granulomatous disease) can be investigated with either nitroblue tetrazolium dye reduction or dichlorofluorescein assay. Chemotaxis is commonly assayed in agarose, and *in vitro* quantitative microbicidal assays can be used to assess the bactericidal capacity of isolated neutrophils and monocytes.

60. An 8-month-old with oculocutaneous albinism and recurrent pyogenic skin and respiratory tract infections likely has what syndrome?

Chédiak-Higashi syndrome is an autosomal recessive disorder characterized by leukocytes containing giant lysosomal granules, abnormal phagocytosis (due to deficient degranulation), and abnormal chemotaxis.

61. What types of infections are commonly seen in children with chronic granulomatous disease?

The neutrophils in these children fail to produce superoxide radicals, which are important in the killing of *Staphylococcus*, gram-negative bacteria, and some fungi. Superficial staphylococcal skin infections, particularly around the nose, eyes, and anus, are common. Severe adenitis, recurrent pneumonia, indolent osteomyelitis, and chronic diarrhea are frequent. Of note, a male child with a liver abscess should be considered to have chronic granulomatous disease until proven otherwise.

62. What is the basis for leukocyte adhesion deficiency (LAD)?

Leukocytes express a functionally related glycoprotein complex on the cell surface with a common β subunit and a cell-specific family of α subunits. LAD, also known as Mac-1 deficiency, is a deficiency of all three members of the β_2 (CD18) subfamily of surface proteins. Affected cells do not migrate properly because they are unable to adhere to endothelial or connective tissue surfaces. Clinically affected children can exhibit delayed umbilical cord separation, persistent leukocytosis, skin infections with little pus formation, impaired wound healing, and severe periodontal disease.

HEMATOLOGY LABORATORY

63. Of the seven red cell parameters given by a Coulter counter, which are measured and which are calculated?

The Coulter counter, the most commonly used automated electronic cell counter, utilizes the impedance principle. A precise volume of blood passes through an narrow aperture and impedes an electrically charged field, and each "blip" is counted as a cell. The larger the red cell, the greater the electric displacement. In a separate chamber, the same volume is hemolyzed and colorimetrically analyzed to determine the hemoglobin concentration.

Measured values
- Red blood cell (RBC) count
- Mean corpuscular volume (MCV)
- Hemoglobin (Hb)

Calculated values
- Mean corpuscular hemoglobin (MCH, in pg/cell) = $(10 \times [Hb/RBC])$
- Mean corpuscular hemoglobin concentration (MCHC, in gm/dl) = $(100 \times [Hb/Hct])$
- Hematocrit (Hct, in %) = $(RBC \times [MCV/10])$
- Red cell distribution width (RDW) = coefficient of variation in RBC size

64. What factors can interfere with electronically derived red cell indices?

1. *Hyperleukocytosis:* Overestimates the hemoglobin determination because of increased turbidity during measurement. Similarly, the MCV and RBC count can be artifactually elevated (usually when WBC count > 50,000/mm^3) because WBCs are counted as RBCs.

2. *Cold agglutinins:* May lower the RBC count, as aggregated collections are counted as a single cell. MCV may thus be artifactually high.

3. *Hyperglycemia:* When hyperglycemia is prolonged, RBCs become hyperosmolar and expand when placed in diluent. This results in an artifactually high MCV and hematocrit.

4. *Hypernatremia:* Similar to hyperglycemia.

5. *Hypertriglyceridemia:* If very elevated, can increase turbidity and result in an artifactually high hemoglobin concentration.

Stockman J: Using electronic RBC counts to diagnose anemia. Contemp Pediatr 6:99, 1989.

65. How does the mean corpuscular volume help provide a quick screen of the possible causes of anemia?

Microcytic: iron deficiency, thalassemias, sideroblastic anemia

Normocytic: autoimmune hemolytic anemia, hemoglobinopathies, enzyme deficiencies, membrane disorders, anemia of chronic disease

Macrocytic: disorders of B_{12} and folic acid metabolism, bone marrow/stem cell failure

66. In addition to an elevated reticulocyte count, what laboratory studies suggest increased destruction (rather than decreased production) of rbcs as a cause of anemia?

1. *Increased serum erythrocyte lactate dehydrogenase (LDH):* More commonly seen in hemolytic diseases, it can be greatly elevated in ineffective erythropoiesis (e.g., megaloblastic anemia).

2. *Decreased serum haptoglobin:* When RBCs lyse, serum haptoglobin binds the released hemoglobin and is excreted. However, up to 2% of the population has congenitally absent haptoglobin.

3. *Hyperbilirubinemia (indirect):* Usually increased with RBC lysis. However, it may also be elevated in ineffective erythropoiesis (e.g., megaloblastic anemia). Additionally, 2% of the population have Gilbert disease. In these patients, acute infection can cause a transient elevation of bilirubin secondary to liver enzymatic dysfunction rather than hemolysis.

67. What is the difference between the direct and indirect Coombs test?

Coombs serum is rabbit anti-human IgG. In the **direct** test, the Coombs serum is added directly to a patient's washed RBCs. The occurrence of agglutination means that the patient's RBCs have been sensitized *in vivo* by antibody. The **indirect** test involves incubating a patient's serum with RBCs of a known type and adding Coombs serum. If *in vitro* sensitization occurs, agglutination will result, indicating antibodies are present against the known blood type. Direct Coombs testing is vital in diagnosing autoimmune hemolytic anemias, while indirect testing is key in blood crossmatching.

68. How is the corrected reticulocyte count calculated?

Because the reticulocyte count is expressed as a percentage of total RBCs, it must be corrected according to the extent of anemia with the following formula: reticulocyte% × (patient Hct/normal Hct) = corrected reticulocyte count. For example, a very anemic 10-year-old patient with a hematocrit of 7% (contrasted with an expected normal hematocrit of 36%) and a reticulocyte count of 5% has a corrected reticulocyte count of 1.0% (5% × 7%/36% = 1%) which is not elevated, as might be seen in severe iron deficiency.

69. What is the significance of targeting on an RBC smear?

Red cell targets on a peripheral smear are caused by excessive membrane relative to the amount of hemoglobin. Therefore, target cells are found when the membrane is increased, as in patients with liver disease, or when the intracellular hemoglobin is diminished, as in patients with iron deficiency or thalassemia trait. Target cells may also be found in patients with certain hemoglobinopathies, such as hemoglobin C and hemoglobin S. In these instances, the target cells are caused by aggregation of the abnormal hemoglobin.

70. In what conditions are Howell-Jolly bodies found?

Howell-Jolly bodies are nuclear remnants found in red cells of patients with **reduced or absent splenic** function and in patients with **megaloblastic anemias**. They are occasionally present in the red cells of premature infants. Howell-Jolly bodies are dense, dark, and perfectly round, and their characteristic appearance makes them easily distinguishable from other red cell inclusions and from platelets overlying red cells.

71. What is the cause of Heinz bodies?

Heinz bodies represent *precipitated denatured hemoglobin* in the red cell. Heinz bodies occur when the hemoglobin is intrinsically unstable, as in hemoglobin Koln, or when the enzymes that normally protect hemoglobin from oxidative denaturation are abnormal or deficient, as in G6PD deficiency. These inclusions are not visible with a routine Wright-Giemsa stain but can be seen readily with methyl violet or brilliant cresyl blue stains.

72. What is the difference between echinocytes and acanthocytes?

These are the two basic types of spiculated RBCs. *Echinocytes* have small uniform projections distributed evenly, while *acanthocytes* have variably sized projections with irregular placement over the cell. *Echinocytes* are seen in healthy premature infants and in patients with uremia, defects in glycolytic metabolism, or microangiopathic hemolytic anemia (rare). *Acanthocytes* are found in patients with severe hepatocellular disease, abetalipoproteinemia, and anorexia nervosa.

Becker PS, Lux SE: Disorders of the red cell membrane. In Nathan DG, Oski FA (eds): Hematology of Infancy and Childhood, 4th ed. Philadelphia, W.B. Saunders, 1993, p 591–592.

73. Of what clinical value is the sedimentation rate?

An elevated erythrocyte sedimentation rate (ESR) is a nonspecific marker for inflammatory disease. The clinical use of the ESR usually exceeds its clinical usefulness. However, the test may be of some value in suggesting the presence of deep-seated infection or collagen vascular disease, particularly in patients with fever of unknown origin. Unfortunately, there are few data to define the predictive value of the ESR in this setting. A better use of the ESR may be the monitoring of the response to therapy in particular infections, such as bacterial endocarditis and osteomyelitis. In these conditions, a falling ESR is considered to be a reliable indicator of the resolution of the inflammatory process.

74. What conditions give a low sedimentation rate?

Low ESRs may be due to a **reduction in the concentration of large proteins** (nephrosis, liver disease, congestive heart failure), **abnormal red cell membrane** (sickle cell disease), or **polycythemia** (cyanotic congenital heart disease). A low ESR, however, has little diagnostic value. In fact, it may create confusion by masking the normally increased ESR that is expected during infection in, for example, a patient with nephrotic syndrome and peritonitis or a patient with sickle cell anemia and osteomyelitis.

HEMOLYTIC ANEMIA

75. What two types of RBC forms are commonly seen on the peripheral smear in patients with hemolytic anemia?

1. *Spherocytes or microspherocytes.* These forms can be seen in any hemolytic anemia that results from a loss of RBC membrane surface area (e.g., Coombs positive hemolytic anemia, DIC, or congenital spherocytosis).

2. *Schistocytes.* These various forms of fragmented RBCs can be seen in microangiopathic hemolytic anemia, a form of intravascular hemolysis from mechanical disruption (e.g., prosthetic heart valves, hemolytic-uremic syndrome, cavernous hemangioma).

76. Which disorder is most commonly associated with an elevated mean cell hemoglobin concentration (MCHC)?

Hereditary spherocytosis. The hyperchromic appearance of spherocytes and microspherocytes is due to loss of surface membrane, an excess of hemoglobin, and mild cellular dehydration. In other hemolytic anemias associated with spherocytosis, the percentage of spherocytes is usually insufficient to raise the MCHC.

77. Name the two most common inherited disorders of red cell membranes.

Hereditary spherocytosis and hereditary elliptocytosis. **Hereditary spherocytosis** is usually inherited in an autosomal dominant pattern. More recently, kindreds with an autosomal recessive form have been described. In approximately 30% of children with hereditary spherocytosis, neither parent has anemia or morphologic alterations of the red cells. Some of these cases may represent new mutations in the child, whereas others may represent the autosomal recessive form of the disease. **Hereditary elliptocytosis** is inherited in an autosomal dominant pattern.

78. How are disorders of red cell membranes diagnosed?

Most membrane disorders can be identified by careful analysis of red cell morphology on the peripheral smear. The characteristic spherocytes, elliptocytes, ovalocytes, or stomatocytes are usually readily apparent. The osmotic fragility test is used frequently to confirm the diagnosis of spherocytosis, since spherocytes are more sensitive to osmotic lysis than normal red cells because of their reduced surface to volume ratio. Most membrane disorders are associated with an abnormality in cation and/or water transport across the red cell membrane. Specific studies of intracellular ion and water content may be useful in diagnosing the more unusual varieties of membrane disorders. Additional studies, available only in research laboratories, include analysis of membrane proteins or the genes associated with these proteins.

79. Why can hereditary spherocytosis present at multiple ages?

The time of presentation of hereditary spherocytosis is largely dependent on the severity of the disease. When hemolysis is brisk, the initial presentation may be jaundice in the neonatal period or signs and symptoms of anemia during early infancy. Some children first present with an aplastic crisis in which the hemoglobin level and reticulocyte count are both low. The latter finding may initially obscure the diagnosis since an elevated reticulocyte count is expected in a hemolytic disorder. Children with less severe hereditary spherocytosis may not be recognized until a routine blood count reveals a low hemoglobin level or until an enlarged spleen is found on examination. Some children with mild disease will escape detection until they are adults and develop gallstones.

80. Why is splenectomy usually curative for hereditary spherocytosis?

In hereditary spherocytosis, an abnormality in the skeletal structure of the red cell membrane allows sodium influx into the RBC followed by water, which swells the cell and decreases its deformability. This problem is accentuated when the RBC reaches the spleen, where conditions are ideal for the destruction of metabolically incompetent red cells. In this case, the increased rate of glycolysis which is needed to compensate partially for the sodium leak is compromised by the low pH and the small amount of available glucose in the spleen. In addition, the poor deformability of the swollen RBC may lead to trapping of the cell in the cords of the spleen and loss of membrane to the surrounding macrophages. This results in a further reduction in the surface to volume ratio of the RBC, leaving the cell even less deformable and more vulnerable to a metabolic or mechanical death in its next trip through the spleen. This prominent role of the spleen in the pathophysiology of the hemolytic anemia in hereditary spherocytosis explains why splenectomy is usually curative.

81. In which settings do isoimmune and autoimmune hemolytic anemia most commonly appear?

Isoimmune:	Red cell antigen incompatibility between mother and fetus
	Transfusion of incompatible blood
Autoimmune:	Idiopathic (most common)
	Infectious (including *Mycoplasma pneumoniae*, infectious mononucleosis, varicella, viral hepatitis)
	Drugs (antimalarials, penicillin, tetracycline)
	Hematologic disorders (Evans syndrome)
	Systemic autoimmune disorders (including systemic lupus erythematosus, dermatomyositis)

Tabbara IA: Hemolytic anemias: Diagnosis and management. Med Clin North Am 76:649–668, 1992.

82. How should children with a suspected immune-mediated hemolytic anemia be evaluated?

Quickly and carefully, as this may be a life-threatening disease. History and physcial examination are key. Typical findings may include rapid onset of pallor, jaundice, dark urine, abdominal pain, splenomegaly, and fever. The laboratory evaluation should include a cbc, reticulocyte count (elevated), evaluation of the peripheral blood smear (possible red cell fragments, spherocytes, polychromasia, and occasionally nucleated rbcs), a direct Coombs test, indirect bilirubin, and if suggested by history, a cold agglutinin titer. Approximately 10% of patients with autoimmune hemolytic anemia are Coombs negative. Thus, patients should be treated for auto-immune hemolytic anemia if the disease is strongly suspected, even if the direct Coombs test is negative.

In children older than 10 years of age, immune hemolytic anemia is more likely to be secondary to an underlying disease rather than the idiopathic or autoimmune IgG-mediated type seen in younger children. Cold agglutinin (IgM) disease is uncommon in pediatric patients, except in the setting of mycoplasmal infection.

83. What are the differences between autoimmune hemolytic anemias caused by "warm" and "cold" antibodies?

Warm: IgG antibodies with maximum activity at 37°C; directed most commonly against the Rh antigens; generally do not require complement for *in vivo* hemolysis; hemolysis is predominantly extravascular with primarily splenic consumption; more likely to be associated with underlying disease (especially SLE in females); splenectomy and immunosuppression often effective.

Cold: IgM antibodies with maximum activity between 0°–30°C; directed most commonly against I or i antigen; intravascular hemolysis via complement activation is common; extravascular hemolysis involves primarily hepatic consumption; more commonly associated with acute infection (e.g., *Mycoplasma pneumoniae*, cytomegalovirus); chronic hemolysis less likely; splenectomy and immunosuppression often ineffective.

84. An 8-year-old black male developed jaundice and very dark urine 24–48 hours after beginning nitrofurantoin for a urinary tract infection. What is the likely diagnosis?

Glucose-6-phosphate dehydrogenase (G6PD) deficiency is the most common hemolytic anemia caused by an RBC enzymatic defect. The enzyme G6PD is a key component of the pentose phosphate pathway, which ordinarily generates sufficient NADPH to maintain glutathione in a reduced state (and thus available for combating oxidant stresses). The deficiency is inherited in an X-linked recessive fashion. In patients who are deficient (most commonly those of African, Mediterranean or Asian ancestry), oxidant stresses, particularly certain drugs, can result in hemolysis.

85. In a patient with G6PD deficiency, why is the initial diagnosis often difficult in the acute setting?

The amount of G6PD enzymatic activity is dependent on the age of the RBC. Older RBCs have the least, reticulocytes the most. In an acute hemolytic episode, the older cells are destroyed first, younger ones may remain, and reticulocytes increase. If erythrocytic G6PD levels are measured at this point, the result may be misleadingly near or above the normal range. If clinical suspicions remain, repeating the test when the reticulocyte count is reduced will give a more accurate measurement.

86. What are the biochemical variants of G6PD deficiency?

The most common form of G6PD deficiency found in the United States is the Gd^A- variant, found in approximately 8–10% of black males. In this variant, the activity of the enzyme falls rapidly as the red cell ages. The measured G6PD activity is reduced but not absent. The Gd^Mediterranean variant has little if any measurable activity. More than 100 other variants of G6PD structure or activity have been described but are rarely identified in patients in the U.S.

87. What are the clinical manifestations of G6PD deficiency

Children with the Gd^A- or the Gd^Mediterranean variants of G6PD deficiency are usually hematologically normal unless exposed to an oxidant stress. Acute intravascular hemolysis may occur in the face of certain drugs such as the antimalarial agent chloroquine, certain toxins such as naphthalene found in many mothballs, or certain viral infections. These hemolytic episodes are characterized by an abrupt fall in hemoglobin level and a rise in reticulocyte count. Hemoglobinuria may be manifested as a positive test for blood by dipstick in the absence of red cells on microscopic analysis. Jaundice may accompany the hemolysis. The red cells have a characteristic appearance during acute hemolytic episodes. The peripheral smear shows blister cells in which the hemoglobin is pushed to one side of the cell, leaving a clear area beneath the membrane on the opposite side. In the Gd^{A-} variant, the hemolytic episode is usually self-limited since the reticulocytes have a normal complement of enzyme activity and are therefore resistant to the oxidant stress of the drug, toxin, or infection. Recovery usually occurs within 48–72 hours. In the Gd^{Mediterranean} variant, acute hemolysis is more common and more severe due to the lower overall level of enzyme activity.

88. Why do children with pyruvate kinase (PK) deficiency tolerate anemia better than children with other anemias?

PK deficiency is an RBC glycolytic enzyme deficiency that most commonly affects those of northern European ancestry. Levels of 2,3-diphosphoglycerate (a glycolytic intermediate) are increased in patients with PK deficiency, and this compound shifts the oxygen dissociation curve to the right. As a result of this shift, oxygen is more readily delivered from the red cells to the tissue. This rightward shift is much greater than is ordinarily found in patients with similar degrees of anemia due to other causes. Thus, some symptoms typically associated with anemia may be less severe or even absent in patients with PK deficiency.

IMMUNODEFICIENCY

89. How do immunoglobulin levels change during the first years of life?
- Due to active placental transport of **IgG**, a full-term baby has a level that is equal to or slightly higher than maternal levels. With an IgG half-life of 21 days, this transported maternal IgG reaches a nadir after 3–4 months. As the infant begins to make IgG, the level begins to rise slowly and reaches adult levels by 6–10 years of age.
- Although a normal baby has very low concentrations of **IgM** at birth, normal adult concentrations are usually achieved by about 1 year of age.
- **IgA** is the last immunoglobulin produced, and adult levels are not reached until adolescence. Because delays in production of IgA are not unusual, the diagnosis of IgA deficiency is difficult to make with certainty in a child < age 2 years.
- **IgD** and **IgE**, both of which are present in low concentrations in the newborn, reach 10–40% of adult concentrations by 1 year of age.

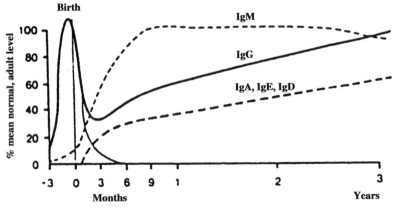

Normal development of serum immunoglobulin levels. (From Hobbs JR: Primary immune paresis. In Adinolfi M (ed): Immunology and Development. Clinics in Developmental Medicine, no. 34. London, Spastics Int Medical Publ./William Heinemann Medical Books Ltd., 1969, pp 114–158; with permission.)

90. Why aren't antibodies produced by the fetus in appreciable quantities?
1. The fetus is in a sterile environment and is not exposed to foreign antigens.
2. The active transport of maternal IgG across the placenta may suppress fetal antibody synthesis.
3. Fetal and neonatal monocyte/macrophages may not process foreign antigens normally.

91. What is the immunologic importance of the major histocompatibility complex (MHC) antigens?
The MHC molecules are part of the immunoglobulin supergene family. These antigens are responsible for the rejection of unrelated tissues following transplantation. Every antigen, both non-self and self, is recognized by T cells in conjunction with MHC molecules. *Class I MHC gene products* (human leukocyte antigens [HLA] A, B, and C) are expressed on every living cell. *Class II MHC antigens* (HLA-D/DR) are expressed in large quantities only on resting B cells, monocyte/macrophages, and activated T cells. *CD4* (helper T cells) recognize foreign antigens in conjunction with Class II molecules, whereas *CD8* (cytotoxic T cells) recognize foreign antigens in association with Class I MHC antigens.

92. What are the four types of hypersensitivity reactions?
Type I   IgE-mediated; immediate or anaphylactic (e.g., urticaria, allergic rhinitis)
Type II Antibody-dependent cytotoxicity (e.g., Goodpasture syndrome, erythroblastosis fetalis)
Type III Immune complex or Arthus reaction (e.g., poststreptococcal glomerulonephritis, serum sickness)
Type IV Delayed hypersensitivity (e.g., contact dermatitis, tuberculin skin testing)

93. What is the normal lymphocytic makeup of the peripheral blood?
Approximately 55–80% of the lymphocytes are T cells, 5–20% are B cells, and 5–20% are natural killer (NK) cells. There are usually a small number of cells that cannot be accounted for using the routine typing reagents.

94. How do natural killer cells differ from other lymphocytes?
NK cells are large granular lymphocytes that lyse tumor or viral-infected target cells. This type of immunity does not require antibody and is not MHC restricted.

95. What are CD antigens?
CD, or cluster designated, antigens are one or more cell-surface molecules, detectable by monoclonal antibodies, that define a particular cell line or state of cellular differentiation.

96. What is the clinical importance of the CD4/CD8 ratio?
The CD4/CD8 ratio is an index of helper to suppressor cells and may be significantly altered in a variety of immunodeficiencies. In normal individuals, the ratio ranges from 1.4–1.8/1.0. In viral infections (particularly HIV), the ratio can be reduced, and in bacterial infections it can be increased.

97. How common are the primary immunodeficiencies?
About 400 new cases of primary immunodeficiency occur annually, for an incidence rate of 1:10,000 (excluding asymptomatic IgA deficiency). The relative prevalences of primary immunodeficiencies are:

B-cell deficiencies (excluding asymptomatic IgA deficiency)	50%
T-cell deficiencies	10%
Combined immunodeficiencies	20–25%
Phagocytic deficiencies	15%
Complement deficiencies	< 3%

Stiehm ER (ed): Immunologic Disorders in Children, 3rd ed. Philadelphia, W.B. Saunders, 1989.

98. How do the clinical characteristics vary between T-cell and B-cell deficiencies?

Variation of Clinical Characteristics between T-cell and B-cell Deficiencies

	T-CELL DEFICIENCIES	B-CELL DEFICIENCIES
Age of onset	Early infancy (4–6 mos)	Usually delayed until > 6 mos of age, coinciding with disappearance of maternal antibody
Type of recurrent infection	Fungal, viral, mycobacterial, opportunistic organisms (e.g., *Pneumocystis carinii*)	Encapsulated bacterial pathogens (with sinopulmonary infections, otitis media, meningitis, sepsis, abscess, osteomyelitis)
Growth	Failure to thrive	Little growth failure
Secondary associations	Increased incidence of malignancy	Increased incidence of allergy and autoimmune disorders

Middleton E Jr, et al (eds): Allergy: Principles and Practice, 4th ed. St. Louis, Mosby, 1993, pp 1037–1044.

99. Which screening tests can be done for evaluation of B-cell immune function?
Quantitative serum immunoglobulin levels (IgG, IgA, IgM, IgE): A combined IgG, IgA, and IgM level < 400 mg/dl suggests immunoglobulin deficiency; > 5000 IU/ml for IgE suggests hyper-IgE syndrome
IgG subclasses
Specific antibodies
   Isohemagglutin titer (anti-A, anti-B): ≤ 1:4 after age 1 suggests specific IgM deficiency
   Tetanus/diphtheria (IgG_1)
   Pneumococcal polysaccharide antigens (IgG_2)
   Viral respiratory agents (IgG_3)
Iseki M, Heiner DC: Immunodeficiency disorders. Pediatr Rev 14:230, 1993.

100. What are the criteria for the diagnosis of IgA deficiency?
   IgA deficiency is relatively common, with a frequency ranging from 1:500 to 1:1000, especially in individuals of European heritage. It is present as an isolated condition if serum IgA is < 5 mg/dl, salivary IgA is absent, and other immunologic indices (IgG, IgM, cellular immunity) are normal.

101. Describe the clinical expression of IgA deficiency.
   The expression is extremely variable, which makes the interpretation of a low IgA level difficult. More than 50% of patients are asymptomatic. Although IgA represents < 15% of total immunoglobulin, it is predominant on mucosal surfaces. Therefore, most patients with symptoms have recurrent diseases involving mucosal surfaces, including otitis media, sinopulmonary infections, and chronic diarrhea. Systemic infections are rare. Patients with IgA deficiency have associated increased risks of atopic diseases (e.g., allergic rhinitis, atopic dermatitis, food allergy), autoimmune diseases (e.g., thyroiditis, pernicious anemia), and rheumatic diseases (e.g., juvenile rheumatoid arthritis, systemic lupus erythematosus). Incidence of infections and chronic illness is increased in individuals who have both IgA deficiency and IgG subclass deficiency.
   Lederman HM: Disorders of humoral immunity. In Oski FA, et al (eds): Principles and Practice of Pediatrics, 2nd ed. Philadelphia, J.B. Lippincott, 1994, p 186.

102. Why is gamma globulin therapy not utilized as a treatment for selective IgA deficiency?
   Unless a patient has a concurrent IgG subclass deficiency (and even in this setting, therapy is controversial), gamma globulin therapy is not indicated and relatively contraindicated because:
   1. The short half-life of IgA makes frequent replacement therapy impractical.
   2. Gamma globulin preparations have insufficient IgA quantities to restore mucosal surfaces.
   3. Patients can develop anti-IgA antibodies with the potential for hypersensitivity complications, including anaphylaxis.

103. What is the significance of IgG subclass deficiencies?

IgG exists in four subgroups (IgG_1, IgG_2, IgG_3, IgG_4), each with functional differences. In response to protein antigens, IgG_1 and IgG_3 subclasses predominate, while IgG_2 and IgG_4 are typically noted with polysaccharide antigens. In the mid-1970s, reports began to appear describing children with recurrent infections (primarily sinopulmonary) who had selective subclass deficiency. Most common was IgG_2, but multiple other combinations have since been described. Patients with selective deficiency and recurrent infection may benefit from polysaccharide–protein conjugate vaccines, prophylactic antibiotics, and, if the infections are severe, intravenous gamma globulin. Considerable debate exists regarding the treatment and clinical importance of subclass deficiencies because:

1. IgG values have a very wide and age-dependent range.
2. Methodologic variability among laboratories is widespread.
3. Specific antibody responses may be more important than absolute subclass quantities.
4. Coexistent immunologic problems (e.g., IgA deficiency) may be present.
5. Subclass deficiencies can be the presenting abnormality in more serious immunologic disorders (e.g., ataxia-telangiectasia, common variable immunodeficiency, chronic mucocutaneous candidiasis, adenosine deaminase deficiency).
6. Some younger patients with subclass deficiencies have immunoglobulin levels that return to normal with maturation.

Shackelford PG: IgG subclasses: Importance in pediatric practice. Pediatr Rev 14:291–296, 1993.

104. In an infant with panhypogammaglobulinemia, how can quantitation of B and T lymphocytes in peripheral blood help distinguish the diagnostic possibilities?

- Normal numbers of T lymphocytes, no detectable B lymphocytes: X-linked agammaglobulinemia (Bruton disease)
- Normal numbers of T and B lymphocytes: transient hypogammaglobulinemia of infancy, common variable immunodeficiency
- Decreased numbers of T lymphocytes, normal or decreased numbers of B lymphocytes: severe combined immunodeficiency
- Decreased CD4 lymphocytes: HIV infection

Lederman HM: Disorders of humoral immunity. In Oski FA, et al (eds): Principles and Practice of Pediatrics, 2nd ed. Philadelphia, J.B. Lippincott, 1994, p 185.

105. Which screening tests are useful for evaluation of a T-cell immunity?

1. *Absolute lymphocyte count:* Although most T-cell immunodeficiencies are not associated with a decreased lymphocyte count, a total count < 1500/mm³ suggests a deficiency.
2. *Chest x-ray* to evaluate the thymic shadow in the newborn infant.
3. *Delayed skin hypersensitivity testing* to recall antigens: 75% of normal children aged 12–36 months will respond to *Candida* skin testing at 1:10 dilution; by 18 months, approximately 90% of normal children will respond to one of a panel of recall antigens (tetanus toxoid, trichophyton, and *Candida*); the younger the child, the less likely the reactivity.
4. *Quantitation of T-cell subsets:* total T cells with < 60% mononuclear cells, helper (CD4) cells < 200/μl, or CD4/CD8 < 1.0 suggests T-cell deficiency.

Middleton E Jr, et al (eds): Allergy: Principles and Practice, 4th ed. St. Louis, Mosby–Year Book, 1993, p 1044.

106. In children with severe combined immunodeficiency (SCID), how often is a family history positive for affected relatives?

50–60%. SCID represents a heterogeneous group of disorders characterized by both humoral and cell-mediated immune dysfunction that can be very profound. SCID can be inherited in both an autosomal recessive and an X-linked form.

Stephan JL, et al: Severe combined immunodeficiency: A retrospective single-center study of clinical presentation and outcome in 117 patients. J Pediatr 123:564–572, 1993.

107. What disease did the "bubble boy" have?

Adenosine deaminase (ADA) **deficiency**. In this form of severe combined immunodeficiency, the lack of ADA results in abnormalities of B-cell and T-cell function and increased susceptibility to infection. The bubble served as a means of minimizing contagion but also promoted social isolation. While bone marrow transplantation has been curative as a treatment, ADA deficiency is the first disease (by initial reports) to be successfully treated by gene therapy (i.e., insertion of functional ADA genes into the patient's autologous cells and infused).

108. An infant with hypocalcemic tetany, a loud murmur, and dysmorphic facies likely has what syndrome?

DiGeorge syndrome (also called DiGeorge sequence or anomaly). The clinical pattern results from maldevelopment of the third and fourth pharyngeal pouches during embryogenesis, resulting in a spectrum of malformations including:
- Cardiac defects: aortic arch anomalies, and conotruncal anomalies, especially truncus arteriosus
- Parathyroid absence or hypoplasia with abnormal calcium homeostasis
- Abnormal facies, including low-set ears, short philtrum, hypertelorism, notched ear pinna, micrognathia, and downslanting palpebral fissures
- Thymic hypoplasia

The thymic maldevelopment is variable in degree and usually results in diminished numbers of T cells. However, clinically significant immunologic abnormalities are often absent.

109. Describe the clinical features of Job syndrome.

Also known as the **hyper-IgE syndrome**, Job syndrome is characterized by:
1. Eczema
2. Recurrent skin infections—boils or abscesses with reduced amounts of inflammation ("cold abscesses")
3. Recurrent sinopulmonary infections
4. Extremely elevated IgE
5. Eosinophilia

Multiple immunologic problems exist, particularly chemotactic abnormalities. The name derives from the Biblical problems of Job: "So went Satan forth from the presence of the Lord and smote Job with boils from the sole of his foot unto his crown."

110. A 26-month-old has ataxia, frequent episodes of sinusitis, and telangiectasias on the bulbar conjunctiva. What is the likely diagnosis?

Ataxia-telangiectasia (to see it is to diagnose it). In this multisystem, autosomal recessive condition, progressive neurologic deterioration is associated with Purkinje cell degeneration of unknown cause. Ataxia is often the first neurologic sign. Telangiectasias develop on the conjunctiva and skin of exposed areas. Variable immunologic deficits involving cellular and humoral immunity exist. There is a high frequency of immunoglobulin isotype deficiencies (especially IgA and IgE deficiency). Up to 10% of patients develop lymphomas.

111. What makes the lymphocyte bare in the bare lymphocyte syndrome?

The *bare lymphocyte syndrome* is characterized by absence of Class I and/or Class II MHC-HLA antigens. Lack of MHC antigens interferes with processes of recognition and cytotoxic defense. The immunologic features are similar to those noted with combined immunodeficiency diseases. There is severe lymphopenia and increased susceptibility to infection, particularly viral.

112. How do patients with complement deficiencies usually present?

While there may be overlap, early complement deficiencies (C1, C4, C2) tend to present with a lupus-like syndrome or vasculitis. Late complement deficiencies (C5–C8) are associated with disseminated neisserial infections, such as recurrent gonococcal arthritis or meningococcal meningitis. C3 deficiency can be associated with both early and late features, such as septicemia or vasculitis.

113. How is the classic complement cascade evaluated?

The primary screening test is the **CH$_{50}$**. It assesses the ability of an individual's serum (in varying dilutions) to lyse sheep RBCs after those cells are sensitized with rabbit IgM anti-sheep antibody. The CH$_{50}$ is an arbitrary unit indicating the quantity of complement necessary for 50% lysis of the RBCs in a standardized setting. Test results are usually expressed as a derived reciprocal of the test dilution needed for 50% lysis. The test is relatively insensitive, as major reductions in individual complement components are necessary before the CH$_{50}$ is altered. Therefore, **C3** and **C4 levels** are often included in the initial screening of a child with a suspected complement deficiency.

114. A 10-year-old with recurrent nonpruritic swelling of the face and arms may have what complement-related abnormality?

C1 esterase inhibitor deficiency, also called hereditary angioneurotic edema (HANE). This inhibitor prevents activation of the complement cascade. Diagnosis is confirmed by direct assay of the inhibitor level. Clinical presentations of this autosomal dominant condition can include:

1. *Recurrent facial and extremity swelling*—acute, circumscribed edema that is not painful, red, or pruritic, clearly distinguishing it from urticaria. Usually self-resolves in 72 hours.

2. *Abdominal pain*—recurrent, often severe, colicky pain, due to interstitial wall edema with vomiting and/or diarrhea; may be misdiagnosed as an acute abdomen.

3. *Hoarseness, stridor*—a true emergency, as death by asphyxiation may occur due to laryngeal edema. Epinephrine, hydrocortisone, and antihistamines are often of only limited benefit, and tracheostomy is needed if there is progression of symptoms.

115. Describe the functions of the various interferons (IFN).

Interferons are glycoproteins that were initially discovered as factors produced by cells during the course of viral infections. Three major types (α, β, γ) have been identified. IFNs α and β are produced by leukocytes and fibroblasts in response to viral infections, and γ is produced by T cells in response to an antigen or mitogen. The effects of interferons on cellular functions are widespread including:

Inhibit	Enhance	Mixed effects
Cell proliferation	Promyelocytic and monoblastic	Erythroleukemic cell differ-
Tumor growth	leukemic cell differentiation	tiation
Fibroblast-adipocyte	Phagocytosis by macrophages	Production of antibodies
differentiation	Accessory cell functions of macro-	Cell-mediated immune
	phages (IFN γ > IFN α, β	phenomena
	Endotoxin-induced interleukin-1	
	secretion by macrophages	
	(IFN γ, α, β)	
	Generation of cytotoxic T	
	lymphocytes	
	Activity of NK cells	
	Expression of class I and II MHC	
	antigens and Fc receptors	

From Stites DP, Terr AI: Review of Basic and Clinical Immunology, 7th ed. Norwalk, CT, Appleton & Lange, 1990, p 93; with permission.

116. What are the indications for interferon therapy?

It is a growing list. Recombinant **IFN** α has been used as adjuvant treatment in multiple conditions including various malignancies (including hairy-cell leukemia), condyloma acuminata, hepatitis (C and D), and large or diffuse hemangiomas. **IFN** β is used experimentally to treat selected tumors. **IFN** γ has a role in a number of infectious (e.g., chronic granulomatous disease, chronic active hepatitis, leishmaniasis), fibrotic (e.g., scleroderma, keloids), and IgE-mediated diseases (e.g., atopic dermatitis, hyper-IgE syndrome).

Gallin JI, et al: Interferon γ in the management of infectious diseases. Ann Intern Med 123:216–224, 1995.

IRON-DEFICIENCY ANEMIA

117. At what age do exclusively breastfed infants become at risk for iron deficiency?

Healthy *term* infants who are exclusively breastfed are at risk for iron deficiency after 6 months of age. The age of risk for exclusively breastfed *premature* infants can be more complicated, particularly for the smaller and sicker infants, and recommendations vary. The lower iron stores of premature infants are more rapidly depleted compared to term babies. As a rule, the smaller the baby, the earlier and greater the amount of iron-supplementation needed. Low-birth-weight babies (1000–1500 gm) may need supplementation (2–3 mg/kg/day) beginning at 2 months of age, and very-low-birth-weight babies (< 1000 gm) perhaps even sooner (2–4 weeks). Of note, multiple transfusions can decrease or delay the need for supplementation because they are an excellent source of iron (1 mg/ml) once the cells have completed their lifespan.

Neu J, et al: Scientifically-based strategies for nutrition of the high-risk low-birth-weight infant. Eur J Pediatr 150:2–13, 1990.

118. Why are infants who begin cow milk at an early age susceptible to iron-deficiency anemia?

Although breast milk and cow milk contain about the same amount of iron (0.5–1.0 mg/l), nonheme iron is absorbed at 50% efficiency from breast milk but only at 10% from cow milk. In addition, cow milk may cause microscopic gastrointestinal bleeding in younger infants due to mucosal injury, possibly from sensitivity to bovine albumin. In older infants, cow milk may interfere with iron absorption from other sources.

Fuchs G, et al: Gastrointestinal blood loss in older infants: Impact of cow milk versus formula. J Pediatr Gastroenterol Nutr 16:4–9, 1993.

Sullivan P: Cow's milk induced intestinal bleeding in infancy. Arch Dis Child 68:240–245, 1993.

119. In which pediatric groups should screening for iron-deficiency anemia be considered?

• Low birth weight
• Consumption of whole cow milk before 7 months of age
• Use of formula not fortified with iron
• Low socioeconomic status
• Exclusive breastfeeding (without solid or formula supplementation) beyond 6 months of age
• Perinatal blood loss
• Teenage females (if menstruation is heavy or with pregnancy)

Oski F: Iron deficiency in infancy and childhood. N Engl J Med 329:190–193, 1993.

120. How common is anemia in teenage athletes?

Frank anemia is uncommon. However, nonanemic iron deficiency may be found in approximately ½ of adolescent female athletes and up to an ⅛ of male athletes, particularly long-distance runners. An adverse effect of this iron deficiency on athletic performance, however, in the absence of anemia has never been conclusively demonstrated. On the other hand, iron depletion (with or without anemia) may be associated with lassitude, decreased concentration ability, and mood swings.

Rowland TW: Iron deficiency in the young athlete. Pediatr Clin North Am 37:1153–1162, 1990.

Ballin A, et al: Iron state in female adolescents. Am J Dis Child 146:803–805, 1992.

121. As iron becomes depleted from the body, what is the progression at which lab tests change?

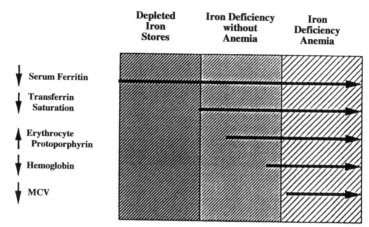

The left end of the line for each test indicates the point at which the result deviates from its baseline. As shown in this diagram, in general, depletion of marrow, liver, and spleen reserves (as represented by ferritin) occurs first, followed by a decrease in transport iron (as represented by transferrin saturation), and finally a fall in hemoglobin and mean cell volume (MCV). The diagram illustrates that absence of anemia does not exclude the possibility of iron deficiency and that iron depletion is relatively advanced before anemia develops.

From Dallman PR, et al: Iron deficiency and related nutritional anemias. In Nathan DG, Oski FA (eds): Hematology of Infancy and Childhood, 4th ed. Philadelphia, W.B. Saunders, 1993, p 427; with permission.

122. How do acute inflammatory states affect tests for iron deficiency?

The *ferritin* level, used to monitor body iron stores, is exquisitely sensitive to inflammation, increasing even with mild upper respiratory infections. Elevations of ferritin may persist for some time. In contrast, *serum iron, transferrin* level, and percent *transferrin saturation* may decrease with infection or inflammation. *Free erythrocyte protoporphyrin* should not be affected by acute inflammation but may increase in chronic inflammatory states. All of these changes increase the difficulty of evaluating iron stores in the patient with acute or chronic inflammation.

123. How is the Mentzer index helpful in the diagnosis of microcytic anemia?

The Mentzer index is mean cell volume (MCV)/RBC count. It helps distinguish between the two leading causes of microcytosis, iron deficiency and thalassemia trait. In the former, there is a decreased RBC count, while in the latter, an increased RBC count. Thus, a Mentzer index > 13 is usually associated with iron-deficiency anemia, while a Mentzer index < 13 is more commonly associated with thalassemia trait. Specific testing is necessary to confirm a diagnosis.

124. How is the red cell distribution width (RDW) helpful in diagnosing microcytic anemia?

The RDW is a quantification of anisocytosis or variation in red cell size. It is derived from the RBC size histogram measured by automated cell counters and is reported as a percentage. In children, normal values range from about 11.5–14.5% but can vary between instruments. Statistically, it is the coefficient of variation of red cell volume distribution. Practically, when elevated in a patient with microcytosis, it suggests that iron deficiency is a more likely cause of anemia than thalassemia trait. Thalassemia trait tends to have values that overlap with normal RDW values. Of note, the combination of an RDW above the normal range with free erythrocyte protoporphyrin > 35 µg/dl is sensitive and specific for iron-deficiency anemia.

Cesana BM, et al: Relevance of red cell distribution width (RDW) in the differential diagnosis of microcytic anaemias. Clin Lab Haematol 13:141–151, 1991.

125. In a child with suspected iron-deficiency anemia, is a therapeutic trial with iron an acceptable diagnostic approach?

If an infant or child is otherwise well, a therapeutic trial of 4–6 mg/kg/day of elemental iron can substitute for additional diagnostic testing (e.g., ferritin, transferrin saturation, free erythrocyte protoporphyrin) since dietary iron deficiency is the most likely cause of microcytic anemia. If the child is iron-deficient, the hemoglobin should rise in about 1 month by > 1 gm/dl. If the hemoglobin does rise, therapy should be continued for an additional 2 months to replenish iron stores. False-positive results can occur if the initial hemoglobin was low due to recent infection (and thus would spontaneously rise).

126. After iron therapy is initiated, how early can a response be detected?

2–5 days: Increase in reticulocyte count

7–10 days: Increase in hemoglobin level

For patients with mild iron-deficiency anemia, the hemoglobin level should be checked after several weeks of therapy. For patients with more severe anemia, it may be useful to check the hemoglobin and reticulocyte levels after a few days to make certain that the hemoglobin has not declined to dangerous levels and that the reticulocyte response is beginning.

127. What foods affect the bioavailability of nonheme iron?

Decreased by: Phosphates, tannates, polyphenols and oxalates found in cereal, eggs, cheese, tea, and as complex carbohydrates.

Increased by: Fructose, citrate, and especially ascorbic acid found in red kidney beans, cauliflower, and bananas. In children with iron deficiency, administration of replacement iron with a vitamin C-fortified fruit juice 30 minutes before a meal makes physiologic sense.

128. What are the indications for parenteral iron therapy?

Clearly documented *noncompliance* with oral iron replacement therapy, *total parenteral nutrition* for severe malabsorption or inflammatory bowel disease, and *bleeding* that exhausts iron stores so rapidly as to make oral iron therapy ineffective.

129. What are the side effects of parenteral iron therapy?

Common side effects include pain and skin discoloration at the site of intramuscular injection. Occasionally reported toxicities include fever, urticaria, headache, malaise, arthralgia, and regional adenopathy. A few patients have had severe, even fatal, anaphylactic reactions. The frequency or seriousness of side effects of parenteral iron strongly argues against its use in children who have not been given an adequate trial of oral iron, even if the trial requires inpatient supervision.

130. What are the differences between pica, geophagia, and pagophagia?

All are clinical markers that suggest the diagnosis of iron deficiency. **Pica** is a more general term indicating a hunger for items not normally consumed as food. The others are more specific. **Geophagia** refers to the consumption of dirt or clay, and **pagophagia**, to excessive consumption of ice. These are distinguished from **cissa**, which is the physiologic craving of pregnancy for unusual food items or combinations (e.g., root beer float with turkey bits, heavy on the garlic sauce).

131. Discuss the relationship between iron deficiency and development in infants and toddlers.

Multiple studies have shown an association between iron deficiency in infants aged 9–24 months and lower motor and cognitive scores and increased behavioral problems when compared with nonanemic controls. Some longer-term studies suggest that the developmental impairments may be long-lasting. Debate remains on whether this relationship is causal and, if so, whether the correction of anemia leads to a reversal of the problems.

Moffatt MEK, et al: Prevention of iron deficiency and psychomotor decline in high-risk infants through use of iron-fortified formula: A randomized clinical trial. J Pediatr 125:527–534, 1994.

132. Why are iron-deficient children at increased risk for lead poisoning?

1. Pica associated with iron deficiency increases likelihood of ingestion of lead-contaminated items.

2. GI absorption of lead may be increased in patients who consume less iron-containing nutrients.

Watson WS, et al: Food iron and lead absorption in humans. Am J Clin Nutr 44:248–256, 1986.

MEGALOBLASTIC ANEMIA

133. Is megaloblastic anemia responsible for most macrocytic anemias in children?

No. Macrocytic anemia can be found in conditions associated with a high reticulocyte count (e.g., hemolytic anemia or hemorrhage), bone marrow failure (e.g., Fanconi anemia, aplastic anemia, Diamond-Blackfan syndrome), liver disease, Down syndrome, and hypothyroidism.

134. What findings on a complete blood count are suggestive of megaloblastic anemia?

Red cells:	Elevated mean corpuscular hemoglobin and mean cell volume (often 106 fl or more) with variability in cell size (anisocytosis) and cell shape (poikilocytosis) due to ineffective erythropoiesis
Neutrophils:	Large and multilobed; occasional neutropenia in more severe anemia
Platelets:	Usually normal, thrombocytopenia in more severe anemia

135. What are the causes of vitamin B_{12} (cobalamin) deficiency in children?

Decreased intake	Decreased absorption
May occur in vegetarians who consume no animal products (or in their breastfed offspring)	Ileal mucosal abnormalities (e.g., Crohn disease)
General malnutrition	Surgical resection of terminal ileum
	Competition for cobalamin in bacterial overgrowth syndromes or infection with fish tapeworm (*Diphyllobothrium latum*)
	Congenital abnormalities of the receptor for vitamin B_{12}–intrinsic factor complex
	Gastric mucosal defects that interfere with secretion of intrinsic factor

136. How does the pathophysiology of juvenile pernicious anemia differ from that of adult pernicious anemia?

Intrinsic factor (a glycoprotein) is released from gastric parietal cells and binds vitamin B_{12} to form a complex that is ultimately absorbed in the terminal ileum. Pernicious anemia is due to lack of intrinsic factor. **Juvenile pernicious anemia** is due most commonly to a congenital inability to secrete intrinsic factor. Since transplacental vitamin B_{12} stores (from non-vegetarian mothers) can last for years, symptoms can be delayed for up to 5 years in children. Gastric acidity and histology are normal, and the cause is unknown. In **adult pernicious anemia**, autoantibodies are produced against gastric parietal cells (resulting in achlorhydria); in addition, there is decreased production of intrinsic factor and, in many cases, antibodies to intrinsic factor are also found. These antibodies are not typically found in children. However, they can cross the placenta and impair cobalamin absorption during the first few weeks of life.

137. How is the Schilling test done?

This is a test to identify the cause of vitamin B_{12} deficiency. Administration of radiolabeled B_{12} by mouth is followed by an intramuscular (IM) dose of unlabeled B_{12}. Urine is collected for 24 hours and assayed for percent excretion of the oral dose (normal, 10–35%). The IM B_{12} is given to saturate tissue B_{12}-binding sites to facilitate excretion of the oral dose. Normal results depend on both the availability of intrinsic factor and undisturbed intestinal absorption. Oral intrinsic factor may also be given if results are abnormal. In pernicious anemia, excretion will normalize with administration of exogenous intrinsic factor, while in disorders of the terminal ileum, urinary excretion remains low even with intrinsic factor since absorption is defective.

138. What are the best dietary sources of folate and B_{12}?

Folate: Rich foods include liver, kidney, and yeast. Good sources include green vegetables (particularly spinach) and nuts. Moderate sources include fruits, bread, cereals, fish, eggs, and cheese. Rice, milk, meat, and poultry are poor sources of folate. Pasteurization or boiling destroys folate.

Vitamin B_{12}: Humans do not manufacture B_{12}; bacterial and fungi do. Animals require it while plants do not. Consequently, our major dietary source of vitamin B_{12} is consumption of animal tissue, milk, or eggs. Seafood, which live on bacterial diets, are also a good dietary source. Of note, B_{12} is required for normal folate metabolism.

139. A 10-month-old fed exclusively goat milk is likely to develop what anemia?

Megaloblastic anemia due to folic acid deficiency. Goat milk contains very little folic acid compared with cow milk. Infants consuming large amounts, especially if not receiving significant supplemental solid foods, are susceptible. In addition, the diagnosis can be complicated by the higher risk of coexistent iron-deficiency anemia in this age group.

PLATELET DISORDERS

140. How can a platelet count be estimated from a peripheral smear?

As a rule, each platelet visible on a high-power microscopic field ($100\times$) represents 15,000–20,000 platelets/mm³. If platelet clumps are observed, the count is usually > 100,000/mm³.

141. What factors can interfere with the automated platelet count?

Since automated cell counters utilize only size to identify platelets, small objects such as red cell fragments, white cell fragments, or leukemic blast fragments may be counted as platelets, falsely elevating the automated count. Conversely, the automated count may be depressed if large or giant platelets are counted as red cells. Inadequate anticoagulation of the sample may also cause a falsely low platelet count. Platelets may also agglutinate in vitro in some patients by EDTA (anticoagulant)-dependent antibodies. In this disorder, the cause of platelet clumping is an IgG or IgM antibody directed against a platelet antigen that is present only in the presence of EDTA.

142. How much does a platelet transfusion raise the platelet count?

0.1–0.2 unit/kg of transfused platelets should raise the platelet count by 40,000/mm³, or 1.0 unit/m² should raise the count by 10,000/mm³. In normal patients, platelet survival time is 7–10 days but is often considerably shorter in thrombocytopenic patients due to a variety of causes.

143. A previously healthy 3-year-old develops mucosal petechiae, multiple ecchymoses, and a platelet count of 20,000/mm³ 2 weeks after a bout of chickenpox. What's his most likely diagnosis?

Acute idiopathic (immune) thrombocytopenic purpura (ITP). ITP is one of the most common bleeding disorders of childhood, and the presentation is postinfectious in about 50% of cases.

144. Describe the natural history of ITP.

With or without medical treatment, 50–60% of patients with acute ITP will have normal platelet counts within 1–3 months of diagnosis and 75% are well after 6 months. By 1 year, only 10% of children with ITP remain thrombocytopenic, and some of the children with chronic ITP still improve as long as 5–10 years after diagnosis. Because of this predominantly benign natural course of ITP, careful consideration is necessary before instituting treatment that is hazardous or irreversible.

145. In a toddler with suspected ITP, what is the significance of a palpable spleen on exam?

Although patients with ITP may rarely have a palpable spleen tip, the presence of splenomegaly in a patient with thrombocytopenia warrants more aggressive evaluation for an associated problem (e.g., collagen-vascular disease, hypersplenism).

146. In patients with suspected ITP, should a bone marrow evaluation be done?

A topic of much debate. A major concern is that without a bone marrow aspiration, the diagnosis of leukemia may be delayed or the course of illness worsened by treatment (such as corticosteroids) that is begun for presumed ITP. However, it is very rare that patients with leukemia present with isolated thrombocytopenia. Local custom will likely prevail regarding the need for bone marrow examination in the setting of "classic" acute ITP, but heightened consideration should be given if: (1) other cell lines are involved, (2) history and physical examination have atypical features (e.g., weight loss, hepatosplenomegaly), and (3) steroid therapy is to be used.

Dubansky A, et al: Isolated thrombocytopenia in children with acute lymphoblastic leukemia: A rare event in a Pediatric Oncology Group study. Pediatrics 84:1068, 1989.

147. When should medical treatment be given for acute ITP without active bleeding?

Because the long-term prognosis of ITP does not appear to be influenced by medical treatment, the management of a newly diagnosed child with ITP and no serious bleeding remains controversial. The principal concern is susceptibility to intracranial bleeding, which occurs in < 1% of affected patients (but can have 30–50% mortality), almost always when the platelet count is < 20,000/mm^3. Prospective studies to evaluate the best ways to minimize this complication will never be done because of the need to enroll > 10,000 subjects to answer that question. Local custom will prevail, but some authorities will treat medically when the platelet count is < 20,000/mm^3 to minimize the chance of intracranial catastrophe and to avoid excessive limitations of physical activity that might otherwise be imposed on a child with ITP.

148. If a child with ITP requires treatment, how does the response to steroids compare with gammaglobulin?

Gammaglobulin: Intravenous immune globulin (IVIG), 0.8–1.0 gm/kg/day, raises the platelet count in approximately 85% of patients. The response usually occurs within 48 hours and persists for 3–4 weeks. Up to 75% of patients will have some degree of limited adverse reaction (e.g., nausea, vomiting, headaches, fever). Gammaglobulin is more expensive than steroids.

Steroids: Steroids are similarly effective, but oral steroids take about twice as long (4 days) to raise the platelet count significantly. The steroid effect may be multifactorial because signs of hemorrhage tend to decrease before the increase in platelets occurs. Side effects of long-term frequent steroid use are multiple.

Blanchette VS, et al: A prospective, randomized trial of high-dose intravenous immune globulin G therapy, oral prednisone therapy, and no therapy in childhood acute immune thrombocytopenic purpura. J Pediatr 123:989–995, 1993.

149. Are platelet transfusions of any value in ITP?

ITP is a disorder of increased platelet destruction rather than decreased production. In some severe cases, the platelet half-life might be as little as 10 minutes (normal 7–10 days). Because the antiplatelet antibody produced by the patient is as "effective" against donor platelets as it is against the patient's own platelets, transfusions usually do not increase the peripheral platelet count. Nonetheless, patients with ITP and life-threatening bleeding may benefit from platelet transfusion, since there may be a local hemostatic effect even in the absence of a demonstrable effect on the peripheral blood platelet count.

150. Which children with ITP are candidates for splenectomy?

Splenectomy improves the platelet count in up to 90% of patients. Since spontaneous remission is common in acute ITP, splenectomy is usually limited to bleeding that is life-threatening and unresponsive to medical therapies. Patients with ITP lasting > 1 year with continued bleeding, severe thrombocytopenia, or with unacceptable restrictions may be reasonable candidates for splenectomy. If possible, splenectomy should be deferred until a child is at least 5 years old to minimize the risk of overwhelming sepsis that can occur in younger splenectomized patients.

151. How does the age of presentation of ITP influence the long-term outcome?

Children with the onset of ITP after age 10 years are more likely to develop chronic ITP, which by definition is persistence > 6–12 months. Chronic ITP is more commonly associated with other underlying problems (e.g., systemic lupus erythematosus, autoimmune thyroid disease, HIV infection), and the likelihood of spontaneous remission is significantly diminished.

152. A 6-month-old boy has an eczema, recurrent pneumonia, and a platelet count of 5000/mm³ with small platelets noted on the blood smear. What condition is likely?

Wiskott-Aldrich syndrome. This X-linked recessive syndrome is characterized by multiple immunologic defects (especially poor B-cell response to polysaccharide antigens and diminished T-cell function) and persistent thrombocytopenia. The small platelet size is a particularly important diagnostic clue.

Rosen FS, et al: The primary immunodeficiencies. N Engl J Med 333:431–440, 1995.

153. What are the inherited disorders of platelet function?

Membrane glycoprotein abnormalities	Granule defects	Metabolic abnormalities
Bernard-Soulier syndrome	Hermansky-Pudlak syndrome	Impaired arachidonic acid release
Glanzmann thrombasthenia	Wiskott-Aldrich syndrome	Cyclo-oxygenase deficiency
	Chédiak-Higashi syndrome	
	Gray platelet syndrome	

Several rare, inherited disorders of platelet function involve membrane receptors or metabolic processes important for platelet aggregation and the formation of a primary platelet plug. In more severe disorders, such as Glanzmann thrombasthenia, bleeding usually occurs early in life. Hemorrhagic manifestations include prolonged bleeding from circumcision, sustained GI bleeding, and oral mucosal bleeding. Platelet transfusions are effective initially, but over time, there is a high risk of alloimmunization to donor platelets.

154. In what conditions in children is thrombocytosis most commonly seen?

- Acute infections (e.g., upper and lower respiratory tract infections)
- Chronic infections (e.g., tuberculosis)
- Iron deficiency anemia
- Hemolytic anemia
- Blood loss
- Medications (including vinca alkaloids, epinephrine, corticosteroids)
- Trauma (with tissue damage)
- Inflammatory disease (e.g., Kawasaki syndrome)
- Malignancy (including chronic myelogenous or megakaryocytic leukemia)
- Chronic renal disease

Yohannan MD, et al: Thrombocytosis: Etiologic analysis of 663 patients. Clin Pediatr 33:340–343, 1994.

155. What level of thrombocytosis requires treatment?

In contrast with adults, a high platelet count in children does not appear to be a cause of significant morbidity. There is no magic platelet count at which treatment of thrombocytosis is warranted. In some centers, aspirin in doses of 60–300 mg daily is administered when the platelet count exceeds $1–1.5 \times 10^6/mm^3$. Early introduction of aspirin therapy may be more important if the patient has other problems that might contribute to hyperviscosity, such as a high WBC count or hemoglobin level.

SICKLE CELL DISEASE

156. Why screen for neonatal sickle cell disease?

Sickle cell disease is often asymptomatic in the first months of life. In the neonatal period, the presence of large amounts of fetal hemoglobin reduces the rate of polymerization of HbS and the sickling of red cells containing this abnormal hemoglobin. As the amount of fetal hemoglobin decreases after age 3–6 months, patients with sickle cell disease are increasingly likely to experience their first clinical manifestations. These can include pneumococcal sepsis and splenic sequestration, which are associated with significant morbidity and mortality.

If a neonate is identified with sickle cell disease, parental education can be given, and early daily prophylactic penicillin initiated. Early detection has been shown to decrease mortality in sickle cell disease.

Vinchinsky E, et al: Newborn screening for sickle cell disease: Effect on mortality. Pediatrics 81:749–755, 1988.

157. When does functional asplenia occur in children with sickle cell disease?

It may begin as early as 5 or 6 months of age and may precede the presence of Howell-Jolly bodies in the peripheral smear. Clinical experience indicates that the period of increased risk for serious bacterial infection parallels the development of functional asplenia. Loss of splenic function usually occurs later in patients with HbSC or HbS β^+-thalassemia than in patients with HbSS.

158. A 4-year-old black male whose spun hematocrit is 25% but whose Coulter-derived hematocrit is 20% is likely to have what condition?

Sickle cell anemia or **iron-deficiency anemia**. Both result in RBCs that are variable in size, misshapen, or poorly deformable. When hematocrits are spun, the regular packed arrangement of the cells is disrupted and the measured column artifactually high. However, since the Coulter derives the hematocrit from the total RBC volume, it usually gives a lower value.

159. Is the finding of a palpable spleen during the exam of a 13-year-old with a sickling disorder unusual?

It is a strong clue to the presence of HbSC or HbS β^+-thalassemia. In HbSS, the spleen is rarely palpable after 5 or 6 years of age.

160. List the morbidities associated with sickle cell disease.

Acute	Long-term
• Vaso-occlusive (painful) crisis	• Renal failure
• Splenic sequestration	• Congestive heart failure
• Severe anemia secondary to aplastic crisis or hemolytic crisis	• Retinal damage
• Acute chest syndrome	• Leg ulcers
• Cerebral infarction or hemorrhage	• Aseptic necrosis of the hip
• Infection	• Respiratory failure

161. A 6-month-old black male has painful swelling of both hands. He has what likely condition?

Hand-foot syndrome, or dactylitis. This common early manifestation of sickling disorders in infants and young children is characterized by painful swelling of the hands, feet, and proximal fingers and toes caused by symmetric infarction in metacarpals, metatarsals, and phalanges. Lack of systemic signs, presence of symmetric involvement, and young patient age help distinguish hand-foot syndrome from the much less common osteomyelitis which may also complicate sickle cell disease.

162. How should a child with a painful crisis be managed?

A painful (or vaso-occlusive) crisis is one of the most difficult and challenging problems in the treatment of sickle cell disease. The mainstays of treatment are fluid therapy to prevent dehydration ($D_5\frac{1}{4}NS$ or $D_5\frac{1}{2}NS$ 1.5–2 times maintenance) and analgesia. Approaches to pain control are notoriously varied and untested. The guiding principles are adequate relief of pain, awareness of drug side effects, and close familiarity with a particular drug, including its usual dose and route of administration. Treatment is considerably easier when the physician is familiar with or inquires of an individual patient's particular pattern of painful episodes and analgesic response.

For outpatients with an acute painful crisis, acetaminophen or acetaminophen and codeine are reasonable choices. Patients with intensely painful crises require hospitalization for opioid (including morphine and meperidine) analgesics, ideally given intravenously. Patient-controlled analgesia (PCA) offers the dual benefit of a constant infusion and intermittent boluses of an analgesic. Within parameters set by the physician, the patient determines the frequency of bolus doses.

Other supplementary agents, including nonsteroidal analgesics (e.g., ketorolac), vasodilators/membrane active agents (e.g., cetiedil citrate), and high-dose methylprednisone, are presently under study. For severe crises unresponsive to standard measures, blood transfusions to reduce the amount of sickle cells to < 40% may be beneficial. Of note, the reasons for the enormous variability in occurrences among sickle cell patients remain unclear. Forty percent never experienced a painful crisis in a 10-year study.

Platt OS, et al: Pain in sickle cell disease: Rates and risk factors. N Engl J Med 325:11–16, 1991.

163. How should children with sequestration crisis be managed?

Acute sequestration crisis represents a true emergency in sickle cell disease and is the second leading cause of death in young children with this hemoglobinopathy. The clinical problem is primarily one of hypovolemic shock due to pooling of blood in the acutely enlarged spleen. The hemoglobin level may drop as low as 1 or 2 gm/dl. The major therapeutic effort should be directed toward **volume replacement** with whatever fluid is handy. In most instances, normal saline or colloid solutions will be adequate until properly cross-matched blood is available. Acute sequestration crisis is one of the few instances in sickle cell disease in which **transfusion** with whole blood is appropriate, since the problem is one of hypovolemia and anemia rather than anemia alone. If whole blood is not available, packed RBCs alone or packed RBCs plus plasma may be an alternative therapy.

164. How is abdominal pain due to a sickle cell crisis distinguished from a surgical abdomen?

Patiently and carefully. Children with this clinical scenario should be treated as if they may have a surgical abdomen, including omission of high dose analgesics, cessation of oral intake, and early surgical consultation. Clinical clues to suggest sickle cell crisis include the presence of bowel sounds, concomitant vaso-occlusive pain elsewhere, and a report by the patient that the pain is typical for his or her previous vaso-occlusive crises. Plain films are indicated to rule out perforation of a viscus in severe cases, and ultrasound may help to identify a localizing source such as cholecystitis or appendicitis. If clinical deterioration occurs with adequate hydration and moderate analgesia, surgical exploration should be strongly considered. Although simple or exchange transfusion preoperatively is recommended to help prevent the development of acute chest syndrome postoperatively, truly emergent surgery should *never* be delayed.

165. What causes "acute chest syndrome" in sickle cell patients?

Acute chest syndrome refers to the constellation of findings (e.g., fever, cough, chest pain, pulmonary infiltrates) that can resemble pneumonia or pulmonary infarction. The exact mechanism is unknown and the cause is likely multifactorial. Various infections (e.g., viral, chlamydial, or mycoplasmal) may initiate respiratory inflammation which ultimately causes localized hypoxia. Increased pulmonary sickling may then result. Rib and other bone infarcts can also occur, and hypoventilation may result from chest splinting. Overly vigorous hydration can lead to pulmonary edema.

Castro O, et al: The acute chest syndrome in sickle cell disease: Incidence and risk factors. Blood 84:643–649, 1994.

166. Why is hydroxyurea beneficial in some patients with sickle cell disease?

Hydroxyurea, a chemotherapeutic agent used in some forms of leukemia, has as one of its side effects the ability to increase fetal hemoglobin production. Cells with higher concentrations of fetal hemoglobin are less prone to sickle. Other agents, including 5-azacytidine, butyric acid analogues, and recombinant human erythropoietin, have also been shown to increase levels of fetal hemoglobin.

Charache S, et al: Effect of hydroxyurea on the frequency of painful crises in sickle cell anemia. N Engl J Med 332:1317–1322, 1995.

167. How common is sickle cell trait in the United States?

Heterozygosity for the sickle gene occurs in about 8% of blacks in the U.S., 3% of Hispanics in the eastern U.S., and a much smaller percentage of individuals of Italian, Greek, Arabic, and Veddah Indian heritage. Of note, 2% of blacks in the U.S. have hemoglobin C trait.

168. Does sickle cell trait have any morbidity?

Under normal physiologic conditions, RBCs in individuals with sickle cell trait contain only 30–40% sickle hemoglobin, which is insufficient to cause sickling. However, in hypoxic settings, sickling may occur. At high altitudes (such as mountain climbing or unpressurized aircraft), splenic infarction is possible. In addition, portions of the kidney may have physiologically low oxygen concentrations which can interfere with function and lead to hyposthenuria and hematuria (usually microscopic and asymptomatic). Higher rates of sudden unexplained death in military recruits have raised questions about the danger of severe, prolonged exertion in patients with sickle trait. However, most authorities place no restriction on activity. Life expectancy is not altered by sickle cell trait.

169. What is the second most common worldwide hemoglobin variant?

Hemoglobin E. This variant is particularly high in the southeast Asian population (especially those of Laotian, Thai, and Cambodian heritage). Heterozygotes are asymptomatic; homozygotes can have a mild microcytic anemia. The most common abnormal findings on a peripheral smear are microcytosis and target cells.

THALASSEMIA

170. What accounts for the variability in clinical expression of the thalassemias?

The thalassemias are a heterogeneous group of disorders due to diminished or absent normal globin chain production. Normally, 4 α-globin genes and 2 β-globin genes are expressed to make the tetrameric globin protein, which then combines with a heme moiety to make the predominant hemoglobin in red cells, HbA (subunits $\alpha_2\beta_2$). Depending on the number of genes that are deleted, the production of polypeptide chains is diminished. In α-thalassemia, deletions of the α-globin gene(s) occur, and in β-thalassemia, deletions of β-globin gene(s) occur. When one class of polypeptide chains is diminished, this leads to a relative excess of the other chain. The result is ineffective erythropoiesis, precipitation of unstable hemoglobins, and hemolysis due to intramedullary RBC destruction.

Clinical heterogeneity results from variability in the number of gene deletions (particularly in α-thalassemia). However, as a rule, the greater the number of deletions, the more severe the symptoms. A large number of point mutations have been identified in various populations which can contribute to the phenotypic diversity. In addition, the inheritance of other thalassemia genes, such as δ or the persistence of fetal hemoglobin, can modify the clinical course.

171. How is the diagnosis of thalassemia made in most clinical laboratories?

Homozygous β-thalassemia is detected by the absence (β^0) or reduction (β^+) relative to HbF ($\alpha_2\gamma_2$ or fetal hemoglobin) in the amount of HbA ($\alpha_2\beta_2$) on hemoglobin electrophoresis. The carrier state for β-thalassemia is characterized by a low mean cell volume (MCV) and, in most instances, an increased level of HbA$_2$ ($\alpha_2\delta_2$) or HbF. The levels of these two hemoglobins are most accurately measured by column chromatography. Estimation or quantitation from electrophoretic patterns is frequently misleading. Alpha thalassemia trait remains a diagnosis of exclusion (low MCV in the absence of an identifiable cause) in the clinical laboratory although the enumeration of missing alpha genes is easily accomplished by molecular techniques.

Testing for Thalassemia

	TEST	
DISORDER	SCREENING	DEFINITIVE
Thalassemia major	cbc Peripheral smear	• Hemoglobin electrophoresis • Globin chain synthesis • Molecular detection of thalassemia mutation
β-Thalassemia trait (thalassemia minor)	cbc MCV	• Hemoglobin electrophoresis • HbA$_2$ • HbF
α-Thalassemia trait	cbc MCV	• α-Gene enumeration by molecular techniques

172. Why is splenomegaly common in thalassemia?

The excess α-globin chains in the red cells of patients with β-thalassemia and the excess β-globin chains in the red cells of patients with α-thalassemia form inclusion bodies on the red cell membranes. These cells are cleared by the spleen because of their diminished flexibility, and the spleen enlarges as a result. The spleen may also enlarge as it attempts to make red cells to compensate for the severe anemia and as it stores iron that accumulates from repeated red cell transfusions.

173. Describe the clinical features of the α-thalassemia syndromes.

Clinical Features in α-Thalassemia

SYNDROME	USUAL GENOTYPE	α GENE NUMBER	CLINICAL FEATURES
Normal	α α/α α	4	Normal
Silent carrier	α –/α α	3	Normal
α-Thalassemia trait	α –/α – α α/– –	2	Mild microcytic anemia
HbH disease	– –/α α	1	Moderate microcytic anemia Splenomegaly Jaundice
Homozygous α-thalassemia	– –/– –	0	Fetal hydrops due to severe anemia

174. What are the clinical features of the β-thalassemia syndromes?

Thalassemia minor: minimal or no anemia (hemoglobin 9–12 gm/dl); microcytosis; elevated rbc count

Thalassemia intermedia: microcytic anemia with hemoglobin usually > 7 gm/dl; growth failure; hepatosplenomegaly; hyperbilirubinemia; and thalassemic facies (i.e., frontal bossing, mandibular malocclusion, prominent malar eminences due to extramedullary hematopoiesis) develop between ages 2–5 years

Thalassemia major (Cooley anemia): severe anemia (hemoglobin 1-6 gm/dl) usually in the first year of life; hepatosplenomegaly; growth failure

175. How can coexistent iron deficiency increase the difficulty of diagnosing β-thalassemia?

β-thalassemia trait is usually diagnosed by hemoglobin electrophoresis, with quantitative hemoglobins revealing elevated HbA_2 and/or HbF levels. Iron deficiency can cause a lowering of HbA_2, masking the diagnosis. With iron replacement, the hemoglobin A_2 will rise to the expected elevated levels in β-thalassemia trait.

176. What are the adverse effects of chronic iron overload in children with thalassemia?

The major cause of morbidity and mortality from transfusional iron overload is related to iron accumulation in the heart, manifested as congestive heart failure, dysrhythmias, and, less frequently, pericarditis. Common iron-induced endocrine abnormalities include delay in growth and sexual development, hypoparathyroidism, and hypothyroidism. Diabetes due to iron overload is irreversible, even with intensive chelation. Excessive hepatic iron storage causes progressive liver fibrosis and cirrhosis, although death from cardiac disease occurs before most patients develop major problems related to liver dysfunction.

Cohen A: Management of iron overload in the pediatric patient. Hematol Oncol Clin North Am 1:521–544, 1987.

177. How do you reduce iron accumulation in children requiring repeated transfusions?

The two most common diseases associated with transfusion-related iron overload are thalassemia major and sickle cell disease. Strategies for reducing iron accumulation include:

1. *Chelation therapy:* Subcutaneous or intravenous deferoxamine has been the standard therapy for transfusional overload. Effective oral iron chelators are under development.

2. *Splenectomy:* Used primarily in thalassemia (and a small subgroup of sickle cell patients) with hypersplenism which results in premature destruction of RBCs.

3. *Diet:* Drinking tea with meals reduces dietary iron absorption and may be most helpful in diseases such as thalassemia intermedia, in which the bulk of excessive iron is dietary in origin.

4. *Erythrocytapheresis:* Automated erythrocytapheresis rather than repeated simple transfusions may markedly reduce transfusional iron loading in sickle cell disease.

10. INFECTIOUS DISEASES

Joseph W. St. Geme, III, M.D., David B. Haslam, M.D., and Mark F. Ditmar, M.D.

ANTI-INFECTIVE THERAPY

1. In prescribing antibiotics for obese children, should the dosage be based on the actual or ideal weight of the child?

As a rule, most antibiotics distribute poorly into fat and fat cells do not metabolize the drug. Therefore, ideal body weight for height is a better determinate of total daily dosage than actual weight.

2. Which antibiotics are contraindicated in hepatic failure?

Antibiotics that are primarily excreted or detoxified in the liver should be avoided or used with extreme caution in patients with impaired hepatic function. Examples of such drugs include chloramphenicol, tetracycline, erythromycin, lincomycin, clindamycin, rifampin, and isoniazid. If these agents are used, their dosage should be modified to account for the diminished excretion. Other drugs that should be used with caution or for which serum levels should be monitored in patients with severe liver disease include metronidazole, ketoconazole, miconazole, nitrofurantoin, and pyrazinamide.

3. How common are rashes related to ampicillin?

Minor reactions to ampicillin are manifested by a morbilliform, erythematous, papular rash that appears about 3 days after initiation of therapy. These rashes are common (7% of ampicillin courses) and are thought to be due to IgM complexes formed with penicilloyl antigens. They resolve spontaneously as IgG-blocking antibodies are formed. Clinical resolution occurs even though ampicillin therapy is continued. Ampicillin rashes should be distinguished from immediate, IgE-mediated hypersensitivity reactions. The latter are rare (1 in every 20,000 courses of drug) and occasionally life-threatening, being manifested by an urticarial rash, shock, bronchospasm, and laryngeal edema. Usually, this form of reaction follows immediately upon exposure to the drug, but a mild form may be delayed from a few hours to a few days.

Boguniewicz M, Leung DYM: Hypersensitivity reactions to antibiotics commonly used in children. Pediatr Infect Dis J 14:221–231, 1995.

4. How are children with allergy to penicillin managed?

Only about 10% of children with a history of adverse reactions to penicillin have an IgE-mediated sensitivity to the drug as demonstrated by a positive skin test. It is imperative, however, that a thorough history be elicited in children with a history of an adverse reaction to penicillin.

Some have advocated skin testing in children with such histories to determine whether a reported adverse reaction to the drug is, in fact, IgE-mediated. There is an approximate 95% sensitivity in skin testing using both Prepen (penicilloyl-polylysine, a major antigenic determinant) and penicillin G. The sensitivity of skin testing is improved when minor determinants of penicillin are included in the skin testing panel. The minor determinant mixtures, however, are not yet commercially available. On the other hand, others advocate a different approach, including alternate antibiotic therapy in patients with a previous adverse reaction to penicillin. If alternative drug therapy would not be satisfactory, penicillin skin testing can then be done.

Skin testing itself poses a risk, including the possibility of anaphylaxis, and should be done by an individual experienced in such procedures and in an appropriate clinical setting. In situations in which penicillin-specific IgE has been demonstrated and in which it is imperative that the patient receive a penicillin drug, desensitization can be done by experienced medical personnel in a clinical setting able to handle emergency situations.

Boguniewicz M, Leung DYM: Management of the patient with allergic reactions to antibiotics. Pediatric Pulmonol 12:113–122, 1992.

5. Are antibiotic-resistant pneumococci more virulent than sensitive strains?

The occurrence of antibiotic-resistant *Streptococcus pneumoniae* is a growing problem in both adult and pediatric infectious disease management. Resistance has been documented to penicillins, cephalosporins, erythromycin, tetracycline, and trimethoprim-sulfamethoxazole. Those persons at most risk for acquiring these resistant strains are hospitalized individuals, those with multiple antibiotic exposures, and either the very young or very old. It does not appear that the resistant strains are more virulent or present with a different type of clinical picture. For severe illness, treatment may require vancomycin plus an extended-spectrum cephalosporin. At-risk children > 2 years should receive the 23-valent pneumococcal vaccine.

Friedland IR, McCracken GH Jr: Management of infections caused by antibiotic-resistant *Streptococcus pneumoniae*. N Engl J Med 331:377–382, 1994.

6. What are the risk factors for infection by penicillin-resistant *S. pneumoniae*?

In children, **day-care attendance** and the **previous use of antibiotics**. The emergence of penicillin resistance in clinical isolates of *S. pneumoniae* is a growing problem in pediatrics, particularly with respect to otitis media and meningitis. On average, up to 25% of pneumococcal strains are not completely susceptible to penicillin.

McCracken GH: Emergence of resistant *Streptococcus pneumoniae*: A problem in pediatrics. Pediatr Infect Dis J 14:424–428, 1995.

7. How do the clinical indications and limitations of first-, second-, and third-generation cephalosporins compare?

First-generation cephalosporins (e.g., cefazolin, cephalexin)

1. Alternative drugs for patients who cannot tolerate penicillins, although there is a 5–10% risk of cross reactivity
2. Prophylaxis in orthopedic and cardiovascular surgery
3. Better *Staphylococcus aureus* coverage compared to second- and third-generation cephalosporins
4. Lack of efficacy against *Haemophilus influenzae* has limited their use

Second-generation cephalosporins (e.g., cefaclor, cefuroxime, cefprozil)

1. Increased spectrum of activity, including many gram-negative organisms (most *H. influenzae* isolates are sensitive)
2. Prophylaxis for intra-abdominal and pelvic surgery (cefoxitin)
3. Improved compliance with oral medications (most with twice-daily dosing)
4. Poor penetration into CSF fluid limits use for CNS infections
5. No antipseudomonal activity

Third-generation cephalosporins (e.g., ceftriaxone, cefotaxime, cefixime, cefpodoxime)

1. Broadest spectrum, including excellent activity against gram-negative bacteria
2. Generally less activity against gram-positive organisms than earlier generations
3. Very high blood and CSF levels achievable in relation to minimum inhibitory concentration for bacterial strains
4. Some with antipseudomonal activity (e.g., ceftazidime)
5. Wide therapeutic index with generally minimal toxicity (similar to previous generations)
6. Some offer single-daily dosing
7. Most expensive

Darville T, Yamauchi T: The cephalosporin antibiotics. Pediatr Rev 15:54–62, 1994.

8. How often should chloramphenicol levels be monitored?

In neonates, chloramphenicol toxicity manifested by circulatory collapse (gray baby syndrome) occurs because hepatic metabolism of the drug is poor. It is necessary to determine serum levels frequently (daily to every other day) to anticipate this complication. The serum chloramphenicol level should be maintained between 10–25 μg/ml. In older children, this syndrome is not seen, and the only common side effect is a reversible bone marrow depression. As a consequence, most experts feel that monitoring drug levels in this population is unnecessary and instead recommend twice weekly blood counts. The fatal aplastic anemia that follows chloramphenicol treatment in 1 in every 20,000–40,000 cases is idiosyncratic and non-dose-dependent and thus cannot be avoided by drug level monitoring.

9. In which patients should the use of trimethoprim-sulfamethoxazole be avoided or used with caution?

Trimethoprim-sulfamethoxazole (TMP-SMX) acts by inhibiting the folic acid pathway of bacteria. Disruption of human folic acid synthesis may occur, affecting rapidly replicating cells, especially in the bone marrow and skin. Avoidance or cautious use is suggested in the following settings:

1. Patients who have not received folate supplementation and who are known or expected to be deficient in folate, including:
   a. Phenytoin use
   b. Therapy with other folate antagonist
   c. Protein-calorie malnutrition
   d. Prematurity
2. Pregnancy
3. Fragile X syndrome
4. Known sensitivity to any sulfonamide
5. Infants ≤ 2 months of age
6. Skin rash that develops while receiving TMP-SMX
7. G6PD deficiency

From Gutman LT: The use of trimethoprim-sulfamethoxazole in children: A review of adverse reactions and indications. Pediatr Infect Dis J 3:355, 1984; with permission.

10. Which antibiotic is most frequently associated with the "red man syndrome"?

A frequent occurrence with the rapid infusion of **vancomycin**, the red man syndrome is characterized by flushing of the neck, face, and thorax. This effect is related to histamine release but not mediated by IgE and therefore does not represent a true hypersensitivity reaction. It can generally be avoided by slowing the rate of drug infusion.

11. What are the other adverse effects of vancomycin?

When vancomycin was introduced, commercial preparations contained as much as 30% of another substance of unknown nature that probably contributed to its toxicity. With the purified preparations now available, adverse reactions are much less common. The most frequent side effects are *fever, chills,* and *phlebitis* at the site of infusion. Maculopapular or diffuse erythematous *rashes* presumed to represent hypersensitivity occur in about 5% of patients. *Neurotoxicity*, manifested by auditory nerve damage and hearing loss, is associated with very high serum concentrations (generally > 80 μg/ml). Nephrotoxicity was relatively common with the early impure preparations but is now uncommon. While vancomycin is no longer appreciably nephrotoxic, there may be some effect on renal function when it is administered concomitantly with other nephrotoxic drugs.

12. Name six steps to follow in order to minimize the emergence of antibiotic-resistant pathogens.

1. Appropriate handwashing to minimize transmission of resistant organisms to other patients.
2. Use narrowest-spectrum antibiotic possible.
3. Minimize empiric use of broad-spectrum antibiotics.
4. Avoid empiric antibiotic treatment for likely viral illnesses.
5. Educate patients on the inappropriateness of antibiotics for viral illnesses.
6. Maintain awareness of the hospital's antibiotic resistance patterns.

Woodin KA, Morrison SH: Antibiotics: Mechanisms of action. Pediatr Rev 15:440–447, 1994.

13. Are any antiviral agents effective in eradicating cytomegalovirus (CMV)?

Both **ganciclovir** and **foscarnet** have activity against CMV. Ganciclovir has been studied more thoroughly and has efficacy in patients with AIDS who have CMV retinitis and in some transplant patients. Foscarnet has been used primarily when an isolate develops resistance to ganciclovir.

CLINICAL ISSUES

14. Name the three stages of pertussis infections.
1. Catarrhal (1–2 wks): upper respiratory tract symptoms
2. Paroxysmal (2–4 wks): severe cough, onset of inspiratory "whoop"
3. Convalescent (1–2 wks): resolution of symptoms

15. What is the most common cause of death in children with pertussis infections?

Ninety percent of deaths are attributable to **pneumonia**, most of which are secondarily infected bacterial pneumonias. These can be easily missed in the paroxysmal phase, when respiratory symptoms are so prominent and usually attributed solely to pertussis. A new spiking fever should prompt a careful search for an evolving pneumonia.

16. Is erythromycin of value in pertussis infections?

If used in the first 14 days of illness or before the paroxysmal stage, erythromycin may eliminate or lessen the severity of symptoms in the paroxysmal stage. If the diagnosis is made after that point, erythromycin should still be given, as it eliminates pertussis carriage in the nasopharynx and may limit the spread of disease. The dose is 50 mg/kg/day for 14 days, not to exceed a total daily dose of 1 gm.

17. Are cold and cough medicines effective in children?

A review of efficacy trials done between 1950 and 1990 concluded that although the cold and cough medications may be of benefit for adults, no evidence existed to show their benefit for children < 5 years of age. The data on older children are inconclusive.

Smith MBH, Feldman W: Over-the-counter (OTC) medication use in children with colds: A critical appraisal. Am J Dis Child 145:403, 1991.

18. Do antibiotics prevent the development of pneumonia after an upper respiratory tract infection (URI)?

Over 90% of URIs are caused by viruses, and children younger than age 5 can experience 3–8 URI episodes per year. Multiple studies have shown that antibiotic treatment of URIs does *not* shorten their course or prevent the development of pneumonia. Antibiotics can cause adverse reactions, and the overuse of antibiotics in inappropriate settings is contributing to the growing problem of antibiotic resistance worldwide.

Gadomski AM: Potential interventions for preventing pneumonia among young children: Lack of effect of antibiotic treatment for upper respiratory infections. Pediatr Infect Dis J 12:115–120, 1993.

19. Sternal edema is classically the sign of what infection?

Mumps.

20. How does Hatchcock's sign help distinguish swelling due to mumps from swelling caused by adenitis?

With a positive Hatchcock's sign, upward pressure applied to the angle of the mandible (ramus) produces tenderness with mumps but no tenderness with adenitis.

21. Why are young girls susceptible to vulvovaginitis?

Because of low levels of estrogen, the vaginal mucosa is thin and more susceptible to irritation and infection. The alkaline pH of the vaginal secretions allows for bacterial growth, and the relatively short distance between the vagina and rectum allows for easy contamination of the vagina with fecal flora.

22. Describe criteria used to diagnose toxic shock syndrome.

The CDC case definition for toxic shock syndrome is as follows:

Temperature > 38.9°C

Rash: diffuse macular erythroderma

Desquamation: particularly of palms and soles 1–2 weeks after onset of illness

Shock with hypotension and poor peripheral perfusion

Multisystem involvement—3 or more of the following:

Gastrointestinal: vomiting or diarrhea at the onset of the illness

Musculoskeletal: severe myalgia or raised creatinine kinase

Mucous membrane: conjunctival hyperemia or oropharyngeal hyperemia

Renal: elevated blood urea or creatinine or pyuria without urinary infection

Hepatic: raised alanine or aspartate transaminases

CNS: alteration of consciousness

Hematologic: < 100×10 platelets/mm^3

Negative results on:

Blood, throat, or CSF cultures (except *Staphylococcus aureus*-positive blood cultures)

No rise in titers to Rocky Mountain spotted fever, leptospirosis, or rubeola antigens

A toxic shock-like syndrome has also been associated with infections due to *Streptococcus pyogenes*. In at least some cases, the pathogenesis of this disease appears to be similar to that caused by *Staphylococcus aureus* in that the group A streptococci can produce either of two toxins with a large degree of homology to the staphylococcal toxic shock syndrome toxin (TSST-1).

Todd JK: Staphylococcal infections. In Behrman RE, et al (eds): Nelson Textbook of Pediatrics, 15th ed. Philadelphia, W.B. Saunders, 1996, pp 749–750.

23. Discuss the distinguishing features of staphylococcal scalded skin syndrome, staphylococcal toxic shock syndrome, and streptococcal toxic shock syndrome.

Distinguishing Features of Staphylococcal Scalded Skin Syndrome, Staphylococcal Toxic Shock Syndrome, and Streptococcal Toxic Shock Syndrome

CLINICAL FEATURES	STAPHYLOCOCCAL SCALDED SKIN SYNDROME	STAPHYLOCOCCAL TOXIC SHOCK SYNDROME	GROUP A STREPTOCOCCAL TOXIC SHOCK-LIKE SYNDROME
Organism	*Staphylococcus aureus* Usually phage group 11, type 71	*Staphylococcus aureus* Usually phage group 1, type 29	Group A streptococci Usually type 1, 3, or 18 Exotoxin A production
Site of infection	Usually focal Mucocutaneous border: nose, mouth, diaper area Sometimes inapparent	Mucous membranes Infected wound or furuncle Sometimes inapparent	Blood, abscess, pneumonia, empyema, cellulitis, necrotizing fasciitis Sometimes inapparent
Skin rash	Tender erythroderma: face, neck, generalized Bullae, no petechiae	Tender erythroderma: trunk, hands, feet Edema of hands, feet	Erythroderma: trunk, extremities
Desquamation	Early, first 1–2 days, generalized	Late, 7–10 days, mostly hands and feet Hyperemia of oral and vaginal mucosa	Late, 7–10 days, mostly hands and feet Hyperemia of oral and vaginal mucosa
Mucous membranes	Normal	Hypertrophy of tongue papillae	Hypertrophy of tongue papillae
Conjunctivae	Normal	Markedly injected	Injected
Course	Insidious, 4–7 days benign, < 1% mortality	Fulminant, shock with secondary multiple organ failure, 10% mortality	Fulminant, shock with early primary multiple organ failure, 30–50% mortality

From Bass JW: Treatment of skin and skin structure infections. Pediatr Infect Dis J 11:154, 1992; with permission.

24. What percentage of cases of toxic shock syndrome are nonmenstrual?

Approximately 10%. The syndrome occurs in the setting of focal staphylococcal colonization or focal infections, including empyema, osteomyelitis, soft tissue abscess, surgical infections, and burns.

Resnick SD: Toxic shock syndrome: Recent developments in pathogenesis. J Pediatr 116:321–325, 1990.

25. What are the biphasic features of leptospiral infection?

Both anicteric and icteric cases of leptospirosis have two phases:

First phase: fever, headache, conjunctivitis, myalgia, abdominal pain; leptospires found in CSF and blood; lasts 4–7 days.

Second phase: phase of immunologic response; leptospires found in urine; lasts 4–30 days
    Anicteric type (90%): rash, meningitis, uveitis
    Icteric type (10%): jaundice, myocarditis, hemorrhage, renal dysfunction

26. In a recovering patient, where in the body do leptospires persist the longest?

The **aqueous humor**. Regions of the eye serve as an immunologic barrier, allowing chronic carriage for months. Some affected patients have recurrent uveitis.

27. What diseases are transmitted by ticks?

Disease	Agent
Lyme disease	*Borrelia burgdorferi*
Relapsing fever	*B. duttonii*
Q fever	*Coxiella burnetti*
Tularemia	*Francisella tularensis*
Rocky Mountain spotted fever	*Rickettsia rickettsii*
Queensland tick typhus	*R. australis*
Boutonneuse fever	*R. conorii*
Asian tick typhus	*R. sibirica*
Colorado tick fever	Arbovirus
Tick-borne encephalitis complex	Arbovirus
Ehrlichiosis	*Ehrlichia chaffeensis, E. equi, E. phagocytophila*
Babesiosis	*Babesia microti, B. divergens, B. bovis*

Adapted from Kaplan SL: Arthropoda. In Feigin RD, Cherry JD (eds): Textbook of Pediatric Infectious Diseases, 3rd ed. Philadelphia, W.B. Saunders, 1992, p 2120; with permission.

28. In the setting of clinical signs and symptoms of an encephalitis, what EEG pattern is suggestive of herpes simplex disease?

Periodic lateralized epileptiform discharges (PLEDs). PLEDs may be seen in other, rarer causes of encephalitis, such as Epstein-Barr virus and slow viruses (i.e., Creutzfeldt-Jakob disease and subacute sclerosing panencephalitis).

29. When is a brain biopsy indicated in children with suspected herpes simplex encephalitis?

Encephalitis due to herpes simplex virus (HSV) is a devastating disease with significant mortality and morbidity. Antiviral therapy is successful only if the disease is diagnosed early. In the past, no single noninvasive method could simply and reproducibly diagnose HSV encephalitis; definitive diagnosis relied on brain biopsy. In recent years, a number of studies have demonstrated that analysis of CSF using the polymerase chain reaction (PCR) allowsrapid and accurate diagnosis. According to Lakeman et al., PCR detects over 98% of cases and may be more sensitive than brain biopsy. When performed with the proper precautions and controls, PCR is also highly specific. With this information in mind, the need for brain biopsy has diminished considerably. Nowadays, brain biopsy should be considered only when (1) PCR is negative and the diagnosis remains obscure; or (2) PCR is positive, but the clinical course is atypical for HSV encephalitis and the response to antiviral therapy is slow.

Lakeman FD, et al: Diagnosis of herpes simplex encephalitis: Application of polymerase chain reaction to cerebrospinal fluid from brain-biopsied patients and correlation with disease. J Infect Dis 171:857–863, 1995.

DeVincenzo JP, Thorne G: Mild herpes simplex encephalitis diagnosed by polymerase chain reaction: A case report and review. Pediatr Infect Dis J 13:662–664, 1994.

30. How long should animals be observed in confinement when rabies is a concern?

When animals are shedding the virus and thus capable of being contagious, they are usually sick within 5 days after the onset of shedding. In some experimental settings, this asymptomatic period can last up to 14 days. The standard in the United States is to confine dogs and cats for 10 days following a suspicious human contact. There has not been a report of a case of rabies transmission by an animal that remained healthy during that time period.

31. What causes visceral larval migrans?

Toxocara canis (a dog helminth) and *T. cati* (a cat helminth) cause this infiltrative granulomatous disease. Clinical features include fever, hepatomegaly, myocardial involvement, retinal disease, and pneumonitis.

32. Other than definitive serologic tests, what two laboratory tests are most suggestive of *Toxocara* infections?

1. Marked eosinophilia (20–90% of peripheral white blood cells)
2. Markedly elevated isohemagglutinin titers (i.e., anti-A and/or anti-B titers in individuals who are not blood type A or B)

33. What is the difference between a felon and a paronychia?

A **paronychia** is an inflammation or infection in the soft tissue adjacent to the nail (*onyx* = *nail*, Greek). A **felon** is an infection (often an abscess) in the fat pad spaces (also known as volar pulp) of the distal phalanx.

34. How quickly do central lines become colonized?

The timing and rate of central line colonization depend on a number of factors. Manipulation of the catheter (e.g., for blood drawing, medication administration, or flushing) and poor handwashing by health care providers are probably most important in increasing the risk of colonization. In general, the likelihood of colonization increases with the length of time the catheter has been in place. Colonization rates have been reported to be < 10% of catheters < 3 days old, approximately 15% for catheters 3–7 days old, and about 20% for catheters in place or > 7 days.

35. What is the most proper medical term for oral thrush?

Acute pseudomembranous candidiasis. Quite a mouthful. Although thrush is sometimes confused with residual formula in the mouth, formula is more easily removed with a tongue blade. When thrush is scraped, small bleeding points often occur on the underlying mucosa.

CONGENITAL INFECTIONS

36. Is total serum IgM an effective screening test for congenital infection?

In a retrospective study of over 5700 infants from whom serum IgM was obtained because of concerns of congenital infection, the diagnostic yield was very low (< 1%) and only 1 infant was diagnosed with a congenital infection that was not specifically suspected prior to screening. Instead of IgM screening, more specific studies are recommended based on the clinical constellation of symptoms and signs.

Mahon BE, et al: Problems with serum IgM as a screening test for congenital infection. Clin Pediatr 33:142–146, 1994.

37. Which congenital infections cause cerebral calcifications?

Cerebral calcifications are most frequently observed in **congenital toxoplasmosis** and **cytomegalovirus** (CMV) infections. Toxoplasmosis often produces dense round calcifications scattered diffusely throughout the white matter of the brain, although it may also present as curvilinear streaks in the basal ganglia. Infants with CMV infections present with periventricular calcifications, but there is considerable overlap between the presentations of these two diseases.

Herpes simplex has also been reported to cause massive bilateral calcifications of the cerebral hemispheres, as has congenital rubella infection (rarely).

38. List the late sequelae of congenital infections.

The late sequelae of chronic intrauterine infections are relatively common and may occur in infants who are asymptomatic at birth. Most sequelae present later in childhood rather than infancy.

Late Sequelae of Chronic Intrauterine Infection

CMV	Hearing loss,* minimal to severe brain dysfunction* (motor, learning, language, and behavioral disorders)
Rubella	Hearing loss,* minimal to severe brain dysfunction* (motor, learning, language and behavioral disorders), autism,* juvenile diabetes, thyroid dysfunction, precocious puberty, progressive degenerative brain disorder*
Toxoplasmosis	Chorioretinitis,* minimal to severe brain dysfunction,* hearing loss, precocious puberty
Neonatal herpes	Recurrent eye and skin infection, minimal to severe brain dysfunction
Hepatitis B virus	Chronic subclinical hepatitis, rarely fulminant hepatitis

* Seen with infections that are subclinical in early infancy.
From Plotkin SA, Alpert G: Pediatr Clin North Am 33:465, 1986; with permission.

39. What is the most common congenital infection?

Congenital CMV infection, which in some large screening studies can occur in up to 1.3% of newborns. However, 90–95% are asymptomatic.

40. Discuss the means of vertical transmission of CMV from mother to infant.

Vertical transmission of CMV from mother to child can occur transplacentally, natally, or postnatally. The first route is associated with more severe complications, but the latter two are probably 5–10 times more common. Natally, maternal cervical secretions are the likely source of infection, whereas postnatally, breast milk is probably the most important source of infection, with saliva and possibly urine also being important routes of transmission.

41. How do complications vary between newborns with CMV infection who are symptomatic versus asymptomatic at birth?

Symptomatic Versus Asymptomatic Complications Between Newborns with CMV Infection

	% OCCURRENCE	
COMPLICATION	92 INFANTS SYMPTOMATIC	267 INFANTS ASYMPTOMATIC
Death	30	0
Microcephaly	48	4
Psychomotor retardation, neuromuscular disorder	70	4
Hearing loss	61	5
Unilateral	30	64
Bilateral	70	36
Stable	43	64
Progressive	57	36
Chorioretinitis or optic atrophy	14	2
Dental defects	27	4
Serious bacterial infections	4	5
Total infants with one or more complications	92	6

From Remington JS, Klein JO (eds): Infectious Diseases of the Fetus and Newborn Infant, 3rd ed. Philadelphia, W.B. Saunders, 1990, p 262; with permission.

42. Which infants with CMV infection have the worst prognosis?
- Neonates born to mothers with primary CMV infection during pregnancy
- Infants with symptoms at birth (particularly those with CNS signs)
- Infants with microcephaly and/or intracranial calcifications
- Neonates with elevated quantitative IgM or with CMV-specific IgM

Overall JC Jr: Viral infections of the fetus and neonate. In Feigin RD, Cherry JD (eds): Pediatric Infectious Diseases, 3rd ed. Philadelphia, W.B. Saunders, 1992, pp 936–937.

43. What is the risk to the fetus if the mother is infected with parvovirus B19 during pregnancy?

The risk of fetal loss appears to be < 10% following a proven maternal infection. However, delayed development of fetal hydrops can occur, and serial fetal ultrasounds should be considered. An elevated maternal serum alpha-fetoprotein level may be a marker for an adverse outcome. The signs of parvovirus infection in adults are not very distinctive but may include fever, a maculopapular rash which is lacelike, athralgia, and/or arthritis.

44. What is the risk that a fetus will develop congenital varicella syndrome if a mother develops chickenpox in the first trimester?

The congenital varicella syndrome consists of a constellation of features, the most typical of which is atrophy of a limb, usually associated with a cicatricial lesion involving the affected limb. Other features include neurologic and sensory defects, as well as eye abnormalities (chorioretiniatis, cataracts, microphthalmia, Horner syndrome). The congenital varicella syndrome usually follows maternal infection in the first trimester, though it may be seen following infection up to 20 weeks into gestation. The largest prospective study reported to date found 4 cases of fetal varicella syndrome in 141 pregnancies, yielding an incidence of < 3%.

Brunell PA: Varicella in pregnancy, the fetus, and the newborn: Problems in management. J Infect Dis 166(suppl):S42–S47, 1992.

45. When should varicella immune globulin be given to a newborn?

Varicella-zoster immune globulin (VZIG) should be given as soon as possible to a newborn whose mother developed varicella from 5 days before to 2 days after delivery. During this period of high risk, the fetus is exposed to high circulating titers of virus without benefit of maternal antibody synthesis. In contrast, if the child's mother develops primary infection > 5 days before delivery, maternal antibody is synthesized and provides passive protection for the fetus. Similarly, if symptoms develop in the child's mother > 2 days after delivery, it is assumed that the fetus was not exposed to maternal viremia.

Other indications for VZIG in the newborn period following varicella virus exposure include prematurity:

1. If the infant is ≥ 28 weeks gestation, VZIG is indicated in infants whose mother has no history of chickenpox.

2. If the infant is < 28 weeks gestation or ≤ 1,000 gm, VZIG should be given regardless of maternal history because little maternal antibody crosses the placenta prior to the third trimester of pregnancy.

Some authors recommend giving VZIG to all infants who are exposed to varicella in the first month of life. However, this is not currently recommended by the American Academy of Pediatrics.

46. Do urogenital mycoplasmas have a role in neonatal disease?

Colonization of the respiratory tract of very-low-birthweight infants during the first weeks of life with *Ureaplasma urealyticum* and/or *Mycoplasma hominis* has been associated with the later development of bronchopulmonary dysplasia. Their relationship to chorioamnionitis and neonatal sepsis remains unclear.

47. If a mother is culture-positive for *Ureaplasma urealyticum* or *Mycoplasma hominis*, what is the likelihood of transmission to the newborn infant?

Vertical transmission occurs in up to 60% of exposed newborns. Risk of transmission is higher in preterm and low-birthweight infants and correlates with prolonged rupture of membranes and maternal fever. Infants delivered by cesarean section over intact membranes have a very low rate of colonization compared to those delivered vaginally.

48. Describe the features of the congenital rubella syndrome.

Rubella virus is a teratogenic agent that induces characteristic congenital abnormalities. Some of these are present only in the neonatal period, while others persist through life. The features of congenital rubella syndrome may be divided into three broad categories:

1. *Transient*—including low birthweight, hepatosplenomegaly, thrombocytopenia, hepatitis, pneumonitis, and radiolucent bone lesions.

2. *Permanent*—including deafness, cataracts, and congenital heart lesions (patent ductus arteriosus > pulmonary artery stenosis > aortic stenosis > ventricular septal defects).

3. *Developmental*—including psychomotor delay, behavioral disorders, and endocrine dysfunction.

The **most characteristic** features of congenital rubella syndrome are congenital heart disease, cataracts, microphthalmia, corneal opacities, glaucoma, and radiolucent bone lesions.

49. Should all pregnant women be screened for herpes simplex virus (HSV) during pregnancy?

Neonatal herpes infections is usually contracted at delivery from contact with genital secretions that contain infectious virus. In most cases, the mother is asymptomatic and has no history of clinical herpes genitalis. Existing data indicate that antepartum cultures of the maternal genital tract fail to predict viral shedding at the time of delivery. As a consequence, routine antepartum cultures are not recommended.

Prober CG, et al: The management of pregnancies complicated by genital infections with herpes simplex virus. Clin Infect Dis 15:1031–1038, 1992.

50. What are risk factors for the development of neonatal herpes infections from mothers with positive cervical cultures?

1. Primary maternal infection at the time of delivery—30–50% of infants delivered to mothers with primary disease will develop a postnatal infection with HSV, but only 3–5% of infants born to mothers with recurrent disease become infected. Of note, distinguishing between primary and recurrent herpes infections by history and clinical exam is often difficult.

2. Prematurity or low birthweight

3. Vaginal delivery

4. Rupture of membranes > 6 hours before birth

5. Fetal scalp monitoring may result in the direct inoculation of the virus into the baby's scalp.

51. Name the three types of clinical presentation of neonatal herpes simplex.

Neonatal herpes simplex can masquerade as a variety of systemic, cutaneous, and ocular disorders. Asymptomatic HSV infections rarely occur in the neonate. Occurring with approximately equal incidence, the three patterns are:

1. Infection localized to the CNS

2. Infection localized to the skin, eye, or mouth

3. Disseminated infection (± CNS involvement) with a picture resembling bacterial sepsis

It is important to note that up to one-third of infants with systemic or CNS infections will present without visible external lesions.

52. Is acyclovir or vidarabine the preferred treatment for neonate HSV infections?

In clinical trials, neither drug has been superior to the other in the treatment of neonatal HSV infection. Acyclovir is felt to be superior in the treatment of HSV encephalitis in older patients.

Vidarabine must be administered in large fluid volumes with the theoretical risk of worsening cerebral edema. Both acyclovir and vidarabine have little toxicity when used in appropriate doses. Prolonged administration of acyclovir may be associated with emergence of drug-resistant virus. Generally, acyclovir has become the preferred drug.

Whitley R, et al: A controlled trial comparing vidarabine with acyclovir in neonatal herpes simplex virus infections. N Engl J Med 324:444–449, 1991.

53. How often does relapse occur after an infant is "successfully" treated for an HSV infection?

After a 10–14-day course of treatment for HSV infection, approximately 35% of acyclovir recipients and 19% of vidarabine recipients suffer a cutaneous relapse. A CNS relapse is less common, but with a higher rate in infants receiving vidarabine. Some babies may suffer subclinical CNS recurrences; however, the efficacy of long-term antiviral chemotherapy has not been proved.

54. In which groups of women is prenatal hepatitis B surface antigen (HBsAg) screening recommended?

In the past, women were screened for HBsAg if they fell into a high-risk group based on ethnic origin, immunization status, or history of exposure to blood products, intravenous drugs, or high-risk partner(s). However, historical information only reveals a portion of HBsAg carriers, and it is recommended that all pregnant women be screened for HBsAg.

55. What precautions are needed during delivery of infants born to women with known active hepatitis A, B, or C?

During delivery, scalp clips and other trauma to infants should be minimized to avoid maternal-fetal transmission of infected blood and fluid. In addition, gastric contents should be removed, and infants should be carefully bathed following delivery. Breast-feeding should be avoided.

For infants born to women with an acute hepatitis B or who test positive for HBsAg, hepatitis B immune globulin (HBIG, 0.5 ml) should be administered as soon as possible following delivery to reduce the risk of infection. In addition, these infants must receive 3 doses of hepatitis B vaccine. The first dose can be given at the same time as HBIG if different sites and syringes are used. The second and third dose are given at 1 and 6 months, respectively.

Neonates born to mothers with active hepatitis A or C infection may receive 0.5 ml of immune serum globulin intramuscularly, although the effectiveness of this approach is not proven. The value of administering the hepatitis A vaccine to these infants is under study.

56. How do the clinical features of early and late congenital syphilis differ?

The manifestations of congenital syphilis are protean and may be divided into early and late findings. Early manifestations occur during the first 2 years of life; late manifestations occur after 2 years of age.

Early and Late Manifestations of Congenital Syphilis

EARLY CONGENITAL SYPHILIS (310 PATIENTS)		LATE CONGENITAL SYPHILIS (271 PATIENTS)	
Hepatomegaly	32%	Frontal boss of Parrot	87%
Skeletal abnormalities	29	Short maxilla	84
Splenomegaly	18	High palatal arch	76
Birthweight < 2500 gm	16	Hutchinson triad	75
Pneumonia	16	Hutchinson teeth	63
Severe anemia, hydrops, edema	16	Interstitial keratitis	9
Skin lesions	15	VIII nerve deafness	3
Hyperbilirubinemia	13	Saddle nose	73
Snuffles, nasal discharge	9	Mulberry molars	65
Painful limbs	7	Higouménakis sign	39
CSF abnormalities	7	Relative protuberance of mandible	26
Pancreatitis	5	Rhagades	7

(Table continued on following page.)

Early and Late Manifestations of Congenital Syphilis (Cont.)

EARLY CONGENITAL SYPHILIS (310 PATIENTS)		LATE CONGENITAL SYPHILIS (271 PATIENTS)	
Nephritis	4	Saber shin	4
Failure to thrive	3	Scaphoid scapulae	0.7
Testicular mass	0.3	Clutton joint	0.3
Chorioretinitis	0.3		
Hypoglobulinemia	0.3		

Adapted from Gutman LT: Syphilis. In Feigin RD, Cherry JD (eds): Pediatric Infectious Diseases, 3rd ed. Philadelphia, W.B. Saunders, 1992, pp 556–557; with permission.

57. What is Hutchinson's triad for late congenital syphilis?
  1. Hutchinson's teeth (screwdriver, peg-shaped teeth)
  2. Interstitial keratitis
  3. Eighth nerve deafness

58. How is the diagnosis of congenital syphilis made?

Criteria for the Diagnosis of Early Congenital Syphilis (Patient < 2 Years)

Clinical
Absolute
1. Specimen from lesions showing *Treponema pallidum* on dark field or histologic exam
Major
2. Positive reagin test of CSF
3. Condyloma lata
4. Osteochondritis, periostitis
5. Snuffles, hemorrhagic rhinitis
6. Bullous lesions, palmar/plantar rash

Serologic
Major
1. Fourfold rise in reagin titer and positive treponemal antibody test
2. Development of positive treponemal antibody test after birth
3. Positive reagin test or treponemal antibody test after 4 months of age
Epidemiologic
Major
1. Untreated early syphilis in the mother within 4 weeks of delivery
2. Mother an untreated contact to lesion syphilis during pregnancy

From Gutman LT: Syphilis. In Feigin RD, Cherry JD (eds): Pediatric Infectious Diseases, 3rd ed. Philadelphia, W.B. Saunders, 1992, p 559; with permission.

The diagnosis of early congenital syphilis is often difficult and is based on clinical, serologic, and epidemiologic considerations. Nontreponemal antigen tests are often used to screen newborn infants for possible congenital infection with *T. pallidum*. Such tests include the rapid plasma reagin (RPR) card test and Venereal Disease Reference Laboratory (VDRL) slide test. Serum from the infant is preferred to cord blood, since cord specimens can produce false-positive results. A nonreactive titer in both the infected mother and infected infant may occur if the mother acquired disease late in pregnancy or in the case of a prozone phenomenon (see Question 59). Alternatively, the mother's titer can be reactive and the infected infant's test nonreactive, depending on the timing of maternal infection. A mother who has been treated adequately for syphilis during pregnancy can still passively transfer antibodies to the neonate, resulting in a positive titer in the infant in the absence of infection. In this circumstance, the infant's titer is usually less than the mother's and reverts to negative over several months.

59. What is the prozone phenomenon?
  Agglutination of an antigen by an antibody requires that the antigen and antibody be present in relative concentrations. When the antibody concentration is far greater than the amount of antigen, agglutination will not occur. This is considered the "prozone" of the dilution range of

the antibody. In some infants with congenital syphilis, serum antibody levels are so high that undiluted serum fails to agglutinate the nontreponemal antigens used to diagnose syphilis (i.e., the VDRL and RPR are nonreactive). To account for the possibility of the prozone phenomenon in infants being evaluated for congenital syphilis, VDRL or RPR titer should be determined with *and* without dilution of the serum.

60. If a pregnant woman is found to have *Chlamydia trachomatis* in her birth canal, what is the most appropriate course of action?

A pregnant women with a known chlamydial infection should be treated with oral erythromycin to reduce or prevent the risk of neonatal chlamydial pneumonia and conjunctivitis. Simultaneous treatment of the male partner(s) with tetracycline or doxycycline should also be undertaken.

61. Explain the derivation of the name *Toxoplasma gondii*.

Toxoplasma gondii is an obligate intracellular parasite. Its name derives from the Greek word *toxon*, which means an arc or bow (referring to the shape of the organism), and from the word *gondi*, which is a North African desert rodent in whose splenic mononuclear cells the parasite was initially observed.

Freij BJ, Sever JL: Toxoplasmosis. Pediatr Rev 12:227, 1991.

62. What is the risk to a fetus following primary maternal *Toxoplasma* infection?

The risk depends on the time during pregnancy that the mother becomes infected. Assuming the mother is untreated, first-trimester infection is associated with a fetal infection rate of approximately 25%, second-trimester infection with a rate > 50%, and third-trimester infection with a rate of roughly 65%. The severity of clinical disease in congenitally infected infants is inversely related to gestational age at the time of primary maternal infection.

63. If a mother does acquire toxoplasmosis during pregnancy, can transmission to the fetus be prevented?

Treatment with spiramycin in the first half of pregnancy or pyrimethamine plus sulfadiazine or trisulfapyrimidines after 20 weeks gestation is recommended. Data from several studies suggest that the incidence of toxoplasmosis can be reduced by 50–60%. The rationale for such treatment is based on the observation that there may be a significant lag period between the onset of maternal infection and infection in the fetus. However, if fetal infection has been established, maternal treatment fails to decrease the likelihood of clinically severe disease.

64. Describe the typical presentation of congenital toxoplasmosis.

As with other congenital infections, the presentations are varied. Presentations range from severe disease (in about 10%) with systemic (fever, hepatosplenomegaly, chorioretinitis) and/or neurologic features (seizures, hydrocephalus, microcephaly) to apparent lack of signs or symptoms. In the latter group, which constitutes about two-thirds of cases, intracranial calcifications are often present, and long-term risks include impaired vision, learning disabilities, mental retardation, and seizures.

65. How can a woman minimize the chance of acquiring a *Toxoplasma* infection during pregnancy?

Measures relate to personal hygiene, food preparation, and exposure to cats.

1. Cook meat to > 150°, smoke it, or cure it in brine.

2. Wash fruits and vegetables before consumption.

3. Avoid touching mucous membranes of mouth and eyes while handling uncooked meat or unwashed fruits or vegetables.

4. Wash hands and kitchen surfaces thoroughly after contact with raw meat or unwashed fruits or vegetables.

5. Prevent access of flies, cockroaches, and other coprophagic insects to fruits and vegetables.

6. Avoid contact with materials that are potentially contaminated with cat feces, such as cat litter boxes, or wear gloves when handling such materials and when gardening.

7. Disinfect cat litter box for 5 minutes with nearly boiling water.

From Wilson CB, Remington JS: Toxoplasmosis. In Feigin RD, Cherry JD (eds): Pediatric Infectious Diseases, 3rd ed. Philadelphia, W.B. Saunders, 1992, p 2068; with permission.

THE FEBRILE CHILD

66. Fever in children—is it friend or foe?

In certain situations, fever is beneficial, and in others it is detrimental. Gonococci and some treponemes are killed at temperatures $\geq 40°C$ ($104°F$), and benefits from fever therapy have been reported in cases of gonococcal urethritis and neurosyphilis. In addition, fever appears to hamper growth of some types of pneumococci and some viruses. Fever also is associated with a decrease in the amount of free serum iron, an essential nutrient for many pathogenic bacteria. Modest fever can accelerate a variety of immunologic responses, including phagocytosis, leukocyte chemotaxis, lymphocyte transformation, and interferon production.

On the other hand, other data indicate that high fever can impair the immune response. In addition, while the metabolic effects of fever are well-tolerated by most children, in some situations these effects may be dangerous. Examples include patients at risk for cardiac or respiratory failure and those with neurologic disease or with septic shock. Fever can precipitate febrile seizures in the susceptible population, children aged between 6 months to 5–6 years.

67. At what temperature does a child have fever?

A simple question without a simple answer. Because body temperatures vary among individuals and age groups and vary daily in an individual (lowest around 4–5 AM and highest in late afternoon and early evening), a precise cutoff point is difficult to determine. In children aged 2–6 years, diurnal variation can range up to $0.9°C$ ($1.6°F$). Infants tend to have a higher baseline temperature pattern, with 50% having daily rectal temperatures $> 37.8°C$ ($100.0°F$); after age 2 years, this elevated baseline falls. In addition, activity and exercise (within 30 min), feeding or meals (within 1 hr), and hot foods (within 1 hr) can cause body temperature elevations. Most authorities agree that in a child age < 3 months, a rectal temperature $> 38°C$ ($100.4°F$) constitutes fever. In infants age 3–24 months, who tend to have a higher baseline, a temperature $\geq 38.33°C$ ($101°F$) likely constitutes fever. In those > 2 years, as the baseline falls, fever more commonly is defined as a rectal temperature $> 38°C$ ($100.4°F$).

68. Where did the popular notion of a normal temperature being 98.6°F originate?

98.6°F was established as the mean healthy temperature in 1868 after > 1 million temperatures from 25,000 patients were analyzed. Ironically, these were axillary temperatures, and the waters of what constitutes normal have been muddied since.

Mackowiak PA, et al: A critical appraisal of 98.6°F, the upper limit of the normal body temperature, and other legacies of Carl Reinhold August Wunderlich. JAMA 268:1578–1580, 1992.

69. How does temperature vary among different body sites?

Rectal	Standard
Oral	0.5–0.6°C (1°F) lower
Axillary	0.8–1.0°C (1.5–2.0°F) lower
Tympanic	0.5–0.6°C (1°F) lower

70. Are tympanic thermometers effective in screening for fever?

Using the rectal temperature as the gold standard, studies have shown varied results—some show good correlation and others poorer correlation. As a rule, the correlation is better with older children. Tympanic thermometers may miss 10–30% of fevers in children < 3 months. Because

Infectious Diseases

fever in these children usually requires more evaluation, many authorities recommend rectal temperatures rather than tympanic ones in this age group.

71. If a tympanic thermometer is used, does the presence of otitis media increase the reading?

Tympanic thermometers work by measuring naturally occurring infrared emissions from the eardrum and surrounding structures. Otitis media causes only a very minor (approximately 0.1°C) difference in the reading. Mastoiditis and external otitis may cause greater differences because of increased local blood flow. Cerumen, which is translucent to infrared emissions, does not affect readings.

72. How should the temperature of young infants be taken?

In infants < 3 months of age, when fever can be more clinically significant, a rectal temperature is the preferred method. Tympanic recordings are much less sensitive in this age group because the narrow, tortuous external canal can collapse, resulting in readings obtained from the cooler canal rather than the warmer tympanic membrane. Axillary temperatures often underestimate fever. The oral route is usually not used until a child is 5–6 years old.

73. Can excessive bundling raise an infant's temperature?

Prospective studies have found mixed results. One study of newborns in a warm environment of 80°F found that rectal temperatures in bundled infants could be elevated above 38°C, the "febrile range." Another study of infants up to age 3 months found that in room temperatures of 72–75°F, the bundling of infants up to 65 minutes did not produce any temperatures rectally > 38°C. A clinical method that may distinguish disease-related fevers from possible environmental overheating has been the "abdomen-toe" temperature differential. A foot as warm as the abdomen suggests an overly warm environment, while a cooler foot suggests fever with peripheral vasoconstriction.

Cheng TL, Partridge JC: Effect of bundling and high environmental temperatures on neonatal body temperature. Pediatrics 92:238–240, 1993.

Grover C, et al: The effects of bundling on infant temperature. Pediatrics 94:669–673, 1994.

74. Does teething cause fever?

Long a doctrine of grandmothers, the association of teething and fever may have some basis in fact. In one study of 46 healthy infants with rectal temperatures recorded for 20 days prior to the eruption of their first tooth, nearly half had a new temperature elevation above 37.5° on the day of the eruption. However, significant temperature elevations should never be ascribed simply to teething. Trust the grandmothers, but verify.

Jaber L, et al: Fever associated with teething. Arch Dis Child 67:233–234, 1992.

75. Do sponge baths reduce fever?

Because fever is the result of an elevated set-point of the thermoregulatory center in the hypothalamus, a critical intervention to reduce temperature is to return the set-point to normal. This effect can be achieved by treatment with any of several drugs, including acetaminophen, ibuprofen, and nonsteroidal antiinflammatory agents. While aspirin has the same effect, it is no longer recommended for routine treatment of fever in children due to its association with Reye syndrome. Provided the set-point has been normalized, external cooling (by sponging with cold, cool, or tepid water) can be effective in reducing fever. Sponging with ice water is most effective but is very uncomfortable. Water in the range of 29.4–32°C (85–90°F) is preferred. Alcohol sponge baths are contraindicated because of the potential for significant absorption of alcohol through the skin.

76. Does a viral infection respond better to antipyretic therapy than a bacterial infection?

Traditional theory had been that a viral illness should respond better to antipyretics than a bacterial infection. However, there is little difference in the pattern of response, and it is of no clinical help.

77. What is occult bacteremia?

The clinically unsuspected finding of bacteria in the blood of patients, usually aged 3–24 months, who are febrile without an apparent focus of infection. This term should be distinguished from *septicemia*—the growth of bacteria in the blood from a child with the clinical picture of toxicity and shock.

78. Is there an association between the degree of fever and the incidence of bacteremia?

In children, the relationship between fever and likelihood of bacteremia has been examined most thoroughly in patients who are febrile yet have no localizing signs on physical examination. In general, the risk of bacteremia in this population increases with the magnitude of fever. In one series, among febrile children < 2 years of age who were seen in a clinic, bacteremia was present only if the rectal temperature was ≥ 38.9°C (102°F). In another series of febrile children seen in a pediatric emergency room, among patients with temperatures > 41.1°C (106°F), the incidence of bacteremia was 13%.

Teele DW, et al: Bacteremia in febrile children under 2 years of age: Results of cultures of blood of 600 consecutive febrile children in a "walk-in" clinic. J Pediatr 87:227–230, 1975.

McCarthy PL, Dolan TF: Hyperpyrexia in children: Eight-year emergency room experience. Am J Dis Child 130:849–851, 1976.

79. What constitutes the Yale Observation Scales?

This set of 6 items of observation and physical signs was designed at Yale to assist in detecting serious illness in febrile children < 24 months. Normal (1 point), moderate impairment (3 points), and severe impairment (5 points) scores are given for *quality of cry, reaction to parental stimulation, state of alertness, color, hydration,* and *response to social overtures.* Scores of ≤ 10 correlate with a low likelihood of serious illness, primarily in infants > 2 months.

McCarthy PL, et al: Observation scales to identify serious illness in febrile children. Pediatrics 70:802–809, 1982.

80. What is the proper way to evaluate and manage febrile illness in infants < 60 days of age?

A very contentious area. On average, about 10% of febrile infants < 2 months of age have serious bacterial infections (bacteremia, meningitis, osteomyelitis, septic arthritis, urinary tract infection, or pneumonia). One-third to one-half of these infections are associated with bacteremia. In the past, the approach to the evaluation and management of febrile young infants has varied. At academic centers, evaluation has included cultures of blood, CSF, and urine, and infants have been hospitalized for presumptive antibiotic therapy. In contrast, many practitioners have been more discriminating in deciding about the extent of evaluation and the need to hospitalize and treat.

In one study, 747 infants between 29–56 days of age with temperatures ≥ 38.2°C were evaluated according to the following "low-risk" criteria:

- Well-appearing infant
- No evidence of focal infection on physical exam
- Total peripheral blood WBC count < 15,000/mm³
- CSF WBC < 8/mm³ and Gram stain negative
- Urinalysis: WBC < 10/high-power field (hpf) and ≤ 3 bacteria on spun specimen
- No pulmonary infiltrate on chest radiograph

Of the 287 infants who met these criteria and were observed without antibiotics, only 1 developed a serious infection (viral meningitis). This study and others suggest that infants who meet low-risk criteria may not require antibiotic therapy, provided the social setting is suitable and close outpatient follow-up is possible.

Currently, infants < 28–30 days are generally hospitalized for empiric therapy, but studies are ongoing to identify low-risk criteria for these patients as well.

Baker MD, et al: Outpatient management without antibiotics of fever in selected infants. N Engl J Med 329:1437–1441, 1993.

Jaskiewicz JA, et al: Febrile infants at low risk for serious bacterial infection: An appraisal of the Rochester criteria and implications for management. Pediatrics 94:390–396, 1994.

81. How should older infants and toddlers (2–36 months of age) with fever and no apparent source be managed?

As with infants < 2 months of age, the management of older children with fever and no identifiable source remains controversial. The basis for this controversy relates to the difficulty in distinguishing viral illness from occult bacteremia and the fear of occult bacteremia leading to more serious infection, especially meningitis. In recent years, consideration of this issue has been influenced by the remarkable success of the *Haemophilus influenzae* vaccination program. In the past, *H. influenzae* occult bacteremia was relatively common and, in ~ 10% of cases, was associated with progression to meningitis. *Streptococcus pneumoniae* now accounts for > 90% of all episodes of occult bacteremia, and *S. pneumoniae* occult bacteremia seldom progresses to meningitis.

Strategies for management of febrile young children aged 2–36 months vary. For patients with temperatures ≥ 39°C, some experts advocate use of a protocol involving:

1. Urine cultures for males < 6 months of age and females < 2 years of age
2. Stool culture if stool has blood or mucus or > 5 WBCs/hpf
3. Chest x-ray if dyspnea, tachypnea, rales, or decreased breath sounds
4. Blood culture
5. WBC count (> 15,000/mm^3 associated with greater risk of occult bacteremia)

Empiric antibiotics (e.g., oral amoxicillin or intramuscular ceftriaxone) are then prescribed pending culture results. Other specialists consider the degree of fever and height of the WBC count to assess the likelihood of bacteremia and the need for empiric antibiotic therapy. Still others advise no testing and no empiric therapy and emphasize that parents be provided with specific information about signs and symptoms that should prompt reevaluation.

Long SL: Antibiotic therapy in febrile children: "Best laid schemes. . . ." J Pediatr 124:585–588, 1994.

Baraff LJ, et al: Practice guidelines for the management of infants and children 0 to 36 months of age with fever without source. Pediatrics 92:1–12, 1993.

Bass JW, et al: Antimicrobial treatment of occult bacteremia: A multicenter cooperative study. Pediatr Infect Dis J 87:48–53, 1993.

82. When are chest x-rays indicated in the febrile young infant?

While some clinicians believe that chest x-rays should be performed in all febrile infants < 2–3 months of age, others reserve this study for infants who have respiratory symptoms or signs, including cough, tachypnea, irregular breathing, retractions, rales, wheezing, or decreased breath sounds. In a study of infants < 8 weeks of age who were admitted with fever, 31% of patients with respiratory manifestations had an abnormal chest x-ray compared with only 1% of asymptomatic infants.

Crain EF, et al: Is a chest radiograph necessary in the evaluation of every febrile infant less than 8 weeks of age? Pediatrics 88:821–824, 1991.

83. Which children with "seizure and fever" need to have a lumbar puncture?

Among pediatric textbooks, physicians, and residency programs, there is little uniformity. The concern is that the seizure might be a manifestation of meningitis. Specific signs of meningitis, such as stiff neck and bulging fontanel, are often lacking in affected patients who are < 12–18 months. Many authorities mandate LPs for children < 18 months who have had a seizure with fever, regardless of clinical appearance. It is a difficult issue to resolve, but unless a child is alert and completely well-appearing at the time of examination, a lumbar puncture should be seriously considered.

The occurrence of a simple febrile seizure as the sole manifestation of meningitis in a child is very unusual. In one retrospective study of 503 children with meningitis, none with bacterial meningitis presented solely with a seizure. Other studies have shown that bacterial meningitis, even in younger children, is nearly always accompanied by some abnormal sign or symptom, particularly lethargy or a toxic appearance.

Green SM, et al: Can seizures be the sole manifestations of meningitis in febrile children? Pediatrics 92:527–534, 1993.

84. Is there a risk in performing a lumbar puncture in a bacteremic infant?

A definitive estimate of this risk in humans is not available. Such an estimate would require a systematic study, taking into account such variables as magnitude of the bacteremia, amount of blood introduced into the CSF, and the patient's immune status. It is unlikely that such a study could ever be performed, and even if it were, its application to individual cases would be impossible. Suffice to say that the risk is small and would never outweigh the risk of not doing a lumbar puncture.

Klein JO, et al: Report of the Task Force on the Diagnosis and Treatment of Meningitis. Pediatrics 78:959–982, 1986.

85. Does changing needles during the collection of blood cultures reduce contamination?

No. Replacing the needle used for venipuncture with a fresh, sterile needle before inoculating the blood into a culture medium resulted in no change in the contamination rate in one study of 303 children. Of note, if the incubation of a blood culture is delayed ≥ 2 hours, the likelihood of positivity may be significantly decreased, especially for *Streptococcus pneumoniae*.

Isaacman DJ: Lack of effect of changing needles on contamination of blood cultures. Pediatr Infect Dis J 9:274–278, 1990.

Roback MG, et al: Delayed incubation of blood culture bottles: Effect on recovery rate of *Streptococcus pneumoniae* and *Haemophilus influenzae* type b. Pediatr Emerg Care 10:268–272, 1994.

86. What are the approximate risks of developing meningitis in a child with a positive blood culture?

Pneumococcus	4%
Haemophilus influenzae type b	7%
Meningococcus	25%

87. In what clincal settings are blood cultures for anaerobic bacteria indicated?

Although routinely obtaining anaerobic blood cultures in pediatric patients is widespread, the yield is very low. As part of a diagnostic evaluation for sepsis, patients with the following are more likely to have a positive anaerobic blood culture:

- Abdominal signs and symptoms
- Debilitation with sacral decubitus ulcers or cellulitis
- Poor dentition, oral mucositis, or chronic sinusitis
- Neutropenic patients on high-dose steroids (in whom abdominal signs and symptoms may be masked)
- Sickle cell disease
- Infants of mothers with prolonged rupture of membranes or amnionitis
- Human bite wounds or crushing trauma

Zaidi AK, et al: Value of routine anaerobic blood cultures for pediatric patients. J Pediatr 127:263–268, 1995.

88. How long should one wait before a blood culture is designated negative?

Bacterial growth is evident in the vast majority of cultures of blood within 48 hours. With the use of conventional culture techniques and subculture at 4 and 14 hours, Pichichero and Todd found that only 4 of 105 cultures that were ultimately positive required > 48 hours of incubation. Using a radiometric technique (Bactec 460), Rowley and Wald reported that 40 of 41 cultures positive for group B *Streptococcus* and 15 of 16 cultures growing *Escherichia coli* were identified within 24 hours. Results with quantitative techniques are similar.

While 48–72 hours is generally sufficient time to isolate common bacteria present in the bloodstream, fastidious organisms may take longer to grow. Therefore, in situations where one suspects anaerobes, fungi, or other organisms with special growth requirements, a longer time should be allowed before designating a culture negative.

Pichichero MD, Todd JK: Detection of neonatal bacteremia. J Pediatr 94:958, 1979.

Rowley AH, Wald ER: Incubation period necessary to detect bacteremia in neonates. Pediatr Infect Dis J 5:540, 1986.

89. How should a child with fever and petechiae be evaluated?

In a patient with fever and petechiae, the most significant concern is serious systemic bacterial infection.

History: Elicit information about exposures, travel, animal contacts, immunizations, and immunologic status.

Physical exam: Vital signs, general appearance, signs of toxicity, evidence of nuchal rigidity, and distribution of the petechiae (patients with systemic bacterial disease rarely have petechiae confined to the area above the nipple line).

Laboratory evaluation: Blood culture, complete blood count with differential and platelet quantitation, prothrombin and partial thromboplastin times, and lumbar puncture.

90. What is the common differential diagnosis of children with fever and petechiae?

Bacterial
  Meningococcemia
  Haemophilus influenzae sepsis
  Staphylococcus aureus sepsis
  Streptococcus pneumoniae sepsis
  Listeria monocytogenes sepsis
  Disseminated gonococcal infection
  Group A streptococcal pharyngitis

Rickettsial
  Rocky Mountain spotted fever
  Ehrlichiosis
Viral
  Enterovirus (esp. coxsackie A9, echovirus 9)
  Epstein-Barr virus
  Cytomegalovirus
  Atypical measles
Parasitic
  Malaria

The most common noninfectious etiologies of fever and petechiae include vasculitis (e.g., Henoch-Schöenlein purpura) and thrombocytopenia with associated fever (e.g., due to acute leukemia).

91. In which type of infection do the Damrosch criteria apply?

The presence of 3 or more of the Damrosch criteria define a poor prognosis for patients with **meningococcal** infection:

1. Presence of petechiae for < 12 hours prior to admission
2. Shock
3. Absence of meningitis (< 20 WBCs in CSF)
4. Normal or low peripheral WBC count
5. Low or normal erythrocyte sedimentation rate

Stiehm ER, Damrosch DS: Factors in the prognosis of meningococcal infection. J Pediatr 68:457–467, 1966.

92. When is fever considered a fever of unknown origin (FUO)?

The definition of FUO, for clinical purposes, is the presence of persistent fever (temperature > 38°C or > 100.4°F) in a child in whom a careful and thorough history, physical examination, and preliminary laboratory data fail to reveal the probable cause of fever. In adults, the duration of a fever to constitute an FUO has classically been ≥ 3 weeks, but in children that duration varies from ≥ 8 days to ≥ 2–3 weeks.

93. What is the eventual etiology of fever in children with FUO?

In a summary of 446 cases, the following causes were identified:

Infection	198	44.4%
Respiratory	102	22.9
Other	97	21.7
Collagen disease	57	12.8
Inflammatory bowel disease	7	1.6
Neoplasm	25	5.6
No diagnosis	48	10.7
Resolved	56	12.6
Miscellaneous	54	12.1

Gartner JC Jr: Fever of unknown origin. Adv Pediatr Infect Dis 7:6, 1992; with permission.

94. How should a child with FUO be evaluated?

FUO is more likely to be an unusual presentation of a common disorder rather than a common presentation of a rare disorder. After obtaining a complete and detailed history and performing a physical examination, one should avoid indiscriminately ordering a large battery of tests. The erythrocyte sedimentation rate (ESR) and the albumin/globulin ratio may be helpful screening tests, with an elevated ESR or a reversal of the ratio suggesting more serious illness. Additional laboratory studies should be directed as much as possible toward the most likely diagnostic possibilities.

95. In children with FUO, how helpful are CT scans and nuclear medicine studies in determining the diagnosis?

Minimally. In a prospective study of 109 patients with FUO, various scanning procedures (e.g., abdominal CT scan, gallium or indium scanning, technetium bone scanning) had very low utility when clinical findings had not suggested a localized process. In addition, bone marrow examination was not found to be routinely indicated in an immunologically normal host if there was no evidence of hematologic abnormalities.

Steele RW, et al: Usefulness of scanning procedures for diagnosis of fever of unknown origin in children. J Pediatr 119:526–530, 1991.

HIV INFECTION

96. When did HIV testing begin of blood intended for transfusion?

Spring of 1985. Patients at greatest risk for transfusion-acquired AIDS are those transfused from 1978 to spring 1985.

97. How is a "western blot" test done?

The western blot is the most sensitive and specific test currently available for detection of HIV antibodies. It is more precise than standard enzyme immunoassays which have a higher incidence of false-positive reactions, but there is a lack of standardization of the western blot among laboratories with resultant variability. The test is also expensive and results may be difficult to interpret.

The western blot is performed as follows: Purified HIV is separated into protein components by electrophoresis on a gel. These components are transferred from the gel to a nitrocellulose membrane (the blot). Serum or plasma is placed over this blot and incubated. Antibodies, if present, bind to the antigen. The antibodies are then illuminated by the addition of an enzyme–anti-IgG complex, which binds to the HIV antibody. A substrate is added which is converted to a colored compound in the presence of bound enzyme. The amount of color produced can be quantified.

98. How common is maternal to infant transmission of HIV?

Virtually all infants born to HIV-seropositive mothers will acquire antibody to the virus transplacentally. However, only 15–40% of these infants will subsequently be diagnosed as being infected with the virus. It appears that most maternal–infant HIV transmission occurs late in pregnancy or during labor and delivery. Clinical trials have shown the benefits of zidovudine in reducing the risk of transmission. In one study, a regimen of zidovudine given antepartum and intrapartum to the mother and subsequently to the newborn for 6 weeks reduced the risk from 25% to 8%.

Connor EM, et al: Reduction of maternal-infant transmission of human immunodeficiency virus type I with zidovudine treatment. N Engl J Med 331:1173–1180, 1994.

99. How is a newborn infant whose mother is infected with HIV confirmed as HIV-positive?

The standard methods used to diagnose HIV infection in older children and adults rely on detection of antibody to HIV by ELISA or western blot. Since maternal antibody may persist well into the infant's second year of life, these techniques are unreliable until approximately 18 months of age. The diagnosis of HIV infection in the newborn therefore usually relies on direct detection of the virus or viral components in the infant's blood or body fluids. Three methods are currently available:

1. *Culture:* A positive culture for HIV from an infant's blood is diagnostic of infection. Sensitivity and specificity surpass 90% in infants > 1 month of age. However, sensitivity may be

as low as 50% in the immediate newborn period, possibly owing to very low levels of viremia in some newborn infants. The technique is labor-intensive and expensive and is currently available only in specialized centers.

2. *Detection of HIV nucleic acid:* The polymerase chain reaction (PCR) allows for enzymatic amplification of minute quantities of RNA or DNA to detectable levels. Hence, HIV nucleic acid sequences may be detected directly from peripheral blood of infected patients. The sensitivity and specificity of PCR are approximately 98% after the first month of life. As with HIV culture, sensitivity of PCR in the neonatal period may be < 50%.

3. *Antigen detection:* An HIV core protein, designated p24 antigen, may be detected from blood by ELISA. The technique is less sensitive than culture and PCR, but the procedure is commercially available and much less costly. Increased sensitivity in detecting the p24 antigen in a newborn can be achieved by dissociating maternal antibody from the antigen.

Miles SA, et al: Rapid serologic testing with immune-complex-dissociated HIV p24 antigen for early detection of HIV infection in neonates. N Engl J Med 328:297–302, 1993.

100. What are the earliest and most common manifestations of AIDS in HIV-infected infants?

The vast majority of infants with congenital HIV infection are asymptomatic at birth, although diffuse lymphadenopathy and hepatosplenomegaly are occasionally found. Previous reports of an "HIV embryopathy," with characteristic dysmorphic features, have not been confirmed in prospective trials. Hence, congenital HIV infection cannot be diagnosed reliably on the basis of clinical manifestations in the newborn period.

The progression from asymptomatic HIV infection to AIDS follows a much more fulminant course in infants who acquire the infection congenitally as compared to those who are infected through other routes. In the United States, most vertically infected infants become ill prior to 1 year of age, with the average age of onset of severe immunodeficiency occurring between 5–10 months of age.

Infants with HIV commonly present with failure to thrive, mucocutaneous candidiasis, hepatosplenomegaly, interstitial pneumonitis, or a combination of these features. Toddlers and older children may present with generalized lymphadenopathy, recurrent bacterial infections, parotitis, or neurologic disease.

Pneumonia due to *Pneumocystis carinii* eventually develops in greater than one-third of patients and may be the presenting symptom in 10% of HIV-infected children. All infants between 4–6 weeks of age who are at risk for HIV infection should receive chemoprophylaxis until the diagnosis is clarified. Another common feature of pediatric AIDS is lymphoid interstitial pneumonitis, a chronic progressive interstitial lung disease which is often associated with EBV infection. Neurologic dysfunction develops in 90% of children with HIV infection. While these manifestations of HIV infection are common, the disease or its complications may affect virtually every organ system.

Prober CG, Gershon AA: Medical management of newborns and infants born to HIV seropositive mothers. Pediatr Infect Dis J 10:684–695, 1991.

Burroughs MH, Edelson PJ: Medical care of the HIV-infected child. Pediatr Clin North Am 38:45–68, 1991.

1994 Revised classification system for human immunodeficiency virus infection in children less than 13 years of age. MMWR 43(RR12):1–10, 1995.

Pizzo PA, Wilfert CM: Preventing *Pneumocystis carinii* pneumonia in human immunodeficiency virus-infected children: New guidelines for prophylaxis. Pediatr Infect Dis J 15:165–168, 1996.

101. What are the common pulmonary diseases in children with AIDS?

Both infectious and noninfectious pulmonary diseases are common presenting complaints in children with AIDS. These include:

- *Pneumocystis carinii* pneumonia
- Cytomegalovirus pneumonia
- Lymphoid interstitial pneumonia
- Infection with *Mycobacterium avium* complex
- Pulmonary candidiasis

102. How is lymphocytic interstitial pneumonitis (LIP) distinguished from *Pneumocystis carinii* pneumonia (PCP)?

LIP is a chronic pulmonary interstitial disease of lymphocytic and plasma cell infiltration of unknown cause that occurs in about 50% of pediatric AIDS patients. Occasionally, there is concomitant hilar adenopathy. The chest x-ray frequently reveals a noduloreticular pattern. LIP is more commonly seen in patients having generalized lymphadenopathy, salivary gland enlargement, and digital clubbing. Compared with PCP, the onset is gradual and tachypnea and hypoxia are late findings. The development of LIP more commonly occurs when risk for opportunistic infection is low (i.e., CD4+ lymphocyte count is not severely decreased). Patients with LIP have considerably longer periods of survival than those with PCP. PCP usually occurs when CD4+ counts are depressed and has a more rapid onset with tachypnea and hypoxia. The chest x-ray usually reveals a diffuse alveolar-interstitial process. LIP may respond to steroids, while PCP is treated with trimethoprim-sulfamethoxazole (or alternatively pentamidine) with the addition of steroids for severe hypoxia.

103. What immunologic abnormalities are seen in children with HIV infection?

Most patients have elevated serum immunoglobulins, and about 10% have hypogamma-globulinemia. Failure to make antibodies to specific antigens (e.g., tetanus toxoid, pneumococcal vaccine) is common. In more advanced infection, there is a decreased ratio of helper-suppressor (CD4/CD8) T cells, absolute lymphopenia, and decreased in vitro mitogenic responses.

104. Describe the major hematologic manifestations of pediatric HIV infection.

Hematologic manifestations of pediatric HIV infection are due to direct cytopathic effects of HIV on marrow precursors, autoantibody production, drug toxicity, or complications of opportunistic infections. Anemia is very common and may be due to bone marrow suppression (due to HIV or zidovudine treatment), chronic infection, or immune hemolysis (HIV). Neutropenia, with or without leukopenia, and often with a relative lymphocytosis, may be caused by HIV, drugs (zidovudine, didanosine, TMP-SMX), or intercurrent infection. Neutrophil functional defects have also been described. Thrombocytopenia may be a presenting finding of HIV infection, emphasizing the importance of HIV testing in patients thought to have idiopathic thrombocytopenia purpura (ITP). Thrombotic thrombocytopenic purpura is more common in adults but has been rarely seen in children with HIV infection. Coagulopathy may be secondary to HIV-induced hepatitis, lupus-like anticoagulants, autoantibodies to clotting factors, or disseminated intravascular coagulation accompanying systemic infection.

Hilgartner M: Hematologic manifestations in HIV-infected children. J Pediatr 119(suppl 1, pt 2):S47–S49, 1991.

105. What special recommendations regarding vaccination should be made for the child infected with HIV?

Vaccination recommendations for the HIV-infected child include some notable contraindications as well as special indications. Inactivated polio vaccine should be substituted for OPV, regardless of clinical stage of the child's disease. BCG vaccination is contraindicated in the United States. However, the World Health Organization recommends that BCG be administered to asymptomatic children infected with HIV who live in areas of the world with a high incidence of tuberculosis. Vaccination with MMR is currently recommended for all children with HIV infection, due to the high incidence of severe wild-type infection in these children. DTP and Hib vaccines should be administered according to the usual schedule. Symptomatic patients should also receive pneumococcal and influenza vaccines. Passive immunization with intravenous gamma-globulin has been demonstrated to decrease the incidence of opportunistic infections in HIV-infected children with CD4 counts > 200.

106. How common is the transmission of HIV from infected children to household contacts?

Extremely rare. Only two case reports clearly implicate an infected sibling as the source of HIV infection. Nevertheless, children with HIV infection should be taught good hygiene and behavior, and their families should be counseled about HIV and its transmission.

Shirley LR, Ross SA: Risk of transmission of human immunodeficiency virus by bite of an infected toddler. J Pediatrics 114:425–426, 1989.

Rogers MF, et al: Lack of transmission of human immunodeficiency virus from infected children to their household contacts. Pediatrics 85:210–214, 1990.

107. Should a classroom teacher be told that a child is HIV-positive?

There is no absolute indication to inform a classroom teacher, nor any other educator, of the child's HIV status. In certain circumstances, the family may find this advisable, and in those instances, the family has the right to do so. No person except the child's physician need be aware of the child's primary diagnosis.

American Academy of Pediatrics: 1994 Red Book: Report of the Committee on Infectious Diseases, 23rd ed. Elk Grove Park, IL, American Academy of Pediatrics, 1994, p 267.

108. Why are HIV-positive hemophiliacs less likely to develop AIDS than HIV-positive homosexual or IV drug abusing populations?

A large study of HIV-infected hemophiliacs demonstrated that the rate of progression from seroconversion to AIDS was most closely linked to age. Patients < 17 years (excluding neonates) had the lowest incidence of deterioration to AIDS within 8 years after seroconversion. In this age group, the rate of progression was lower than that found in children infected through other means. In contrast, adult hemophiliacs infected with HIV develop AIDS at approximately the same rate as adults infected with HIV through other routes. The reason for the slower deterioration in immune status in hemophiliac children is not completely understood, though there is some evidence that viral replication may be inhibited in this cohort of children.

Goedert JJ, et al: A prospective study of human immunodeficiency virus type 1 infection and the development of AIDS in subjects with hemophilia. N Engl J Med 321:141–148, 1989.

109. What is the mechanism of action of zidovudine?

Zidovudine, formerly called azidothymidine or AZT, is a nucleoside analogue that is converted by cellular enzymes to an active triphosphate form which competitively inhibits viral reverse transcriptase (the enzyme that allows viral RNA to make copies of itself into complementary DNA). Zidovudine incorporates itself into the viral DNA and codes for chain termination.

IMMUNIZATIONS

110. Why is the buttocks a poor location for intramuscular injections in infants?

The gluteus maximus is not a good choice for injections because:

1. The gluteus is incompletely developed in some infants.

2. There is potential for injury to the sciatic nerve or superior gluteal artery if the injection is misdirected.

3. Some vaccinations, particularly those for rabies and hepatitis B, may be less effective if injected into fat.

If injections into the buttocks are given to older children, the proper site is the gluteus medius in the upper outer quadrant, rather than the gluteus maximus which is more medial.

Lawton EL, Hayden GF: Immunization, medication and tuberculin skin test administration procedures. In Lohr JA (ed): Pediatric Outpatient Procedures. Philadelphia, J.B. Lippincott, 1991, pp 25–26.

111. Should premature babies receive immunization based on postconceptional age or chronologic age?

Premature babies should be immunized based on postnatal **chronologic** age. If a premature infant is still in the hospital at 2 months of age, then DTP vaccine should be given. However, oral poliovirus vaccine (OPV) should be deferred until discharge to minimize the possibility of exposing other infants to a live vaccine that might be spread by stools. The rest of the immunization schedule for premature infants should be the same as for babies delivered at term.

112. Should there by any change in the immunization schedule for children with cerebral palsy?

No. In particular, patients with static cerebral palsy should receive immunization against pertussis at the normally recommended times. If cerebral palsy is associated with a neurologic disorder that is evolving, then vaccination with pertussis vaccine should be withheld until the condition is in a stable phase. The decision to proceed with pertussis vaccination in these instances may often require discussion with a pediatric neurologist.

113. Which vaccines are egg-embryo-based vaccines?

Of the more common immunizations administered to children, influenza, measles, and mumps vaccine preparations are grown in chick embryo fibroblast culture. In contrast, rubella vaccine preparations are grown in human diploid cell cultures. Hence, when administered alone, the rubella vaccine is free of egg protein. However, this is not so when the measles, mumps, and rubella vaccines (i.e., MMR) are administered in combination.

114. Discuss the relative merits of OPV and IPV.

Both the live oral poliovirus (OPV or Sabin) vaccine and the inactivated poliovirus (IPV or Salk) vaccine are effective in preventing poliomyelitis. OPV is currently the vaccine of choice because it induces intestinal immunity, is simple to administer, and is well accepted by patients. In addition, OPV vaccination results in immunization of some contacts of vaccinated persons, a phenomenon referred to as herd immunity. Finally, OPV has essentially eliminated infection due to wild-type polioviruses in the United States.

OPV should not be administered to patients or family contacts who have immune dysfunction, to unimmunized adults, or to pregnant women. IPV is indicated in these situations. IPV is generally not as well accepted as OPV because of the requirement for intramuscular injection. Nevertheless, the inactivated vaccine currently in use is highly immunogenic. After three doses with IPV, the seroconversion rate is equal to that following OPV.

115. After an individual has received the OPV, how long does the virus persist?

It persists in the throat for 1–2 weeks and may persist in the stool for up to 2 months. In immunodeficient patients, viral excretion may be much longer.

116. What are the absolute and relative contraindications to pertussis immunization?

The following adverse effects, occurring after a previous pertussis immunization, form contraindications to subsequent pertussis vaccination.

Absolute contraindications
1. Immediate anaphylactic reaction
2. Encephalopathy within 7 days of vaccination

Relative contraindications
1. Convulsion within 3 days of vaccination
2. Persistent, severe, inconsolable screaming or crying for ≥ 3 hours within 2 days of vaccination
3. Collapse or shock-like state within 2 days of vaccination
4. Fever ≥ 40.5°C (104.9°F), unexplained by another cause, within 2 days of vaccination.

The relative contraindications were once considered absolute contraindications to pertussis immunization, but these are now considered precautions. When there is a contraindication to pertussis immunization, DT vaccine should be administered instead.

117. How common are side effects from the DTP immunization?

With the use of the whole-cell DTP vaccine, approximately 40–50% of infants develop fretfulness and redness, swelling, and tenderness at the injection site. About 50% develop fever > 38°C (100.4°F), but no more than 0.5% develop fever > 40.5°C (104.9°F). The acellular pertussis vaccines (DTaP), licensed in the United States in 1993, have much lower incidences of local and systemic reactions, including fever.

118. How often do major neurologic complications or death occur from pertussis vaccine?

The only case-controlled study addressing this issue was the National Childhood Encephalopathy Study (NCES), which was conducted in England from 1976–1979. This study reported that DTP vaccination was temporally related to the development of acute encephalopathy in approximately 1 in 110,000 doses. About one-third of these children had permanent brain damage. This figure formed the basis for previous estimates of a 1 in 310,000 incidence of permanent neurologic deficits following DTP vaccination. However, an expert panel, after reevaluation of these data, concluded that limitations of the study design and the small number of cases precluded valid interpretation regarding the incidence of permanent brain damage following DTP vaccination. Additional studies have not provided evidence to support a causal association between DTP vaccination and permanent neurologic injury.

The Committee on Infectious Diseases of the American Academy of Pediatrics concluded that according to current data, the DTP vaccine has not been proved to be a cause of brain damage. The Committee also stated that while the data do not disprove the association, if brain damage does result from DTP vaccination, the occurrence must be exceedingly rare.

Committee on Infectious Diseases: The relationship between pertussis vaccine and central nervous system sequelae: Continuing assessment. Pediatrics 97:279–281, 1996.

119. How long does protection against pertussis last after infection versus immunization?

Vaccine-induced immunity is of relatively short duration. In patients exposed to a sibling with pertussis, protection against infection was found to be approximately 80% for the first 3 years after vaccination, dropping to 50% at 4–7 years. By 11 years following vaccination, protection was virtually absent. It is hypothesized that subclinical infection during the period of waning immunity may be a factor in prolonging protection following immunization in some instances.

Protective immunity following natural infection with *Bordetella pertussis* is long-lasting. In addition, the immunity induced by natural infection appears to provide better protection than that induced by vaccination, even in the first 3 years following vaccination.

Wardlaw AC, Parton R (eds): Pathogenesis and Immunity in Pertussis. New York, John Wiley & Sons, 1988, p 284.

120. At what age should a child not receive pertussis vaccine?

The vaccine should not normally be given to children > 7 years of age. There is an increased incidence of localized reactions to the vaccine in older children and adults, and pertussis is usually a mild illness when it occurs past early childhood. In general, postexposure antimicrobial prophylaxis is preferred to vaccination in this setting. However, in rare instances, it may be advisable to immunize certain older individuals. For example, during an epidemic when unknown exposures may occur with increased frequency, patients with chronic lung disease should be immunized. The monovalent pertussis vaccine should be used in this circumstance if available, and the dose is half (0.25 ml) the normally recommended dose. Alternatively, an acellular vaccine can be used.

121. What is the difference between the pediatric (DT) and adult (Td) types of diphtheria and tetanus toxoid vaccines?

The **DT vaccine** contains standard doses of diphtheria and tetanus toxoids and should be used to immunize all children < 7 years old when pertussis vaccination is not required or is contraindicated. The **Td vaccine** contains a much smaller dose of diphtheria toxoid with standard tetanus toxoid dose. It should be used to immunize children > 7 years old and adults and is less likely to produce the severe reactions seen in older individuals given the higher dose. Td may be used when tetanus toxoid is required for wound management, as a booster is required every 10 years to ensure continuing diphtheria and tetanus immunity in adulthood.

122. If a pregnant woman is given the rubella vaccine in her first trimester, what is the risk to the fetus?

There is a theoretical risk that congenital rubella infection will occur. The Centers for Disease Control and Prevention has collected information from > 200 susceptible women who received the present rubella vaccine during the first trimester and found that 2% of the infants born to these women had subclinical infection but none had congenital defects. Based on these data, the maximum risk of congenital rubella associated with first-trimester vaccination is estimated to be 1.4%.

123. What are the contraindications to MMR vaccination?

1. *Intercurrent illness.* In general, low-grade fever or afebrile upper respiratory tract symptoms in an otherwise well child are not considered contraindications to MMR vaccination. However, more serious illness should prompt a delay in immunization until the child recovers.

2. *Immunodeficiency.* This includes primary immunodeficiencies, those associated with malignancies, and treatment with immunosuppressive drugs and radiation. Withhold the vaccine for at least 3 months after cessation of immunosuppressive therapy. MMR vaccination is currently recommended for both symptomatic and asymptomatic patients with HIV infection because wild-type measles infection may be fatal in these patients.

3. *Allergies.* Because the MMR vaccine contains trace amounts of neomycin and egg products, previous anaphylactic reaction to neomycin is an absolute contraindication to MMR administration. Similarly, patients with a history of anaphylactic reaction following egg ingestion should be vaccinated with extreme caution after skin testing. Milder allergic reactions to either of these agents are not a contraindication to MMR administration.

4. *Passive immunity.* Administration of immune globulin, whole blood, or other antibody-containing blood products may interfere with response to MMR if given within 3 months prior to vaccination. If MMR is given in this circumstance, either documentation of seroconversion or revaccination 3 months later is recommended.

5. *Pregnancy.* There is no evidence that MMR vaccine administered during pregnancy injures the developing fetus, but due to theoretical concerns, the vaccine should not be administered to women who are pregnant or contemplating pregnancy within 3 months.

6. *Personal or family history of convulsions.* Children with a personal or immediate-family history of seizures have an increased risk of seizures after measles vaccination. However, such history is not a contraindication to vaccination but rather should serve to alert the family and physician of the possibility

124. When was inactivated (killed) measles vaccine used?

1963–1968. About 1.8 million doses were given.

125. Why is it recommended that all infants be immunized with hepatitis B vaccine rather than only high-risk populations?

Efforts to define and target high-risk teenage and adult groups (e.g., intravenous drug abusers, individuals with multiple heterosexual partners, homosexual men) did not decrease the incidence of the disease. In as many as 60% of teenagers who acquire the disease, no risk factor is known. The magnitude of the problem is huge. It is estimated that each year, there are 200,000–300,000 acute hepatitis B infections and 5000 deaths from chronic liver disease due to hepatitis B and that there are now 1,000,000 individuals in the U.S. who are chronic carriers. About 15% of infections develop before adulthood, but these account disproportionately for nearly 40% of chronic carrier cases.

Because of the perceived problems of compliance and cost, universal immunization was recommended for infants as well as continued immunization for high-risk groups. With this system, the major impact will not be realized for 20 years or more.

Hall CB, Halsey NA: Control of hepatitis B: To be or not to be? Pediatrics 90:274–277, 1992.

126. Who should receive the pneumococcal vaccine?

The vaccine is poorly immunogenic in children < 2 years of age. Therefore, only children 2 years of age or older who have increased risk for pneumococcal infection or who are at increased risk for severe disease when infected with pneumococcus should receive the vaccine.

High-risk groups include children with sickle cell anemia, anatomic asplenia, nephrotic syndrome, and Hodgkin disease undergoing therapy. Parents of these children should be aware that the vaccine does not provide complete protection and that these children still require prompt medical attention for febrile illness. There are insufficient data available to assess the need for and efficacy of the vaccine among other high-risk children, such as those with organ transplants and chronic disease including heart failure, pulmonary disease, renal failure, diabetes, and immunodeficiency. Children in the latter group with immunoglobulin deficiencies are better treated with immunoglobulins. Children 2 years of age or older with HIV infection are now generally vaccinated.

127. What are the pediatric indications for the influenza vaccine?

Two types of killed influenza vaccine are available: the split vaccine is used for children < 12 years of age, and the whole virus vaccine is used for older children and adults. Each year in the autumn, a new preparation is made, aimed to cover the expected antigenic types for the winter season. Vaccination should be undertaken each year as soon as possible after the vaccine becomes available. When the vaccine is given for the first time, two doses are given, 1 month apart; in subsequent years, the same patient should be given only one dose. The vaccine is not recommended for children < 6 months of age. Children at high risk for severe influenza infection who should be vaccinated include those with:

1. Chronic lung diseases, e.g., moderate to severe asthma or bronchopulmonary dysplasia
2. Congenital heart disease causing significant hemodynamic disturbance
3. Hemoglobinopathies including sickle cell disease
4. Treatment with immunosuppressive drugs

Other groups who should be strongly considered for vaccination include:

1. Children with chronic renal failure, diabetes mellitus, or other metabolic disorders
2. Children receiving chronic aspirin therapy (who may therefore be at increased risk for developing Reye syndrome following influenza)
3. Individuals in contact with high-risk children, such as household and family members and hospital and nursery personnel (and conversely, children who are in contact with high-risk adults)
4. Children living in institutions, colleges, or boarding schools or attending daycare

128. Under what circumstances should meningococcal vaccine be given?

Patients who have functional or anatomic asplenia or complement deficiency and who are ≥ 2 years of age should be given the vaccine. Revaccination after 2–3 years may be useful. The quadrivalent vaccine available in the United States includes antigen from four serogroups: A, C, Y, and W-135. Most infections in children, however, are due to group B meningococci, against which there is no effective vaccine at present. The current vaccine may be used to control outbreaks due to other meningococcal serotypes and can also be used as an adjunct to chemoprophylaxis of contacts. The vaccine might also be beneficial to persons traveling to areas of epidemic or hyperendemic disease. It is given to all American military recruits.

129. When is rabies human diploid cell vaccine (HDCV) administered?

Pre-exposure vaccination is recommended for individuals at high risk for contact with rabies, such as veterinarians, animal handlers, cave explorers, hunters exposed to rabid animals, and persons living in or visiting areas of countries where the risk of rabies exposure is high. HDCV is also used as a prophylactic regimen in all persons who have been exposed to rabies. Those who have not previously received HDCV should also be given human rabies immune globulin as soon as possible after the exposure.

130. Which vaccines have proven severe side effects?

In most vaccine-related adverse events, the evidence is inadequate to accept or reject a causal relationship (which in the past lead to an explosion of lawsuits). The Institute of Medicine of the National Academy of Sciences, reviewing all available literature on adverse vaccine-related events, identified a few likely causal relationships:

1. Diphtheria/tetanus toxoid and brachial neuritis
2. Diphtheria/tetanus toxoid and anaphylaxis
3. Measles vaccine and anaphylaxis
4. Measles vaccine and death from measles-strain viral infection (all in immunocompromised individuals)
5. Oral polio vaccine and Guillain-Barré syndrome
6. Oral polio vaccine and poliomyelitis and death from polio vaccine-strain viral infection (primarily in immunocompromised individuals)
7. Hepatitis B vaccine and anaphylaxis

Stratton KR, et al: Adverse events associated with childhood vaccines other than pertussis and rubella: Summary of a report from the Institute of Medicine. JAMA 271:1602–1605, 1994.

INFECTIONS WITH RASH

131. What is the traditional numbering of the "original" six exanthemas of childhood?

First disease	measles (rubeola)
Second disease	Scarlet fever
Third disease	Rubella
Fourth disease	Filatov-Dukes disease (described in 1900 and was felt to be a distinct scarlatiniform type of rubella; no longer used)
Fifth disease	Erythema infectiosum
Sixth disease	Roseola infantum (exanthem subitum)

132. What is "atypical" about atypical measles?

1. It occurs primarily in patients who have received inactivated measles vaccine.
2. Koplik spots are unusual.
3. Rash begins on distal extremities and spreads toward head (in typical measles, the exanthem spreads from head to feet).
4. Conjunctivitis and coryza are not part of prodrome.
5. Hepatosplenomegaly is more common.

Cherry JD: Measles. In Feigin RD, Cherry JD (eds): Textbook of Pediatric Infectious Diseases, 3rd ed. Philadelphia, W.B. Saunders, 1992, pp 1599–1600.

133. Why has the incidence of measles been rising?

In 1989 and 1990, the incidence of measles in the United States was increased more than 5-fold over previous years. Greater than 26,000 cases were reported in 1990. The largest increase in measles incidence has occurred in children under 4 years of age.

The reason for the resurgence in measles is not completely understood. The main cause cited is the failure to vaccinate children at the recommended age—70% of cases of measles occur in unvaccinated children, and many cases are from inner-city populations, where vaccination rates may be as low as 50%. The reasons for low vaccination rates include (1) missed opportunities for administration of vaccine, such as minor illness; (2) inadequate access to medical care; and (3) inadequate public awareness of the importance of vaccination.

Vaccine failure accounts for most of the remaining cases of measles, though primary failure occurs in only ~ 5% of children vaccinated at an age of ≥ 15 months. Waning antibody titer following vaccination (secondary vaccine failure) was responsible for most cases of measles prior to 1987. As a consequence, the incidence of measles increased initially in adolescent children. This cohort has presumably served as a reservoir for spread of the epidemic into communities where measles vaccination was inadequate.

National Vaccine Advisory Committee: The measles epidemic: The problems, barriers, and recommendations. JAMA 266:1547–1552, 1991.

134. Why is post-measles blindness so common in underdeveloped countries?

As many as 1% of all cases of measles in underdeveloped regions result in blindness. In contrast, measles keratitis in developed countries is usually self-limited and benign. There are two principal reasons:

1. Vitamin A deficiency—Vitamin A is needed for corneal stromal repair, and a deficiency allows epithelial damage to persist or worsen. Many malnourished children have accompanying vitamin A deficiency, and vitamin A supplements may be of benefit during active illness.

2. Malnutrition may predispose to corneal superinfection with herpes simplex virus.

135. How common is human herpesvirus type-6 (HHV-6) infection in children?

Infection with HHV-6 is ubiquitous and occurs with high frequency in infants, 65% of whom have serologic evidence of primary infection by their first birthday. In addition to typical cases of **roseola**, HHV-6 infection may be associated with a number of common pediatric problems such as "fever without localizing findings," nonspecific rash, and EBV-negative mononucleosis. In a study by Hall and coworkers, up to one-third of all febrile seizures in children age < 2 years were due to HHV-6 infections. On rare occasions, the virus has been associated with fulminant hepatitis, encephalitis, and a syndrome of massive lymphadenopathy called Rosai-Dorfman disease.

Pruksananonda P, et al: Primary human herpesvirus-6 infection in young children. N Engl J Med 326:1445–1450, 1992.

Hall CB, et al: Human herpesvirus-6 infection in children. N Engl J Med 331:432–438, 1994.

136. Name the etiologic agents of exanthem subitum (roseola infantum).

Multiple agents are likely. HHV-6 was discovered in 1986, and in 1988, Japanese investigators isolated it from four children with exanthem subitum. In 1994, human herpesvirus type 7 (HHV-7) was also isolated in children with the clinical features of roseola.

Tanaka K, et al: Human herpesvirus-7: Another causal agent for roseola (exanthem subitum). J Pediatr 125:1–5, 1994.

137. What are the typical features of roseola?

Most children have an abrupt onset of high fever (> 39°C) with no prodrome. Fever usually lasts 3–4 days but can range from 1–8 days. Within 24 hours of defervescence, a discrete erythematous macular or maculopapular rash appears on the face, neck, and/or trunk. Erythematous papules (Nagayama spots) may be noted on the soft palate and uvular base in two-thirds of patients. Other common features on exam include mild cervical lymph node enlargement, edematous eyelids, and bulging of the anterior fontanel in infants. A variety of symptoms may accompany the fever, including diarrhea, cough, coryza, and headache.

Asano Y, et al: Clinical features of infants with primary human herpesvirus-6 infection (exanthem subitum, roseola subitum). Pediatrics 93:104–108, 1994.

138. What is the spectrum of disease caused by parvovirus B19?

- Erythema infectiosum (most common; a childhood exanthem, also called fifth disease or slapped cheek disease because of the classic appearance of the rash)
- Arthritis and arthralgia (most common in adults)
- Intrauterine infection with hydrops fetalis
- Transient aplastic crisis in patients with underlying hemolytic disease (e.g., sickle cell anemia, hereditary spherocytosis, thalassemia, G6PD deficiency, pyruvate kinase deficiency)
- Persistent infection with chronic anemia in patients with immunodeficiencies

In addition, infection may be asymptomatic.

139. Describe the characteristic rash of Rocky Mountain spotted fever.

- Usually seen by third day of illness (5–11 days after tick bite)
- Initially blanching red macules which become petechial
- Begins on wrists and ankles and spreads to extremities and trunk within hours
- Involves palms and soles

140. Why has the Weil-Felix test fallen out of favor?

This study had been used as a diagnostic test for Rocky Mountain spotted fever (RMSF). It is based on the fact that rickettsiae share some common antigens with some *Proteus* strains. In the appropriate clinical setting, rising or elevated antibody titers to these *Proteus* strains suggest RMSF. However, titers may also be elevated in patients with leptospirosis, brucellosis, *Borrelia* infections, typhoid fever, and serious liver disease. Until a rapid microbiologic test is available for RMSF, more specific serologic testing is recommended to diagnose this infection.

141. How long after exposure to chickenpox (varicella) do symptoms develop?

99% develop symptoms between 11–20 days following exposure.

142. Should "well" children with varicella be treated with acyclovir?

Studies have shown that oral acyclovir therapy (20 mg/kg, up to 800 mg) four times daily for 5 days, initiated within 24 hours after the onset of rash, decreases the maximum number of lesions by 15–30%, shortens the duration of the development of new lesions, and shortens the duration of fever by 1 day. The Committee on Infectious Diseases of the AAP opted not to recommend acyclovir for routine use in uncomplicated varicella for otherwise healthy children under age 13 because of "marginal therapeutic effect, the cost of the drug, feasibility of drug delivery in the first 24 hours of illness, and the currently unknown and unforeseen possible dangers of treating as many as 4 million children each year." Of note, the varicella vaccine is now recommended for routine use in children.

Committee on Infectious Diseases: Use of oral acyclovir in otherwise healthy children with varicella. Pediatrics 91:674–676, 1993.

143. What is the risk of varicella-associated complications in normal children 1–14 years old?

More than 3.5 million cases of chickenpox occur in the United States each year, with the great majority occurring in children < 14 years of age. The most common complications include secondary bacterial skin infections (generally due to streptococci or staphylococci), neurologic syndromes (cerebellitis, encephalitis, transverse myelitis, and Guillain-Barré syndrome), and pneumonia. Thrombocytopenia, arthritis, hepatitis, glomerulonephritis, and Reye syndrome occur less commonly.

The frequency of these complications in normal children is not known precisely, but it is estimated to be low on the basis of hospitalization and mortality data. In particular, approximately 4500 otherwise-normal children are hospitalized in the U.S. each year because of chickenpox. In normal children, the death rate due to varicella averages about 1 in 50,000 cases.

Preblud SR: Varicella: Complications and costs. Pediatrics 78:728–735, 1986.

144. How common are second episodes of varicella?

Approximately 1 in 500 cases. They are more likely to occur when the first episode is subclinical or very mild and/or when it develops in a young infant.

Gershon A: Second episodes of varicella: Degree and duration of immunity. Pediatr Infect Dis J 9:306, 1990.

145. In children with herpes zoster, what is the distribution of the rash?

Compared with adults who most commonly have lesions in the lower thoracic and upper lumbar regions, children may have more cervical and sacral involvement with resultant extremity and inguinal lesions.

50% Thoracic
20% Cervical
20% Lumbosacral
10% Cranial nerve

If there are lesions on the tip of the nose, herpes zoster keratitis is more likely because of possible involvement of the nasociliary nerve. When the geniculate ganglion is involved, there is risk of developing the Ramsay Hunt syndrome, which consists of ear pain with auricular and periauricular vesicles and facial nerve palsy.

146. Who gets herpes gladiatorum?

Herpes gladiatorum is a term used for ocular and cutaneous infection with herpes simplex virus type 1 occurring in **wrestlers** and **rugby players**. The infection is transmitted primarily by direct skin-to-skin contact and is endemic among high school and college wrestlers.

147. When did the World Health Organization certify that smallpox had been globally eradicated?

1980.

LYMPHADENITIS/LYMPHADENOPATHY

148. What are the causes of lymphadenitis in normal, otherwise healthy children?

In order of frequency:
1. *Staphylococcus aureus*
2. Group A β-hemolytic streptococci
3. Cat scratch disease
4. *Mycobacterium tuberculosis*
5. Atypical mycobacteria

149. Which children with lymphadenopathy or lymphadenitis should be considered for biopsy or aspiration?

Tissue diagnosis should be sought when:
• Malignancy is a consideration, i.e.:
     In all children with supraclavicular adenopathy
     In all children with nodes fixed to skin or deep tissue
     In children with persistent fever and weight loss without a specific diagnosis
• Atypical mycobacteria is suspected
• Patient fails to respond to antimicrobial agents specific for common etiologic agents

Many authorities suggest biopsy of all nodes remaining enlarged after 3 months of observation. Earlier biopsy should be considered if the nodes demonstrate continued growth.

Knight PJ, et al: When is lymph node biopsy indicated in children with enlarged peripheral nodes? Pediatrics 69:341, 1982.

150. An intensely erythematous but nontender submandibular or tonsillar node is most suggestive of what infectious process?

Nontuberculous mycobacterium infection.

151. How is the diagnosis of nontuberculous mycobacterial disease made?

In children, infection with nontuberculous mycobacterial (NTM) most commonly takes the form of localized lymphadenitis. The submandibular or preauricular glands are most often affected. Suggestive clinical features include adenopathy with minimal warmth and tenderness, positive (indurated) Mantoux skin test (often < 10 mm), and negative chest x-ray. Skin test antigens specific for NTM are of limited usefulness due to cross-reactivity with antigens of *M. tuberculosis*. Definitive diagnosis of NTM infection depends on culture of the organism from infected tissue. Histopathologic examination of the tissue cannot adequately differentiate the organism from *M. tuberculosis*.

Less common forms of disease due to NTM include pulmonary and disseminated infection. These occur almost exclusively in debilitated patients, particularly patients with AIDS, in whom *M. avium* complex infections have become prevalent. On occasion, children with cystic fibrosis may develop symptomatic pulmonary disease due to NTM. In these forms of infection, the diagnosis relies on culture of the organism from the relevant body site, such as sputum or blood.

152. Swollen, tender pectoral nodes are most suggestive of what infection?

Cat scratch disease.

153. What is the etiologic agent of cat scratch disease?

Serologic studies along with culture and PCR testing of infected tissues indicate that most, if not all, cases of cat scratch disease are caused by a gram-negative bacterium, *Bartonella henselae*. This organism was first isolated in 1991 and has also been associated with bacillary angiomatosis and peliosis hepatis, which occur primarily in adults with HIV infection.

154. Describe the types of presentation of cat scratch disease.

Cat scratch disease (CSD) is characterized by chronic regional lymphadenitis. In the typical case, an otherwise healthy child or adolescent presents with regional lymphadenopathy of several days' duration. The lymph nodes most commonly involved are axillary, epitrochlear, cervical, submandibular, inguinal, and preauricular. Enlarged pectoral nodes, a rare occurrence in any infectious disease, are highly suggestive of CSD. A history of cat exposure, particularly kittens, is obtained in up to 90% of patients.

Parinaud oculoglandular syndrome is a less common presentation of CSD. The syndrome is characterized by granulomatous lesions on the palpebral conjunctiva associated with swelling of ipsilateral preauricular nodes. Direct eye rubbing after contact with a cat is the presumed mode of inoculation.

Rarely, CSD may manifest as thrombocytopenic or nonthrombocytopenic purpura, osteolytic lesions, granulomatous lesions of the liver or spleen, or atypical pneumonia. One of the most disturbing presentations is encephalitis, which is associated with convulsions in > 80% of patients. The prognosis for full neurologic recovery, however, is excellent. Other neurologic presentations include polyneuritis, myelitis, or neuroretinitis. Finally, a systemic form of CSD with high fever, suppurative lymphadenitis, and severe constitutional symptoms has been described.

Shinal EA: Cat-scratch disease: A review of the literature. Pediatr Dermatol 7:11–18, 1990.
Klein JD: Cat-scratch disease. Pediatr Rev 15:348–353, 1994.

155. Discuss the natural history of cat scratch disease.

In nearly all cases, lymphadenitis due to CSD resolves within several weeks to months from its onset. On occasion, the nodes suppurate, necessitating aspiration to prevent spontaneous drainage. Incision and drainage is generally not recommended, as this therapy may be associated with a higher incidence of chronic drainage and fistula formation. Excision of the nodes may be required in cases when repeated aspiration is unsuccessful or if the diagnosis is in question.

The use of antibiotics in uncomplicated CSD is controversial, as commonly used antibiotics are not efficacious and most patients recover spontaneously. Some antimicrobial agents appear to offer benefit, however, and may be useful in severe forms of the disease. Trimethoprim-sulfamethoxasole, ciprofloxacin, gentamicin, and rifampin have shown some benefit in uncontrolled clinical studies.

156. What are the common presentations for Epstein-Barr virus (EBV) infections?

EBV infections are frequently asymptomatic in young children. In adolescents and young adults the exact ratio of symptomatic to asymptomatic infections is unclear, but the classic illness is that of infectious mononucleosis:

Clinical	fever, pharyngitis, lymphadenopathy (75–95%); splenomegaly (50%)
Hematologic	> 50% mononuclear cells, > 10% atypical lymphocytes
Serologic	transient appearance of heterophile antibodies; emergence of permanent antibodies to EBV

A wide variety of symptoms (e.g., malaise, headache, anorexia, myalgias, chills, nausea) can also occur. Neurologic presentations are rare but can include encephalitis, meningitis, myelitis, Guillain-Barré syndrome, or cranial or peripheral neuropathies.

157. How was the monospot test developed?

In 1932, Paul and Bunnell observed that patients with infectious mononucleosis coincidentally made antibodies to sheep RBCs. The monospot test evolved from that discovery and uses rapid slide agglutination to identify patients with antibodies to foreign proteins, the so-called heterophile antibodies. Horse or beef RBCs are now more commonly used because they are more sensitive than sheep RBCs to agglutination. Heterophile antibodies can also occur in serum sickness and as a normal variant. If there is clinical confusion, differential absorption can pinpoint the cause. Normal variant heterophile antibodies do not react with beef RBCs. Heterophile antibodies in infectious mononucleosis do not react with guinea pig kidney cells, whereas those of serum sickness do.

Durbin WA, Sullivan JL: Epstein-Barr virus infections. Pediatr Rev 15:63–68, 1994.

158. How common are heterophile antibodies in infectious mononucleosis?

In classic infectious mononucleosis with fever, tonsillopharyngitis and lymphadenopathy, 75% of older children and adolescents have heterophile antibodies by the end of the first week of illness and 85–90% by the third week. These percentages are much lower in infants and young children, and false-negative screening with the monospot test is common in these groups as well as in patients without classic infectious mononucleosis.

159. What is the natural course of serologic responses to EBV infection?

A variety of distinct EBV antigens, including viral capsid antigen (VCA), early antigen (EA), and nuclear antigen (EBNA), can elicit antibody responses. Acute infection is best characterized by the presence of anti-VCA-IgM.

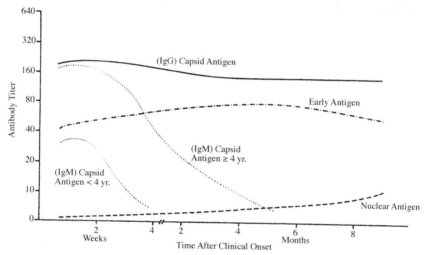

From Sumaya CV: Infectious mononucleosis. In Oski FA, et al (eds): Principles and Practice of Pediatrics, 2nd ed. Philadelphia, J.B. Lippincott, 1994, p 1316; with permission.

160. When are steroids indicated in children with EBV infection?

For the relief of respiratory obstruction due to enlarged tonsils. Some authorities have also advocated their use in severe autoimmune hemolytic anemia, aplastic anemia, neurologic complications and severe life-threatening infections, such as liver failure.

161. What other organisms can cause an infectious mononucleosis-like picture?

Cytomegalovirus, *Toxoplasma gondii*, human herpes virus-6, adenovirus, HIV, and rubella.

162. What are the clinical presentations of acquired cytomegalovirus (CMV) infection?

When it is symptomatic, acquired CMV infection in normal hosts produces fever, malaise, and nonspecific aches and pains. The peripheral blood smear reveals an absolute lymphocytosis and many atypical lymphocytes. In contrast to EBV-infectious mononucleosis, lymphadenopathy and tonsillitis are not prominent. Liver involvement is very common and liver function tests reveal abnormalities. Like EBV disease, CMV mononucleosis can persist for several weeks.

MENINGITIS

163. What are the most common signs and symptoms of meningitis in infants aged < 2 months?

In general, the findings in neonates and young infants with meningitis are minimal and often subtle. Fever occurs in approximately one-half of infected infants, seizures in about 40%, and increasing irritability in about one-third. Lethargy, respiratory distress, disinterest in feeding, and vomiting or diarrhea are frequent nonspecific manifestations of meningitis in this patient group. On physical exam, approximately one-third of newborns and young infants have a bulging fontanel.

Feigin RD, et al: Diagnosis and management of meningitis. Pediatr Infect Dis J 11:785–814, 1992.

164. Which occurs more commonly, aseptic or bacterial meningitis?

Aseptic meningitis. Prior to the availability of the *Haemophilus influenzae* vaccine, two-thirds of meningitis cases were aseptic and one-third bacterial. The percentage of aseptic cases is likely to go even higher.

165. Should CT scans be done prior to a lumbar puncture (LP) in the evaluation of possible meningitis?

CT scans are not routinely indicated prior to an LP unless there are:

1. Signs of herniation (rapid alteration in consciousness, abnormalities of pupillary size and reaction, absence of oculocephalic response, fixed oculomotor deviation of eyes)
2. Overwhelming shock or sepsis
3. Papilledema
4. Abnormalities in posture or respiration
5. Generalized seizures (especially tonic) which are often associated with impending cerebral herniation
6. Any condition mimicking bacterial meningitis (e.g., intracranial mass, lead intoxication, tuberculous meningitis, Reye syndrome)

Haslam RH: Role of CT in the early management of bacterial meningitis. J Pediatr 119:157–159, 1991.

166. What is the range of values found in CSF of infants and children who do not have meningitis?

CSF Values Found in Infants and Children without Meningitis

	WBCs/mm³	PROTEIN (mg/dl)	CSF/BLOOD GLUCOSE (%)
Newborn infants			
Preterm	0–29	65–150	55–105
Term	0–32	20–170	44–248
Infants and children	0–6	15–45	60–90

From McCracken GH: Current management of bacterial meningitis in infants and children. Pediatr Infect Dis J 11:170, 1992; with permission.

167. If bloody CSF is collected during a lumbar puncture, how is CNS hemorrhage distinguished from a traumatic artifact?

More commonly, the blood is due to traumatic rupture of small venous plexes that surround the subarachnoid space, but pathologic bloody fluid can be seen in multiple settings (e.g., subarachnoid hemorrhage, herpes simplex meningoencephalitis). Distinguishing features that suggest pathologic bleeding include:

1. Bleeding that does not lessen during collection of multiple tubes
2. Xanthochromia of the CNS supernatant
3. Crenated RBCs noted microscopically

168. How do the CSF findings vary in bacterial, viral, fungal, and tuberculous meningitis in children beyond the neonatal period?

Although a large overlap is possible (e.g., bacterial meningitis can be associated with a low WBC count early in the illness, or viral meningitis can be associated with a predominance of neutrophils early in the illness), the usual findings are:

Typical Findings in Bacterial, Viral, Fungal, and Tuberculous Meningitis

CSF FINDINGS	BACTERIAL	VIRAL	FUNGAL/TUBERCULOUS
WBC/mm³	> 500	< 500	< 500
PMNs	> 80%	< 50%	< 50%
Glucose (mg/dl)	< 40	> 40	< 40
CSF/blood ratio	< 30%	> 50%	< 30%
Protein (mg/dl)	> 100	< 100	> 100

Adapted from Powell KR: Meningitis. In Hoekelman RA, et al: (eds): Primary Pediatric Care, 2nd ed. St. Louis, Mosby, 1992, p 1354; with permission.

169. How is a traumatic lumbar puncture interpreted?

To interpret the number of WBCs in the CSF following a traumatic lumbar puncture, a correction factor is needed:

$$\text{True WBCs (CSF)} = \text{Actual WBCs (CSF)} - \text{WBCs (blood)} \times \frac{\text{RBCs (CSF)}}{\text{RBCs (blood)}}$$

Ashwal S, et al: Bacterial meningitis in children: Current concepts of neurologic management. Curr Probl Pediatr 24:267–284, 1994.

170. When is the best time to obtain a serum glucose level in an infant with suspected meningitis?

Because the stress of a lumbar puncture can elevate serum glucose, the serum sample is ideally obtained just before the lumbar puncture. When the blood glucose level is acutely elevated, it can take at least 30 minutes before there is equilibration with the CSF.

171. Is intracranial pressure elevated in patients with meningitis?

In acute bacterial meningitis, pressure is elevated in up to 95% of cases. Elevations are also commonly seen in tuberculous and fungal meningitis. The extent of elevation in viral meningitis is less well studied.

172. How often does bacterial meningitis present in younger patients with normal findings on the initial CSF examination?

In up to 3% of cases in children aged 3 weeks to 18 months with positive bacterial cultures of the CSF, the initial CSF evaluation (i.e., cell count, protein and glucose concentrations, and Gram stain) can be normal.

Polk DB, Steele RW: Bacterial meningitis presenting with normal cerebrospinal fluid. Pediatr Infect Dis J 6:1040–1042, 1987.

173. Does antibiotic therapy prior to lumbar puncture affect CSF indices?

In most cases of bacterial meningitis, a few doses of antibiotic will not markedly alter the CSF. Gram stain usually still demonstrates bacteria with typical staining properties, and chemistry values and cell counts are abnormal. Even when children have received appropriate antibiotic therapy for 44–68 hours, chemical and cytologic analysis of the CSF generally still reflects a bacterial process. Among patients with *Haemophilus influenzae* meningitis who have received oral antibiotic therapy prior to lumbar puncture, CSF cultures will often grow the organism. In contrast, there is a tendency for oral therapy to sterilize the CSF of children with pneumococcal or meningococcal disease.

174. What are the most common organisms responsible for bacterial meningitis?
0–2 months
- *Escherichia coli*
- Group B streptococci
- *Listeria monocytogenes*
- Miscellaneous Enterobacteriaceae
- *Haemophilus influenzae* (nontypable and type b)
- Coagulase-negative staphylococci (in hospitalized preterm infants)

2 months–6 years
- *Streptococcus pneumoniae*
- *Neisseria meningitidis*
- *Haemophilus influenzae*

6–18 years
- *Streptococcus pneumoniae*
- *Neisseria meningitidis*

The incidence of *H. influenzae* meningitis has fallen dramatically with the introduction of effective vaccines.

175. How often is meningitis associated with facial cellulitis?
In cases of facial cellulitis occurring after trauma, the etiology is usually group A *Streptococcus* or *Staphylococcus aureus*, and associated systemic disease is rare. In contrast, in the absence of trauma, facial cellulitis in unimmunized children is generally caused by *Haemophilus influenzae* type b. Most of these patients are bacteremic, and approximately 10% have concomitant meningitis.

176. Why is *Haemophilus influenzae* type b more virulent than nontypable *Haemophilus* strains?
Typable *H. influenzae* exhibits a polysaccharide capsule. This is thought to enhance virulence by inhibiting phagocytosis, but it is likely that other factors are involved in determining the virulence of *H. influenzae* as well.

177. What are the drugs of choice for treating bacterial meningitis?

Drugs of Choice for Treating Bacterial Meningitis*

ORGANISM	DRUGS OF CHOICE
Streptococcus pneumoniae	Penicillin, third-generation cephalosporin,[†] vancomycin[†]
Neisseria meningitidis	Penicillin, third-generation cephalosporin, chloramphenicol
Haemophilus influenzae type b	Third-generation cephalosporin, ampicillin, chloramphenicol
Listeria monocytogenes	Penicillin or ampicillin plus aminoglycoside
Streptococcus agalactiae	Penicillin, ampicillin (plus gentamicin for 3–5 days)
Escherichia coli	Aminoglycoside, third-generation cephalosporin, imipenem

*Definitive treatment should be determined by antibiotic susceptibility testing.
[†] Combination of third-generation cephalosporin plus vancomycin for pneumococcal isolates resistant to third-generation cephalosporins (MIC > 0.5).

178. How quickly is the CSF sterilized in children with meningitis?
In successful therapy, the CSF is usually sterile within 36–48 hours of initiation of antibiotics.

179. How long after treatment has been initiated must individuals with meningitis remain in respiratory isolation?
24 hours. Respiratory isolation is recommended for patients with suspected *Haemophilus influenzae* type b or meningococcal meningitis but can be discontinued after 24 hours of therapy.

Lodes   *ER dep.*

180. What is the accepted duration of treatment for bacterial meningitis?

The duration of antibiotic treatment is based on the causative agent and clinical course. In general, a minimum of 5 days of therapy is required for meningococcal meningitis, 7–10 days for *Haemophilus influenzae* meningitis, and 10 days for pneumococcal meningitis. Disease due to group B streptococci or *Listeria monocytogenes* should be treated for 14–21 days, and meningitis caused by gram-negative enteric bacilli should be treated for a minimum of 21 days after the CSF has become sterile. Among patients with complications such as brain abscess, subdural empyema, delayed CSF sterilization, persistence of meningeal signs, or prolonged fever, the duration of therapy may need to be extended and should be individualized.

181. What is the role of corticosteroids in the treatment of bacterial meningitis?

The inflammatory response plays a critical role in producing the CNS pathology and resultant sequelae of bacterial meningitis. A series of studies have suggested that treatment with dexamethasone reduces the incidence of hearing loss and other neurologic sequelae in infants and children with *Haemophilus influenzae* meningitis. According to these studies, dexamethasone therapy should be started before initiation of antibiotic therapy and should be administered intravenously in a dose of 0.15 mg/kg. Doses should be repeated every 6 hours to complete 16 doses over 4 days. The primary side effect associated with this regimen of dexamethasone is gastrointestinal bleeding, but this complication has been observed in < 1% of patients. The role of steroids in meningitis due to other bacterial pathogens remains under study. Most experts advise against steroids for neonatal meningitis.

Prober CG: The role of steroids in the management of children with bacterial meningitis. Pediatrics 95:29–31, 1995.

182. Should children receiving therapy for bacterial meningitis be retapped?

It is widely agreed that retapping is advisable in the child who shows no clinical response to therapy in 24–48 hours as well as in the child with meningitis due to penicillin-resistant *Streptococcus pneumoniae*. When the patient's management and course of illness are uncomplicated, repeat CSF examination either during or at the completion of therapy is unnecessary. An exception is neonatal meningitis, in which retapping to confirm sterilization is recommended because of the greater difficulty in tracking the infant's clinical course and because of the variable response of the immature neonatal immune system. Furthermore, time to sterilization correlates inversely with prognosis.

183. In a patient with meningitis, what are the indications for a CT scan or MRI?

CT scan and MRI are especially useful in identifying intracranial complications of bacterial meningitis, such as subdural collections of fluid (including subdural empyema), brain abscess, cerebrovascular thrombosis, and hydrocephalus. The following suggest the presence of an intracranial complication and should prompt a neuroimaging study: (1) prolonged obtundation, (2) prolonged irritability, (3) seizures developing after the third or foruth day of therapy, (4) focal seizures, (5) focal neurologic deficits, (6) increasing head circumference, (7) persistent elevation of CSF protein or neutrophil count, and (8) recurrence of disease.

In cases of neonatal meningitis caused by *Citrobacter diversus*, brain abscess should be anticipated, and a CT scan or MRI performed early in the course. In these patients, repeat scans are useful to monitor the response to antibiotic therapy and determine the need for surgical intervention.

Lin T-Y, et al: Fever during treatment for bacterial meningitis. Pediatr Infect Dis J 3:319–332, 1984.

184. How common is persistent or recurrent fever in meningitis?

Fever persists for at least 5 days in most children with meningitis. It lasts for 5–9 days in 10–15% of cases and for 10 or more days in another 10–15% of patients. Fever that returns after a minimum of 24 hours of afebrile temperatures is considered recurrent fever and occurs in approximately 15% of patients.

Lin T-Y, et al: Fever during treatment for bacterial meningitis. Pediatr Infect Dis J 3:319–332, 1984.

185. What are the most common causes of prolonged fever in meningitis?
1. Disease at other foci (e.g., arthritis)
2. Nosocomial infection
3. Thrombophlebitis (related to intravenous catheters and infusates)
4. Sterile or infected abscesses from intramuscular injections
5. Drug fever

Subdural effusions have also been associated with prolonged fever, but these occur commonly among children with meningitis and are probably not a cause of fever.

186. How should prolonged fever during treatment for meningitis be managed?
Patients who remain febrile for > 5 days and who are irritable or have persistent neck stiffness should undergo a repeat lumbar puncture. Similarly, children who appear well yet have fever for ≥ 10 days should also undergo repeat lumbar puncture. If the CSF examination reveals a protein concentration > 100 mg/dl or a substantial number of neutrophils, persistent infection is a possibility. Studies should be obtained to exclude an abscess or resistant isolate. If the CSF values are approaching normal, antibiotic therapy can usually be discontinued at the usual time. In this situation, nosocomial viral infection or drug fever would be likely.

187. How commonly are subdural effusions noted in bacterial meningitis?
Subdural effusions are common in bacterial meningitis and should be considered part of the disease rather than a complication. Estimates of their incidence vary from 10–50%. The incidence is highest in younger infants and in patients with *Haemophilus influenzae* meningitis. Most authorities now agree that routine tapping of subdural effusions is unnecessary. Removal of fluid is reserved for patients showing signs of increased intracranial pressure or focal neurologic signs.

188. If a child develops bacterial meningitis, what should the parents be told about long-term outcomes?
In children beyond the newborn period, sequelae such as spasticity, paralysis, ataxia, seizures, school problems, and visual and hearing disorders can persist. Hydrocephalus is very rare. In a meta-analysis evaluating the three main bacterial causes of meningitis, disease due to *Streptococcus pneumoniae* was associated with considerably more mortality and morbidity than was infection caused by *Neisseria meningitidis* or *Haemophilus influenzae*. Among patients with pneumococcal meningitis, 17% had mental retardation, 12% had spasticity, 14% had a seizure disorder, and 15% had profound deafness. Mortality was as high as 15%.

Baraff LJ, et al: Outcomes of bacterial meningitis in children: A meta-analysis. Pediatr Infect Dis J 12:389–394, 1993.

189. How should contacts of children with *Neisseria meningitidis* disease be managed?
Antibiotic prophylaxis (rifampin, ceftriaxone, or, if the isolate is known to be sensitive, sulfisoxazole) is indicated in household, daycare, or nursery school contacts of active cases. Only those medical personnel who have had intimate contact with the patient (e.g., through intubation or mouth-to-mouth resuscitation) need to receive antibiotic prophylaxis. Surveillance cultures of contacts should not be performed to determine the need for prophylaxis; the most important aspect of prophylaxis is close clinical surveillance of contacts for fever or malaise. Because secondary cases can occur weeks following identification of the index case, vaccination should be considered if the organisms is of a serogroup contained in the vaccine (i.e., groups A, C, Y, W-135).

Committee on Infectious Diseases: Meningococcal disease prevention and control strategies for practice-based physicians. Pediatrics 97:404–412, 1996.

190. Name the most common cause of aseptic meningitis.
Aseptic meningitis consists of clinical and laboratory indications of inflammation of the meninges (e.g., CSF pleocytosis and increased protein) without evidence of bacterial infection on Gram stain or culture. Over 80% of cases are caused by **enteroviruses** (i.e., various types of coxsackievirus A and B, enterovirus, echovirus, and, rarely, poliovirus).

OCULAR INFECTIONS

191. What are the most common infectious causes of conjunctivitis by age?

< 2 days	Chemical (silver nitrate)
2 days–2 wks	*Chlamydia trachomatis* (inclusion blennorrhea)
	Neisseria gonorrhoeae
	Escherichia coli and other gram-negative bacilli
2 wks–3 mos	*C. trachomatis*
	Viral
	N. gonorrhoeae
	Staphylococcus aureus
	Streptococcus species
	E. coli and other gram-negative bacilli
> 3 mos	Viral
	Allergic
	Bacterial (any of the above)

From Diamond GR: Red eye. In Fleischer G, Ludwig S (eds): Textbook of Pediatric Emergency Medicine. Baltimore, Williams & Wilkins, 1983, p 229; with permission.

192. Can bacterial conjunctivitis be distinguished from viral conjunctivitis on clinical grounds alone?

Classically, bacterial conjunctivitis is more commonly seen in infants and young children with the discharge being mucopurulent or purulent. Viral conjunctivitis presents with a serous exudate in children of all ages. Bacterial infections are commonly associated with otitis media, and otoscopy should be done on all patients. However, clinical findings can overlap. Both bacteria and viruses can cause unilateral or bilateral symptoms.

Common bacterial etiologies of conjunctivitis include nontypable *Haemophilus influenzae*, *Streptococcus pneumoniae* and *Moraxella catarrhalis*. Staphylococcal species frequently grow in cultures but usually are not a primary cause of the pathology. Aside from culture, the best way to distinguish the culprit is by Giemsa stain of a conjunctival scraping. Neutrophils predominate in bacterial infections, lymphocytes in viral infections, and eosinophils in allergic conjunctivitis.

Weiss A: Acute conjunctivitis in childhood. Curr Probl Pediatr 24:4–11, 1994.

193. What is keratoconjunctivitis?

Keratoconjunctivitis is an inflammatory process that involves both the conjunctiva and cornea. Superficial inflammation of the cornea occurs commonly in association with viral and bacterial conjunctivitis, particularly in adults. Hence, many cases of conjunctivitis are more correctly termed keratoconjunctivitis.

Epidemic keratoconjunctivitis is caused by adenovirus serotypes 8, 19, and 37. Some organisms, including *Pseudomonas aeruginosa*, *Neisseria gonorrhoeae*, and herpes simplex virus have a propensity to cause more severe infection of the cornea. Infection due to these pathogens must be recognized early in order to prevent corneal scarring with subsequent vision loss.

194. Are topical antibiotics effective in treating acute conjunctivitis?

Topical antibiotics have been demonstrated to speed eradication of the organism and to shorten the duration of symptoms in most cases of bacterial conjunctivitis. However, there are several notable exceptions. Topical therapy for chlamydial conjunctivitis is generally ineffective in adults and should never be used as sole therapy in the neonate because of the high likelihood of concomitant respiratory tract colonization (which may eventually progress to pneumonia). Viral conjunctivitis, of course, does not respond to topical antibiotics. Finally, infections due to *Neisseria gonorrhoeae*, *Pseudomonas*, *Haemophilus influenzae* type b, and possibly *N. meningitidis* require systemic therapy to prevent the serious complications seen with these organisms.

195. What is the best method of prophylaxis for ophthalmia neonatorum?

Previously, gonococcal ophthalmia was the most common cause of neonatal conjunctivitis. With the use of 1.0% silver nitrate drops, the rate of this illness dropped to 0.03%. However, silver nitrate drops frequently cause a chemical conjunctivitis (which resolves by about 4 days) and are not completely effective against *Chlamydia*, which is now the predominant etiology of neonatal conjunctivitis. Erythromycin 0.5% ophthalmic ointment and tetracycline 1.0% ophthalmic ointment are now also used in the U.S., although their efficacy in preventing chlamydial disease remains unclear. Worldwide, other methods are utilized. In one large study of > 3000 infants in Kenya, 2.5% povidone-iodine ophthalmic solution was a more effective prophylaxis against neonatal conjunctivitis than silver nitrate drops or erythromycin ointment, and it was considerably cheaper.

Isenberg SJ: A controlled trial of povidone-iodine as prophylaxis against ophthalmia neonatorum. N Engl J Med 332:562–566, 1995.

196. Describe the recommended therapy for gonococcal ophthalmia neonatorum.

Gonococcal ophthalmia neonatorum is a serious disease with the potential for blindness and should be treated with a parenteral antibiotic. Initial therapy should include a third-generation cephalosporin (e.g., ceftriaxone, 25–50 mg/kg once daily, or cefotaxime, 50–100 mg/kg/day divided every 12 hrs). If the isolate is subsequently found to be sensitive to penicillin, crystalline penicillin G may be substituted. Eye irrigation with buffered saline should be instilled until the discharge resolves. In the absence of disseminated disease, the recommended duration of parenteral therapy is 7 days. Some studies have demonstrated the efficacy of a single dose of intramuscular ceftriaxone in infants with localized disease. However, this approach is not currently recommended.

The diagnosis of gonococcal ophthalmia should prompt a thorough search for disseminated gonococcal infection. Careful physical examination should be performed, and blood and CSF should be obtained for culture. In infants who fail to respond adequately to therapy, simultaneous infection with *Chlamydia trachomatis* should be considered.

197. Can newborns with chlamydial conjunctivitis be treated with topical therapy alone?

Newborns diagnosed with chlamydial conjunctivitis should receive systemic therapy with an oral antibiotic. Topical therapy will not eradicate the organism from the upper respiratory tract and fails to prevent development of chlamydia pneumonia. Erythromycin estolate (10 mg/kg/dose every 8–12 hrs) or erythromycin ethylsuccinate (10 mg/kg/dose very 6 hrs) should be given for 2–3 weeks. Close follow-up is indicated thereafter to ensure the absence of relapse.

198. Are ophthalmic solutions better than ophthalmic ointments in eradicating conjunctivitis?

Ophthalmic ointments are usually preferred in infants and young children because they can be instilled more reliably and remain in the eye for a longer time. In older children, ophthalmic solutions may be preferred to prevent blurring of vision which occurs with ointments. In general, the efficacy of ophthalmic ointments is presumed to be superior to solutions. However, several antibiotics are available in high concentration solutions. These "fortified" formulations have not been prospectively compared to other preparations but are widely used because of their presumed enhanced efficacy.

199. What are the side effects of neomycin in eye ointment preparations?

Neomycin eye ointment may cause a localized contact dermatitis. Less commonly the medication may sensitize individuals and lead to rash or other systemic reactions upon reexposure to neomycin. Anaphylactic reactions are rare, but if they occur, the subsequent use of MMR vaccine is contraindicated, as it contains this antibiotic.

200. Name the most common cause of the Parinaud oculoglandular syndrome.

This granulomatous or ulcerating conjunctivitis is accompanied by prominent preauricular or submandibular adenopathy. The most common cause is cat scratch disease, but other causes include tularemia, sporotrichosis, tuberculosis, syphilis, and Lyme disease.

201. What comprises the clinical triad of Behçet syndrome?
1. Recurrent aphthous stomatitis
2. Vulvar ulcerations (painless, but may lead to marked scarring)
3. Ocular inflammation (especially uveitis)
The etiology is unclear, but an autoimmune basis is suspected.

202. How is orbital cellulitis distinguished from periorbital (or preseptal) cellulitis?
   Periorbital cellulitis is inflammation/infection in the tissues anterior to the eyelid septum. **Orbital cellulitis** is a deeper and more dangerous extension into the orbit which may lead to abscess formation and/or cavernous sinus thrombosis. Clinically, the most important evaluations are ocular mobility (e.g., extraocular muscle function), pupillary reflex, visual acuity, and changes in globe position (e.g., proptosis). In periorbital cellulitis, these aspects are normal. Abnormalities in any of these four areas suggest the deeper infection of orbital cellulitis, mandating radiologic evaluation (usually CT scan of the orbit) and possible surgical drainage. Significant eyelid swelling may occur in both types, making visualization of the globe difficult. However, an adequate exam usually can be obtained using eyelid retractors. Although most cases are unilateral (90%), evaluation of the unaffected eye may be helpful. Occasionally, a reflex sympathetic response of abnormal ocular mobility occurs in the unaffected eye, suggesting the deeper infection.

203. What is the difference between hordeolum, stye, and chalazion?
   Clinically, very little. For anatomic and pathologic purists, there are moderate differences. The sebaceous and apocrine sweat glands of the eyelid consist of those that drain near the eyelash follicle (glands of Moll and Zeis) and those that drain nearer the conjunctiva (meibomian glands).
   Hordeolum—purulent, usually staphylococcal infection of these glands; external hordeolum on skin side if Moll or Zeis involved, and internal hordeolum on conjunctival side if meibomian; red, swollen, tender; a mini-abscess.
   Stye—an external hordeolum
   Chalazion—initially a noninflamed lipogranulomatous swelling in the meibomian gland which readily can become superinfected; an internal hordeolum; more likely to be chronic and require excision.
   No matter what the name, all are treated with warm compresses and topical antibiotic drops and usually resolve within 7 days.

OTITIS MEDIA

204. How commonly does cerumen obscure the diagnosis of otitis media?
   Secreted by sebaceous and apocrine glands at the base of hair follicles in the outer third of the ear, cerumen comes in all forms—wet and brown in blacks and whites, and dry and flaky in Orientals. Surprisingly, as many as 50% of white children have no obvious cerumen seen on inspection. When otitis media is part of a differential diagnosis (as in unexplained fever), cerumen must be removed to allow visualization of the tympanic membrane. As many as 30% of cases of otitis media are obscured by this waxy roadblock. Unfortunately, lack of pain is not a helpful clue in diagnosis in that 15–20% of children with otitis media do not have ear pain. The old tale of otitis media being associated with soft wax (from melting by the "hot ear") is unfounded, with that finding occurring in only 10% of cases.
   Schwartz RH: et al: Cerumen removal: How necessary is it to diagnose acute otitis media? Am J Dis Child 137:1065–1068, 1983.

205. Is ear pulling a reliable sign of infection?
   In the absence of other signs or symptoms (e.g., fever, upper respiratory infection symptoms), ear pulling alone is a very poor indicator of acute otitis media.
   Baker RB: Is ear pulling associated with ear infection [letter]? Pediatrics 90:1006–1007, 1992.

206. How often will acute otitis media resolve spontaneously without antibiotics?
Overall, roughly **60%**. It is this high rate of spontaneous improvement that confounds the comparison of drug treatments. Of note, infection due to *Streptococcus pneumoniae* is unlikely to resolve without specific antibiotic treatment (in only 20% of cases).
McCracken GH Jr: Considerations in selecting an antibiotic for treatment of acute otitis media. Pediatr Infect Dis J 13:1054–1057, 1994.

207. Should all children with acute otitis media be treated with antibiotics?
Because of the high rate of spontaneous improvement, some suggest that children (especially those over 2 years of age) may not routinely require antibiotic therapy for uncomplicated otitis media. However, placebo-controlled trials have demonstrated that treatment with an antimicrobial agent shortens the duration of symptoms. Moreover, several studies demonstrate that the use of an antibiotic that is ineffective against the patient's middle ear pathogens is associated with a higher incidence of therapeutic failure. The argument for routine use of antimicrobial agents in otitis media is strengthened by the rare but potentially fatal complications of untreated otitis media. In the pre-antibiotic era, 3% of cases of otitis media were associated with intracranial complications, such as mastoiditis, meningitis, or lateral sinus thrombosis. Since the availability of antimicrobial therapy, the incidence of intracranial complications has decreased to approximately 0.15%. Because of this potential for complications, watchful waiting is not presently recommended.
Berman S: Otitis media in children. N Engl J Med 332:1560–1565, 1995.
Rosenfeld RM:What to expect from medical treatment of otitis media. Pediatr Infect Dis J 14:731–738, 1995.

208. Following an acute episode of otitis media, how long does the middle ear effusion persist?
Approximately 70% of patients will continue to have an effusion at 2 weeks, 40% at 1 month, 20% at 2 months, and 5–10% at 3 months.

209. Name the most common viral and bacterial agents causing otitis media.
Tympanocentesis yields positive bacterial cultures in 65–90% of cases of acute otitis media. Virus or viral antigen is detected from middle ear fluid in 10–25% of cases. The significance of virus in the middle ear fluid is debated, though it seems clear that concomitant viral infection may prolong the course of bacterial otitis media and lead to treatment failures.

Common Bacteria and Viruses Identified in Middle Ear Fluid

BACTERIAL ISOLATES		VIRAL ISOLATES	
Streptococcus pneumoniae	43%	Respiratory syncytial virus	7%
Moraxella catarrhalis	21%	Rhinovirus	3%
Haemophilus influenzae	18%	Influenza virus	2%
Streptococcus pyogenes	4%	Adenovirus	2%
Other	4%	Parainfluenza virus	2%

Values are the percent of total aspirates.
Adapted from Ruuskanen O, et al: Viruses in acute otitis media: Increasing evidence for clinical significance. Pediatr Infect Dis J 10:425–427, 1991.
Del Beccaro MA, et al: Bacteriology of acute otitis media: A new perspective. J Pediatr 120:81–84, 1992.

210. What percentage of otitis media is caused by ampicillin-resistant organisms?
About 25% of *Haemophilus influenzae* and 75% of *Moraxella catarrhalis* infections produce β-lactamases (subject to local variation). Thus, it can be estimated that about 20% of cases of otitis media, in an average location, will be resistant to ampicillin. Precise knowledge of local resistance patterns is a far better guide.

211. What are the indications for tympanocentesis?
1. A "toxic" appearing child
2. Unsatisfactory response to antibiotics

3. Any suppurative complication
4. Immunosuppressed host
5. Newborn infant in whom the usual bacterial pathogens may not be the causative agents

212. When is operative intervention indicated in children with mastoiditis?

Most children with mastoiditis will need a conduit for pus to drain. The surgical approach to establishing such a conduit may be as simple as a tympanostomy tube. Posterior auricular fluctuance should be drained, and the procedure should be hastened if signs of neurologic involvement are detected.

213. Describe the immediate and long-term complications of otitis media.

The most dangerous immediate complications of acute otitis media involve local suppurative spread to structures within the temporal bone and beyond into other compartments of the cranial vault: mastoiditis, labyrinthitis, facial nerve paralysis, osteomyelitis, epidural abscess, lateral sinus thrombosis, otic hydrocephalus, meningitis, and brain abscess. Fortunately, in the antibiotic era, these complications have become rare. Other complications include perforation of the tympanic membrane, tympanosclerosis, fixation of the ossicles, cholesteatoma, chronic otitis media, and hearing loss. There is evidence that repeated bouts of otitis media may have adverse effects on speech development, language acquisition, and cognitive abilities.

214. When should prophylactic antibiotics be considered in children with recurrent otitis media?

Strategies vary, but a common approach is to initiate prophylactic treatment in a child with 3 episodes of otitis in 6 months or 4 in 1 year. The younger the child, the more likely is recurrence. Some experts have suggested more stringent criteria because of concerns about the emergence of resistant bacteria.

Several studies have demonstrated that chronic use of an oral antimicrobial can decrease the incidence of recurrence. Amoxicillin (20 mg/kg once daily) and sulfonamides have been studied most widely, though trimethoprim-sulfamethoxasole and erythromycin have also been found to be effective. However, the efficacy of prophylactic antibiotics is marginal in most studies, regardless of the agent.

Paradise JL: Antimicrobial prophylaxis for recurrent otitis media. Ann Otol Rhinol Laryngol (Suppl)33:155, 1992.

Paradise JL: Managing otitis media: A time for change. Pediatrics 96:712–715, 1995.

215. What are the indications for myringotomy tubes?

Myringotomy tubes are most commonly inserted for the treatment of otitis media with effusion (OME) or for prophylaxis against recurrent otitis media. OME, also known as serous otitis media, secretory otitis media, or "glue ear," is defined as the presence of fluid in the middle ear in the absence of acute inflammation. It is felt to be a sequela of acute otitis media and is the most common cause of hearing deficit in children. A child with fluid persisting in both middle ears ≥ 3 months should undergo hearing evaluation. Tympanostomy tube placement has been shown to improve hearing in children with OME during the initial 6 months after the procedure. The benefits are less marked thereafter, partially due to extrusion of the tubes. Myringotomy tube placement may be complicated by sclerosis, retraction, or atrophy of the eardrum. Hence, some recommend a trial of chronic antibiotic therapy prior to insertion of the tubes.

Myringotomy tube placement has also been demonstrated to be effective in decreasing the incidence of recurrent otitis media in the "otitis-prone" child. As with prophylactic antibiotic therapy, the benefit of tube placement is modest and must be weighed against the risk of complications. Therefore, in the child with recurrent otitis media or secretory otitis media, a trial of long-term antimicrobial therapy appears justified. If this therapy is ineffective, then tympanostomy tube placement is a reasonable option.

Otitis Media Guideline Panel: Managing otitis media with effusion in young children. Pediatrics 94:766–772, 1994.

216. Should a child with tympanostomy tubes be allowed to swim?

Controlled studies have shown that the rate of otorrhea is similar between nonswimmers (15%) and surface swimmers (20%) without earplugs. If diving or underwater swimming is planned, fitted earplugs are recommended. Bath water with shampooing does seem to cause inflammatory changes in the middle ear; if head dunking is anticipated, ear plugs should be used.

Isaacson G, Rosenfeld RM: Care of the child with tympanostomy tubes: A visual guide for the pediatrician. Pediatrics 93:924–929, 1994.

217. Is pneumococcal vaccine useful for prevention of otitis media?

Streptococcus pneumoniae is the most common pathogen identified in studies of the bacteriology of acute otitis media in children. Vaccination against pneumococcus might therefore be expected to decrease the incidence of otitis media. Unfortunately, this is not the case with the currently available vaccine which utilizes purified capsular polysaccharides from 23 pneumococcal serotypes. The polysaccharides are poor immunogens in young infants, and this is especially true for the serotypes that are most commonly associated with otitis media. Future vaccines will likely be modified so that the capsular polysaccharide will be conjugated to a protein antigen, a strategy that has proved successful in the development of vaccines against *Haemophilus influenzae* type b.

Anderson P, Betts R: Human adult immunogenicity of protein-coupled pneumococcal capsular antigens of serotypes prevalent in otitis media. Pediatr Infect Dis J 8:S50–S53, 1989.

218. A child with the acute onset of ear pain and double vision likely has what condition?

Gradenigo syndrome is an acquired paralysis of the abducens muscle with pain in the area served by the ipsilateral trigeminal nerve. It is caused by inflammation of the sixth cranial nerve in the petrous portion with involvement of the gasserian ganglion. The inflammation is usually due to infection from otitis media or mastoiditis. Symptoms may include weakness of lateral gaze on the affected side, double vision, pain, photophobia, tearing, and hyperesthesia.

PHARYNGEAL/LARYNGEAL INFECTIONS

219. Can group A streptococcal pharyngitis be diagnosed clinically?

Streptococcal pharyngitis is a disease with variable clinical manifestations. Clues suggesting streptococcal disease include the abrupt onset of headache, fever, and sore throat with subsequent physical findings of tender cervical lymph nodes, exudate over the tonsils, and palatal petechiae. The presence of concurrent conjunctivitis, rhinitis, or cough suggests a viral process. The physical findings are by no means diagnostic. Even the most skilled clinician cannot exceed an accuracy rate of about 75%. Antigen testing and/or a throat culture is essential for confirming streptococcal infection.

220. What is the rationale for treatment of group A streptococcal pharyngitis?

- To prevent acute rheumatic fever. Even with the marked decline in incidence of acute rheumatic fever in the United States, it is still prevalent in much of the world.
- In comparison with placebo, penicillin can shorten the course of illness, relieve headache and sore throat, and reduce the frequency of tender cervical lymph nodes.
- To reduce the spread of infection and prevent suppurative complications.
- Some cases of acute glomerulonephritis may also be prevented.

221. Should all children with a positive culture for group A streptococci be treated?

Symptomatic children whose throat cultures yield group A β-hemolytic streptococci should be treated. There is a growing conviction among experts that asymptomatic children who are merely carrying streptococci should not be treated. An easy way to avoid the quandary is not to culture such children and sow the seeds of "streptococcal neurosis" in the family. This policy precludes the reculturing of asymptomatic children who have completed treatment for sore throats.

An exception to the general rule of leaving asymptomatic carriers alone would be a carrier in household contact with a patient with rheumatic fever.

Dajani A, et al: Treatment of acute streptococcal pharyngitis and prevention of rheumatic fever: A statement for health professionals. Pediatrics 96:758–764, 1995.

222. How does one differentiate a patient with a sore throat who is a streptococcal carrier with an intercurrent viral pharyngitis from one who is having repeated episodes of group A β-hemolytic streptococcal (GABHS) pharyngitis?

Streptococcal carrier:
- Signs and symptoms of viral infection (rhinorrhea, cough, conjunctivitis, diarrhea)
- Wrong season (streptococcal illness usually occurs in winter and early spring)
- Little clinical response to antibiotics (sometimes difficult to assess because of self-resolving nature of viral infections)
- GABHS present on culture between episodes
- No serologic response (i.e., anti-streptolysin O, anti-deoxyribonuclease)
- Same serotype of GABHS

Recurrent GABHS:
- Signs and symptoms consistent with GABHS
- Seasonal clustering
- Marked clinical response to antibiotics
- No GABHS between episodes
- Positive serologic response
- Different serotypes of GABHS

Gerber MA: Treatment failures and carriers: Perception or problems? Pediatr Infect Dis J 13:576–579, 1994.

223. What are the acceptable alternative therapies for streptococcal pharyngitis?

Except in penicillin-allergic patients, **penicillin V** is the drug of choice as there have been no documented reports of Group A streptococcal resistance to penicillin. IM **benzathine penicillin** has the advantage of guaranteed compliance but the disadvantage of being painful. Oral **penicillin VK** for 10 days is a good alternative. **Erythromycin** is the most widely recommended agent for penicillin-allergic patients, although many such patients will tolerate **cephalosporins, clarithromycin,** and **clindamycin.** Sulfonamides and trimethoprim-sulfamethoxazole are not appropriate. Similarly, 20–40% of *Streptococcus pyogenes* isolates are resistant to tetracyclines.

224. When can children treated for positive streptococcal throat cultures return to school or daycare?

Although clinical improvement can precede culture negativity, one study found that 85% of patients became culture-negative after treatment for 24 hours. Very few became negative within 14 hours after a single dose of antibiotic. To minimize contagion, a full 24 hours of antibiotic therapy (slightly longer if erythromycin is used) appear to be warranted before a return to school or daycare.

Snellman LW, et al: Throat cultures for group A streptococci. Pediatrics 91:1166–1170, 1993.

225. After completion of therapy for streptococcal pharyngitis, is a reculture necessary?

In the past, many clinicians advocated repeat throat cultures to ensure that group A streptococci had been eradicated. However, it now appears that upper respiratory tract carriers will continue to harbor streptococci after seemingly appropriate treatment. In most cases, persistent carriage is inconsequential and can be ignored. Exceptions include when there is a rheumatic individual in the household or epidemic streptococcal disease in the community. Treatment with either clindamycin or the combination of rifampin and penicillin appears to be most effective in eradicating the carrier state.

226. How long after the development of streptococcal pharyngitis can treatment be initiated and still effectively prevent rheumatic fever?

Treatment should be started as soon as possible, but little is lost in waiting for throat culture results to establish the diagnosis. Although such a delay is not desirable, significant reduction in the occurrence of rheumatic fever can still be achieved when therapy is delayed as long as 1 week.

227. What is the difference between herpangina and Ludwig's angina?

Herpangina is a common viral infection during the summer and fall characterized by posterior pharyngeal, buccal, and palatal vesicles and ulcers. Coxsackieviruses A and B and echoviruses are the most common causative agents. In young children, it is often accompanied by a high fever (103–104°F). Herpangina is distinguished from herpes simplex infections of the mouth, which are more anterior and involve the lips, tongue and gingiva.

Ludwig's angina is an acute diffuse infection (usually bacterial) of the submandibular and sublingual spaces with brawny induration of the floor of the mouth and tongue. Airway obstruction may occur. The infections usually follow oral cavity injuries or dental complications (e.g., extractions, impactions).

228. What is quinsy?

Peritonsillar abscess (from Lower Latin for an inflammation of the throat).

229. How is peritonsillar abscess distinguished from peritonsillar cellulitis?

A peritonsillar abscess is diagnosed when a discrete mass is palpated. The bulging abscess causes displacement of the uvula. Trismus more commonly occurs in the setting of abscess than simple cellulitis, which is characterized by signs of diffuse inflammation only.

230. What x-ray features suggest the diagnosis of a retropharyngeal abscess?

When a patient's neck is extended, a measurement of the retropharyngeal space exceeding two times the diameter of the C2 vertebra suggests an abscess. Pockets of air in the space also suggest abscess. The retropharyngeal space extends to T1 in the superior mediastinum, so empyema or mediastinitis is also possible whenever a retropharyngeal abscess is identified.

231. Which age group is most susceptible to retropharyngeal abscess?

This disease is most common between **ages 1–6**. There are several small lymph nodes in the retropharyngeal space which usually disappear by age 4 or 5. These lymph nodes drain the posterior nasal passages and nasopharynx, and they may become involved if those sites are infected.

232. What are the indications for removing the tonsils and adenoids?

Although the presence of tonsils and adenoids is no longer a reason to remove them, neither is their presence a dictum to keep them. Bluestone and colleagues have written extensively on this subject and divide indications into definite and relative:

Definite	Relative
• Obstructive tonsils/adenoids (i.e., causing obstructive apnea or cor pulmonale)	• Peritonsillar abscess
• Malignancy	• Recurrent documented tonsillitis
• Persistent or recurrent tonsillar hemorrhage	• Chronic otitis media with effusion

Although few will quibble with the absolute indications, the relative ones tend to generate vigorous discussion and may break up friendships. In the classic study by Paradise et al., tonsillectomy did reduce the number of episodes of tonsillitis for the first few years following surgery compared to the nonsurgical controls. However, some children in the nonsurgical group also had decreased tonsillitis in that 2-year period. Because entry criteria regarding the number and frequency of infections were strict, extrapolation to individuals with undocumented or less-frequent infections is not warranted. The question boils down to whether, in your clinical opinion, the likely 2-year improvement in symptoms warrants the risk and cost of tonsillectomy. Remember, "the lesser the indication, the greater the complication."

Bluestone CD: Current indications for tonsillectomy and adenoidectomy. Ann Otol Rhinol Laryngol 101:58–64, 1992.

Paradise JL, et al: Efficacy of adenoidectomy for recurrent otitis media in children previously treated with tympanostomy-tube placement. JAMA 263:2066–2073, 1990.

233. How should children with epiglottitis be managed?

Acute epiglottitis is a medical emergency, and all children should be assumed to have a critical airway, i.e., capable of imminent occlusion. Because of the risk of airway obstruction upon agitation, the patient should be allowed to remain with parents, free from restraint, and examined as delicately as possible. If necessary, this may be done from a distance and always without inspection of the oropharynx because of the risk of provoking obstruction. Continuous observation regardless of the setting (e.g., radiology suite), avoidance of supine positioning, and arrangements for intensive care admission are mandatory. Ideally, direct visualization of the epiglottis is done in an operating room, and at that time, prophylactic or therapeutic intubation can be performed.

Previously, > 90% of cases were caused by *Haemophilus influenzae* type b. However, because of the routine use of Hib vaccines in infants, the incidence of epiglottitis has decreased dramatically, and greater numbers of cases are now due to group A streptococci.

234. How is epiglottitis distinguished clinically from croup?

Clinical Distinctions Between Croup and Epiglottitis

CROUP	EPIGLOTTITIS
Age	
Younger (6 mos–3 yrs)	Older (3–7 yrs)
Onset of stridor	
Gradual (24–72 hrs)	Rapid (8–12 hrs)
Symptoms	
Prodromal URI	Minimal rhinitis
Harsh, brassy cough	Little coughing
Hoarseness	Muffled voice
Slightly sore throat	Pain in throat
Signs	
Mild fever	High fever (> 39°C)
Not toxic	Toxic appearance
Variable distress	Severe distress; sits upright; may drool
Harsh inspiratory stridor	Low-pitched inspiratory stridor
Expiratory sounds uncommon	May have a low-pitched expiratory sound
Radiology	
Subglottic narrowing	Edema of epiglottis and aryepiglottic folds (positive "thumb" sign)

235. What is the cause of severe pulmonary edema in a child who has been recently intubated for epiglottitis?

This is a fairly common clinical scenario. Two explanations have been suggested for the development of pulmonary edema.

1. With severe upper airway obstruction, the intrathoracic pressure swings may become very great with negative pressures as high as 70–80 cm H_2O. This hydrostatic gradient far exceeds the oncotic pressure of plasma, and water tends to move into the lung interstitium.

2. A better explanation is that the negative intrathoracic pressure causes an increased venous return to the heart, with an increase in pulmonary vascular volume and impaired left ventricular ejection fraction. This could cause an increase in the ultrafiltration of fluid into the interstitium,

which is masked during the period of obstruction by the very positive pressures that develop during exhalation. After relief of the obstruction, the patient's own PEEP is removed and the pulmonary edema may become apparent. Pulmonary edema is manifested by pink, frothy secretions when the child is intubated. These secretions may be dispersed by nebulized ethyl alcohol to break up the foam if it is causing airway obstruction.

Kanter RK, Watchko JF: Pulmonary edema associated with upper airway obstruction. Am J Dis Child 138:356–358, 1984.

236. What are the criteria for admission of a child with viral croup?

1. Clinical signs of impending respiratory failure: marked retractions, depressed level of consciousness, cyanosis, hypotonicity, and diminished or absent inspiratory breath sounds

2. Laboratory signs of impending respiratory failure: $PCO_2 > 45$ mm Hg, $PaO_2 < 70$ mmHg in room air

3. Clinical signs of dehydration

4. Social considerations: unreliable parents, excessive distance from hospital

5. Historic considerations: high-risk infant with history of subglottic stenosis, prior intubations

6. Debatably, previous administration of racemic epinephrine (see next question)

237. If a child has received racemic epinephrine as a treatment for croup, is hospitalization required?

Previous dogma has been that children treated in this fashion should be hospitalized to observe for potential rebound effects of worsening mucosal edema and airway obstruction, regardless of how they appear clinically. A number of studies have shown that children who are free of significant stridor or retractions at rest 3 hours after the administration of racemic epinephrine may be safely discharged if adequate follow-up is assured. In most of these studies oral or IM dexamethasone (0.6 mg/kg) was also administered. The issue of the safety of outpatient use of racemic epinephrine continues to be debated.

Ledwith CA, et al: Safety and efficacy of nebulized racemic epinephrine in conjunction with oral dexamethasone and mist in the outpatient treatment of croup. Ann Emerg Med 25:331–337, 1995.

238. Is a cool mist vaporizer truly of benefit in croup?

The usual advice given for home management of croup consists of placing a child in a steamy bathroom or the breathing of outside cold night air followed by cool mist vaporizer (or humidifier) therapy. The theory is that the coolness serves as a vasoconstrictor and the mist serves to thin respiratory secretions. However, it remains a time-honored but largely unproven therapy. One small study found no differences between control and mist-treated infants. The calming effects of being held by a parent during the mist treatment may have greater impact.

Bourchier D, et al: Humidification in viral croup: A controlled trial. Aust Paediatr J 20:289, 1984.

239. Are steroids efficacious in croup?

The use of corticosteroids (including intramuscular dexamethasone, oral prenisolone, and nebulized budesonide) has been shown to be beneficial in patients hospitalized for croup. In particular, corticosteroid treatment reduces the incidence of intubation and results in more rapid respiratory improvement. For milder outpatient cases of croup, it is uncertain whether treatment will prevent hospitalization and prolonged emergency room visits with acceptably few adverse side effects for what is usually a self-limited condition. At present, intramuscular dexamethasone at a dose of 0.3–0.6 mg/kg is commonly used on an outpatient basis.

Klassen TP, et al: Nebulized budesonide for children with mild-to-moderate croup. N Engl J Med 331:285–289, 1994.

Cruz MN, et al: Use of dexamethasone in the outpatient management of acute laryngotracheitis. Pediatrics 96:220–223, 1995.

240. What is meant by pseudomembranous croup?

This older term was used for what is now more commonly referred to as **bacterial tracheitis** (membranous croup historically was diphtheria). Bacterial tracheitis has also been called nondiphtheritic laryngitis and membranous laryngotracheobronchitis. It is a bacterial infection, usually caused by *Staphylococcus aureus*, that occurs following a viral respiratory tract infection such as croup or following trauma to the neck or trachea. Its clinical presentation is similar to that of severe croup or epiglottitis. As a consequence, a lateral neck film is often obtained to rule out epiglottitis and sometimes reveals narrowing of the trachea from a thick, purulent exudate which can extend into both mainstem bronchi.

Donnelly BW: Bacterial tracheitis: A report of eight new cases and a review. Rev Infect Dis 12:729–735, 1990.

241. What characterizes spasmodic croup?

Spasmodic croup is a poorly understood cause of recurrent stridor, most commonly occurring in children ages 1–3 years, that resembles acute infectious laryngotracheobronchitis in many aspects. Unlike infectious croup, however, a prodrome of upper respiratory symptoms is often minimal or absent, and the patient is usually afebrile. The onset is sudden, typically at night, with inspiratory stridor and a brassy cough that responds to therapies used for infectious croup (e.g., cool mist, racemic epinephrine, corticosteroids). Recurrence is common. The pathogenesis is unclear, but an allergic and hypersensitivity component is suspected. For the rare patient who requires intubation, the pale and boggy mucosa of allergy is typical rather than the inflamed swelling of a primary infection.

SINUSITIS

242. When do the sinuses develop during childhood?

The maxillary and ethmoid sinuses are present at birth. Pneumatization of the sphenoid sinuses begins at approximately 2–3 years of age and is usually complete by about age 6. Frontal sinus pneumatization varies considerably, beginning around 3–7 years and finishing by age 12.

243. What percentage of teenagers do not have frontal sinuses when x-rays are obtained?

Frontal sinus pneumatization is absent in approximately 10% of the normal population.

244. List the predisposing factors for development of chronic sinusitis.

Allergic rhinitis, anatomic abnormalities (e.g., polyps, enlarged adenoids), impairment of mucociliary clearance (e.g., cystic fibrosis, primary ciliary dyskinesia), foreign bodies (e.g., nasogastric tube), and abnormalities in immune defense.

245. How often is sinus tenderness elicited in radiologically proven cases of sinusitis?

In acute sinusitis, sinus tenderness is demonstrable only 20% of the time, and in chronic sinusitis, almost never.

246. Is transillumination helpful in diagnosing sinusitis in children?

In general, transillumination of the sinuses is of limited value in the diagnosis of acute sinusitis in young children. One controlled trial demonstrated the technique to be of no use. However, clinicians experienced with the technique may find transillumination beneficial in the diagnosis of maxillary or frontal sinusitis in children > 10 years of age. It is recommended that interpretation be confined to the extremes of either normal transmission or no transmission of light through the sinuses.

Wald ER: Sinusitis in children. N Engl J Med 326:319–324, 1992.

247. Which radiographic views should be obtained in evaluating sinusitis?

In children younger than age 6, only the maxillary and ethmoid sinuses are clinically important, and 80% of children in this age group with acute sinusitis will have both sets of sinuses involved. Caldwell (anteroposterior) and Waters (occipitomental) views are necessary to assess these sinuses. To evaluate the frontal and sphenoid sinuses in older children, a lateral view should be ordered.

Wald ER: Radiographic sinusitis: Illusion or delusion? Pediatr Infect Dis J 12:792–793, 1993.

248. What constitutes an abnormal sinus x-ray?
  1. Complete opacification of a sinus cavity
  2. Mucosal thickening of at least 4 mm
  3. Presence of an air-fluid level

In general, sinus films are both sensitive and specific in patients suspected to have acute sinusitis clinically. Correlation with bacterial disease is also good. For example, if a patient has symptoms consistent with acute sinusitis (e.g., persistent nasal discharge of at least 10 days' duration and fever) and an abnormal sinus x-ray, a maxillary sinus aspirate for pathologic bacteria will be positive 70% of the time. It is noteworthy that in children < 1 year of age and in all cases of chronic sinusitis, the utility of x-rays is quite limited.

249. When should CT scans be considered in diagnosing sinusitis?
Scenarios that might warrant use of CT include:
  1. Complicated sinus disease with either orbital or CNS abnormalities
  2. Multiple recurrences
  3. Prolonged symptoms unresponsive to treatment in which anatomic abnormalities might be present and sinus surgery contemplated
  Wald ER: Chronic sinusitis in children. J Pediatr 127:339–347, 1995.

250. Which organisms are responsible for acute and chronic sinusitis in the pediatric age group?

In acute, uncomplicated sinusitis, the etiologic organisms closely parallel those associated with acute otitis media: *Streptococcus pneumoniae*, *Haemophilus influenzae*, and *Moraxella catarrhalis*. *Staphylococcus aureus* is rather rare. In nosocomial infections, gram-negative organisms are frequently recovered, whereas in the child with dental disease, anaerobes must be considered. Mucormycosis is also a concern in the immunosuppressed patient. *Pseudomonas* must always be considered in the patient with cystic fibrosis. While viruses may be responsible for the initiation of sinusitis, symptoms are invariably associated with bacterial superinfection. The precise role of bacterial infection in chronic sinusitis is unknown; where studies have been done, the same bacteria implicated in acute infection have been found.

251. For how long should sinus infections be treated?
Duration of therapy for acute sinusitis in children has not been studied systematically. Two approaches are suggested in the literature:
  1. The patient is treated with amoxicillin for a full 10–14 days. If symptoms persist, than an additional course with a β-lactamase-resistant antibiotic is implemented.
  2. More recently, due to the increasing number of β-lactam-resistant organisms found in acute sinusitis, investigators have suggested using a β-lactamase-resistant antibiotic from the outset. There is continued 7–10 days beyond resolution of symptoms. The total duration of therapy is therefore 2–3 weeks.

TUBERCULOSIS

252. Who should be screened for tuberculosis?
Previously, routine periodic screening with multiple puncture tests was a norm for the entire population of children. Routine screening of low-risk children in low-prevalence areas is no longer advised. Asymptomatic children living in high-prevalence areas should be considered for periodic testing (e.g., ages 4–6 and 11–16). In addition, testing with the Mantoux (purified protein derivative or PPD) test is recommended for high risk groups:
  • Contacts of adults with infectious TB
  • Those who are from, or have parents from, regions of the world with a high prevalence of TB
  • Those with abnormalities on chest x-ray suggestive of TB
  • Those with clinical evidence of TB
  • HIV-seropositive children

- Those with immunosuppressive conditions
- Those with other medical risk factors: diabetes mellitus,chronic renal failure, malnutrition
- Incarcerated adolescents
- Children frequently exposed to adults who are HIV-infected, homeless, users of intravenous and other street drugs, poor and medically indigent city dwellers, residents of nursing homes, migrant farm workers

From Committee on Infectious Diseases: Update on tuberculosis skin testing of children. Pediatrics 97:283, 1996; with permission.

253. When are various strengths of PPD used?

The standard strength of PPD, designated intermediate strength, is 5 tuberculin units (TU). This strength is used for routine skin test screening (Mantoux test). PPD is also available in dose strengths of 1 (first strength) or 250 units (second strength). The 1-TU strength is used only in patients who are suspected of having intense tuberculin skin test reactivity. The 250-TU strength is occasionally used in individuals who have skin test negativity with 5 units when one wants to determine whether reactivity will occur with much higher strength. A positive reaction at 250-unit strength may indicate infection either with *Mycobacterium tuberculosis* or nontuberculous mycobacteria.

254. How is the Mantoux (PPD) test interpreted in children?

The Mantoux test is interpreted in the context of clinical signs and symptoms and epidemiologic risk factors (e.g., known exposure). All reactions ≥ 15 mm are considered positive. Reactions of ≥ 5 mm or ≥ 10 mm may be positive depending on the following factors:

Reaction ≥ 5 mm
- Children in close contact with known or suspected infectious cases of TB
  Households with active or previouslyactive cases if treatment cannot be verified as adequate before exposure, was initiated after period of child's contact, or reactivation is suspected
- Children suspected to have tuberculous disease
  Chest x-ray consistent with active or previously active TB
  Clinical evidence of TB
- Children with immunosuppressive conditions or HIV infection

Reaction ≥ 10 mm
- Children at increased risk of dissemination
  Young age (< 4 years)
  Other medical risk factors: diabetes mellitus, chronic renal failure, malnutrition
- Children with increased environmental exposure
  Born or whose parents were born in high-prevalence regions of the world
  Frequently exposed to adults who are HIV-infected, homeless, users of intravenous and other street drugs, poor and medically indigent city dwellers, residents of nursing homes, incarcerated or institutionalized persons, and migrant farm workers
- Travel and exposure to high-prevalence regions of the world

From Committee on Infectious Disease: Update on tuberculosis skin testing of children. Pediatrics 97:283, 1996; with permission.

255. What are the reasons for false-negative skin testing with PPD?

- Testing during incubation period (2–10 weeks)
- Problems with administration technique
- Severe systemic TB infection (miliary or meningitis)
- Anergy, immunosuppression, malnutrition, or immunodeficiency
- Concurrent infection: measles, varicella, HIV, Epstein-Barr virus, *Mycoplasma*, mumps, rubella
- Recent viral immunization (measles)

From Callahan CW: Tuberculosis. In Schidlow DV, Smith DS (eds): A Practical Guide to Pediatric Respiratory Diseases. Philadelphia, Hanley & Belfus, 1994, p 107; with permission.

256. Why is a multiple puncture test (tine test) not considered an ideal test for tuberculosis?

1. The exact dose of antigen (either PPD or old tuberculin) cannot be standardized, making interpretation imprecise. Any positive test must be confirmed with a Mantoux test.

2. In a patient with a positive tine test, the need for follow-up Mantoux test can lead to a booster phenomenon if the patient has had a previous BCG vaccine or infection with nontuberculous mycobacteria. Interpretation can be confusing.

3. Significant variability exists in false-negative and especially false-positive rates.

4. The use of tine tests has led to parental reporting, which can be very unreliable.

Starke JR, Correa AG: Management of mycobacterial infection and disease. Pediatr Infect Dis J 14:455–470, 1995.

257. How should patients with a positive tuberculin test be evaluated?

The evaluation of a child with a positive tuberculin skin test begins with a thorough history and physical examination. *History* should search for clues suggestive of active infection, such as recurrent fevers, weight loss, adenopathy, or cough. A history of recurrent infections, either in the patient or a family member, may be suggestive of HIV infection, a risk factor for infection with *Mycobacterium tuberculosis*. Information from previous tuberculin skin testing is invaluable.

Epidemiologic information includes an evaluation of possible exposure to TB. A family history is obtained, including questions pertaining to chronic cough or weight loss in a family member or other contact. Travel history as well as current living arrangements should be elucidated. If the patient has immigrated to North America, a history of BCG vaccination should be ascertained.

Physical exam must be thorough and should focus on pulmonary, lymphatic, and abdominal systems. Examination should corroborate the history of BCG vaccination.

Laboratory evaluation, including a chest x-ray with a lateral film is the next stage. Family members and close contacts should undergo skin testing. In certain circumstances, chest x-rays should be performed on the child's contacts.

If there are no clinical or radiographic features suggestive of active TB, then no further evaluation is warranted, and the child is treated as having asymptomatic infection with *M. tuberculosis*. A single antituberculous agent is prescribed for 9 months' duration. If any of the preceding evaluation suggests active infection, samples of sputum or gastric aspirate, urine, and other appropriate sites (such as lymph node tissue) should be obtained for mycobacterial culture and Ziehl-Neelsen or auramine-rhodamine staining. The child is begun on combined antituberculous medications while awaiting culture results, and an aggressive search for the source of the child's infection is initiated.

258. In a younger child suspected of having tuberculosis, how should gastric aspirates be obtained?

Because younger children rarely produce sputum, gastric aspirates are a better source for potential culture of mycobacteria. They yield the organism in up to 40% of cases. The aspirate should be obtained early in the morning as the child awakens to sample overnight accumulations of respiratory secretions. The sample should be collected in a saline-free fluid, and the pH neutralized if there will be a delay in processing.

259. How have treatment courses for tuberculosis changed in recent years?

Recommendations for the treatment of active TB in children have evolved over the past several years. Previously, at least 9 months of therapy were suggested for uncomplicated pulmonary disease. Studies in adults and children have demonstrated that 6 months of combined antituberculous therapy (short-course therapy) is as effective as 9-month therapy. To date, the combined results of nine studies in pediatric patients have demonstrated the efficacy of 6-month therapy to be > 95%.

The current standard regimen for active TB in children consists of 2 months of daily isoniazid, rifampin, and pyrazinamide, followed by 4 months of isoniazid and rifampin (daily or twice weekly if directly observed). Meningitis, disseminated disease, and bone or joint infections are treated for 1 year. Asymptomatic infection is treated for 9 months with a single agent (isoniazid, unless the organism is known to be resistant).

These recommendations must be modified in situations when the patient is at risk of having a drug-resistant strain (e.g., an adult contact with a resistant organism or a local endemic pattern of high resistance). In this instance, a fourth medication, such as ethambutol or streptomycin, is added until the results of susceptibility testing are available.

260. Why are multiple antibiotics used in treating tuberculosis?

Two features of *Mycobacterium tuberculosis* make the organism difficult to eradicate once infection has been established. First, mycobacteria replicate slowly and may remain dormant for prolonged periods, but are susceptible to drugs only during active replication. Second, drug-resistant organisms exist naturally within a large population, even prior to the initiation of therapy. These features render the organism, when present in significant numbers, extremely difficult to eradicate with a single agent. Indeed, the ability to cure patients with asymptomatic infection with a single agent is based on the presence of a small number of organisms that are exposed to a bactericidal antibiotic for an extended period of time.

Starke JR: Multidrug therapy for tuberculosis in children. Pediatr Infect Dis J 9:785–793, 1990.

261. What are the side effects of rifampin?

Rifampin commonly causes an orange discoloration of tears and urine. Contact lenses may be permanently discolored or destroyed. Less common adverse effects include allergic or hypersensitivity reactions, hepatotoxicity, and a flu-like syndrome that occurs particularly with intermittent administration. Hepatotoxicity is unusual in previously health children. Adolescent and adult patients should be warned that rifampin may decrease the efficacy of oral contraceptives and may antagonize the effects of oral anticoagulants.

262. Why is pyridoxine supplementation given to patients who are receiving isoniazid?

Isoniazid interferes with pyridoxine metabolism and may result in peripheral neuritis or convulsions. Administration of pyridoxine is generally not necessary for children who have a normal diet, as they have adequate stores of this vitamin. Children or adolescents with diets deficient in milk or meat should receive pyridoxine supplementation during isoniazid therapy, as should breast-fed infants and pregnant women.

Committee on Infectious Diseases: Chemotherapy for tuberculosis in infants and children. Pediatrics 89:161–165, 1992.

263. How effective is BCG vaccination?

The bacille Calmette-Guérin (BCG) vaccines are among the most widely used in the world at present and are also perhaps the most controversial. The difficulties stem from the marked variation in reported efficacy of BCG against *Mycobacterium tuberculosis* and *M. leprae* infections. Depending on the population studied, efficacy against tuberculosis has ranged from 0–80%. Similarly, the efficacy against leprosy has ranged from 20–60% in prospective trials.

The vaccines were derived from a strain of *M. bovis* in 1906 and were subsequently dispersed to several laboratories around the world, where they were propagated under nonstandardized conditions. Hence, the vaccines in use today cannot be considered homogeneous. The marked variation in observed efficacy is poorly understood, though it may relate partially to variation among the vaccine strains.

264. Is there any indication for BCG use in the United States?

BCG is rarely used and the efficacy of the current vaccine is unknown. It is given primarily to tuberculin-negative individuals who are in close contact with active cases of untreated or ineffectively-treated pulmonary tuberculosis. It may be considered for groups with an excessive rate of new infections or when the usual methods of treatment have failed or are not feasible. BCG is a live vaccine and should not be used in individuals with primary immunodeficiencies, symptomatic HIV infection, or on steroids.

265. How do you tell the difference between the scar from smallpox vaccination and the scar of BCG vaccination?

The scar due to BCG vaccination is a round, slightly depressed area with irregular edges, 4–7 mm in diameter. Occasionally it is raised. The scar resulting from smallpox vaccination is often irregular in shape, larger, and less likely to be associated with keloid scar formation.

Fine PEM, et al: The distribution and implications of BCG scars in northern Malawi. Bull WHO 67:35–42, 1989.

266. How does BCG immunization influence tuberculosis skin testing?

BCG vaccination induces cell-mediated immunity against the antigens found in PPD. The area of induration ranges from 3–19 mm in diameter following skin testing, and the size of the reaction depends on the time since BCG vaccination, patient age, and frequency of tuberculin testing. In general, skin test reactivity decreased with time. As a rule, up to 1 year after the vaccination, a reaction of up to 15 mm can occur. After 3 years, the reaction should not be > 10 mm. Any reaction > 15 mm should not be attributed solely to BCG regardless of the duration of time elapsed since vaccination.

267. Why do children with tuberculosis rarely infect other children?

TB is transmitted via infected droplets of mucus that become airborne when an individual coughs or sneezes. Compared with adults, children with TB have factors that minimize their contagiousness:

1. Low density of organisms in sputum
2. Lack of cavitation or extensive infiltrates on chest x-ray
3. Lower frequency of cough
4. Lower volume and higher viscosity of sputum
5. Shorter duration of respiratory symptoms

Starke JR: Childhood tuberculosis during the 1990s. Pediatr Rev 13:343–353, 1992.

268. In addition to tuberculosis, what other airborne microbes can cause respiratory disease?

Airborne Microbial Diseases

DISEASE	AIRBORNE SOURCE
Aspergillosis	Conidiaspores from decaying vegetation and soil
Brucellosis	Aerosolized from carcasses of domestic and wild animals
Chickenpox	Aerosolized from respiratory secretions
Coccidioidomycosis	Arthroconidia from soil and dust
Cryptococcosis	Aerosolized from bird droppings
Histoplasmosis	Conidiaspores from bat or bird droppings
Legionnaire disease	Aerosolized contaminated water, especially air-conditioning cooling towers
Measles	Aerosolized respiratory secretions
Mucormycosis	Spores from soil
Psittacosis	*Chlamydia psittaci* from birds
Q fever	*Coxiella burnetii* from a variety of farm and other animals
Tularemia	Aerosolized from multiple wild animals, especially rabbits
Viral Nasopharyngitis, bronchiolitis, pneumonia	Aerosolized respiratory secretions

11. METABOLISM

Gerard T. Berry, M.D.

AMINO ACID DISORDERS

1. What is the risk to the fetus of a mother known to have phenylketonuria (PKU)?
Hyperphenylalaninemia during pregnancy can result in a variety of fetal malformations and long-term sequelae, including microcephaly, mental retardation, growth retardation, cardiac defects, and skeletal malformations. The risk of injury to a fetus increases with the maternal phenylalanine level. For mothers with classic PKU who are not on a phenylalanine-restricted diet, the risk of significant fetal injury is essentially 100%. For untreated mothers with milder variants of PKU (blood phenylalanine levels of 10–20 mg/dl), the risk is 10–20%.

2. Why is vitamin C given to newborn premature infants with a positive PKU test?
The most common cause of an abnormal PKU blood screening test in premature infants is hyperphenylalaninemia secondary to transient tyrosinemia of the newborn. Transient tyrosinemia appears to be caused by inadequate activity of *p*-hydroxyphenylpyruvic acid dioxygenase, a vitamin-C-dependent enzyme in the tyrosine degradative pathway. Administration of vitamin C increases the activity of the enzyme and facilitates metabolism of both tyrosine and its precursor, phenylalanine.

3. What are the varieties of hyperphenylalaninemia?

Types of Hyperphenylalaninemia

DISORDER	BLOOD PHENYLALANINE LEVEL (MG/DL)	ENZYME DEFECT	THERAPY
Classic phenylketonuria	> 20	Phenylalanine hydroxylase	Diet
Atypical phenylketonuria	12–20	Phenylalanine hydroxylase	Diet
Persistent mild hyper-phenylalaninemia	2–12	Phenylalanine hydroxylase	Diet
Transient hyperphenyl-alaninemia	2–20	Unknown	None
Transient tyrosinemia	2–12	? *p*-OH-phenylpyruvic acid dioxygenase deficiency ? Secondary to low vitamin C	Vitamin C, low-protein formula
Dihydropteridine reductase deficiency	12–20	Dihydropteridine reductase	Dopa, OH-tryptophan, tetrahydrobiopterin
Biopterin synthesis defects	12–20	Dihydrobiopterin synthetase, GTP-cyclohydrolase, 6-pyruvoyl tetrahydrobiopterin synthetase	Dopa, OH-tryptophan, tetrahydrobiopterin

4. Which children with PKU require treatment?
In addition to classic PKU, for which blood phenylalanine levels typically are > 20 mg/dl with unrestricted protein intake, several variant forms of PKU also have blood levels of phenylalanine that are persistently elevated above the normal range (< 2 mg/dl). Long-term follow-up studies indicate that phenylalanine levels > 10 mg/dl require some limitation of dietary phenylalanine intake.

5. What is the outcome for children with PKU treated in early infancy?

Theoretically, all complications of classical PKU can be prevented by (1) limitation of dietary phenylalanine to only the amount required for growth and (2) provision of adequate dietary tyrosine, which cannot be synthesized from phenylalanine by phenylalanine hydroxylase. The mean IQ of children who are treated from birth is only slightly lower than those of their unaffected siblings. Increasingly severe cerebral injury occurs when institution of dietary treatment is delayed after birth or if the diet is poorly managed after diagnosis.

6. What is the clinical significance of transient tyrosinemia in the newborn infant?

Neonates (especially premature infants) with transient tyrosinemia have been reported to be more lethargic than normal infants and to feed poorly. Controversy remains about the long-term significance of transient tyrosinemia and whether treatment with vitamin C and/or protein restriction is required. Two reports suggest that these infants are at increased risk for mild neurologic and developmental abnormalities during later childhood, but a definitive study has yet to be performed. A bias of ascertainment (i.e., sick premature infants) may explain these findings. Nevertheless, when hypertyrosinemia is found in an infant, a reasonable attempt should be made to restore the tyrosine and phenylalanine levels to normal with vitamin C and/or protein restriction.

7. Describe the characteristic clinical signs of alkaptonuria.

In alkaptonuria, incomplete metabolism of tyrosine and phenylalanine results in an increased concentration of homogentisic acid in blood and urine. Features include:
1. Dark urine on exposure to air (e.g., in a diaper)
2. Ochronosis (grayish discoloration of connective tissue)
3. Degenerative arthritis
4. Valvulitis and aortic degeneration

8. What physical findings help differentiate homocystinuria from Marfan syndrome?

Characteristic	Marfan Syndrome	Homocystinuria
Lens dislocation	Usually upward	Usually downward
Cornea, sclera	Flattened cornea, bluish sclera	Normal
Body habitus and skeleton	Tall, arachnodactyly, pectus deformity	Tall, arachnodactyly, pectus deformity
Joints	Markedly hyperextensible	Normal or mildly contracted, ankle eversion
Skin	Hyperextensible, striae, livedo reticularis	Eczema, malar flush
Hair	Normal	Thin, dry, reddish
Heart	Mitral valve prolapse and regurgitant aortic murmurs common	Mitral valve prolapse in some
Peripheral vasculature	Often severe varicosities	Diabetic-like peripheral vascular disease
Intelligence	Normal	Mental defect in 50–60%, frank psychosis in some
Inheritance	Autosomal dominant; sibs, one parent, and other generations affected	Autosomal recessive; parents unaffected but may be consanguineous
Other	Emphysema, pneumothorax	Hepatomegaly, osteoporosis

9. Why are patients with homocystinuria at risk for thrombotic disease?

Most evidence points to direct endothelial damage by homocysteine, exposing surfaces that activate platelet aggregation and thrombus formation. Homocysteine forms disulfide adducts with free cysteine and interferes with the formation of cysteine–cysteine disulfide bonds in proteins found in the vascular wall and suspensory connective tissue of the lens. The functions of many other proteins, such as protein C and coagulation factor VII, are also affected and may contribute to the vascular lesions that often develop in this disease.

10. Explain the difference between cystinuria and cystinosis.

Cystinuria is a defect of renal tubular and (in some) intestinal transport of dibasic amino acids (cystine, lysine, arginine, ornithine), named for the formation of renal stones from the least soluble amino acid, cystine. Clinical symptoms are limited essentially to those caused by chronic renal lithiasis—recurrent infection, obstruction, renal colic, hypertension, and renal failure. Abnormal growth or other complications attributable to low body cystine or other dibasic amino acid occur rarely, if ever.

Cystinosis is a lysosomal storage disease caused by defective lysosomal transport of cystine. In classic infantile nephropathic cystinosis, most clinical abnormalities are attributed to renal Fanconi syndrome present in almost all affected individuals. The biochemical characteristics are hyperchloremic metabolic acidosis from excessive bicarbonaturia, hypophosphatemia, glucosuria, and generalized aminoaciduria. The presenting clinical problems are growth failure, rickets, photophobia, and pigmentary retinopathy. Eventually, glomerular dysfunction progresses to renal failure, usually by age 10 in the classic form. Milder "adolescent" and "adult" forms of cystinosis are also known.

11. What entity classically causes the "blue diaper syndrome"?

Blue discoloration of the diaper is caused by **intestinal malabsorption** of the **amino acid tryptophan** as an apparently isolated defect of intestinal amino acid transport. Malabsorbed tryptophan is converted by colonic bacteria to indican, which causes blue staining of the diaper on exposure to air. Patients with tryptophan malabsorption may develop hypercalciuria, nephrocalcinosis, and failure to thrive. Curiously, patients with Hartnup disease, an inborn error of intestinal and renal transport of all neutral amino acids including tryptophan, do not develop the blue diaper syndrome despite intestinal malabsorption of tryptophan and conversion to indican and other indoles. Blue discoloration of diapers also has several nonmetabolic causes—methylene blue administration, food colorings, amitriptyline or triamterene ingestion, copper poisoning, and *Pseudomonas* urinary tract infections (bluish green).

CARBOHYDRATE DISORDERS

12. Name the three types of galactosemia.
- Galactose-1-phosphate uridyltransferase deficiency (classic galactosemia)
- Galactokinase deficiency
- Uridine diphosphogalactose epimerase deficiency

13. List the most common clinical findings in children with classic galactosemia.
Acute
- Poor feeding, vomiting, diarrhea
- Poor growth
- Jaundice, severe or prolonged; early in course of neonatal-onset disease, unconjugated bilirubin predominates
- Liver dysfunction—coagulopathy and elevated serum transaminases
- Hypoglycemia
- Cataracts
- *Escherichia coli* sepsis (50%)
Chronic
- Developmental disability, especially language
- Gastrointestinal symptoms following lactose ingestion
- Ovarian failure or hypofunction

14. What are the pathogenic mechanisms responsible for the clinical manifestations of galactosemia?

Increased levels of several metabolites of galactose are believed (but, in most cases, not proved) to cause injury in galactosemia:

Galactose-1-phosphate	Renal Fanconi syndrome
	Hepatocellular disease
	Decreased RBC survival leading to indirect hyperbilirubinemia
Galactitol (dulcitol)	Cataracts
	? Pseudotumor cerebri
Unknown	Ovarian failure
	Mental retardation or cognitive deficits
	Ataxia, dystonia, neurodegenerative disease

Some experts also speculate that abnormal glycoconjugate synthesis employing UDP-galactose may play a role in pathogenesis, but experimental evidence is limited.

15. What is the long-term outcome for children with classic galactosemia treated early in infancy?

Children with classic galactosemia who are treated from birth with galactose-free diets are spared the acute complications of galactosemia. However, ovarian insufficiency, which occurs in most affected females, may be caused by prenatal influences on ovarian development. In a few individuals, significant CNS disease (ataxia, dystonia, tremor) may develop late in childhood and progress despite excellent dietary management. In addition, minor neurologic problems, such as learning disabilities and speech disorders, occur in most patients despite strict observance of a galactose-free diet.

16. What is the earliest metabolic derangement seen in hereditary fructose intolerance?

Hypophosphatemia is the most characteristic metabolic derangement in hereditary fructose intolerance (hepatic aldolase B deficiency). Hypophosphatemia can occur within a few minutes of ingestion of fructose and before clinical symptoms appear and is usually followed by hyper-transaminasemia. Somewhat slower in evolution are **hypoglycemia** and severe **gastrointestinal distress**. Rapid hepatic uptake of inorganic phosphate for phosphorylation of fructose is probably the major factor causing the hypophosphatemia, but other factors, such as hyperphosphaturia, may contribute.

17. Does fructose produce any adverse effects?

Ingestion of excessive amounts of fructose in a normal individual can lead to lactic acidosis, hyperuricemia, and dental caries. Individuals with hereditary fructose intolerance who avoid all sources of fructose have a notable lack of dental caries.

18. What is the long-term outcome for children with hereditary fructose intolerance treated in infancy?

Most individuals with hereditary fructose intolerance (many of whom have self-selected a sucrose- and fructose-free diet) have normal health, growth, and intelligence. However, a few individuals under apparently good dietary management develop growth retardation because of sensitivity to very small amounts of fructose in the diet. Others on "fructose-free" diets develop seizures and deafness, but the relationship of these abnormalities to abnormal fructose metabolism or to possible unidentified dietary sources of fructose is uncertain.

19. Name the major natural sources of fructose ("fruit sugar") in the human diet.

- Most fruits and vegetables
- Sucrose (beet or cane sugar) = glucose-fructose disaccharide
- Molasses and many other natural sweeteners
- Processed corn sugar ("high-fructose" corn syrup)

• D-Sorbitol (artificial sweetener, oxidized to fructose in the liver)
• Some medications, especially liquid preparations (from sucrose)

20. What are the characteristic EKG findings in Pompe disease (type II glycogen storage disease)?
Gigantic QRS complexes in all leads and an abnormally short P-R interval.

21. Why do patients with von Gierke (type I glycogen storage) disease develop bleeding tendencies?
A platelet defect, presumably secondary, occurs in many patients with type I glycogen storage disease (glucose-6-phosphatase deficiency). Platelets from these patients show impaired release of ADP in response to collagen and epinephrine. The cause is unknown.

22. Which two glycogen storage diseases affect primarily muscle?
McArdle disease (type V with deficient muscle phosphorylase) and **Tarui disease** (type VII with deficient muscle phosphofructokinase). Clinically, they are similar, with increasing fatigue and cramps after exercise. Myoglobinuria may be noted. Since both enzyme deficiencies result in blockage of the glycolytic pathway, lactate will not rise after exercise as is normal. Definitive diagnosis is made by muscle biopsy with direct enzyme measurement.

CLINICAL ISSUES

23. Which metabolic diseases can present as sudden infant death syndrome (SIDS) or an acute life-threatening event (ALTE)?
• Fatty acid oxidation defects
• Some organic acidemias
• Defects of aldosterone and glucocorticoid metabolism
Although early reports suggested that medium-chain acyl-CoA dehydrogenase deficiency may be especially common among SIDS deaths, this claim has not been supported by several large population studies that used strict diagnostic criteria for SIDS.

24. What causes neonatal hyperammonemia?
1. Congenital urea cycle defects
2. Organic acidemias (particularly methylmalonic aciduria, propionic acidemia, isovaleric acidemia)
3. Other causes: idiopathic transient hyperammonemia (THAN), hypercatabolic states, excessive dietary protein, severe hepatocellular disease, neonatal hemochromatosis, urinary tract infection with urea-splitting organisms (e.g., *Proteus*)

25. Why do organic acidemias cause neonatal illness?
The mitochondrion is the cell's powerhouse. Body tissues that demand a major expenditure of energy are especially vulnerable to an interruption of their energy supply secondary to disturbed mitochondrial function. As such, brain, muscle, heart, liver, and the GI and renal transport systems fail predominantly due to clinical disorders of the mitochondrion. A variety of conditions can abruptly embarrass mitochondrial function and result in a multisystem crisis. In the newborn, organic acidemia may produce an acute form of encephalopathy manifested initially as feeding intolerance, vomiting, and lethargy, which progresses rapidly to coma, seizures, flaccid paralysis, respiratory depression, reduced gag reflex, and ultimately death. These signs are not specific for mitochondrial failure but suggest overwhelming, widespread CNS dysfunction. Their differential diagnosis includes sepsis, meningitis, intracranial hemorrhage, stroke, or any catastrophic neurologic illness. Neonates with hyperammonemia due to urea-cycle enzyme defects manifest comparable signs; cerebral edema is usually detected and is thought to be the cause of death.

26. How do patients with urea-cycle defects present?

1. Neonatal catastrophe—masquerading as sepsis neonatorum
   - Seizures, hypertonicity, vomiting, coma, death
   - Extreme elevations of NH_3: > 1000 µg/dl
2. Subacute presentation in infancy
   - Recurrent vomiting and growth failure
   - Intermittent ataxia
   - Seizures, mental retardation, developmental regression
3. Presentation later in childhood
   - Psychomotor retardation
   - Intermittent ataxia
   - Vomiting, protein intolerance—history of poor feeding during infancy
   - Overt symptoms after mild illness
4. Asymptomatic variant
   - Usually shows amino acid abnormality without hyperammonemia

From Cohn RM, Roth KS (eds): Metabolic Disease: A Guide to Early Recognition. Philadelphia, W.B. Saunders, 1983, p 138; with permission.

27. What are the treatments of choice for urea-cycle disorders?

Acute
- Continuous arteriovenous hemofiltration or hemodialysis
- Induced anabolism with high-concentration glucose infusions ± insulin
- Aggressive treatment of fevers
- Correction of amino acid deficiencies to prevent secondary catabolism
- Sodium benzoate and sodium phenylbutyrate to increase ammonia excretion via alternate pathways
- Arginine for excretion of ammonia as argininosuccinic acid in argininosuccinic aciduria

Maintenance
- Low-protein diet with supplemental essential amino acids
- Avoidance of fasting or other catabolic stress
- Sodium benzoate, sodium phenylbutyrate
- Supplementation with specific urea-cycle amino acids to prevent a deficiency state (and subsequent catabolism) or to enhance ammonia excretion (e.g., arginine in argininosuccinic aciduria)

28. What is the source of the organic acids in children with organic acidemias?

Most organic acidemias are actually due to defects in amino acid metabolism, but the enzymatic defects occur far down the catabolic pathway so that the amino groups have been removed (e.g., methylmalonic acidemia is a downstream abnormality in metabolism of valine and isoleucine). Organic acidemias due to primary abnormalities in organic acid metabolism, such as lactic acidemia and dicarboxylic aciduria, also occur.

29. In what ways can patients with organic acidemias present?

Neonatal catastrophe
- Acidosis (anion gap)
- Hypoglycemia, hyperammonemia
- Ketosis and ketonuria
- Unusual odor
- Tachypnea
- Neurologic findings
- Neutropenia, anemia, thrombocytopenia

Failure to thrive and vomiting during first year of life
- Deterioration with infection or diarrhea
- Vomiting

- Progressive delay in psychomotor development, acute or worsening extrapyramidal disease
- Acidosis—usually seen with exacerbations but is occasionally persistent
- May be history of protein intolerance leading to symptoms
- Neurologic symptoms with exacerbations
Onset after first year of life
- Episodes of ketoacidosis following a minor infection
- May be lethargy, seizures, or coma with such attacks

From Cohn RM, Roth KS (eds): Metabolic Disease: A Guide to Early Recognition. Philadelphia, W.B. Saunders, 1983, p 360; with permission.

30. How are the organic acidemias diagnosed?

Gas chromatography of a urine specimen can identify the abnormality in 80–90% of cases. However, combined gas chromatographic–mass spectrometric analysis should be performed to confirm the identity. The renal tubule does not effectively reabsorb organic acids, and consequently urine has been preferred to blood for evaluation. For screening purposes, though, the relatively new technique of dual-tandem mass spectrometric analysis of carnitine-esters in blood may indirectly enhance the capability to diagnose organic acidemias (see question 31).

31. Why does secondary carnitine deficiency develop in the organic acidemias?

In most organic acidemias, the deficient enzyme resides in the mitochondrion, and its substrate is the CoA derivative of the organic acid, e.g., propionyl-CoA in propionic acidemia. Accumulation of the CoA substrate leads to esterification with carnitine within the mitochondrion, e.g., propionylcarnitine. Excess formation of such a carnitine-ester, detectable in blood and urine, can lead to free carnitine deficiency.

32. A 19-month-old boy with failure to thrive, spasticity, choreoathetosis, and compulsive self-mutilating behavior probably has what metabolic abnormality?

Lesch-Nyhan syndrome, an X-linked recessive trait, due to complete deficiency of hypoxanthine-guanine phosphoribosyl transferase (HGPRT). This enzyme is involved in the reutilization of purine bases following degradation of their corresponding nucleotides, and without it, uric acid is excessively produced. Urine crystalluria (described by mothers as yellow-red sand in the diaper) may be noted in the newborn period.

Although affected infants (always male) may appear normal at birth, hypotonia, frequent vomiting, and delayed motor development are usually recognized in the first few months. Evidence of extrapyramidal dysfunction—dystonia, chorea, and athetosis—usually appears in the second 6 months of life. Between the first and second year, the evolution of spasticity and dysarthria often suggests the diagnosis of cerebral palsy. After 18 months, the compulsive self-destructive behavior usually develops; common manifestations include lip mutilation, finger-biting, and head-banging. Whereas serum uric acid levels may occasionally be normal in infancy, the uric acid/creatinine ratio in urine is pathologically elevated in affected children. Milder deficiencies of the enzyme may present as only spasticity and/or extrapyramidal disease without self-mutilation.

33. What is the etiology of Reye syndrome?

The cause remains unknown. Pathologically, the disease is characterized by widespread mitochondrial failure, which leads to the characteristic findings of acidosis, hyperammonemia, and hypoketotic hypoglycemia. Liver biopsy reveals fatty infiltration, minimal inflammation, and ultrastructural changes in mitochondria.

34. Describe the biphasic course of Reye syndrome.

Prodrome: mild upper respiratory illness or various viral illnesses (including influenza A and B, varicella, adenovirus, Epstein-Barr virus, herpes zoster, rubeola, mumps)

Acute: pernicious vomiting, afebrile; progression in some to encephalopathy with delirium, stupor, seizures, coma

35. Why is the incidence of Reye syndrome decreasing?
The specific explanation is unknown. However, the more limited use of aspirin may be one key factor in the virtual disappearance of Reye syndrome in the United States. Several case-control studies have identified a statistical association between aspirin use during an antecedent viral illness and the development of Reye syndrome. Although the etiologic role of aspirin has not been proved, both the use of aspirin in young children and the incidence of Reye syndrome decreased during the 1980s. By 1984, the median age of patients with this diagnosis had increased, a change that may reflect less aspirin use in young children.

36. Should children with influenza and chickenpox avoid using Pepto-Bismol?
Pepto-Bismol contains bismuth subsalicylate, and it is unclear if subsalicylate and the acetylsalicylic acid found in aspirin pose similar risks for the development of Reye syndrome. Because of the theoretic risks, the CDC advises against the use of bismuth subsalicylate during chickenpox and flu-like illnesses.

37. Which diseases can present with a clinical picture mimicking Reye syndrome?
• CNS infections (meningitis, encephalitis)
• Hemorrhagic shock with encephalopathy
• Toxin/drug ingestion (valproic acid, salicylates, hypoglycin A)
• Metabolic disease:
 Urea-cycle defects (carbamyl phosphate synthetase, ornithine transcarbamylase)
 Organic acidemias (3-hydroxy-3-methyl glutaric acidemia)
 Fatty acid oxidation defects (short-, medium-, and long-chain acyl-CoA dehydrogenase deficiency)
• Systemic carnitine deficiency
Adapted from Balistreri W: Liver disease associated with systemic disorders. In Behrman RE (ed): Nelson's Textbook of Pediatrics, 14th ed. Philadelphia, W.B. Saunders, 1992, p 1020.

38. When visiting the Caribbean, should you accept a gift of unripe fruit from the ackee tree?
Just don't eat it. The fruit contains hypoglycin A, the toxin responsible for Jamaican vomiting sickness. The disease can be fatal and begins with vomiting and hypoglycemia that can progress to hepatic steatosis and coma. The disease may resemble Reye syndrome.

39. Which metabolic diseases are responsive to pyridoxine (vitamin B$_6$)?
• Homocystinuria
• Oxaluria
• Cystathioninuria
• Pyridoxine-dependent seizures (possible deficiency of glutamate decarboxylase)
• β-Alaninemia

40. What are the causes of hyperuricemia?
Overproduction
• Hypoxanthine-guanine phosphoribosyl transferase (HGPRT) deficiency (Lesch-Nyhan syndrome)
• Hypercatabolic states (e.g., severe anoxia, leukemia, tumor lysis)
• Fatty-acid β-oxidation defects
• Hereditary fructose intolerance
• Glycogen storage diseases
• Reye syndrome
Toxin or drug-induced
• Ethanol poisoning
• Lead intoxication
• Diuretics (most)
• Aspirin
• Nicotinic acid
• Radiocontrast agents
• Chronic ingestion of acids

Other
- Cystinosis, Fabry disease, oxalosis due to renal insufficiency
- Hypo- or hyperparathyroidism
- Hypothyroidism
- High meat or fructose diets

41. List the inherited disorders of neurotransmitter metabolism.

Disease	Neurotransmitter	Presentation
Pyridoxine-dependent neonatal seizures (possible glutamate decarboxylase deficiency)	GABA	Neonatal seizures, mental retardation
Defects of biopterin synthesis (variant phenyl-ketonuria)	Dopamine Serotonin	Hypotonia, seizures, severe mental retardation
4-Hydroxybutyric aciduria (metabolite of GABA)	GABA	Hypotonia, seizures, mental retardation

42. What is the metabolic defect in Wilson disease?

Wilson disease is an autosomal recessive **defect of copper metabolism** for which the primary biochemical lesion remains unknown. The defective gene resides on the long arm of chromosome 13. The major biochemical abnormalities include low serum ceruloplasmin, decreased incorporation of copper into ceruloplasmin, increased urinary copper excretion, and markedly increased levels of copper in many tissues, notably the liver, basal ganglia, and cornea (Kayser-Fleischer rings). A cardinal feature is the high amount of free copper circulating in plasma unbound to ceruloplasmin.

43. What are the common clinical presentations of Wilson disease?

Hepatic/hematologic
- Jaundice and hepatitis
- Cirrhosis
- Fulminant hepatic failure
- Hemolytic anemia

Neurologic
- Psychiatric disturbance
- Tremor, extrapyramidal movement disorder
- Intellectual and behavioral deterioration
- Convulsions

44. How is the diagnosis of Wilson disease confirmed?

The combination of markedly increased copper levels in a liver biopsy specimen (> 400 µg/gm wet weight), low serum ceruloplasmin, and increased urinary copper excretion strongly suggests classic Wilson disease but is not absolutely diagnostic. The additional finding of Kayser-Fleischer rings is nearly pathognomonic of Wilson disease; however, their absence, especially in children, does not rule out the disease, and copper deposits in the cornea may also rarely be seen in other severe liver diseases, such as Indian biliary cirrhosis. The most specific diagnostic test is the demonstration of the slow rate of disappearance of radiolabeled copper from the bloodstream. Newer methods include measurement of radioactive copper uptake and retention by cultured fibroblasts, which is increased in Wilson disease.

45. Is there a treatment of choice for Wilson disease?

D-**Penicillamine**, a copper-chelating agent, is the drug of choice. Another copper-chelating drug, trientine, has been used successfully in patients with Wilson disease who have discontinued penicillamine because of hypersensitivity reactions. Zinc sulfate, which inhibits intestinal copper absorption, has also been used for therapy.

46. Describe the two main clinical features of the porphyrias.

The porphyrias are inborn errors in heme biosynthesis with overproduction of heme precursors. About 15% of heme is synthesized in the liver and the remainder in bone marrow. The precursors vary in their solubility, tissue depositions, and photosensitivity. Two main categories of presentations predominate:

Neurovisceral Symptoms
- Abdominal pain and vomiting
- Constipation or diarrhea
- Muscle weakness
- Mental status changes
- Peripheral nerve disease
- Hypertension and/or tachycardia
- Convulsions
- Bulbar paralysis
- Fever

Photosensitivity Skin Lesions
Acute
- Edematous skin plaques
- Bullae and vesicle formation
- Urticaria
- Purpura
Chronic
- Scarring, erosions, thickening
- Hypertrichosis
- Sensitivity to trauma
- Hyperpigmentation

47. How are the porphyrias classified?

Disease	Neurovisceral Attacks	Photo-sensitivity	Hepatic Disease	Hemolytic Anemia	Age of Onset	Inheritance
Erythropoietic porphyrias						
Erythropoietic porphyria	–	++++	–	++	Childhood	AR
Erythropoietic protoporphyria	–	++	±	–	Childhood	AD
Hepatic porphyrias						
Acute intermittent porphyria	++++	–	+	–	Postpubertal	AD
ALA dehydratase deficiency porphyria	++++	–	–	–	Postpubertal	AR
Porphyria variegata	++	++	–	–	Postpubertal	AD
Hereditary coproporphyria	++	+	±	–	Postpubertal	AD
Porphyria cutanea tarda*	–	+++	++†	–	Adult	Sporadic, some AD

AR—autosomal recessive; AD—autosomal dominant; ALA—α-aminolevulinic acid.
* AR form is hepatoerythropoietic porphyria and is characterized by childhood onset of severe photosensitivity.
† Probable contributing cause (e.g., alcoholic liver disease) rather than primary manifestation of porphyria.

48. Why are females more commonly affected by clinical problems of porphyria than males?
In the biosynthesis of heme, the rate-limiting step involves the first enzyme, ALA-synthase. When this enzyme is stimulated, additional precursors accumulate downstream at the point of specific enzyme blocks. Estrogen is an important inducer of ALA-synthase, and this appears to be the key reason for the greater problems encountered by females. For example, symptoms of acute intermittent porphyria are rare before puberty and oral contraceptives often cause exacerbations.

49. What accounts for the varying clinical features of the mucopolysaccharidoses?
Mucopolysaccharidoses are examples of storage disorders of lysosomes, which are intracellular organelles that degrade structural macromolecules. If enzymes are deficient, metabolites predominantly accumulate in the tissues that are primarily responsible for their degradation.

Mucopolysaccharide	Site of Accumulation
Heparan sulfate	CNS
Dermatan sulfate	Bone, viscera (esp. liver)
Keratan sulfate	Bone
Chondroitin sulfate	Cartilage

50. Describe the radiographic features that characterize the mucopolysaccharidoses.
A constellation of x-ray findings, termed **dysostosis multiplex**, is found:
1. Skull: enlarged and elongated with a thickened calvaria
2. Sella turcica: shaped like a wooden-shoe or boot

3. Vertebral bodies (especially lower thoracic and upper lumbar): hypoplasia of anterosuperior areas resulting in "beaked" appearance; in Morquio syndrome, platyspondylisis (flattening of vertebral bodies with surface irregularities)
4. Ribs: thickened (except at spinal insertion), "oar shaped"
5. Metacarpals: "baby-bottle" appearance with proximal narrowing and distal widening
6. Humerus, ulna: distal angulation
7. Pelvis: flaring of iliac bones, shallow acetabulum, progressive coxa valga
8. Long bones: shortened, thickened

51. Can a metabolic disease in the fetus have an adverse effect on the mother?

Long-chain 3-hydroxyacyl-CoA dehydrogenase deficiency, a fatty-acid oxidation defect in the fetus, can cause acute fatty liver of pregnancy in the mother.

52. An 8-month-old presents with vomiting, lethargy, hypoglycemia, and no ketones on urinalysis. What condition is likely?

Medium-chain acyl-CoA dehydrogenase deficiency (MCAD). Disorders of fatty-acid oxidation and deficiency of carnitine (the principal transporter of fatty acids into mitochondria) can result in maladaptation to fasting periods during intercurrent illnesses. Hypoketotic hypoglycemia results from the inability to utilize fatty acids, which are the primary source of ketones. MCAD affects 1:5000–1:10,000 live births in families of Northern European ancestry, and the clinical presentation varies from asymptomatic to detection by family screening to severe vomiting, encephalopathy, coma, and death. This latter picture occurs in 25% of patients with their first episode and may be confused with Reye syndrome or SIDS.

53. What common laboratory abnormalities are found in disorders of mitochondrial fatty-acid oxidation?

- Hypoketotic hypoglycemia
- Abnormal urinary dicarboxylic aciduria (metabolites of fatty acids)
- Hypocarnitinemia
- Abnormally increased urinary acylglycines (e.g., suberylglycine)
- Increased plasma or urinary acylcarnitines (e.g., octanoylcarnitine)
- Abnormal plasma free fatty acid levels
- Specific mutations on DNA analysis

54. How are fatty acid oxidation disorders treated?

Avoidance of prolonged fasting.

If oral intake is limited, provide adequate IV glucose in excess of basal hepatic glucose production (6 mg/kg/min for newborns, 2 mg/kg/min for adults).

If the defect affects only long-chain fatty-acid metabolism, limit dietary fat and/or provide only medium-chain fatty acids (C6–C10) in addition to minimal amounts of essential fatty acids.

If carnitine levels are low, oral L-carnitine can be used to restore levels to normal (but the benefits are questionable).

55. A 3-month-old has hypotonia, hepatomegaly, a high forehead with flat facies, and increased serum very-long-chain fatty acids. What condition is likely?

Zellweger (cerebrohepatorenal) **syndrome.** This disorder is due to a defect in assembly of the peroxisome, which is an intracellular organelle involved in various metabolic functions, including lipid metabolism and oxidation of very-long-chain fatty acids.

56. What is "Lorenzo's oil"?

This mixture of oleic and erucic acids has been used to treat adrenoleukodystrophy, an X-linked peroxisomal disease characterized by progressive demyelination. Levels of very-long-chain fatty acids are elevated due to an oxidation defect. Lorenzo's oil, popularized in a Hollywood movie, can normalize plasma fatty-acid levels, but does not alter the clinical course of the disease.

Aubourg R, et al: A 2-year trial of oleic and erucic acids (Lorenzo's oil) as treatment of adreno-myeloneuropathy. N Engl J Med 329:745–751, 1993.

57. Is the Smith-Lemli-Opitz syndrome, a congenital disorder with multiple malformations, an example of an inborn error of metabolism?

Yes. The disease, inherited as an autosomal recessive trait, is caused by a defect in cholesterol biosynthesis which leads to organ dysgenesis in the fetus. As a consequence of an enzyme deficiency, 7-dehydrocholesterol cannot be converted to cholesterol.

58. Do all patients with mutations of mitochondrial DNA show a persistent lactic acidosis?

No, but many do, because impaired electron transport chain function is usually the result of these mutations. Because more than one copy of mitochondrial DNA, inherited solely from the mother, is contained in a mitochondrion and there are thousands of mitochondria per cell, the systemic nature of the disease process in a particular patient depends on the number of cells in a tissue with a critical number of diseased mitochondria, the metabolic demands of the tissue, its replicative capacity, and probably other unknown factors. If the mitochondrial DNA mutational burden is high in muscle, brain, or liver, whole body oxidative metabolism will be impaired, and the patient will manifest a lactic acidosis. However, the expression of severe disease in the absence of a lactic acidosis may occur because of limited regional involvement in an organ such as the brain.

59. Are the diseases due to mitochondrial DNA mutations limited to familial inheritance patterns with transmission from mother to all children?

No. There are sporadic cases, and while in the familial forms transmission of mutated mitochondrial DNA to offspring must be 100%, the expression of disease may be < 100%. Examples of sporadic disease include Kearns-Sayre syndrome and acquired zidovudine-induced mitochondrial myopathy, and these are usually associated with DNA deletions. The MELAS (mitochondrial encephalopathy with lactic acidosis and strokes) syndrome is associated with a maternal inheritance pattern and, like most of these familial disorders, is secondary to a single base mutation in mitochondrial DNA.

GENERAL CONCEPTS

60. How are inborn errors of metabolism diagnosed prenatally?

Virtually all can be diagnosed prenatally using a number of different techniques.

• The most common procedure is enzyme analysis of cultured fibroblasts (obtained by chorionic villus sampling or aminocentesis) for the metabolic defect in question (e.g., measure hexosaminidase A activity from cultured amniotic fluid cells in a fetus at risk for Tay-Sachs disease).

• Measuring the concentration of substrate which accumulates in excess due to a specific metabolic block (e.g., measure 17-hydroxyprogesterone in amniotic fluid from a fetus at risk for 21-hydroxylase deficiency congenital adrenal hyperplasia).

• Molecular genetic investigation for direct gene analysis or familial linkage studies (e.g., linkage studies in a fetus at risk for ornithine transcarbamylase deficiency, a lethal X-linked urea-cycle defect).

61. Which inborn errors of metabolism can cause rickets?

Any condition that causes a phosphaturic state:

1. Cystinosis
2. Galactosemia
3. Wilson disease
4. Hereditary fructose intolerance
5. Hereditary tyrosinemia

62. In what settings should inborn errors of metabolism be suspected?

1. Onset of symptoms correlating with dietary changes
2. Loss or leveling of developmental milestones

3. Patient with strong food preferences or aversions
4. Parental consanguinity
5. Unexplained sibling death, mental retardation, or seizures
6. Unexplained failure to thrive
7. Unusual odor
8. Hair abnormalities, especially alopecia
9. Microcephaly or macrocephaly
10. Abnormalities of muscle tone
11. Organomegaly
12. Coarsened facial features, thick skin, limited joint mobility, hirsutism

63. What inborn errors of metabolism commonly cause acidosis during the neonatal period?

Severe metabolic acidosis in the neonatal period is more often caused by sepsis or cardiac defects than inborn errors of metabolism, but they do occur. Disorders of pyruvate metabolism, gluconeogenesis, and branched-chain amino acid catabolism are the most common inherited metabolic diseases causing metabolic acidosis in the newborn. In addition, metabolic acidosis with a normal anion gap occurs in disorders that impair renal uptake of bicarbonate or secretion of hydrogen ion. **Ketonuria** with acidosis in the newborn period is an especially important sign of an inborn error of metabolism and should be assumed to be caused by a metabolic disease until proved otherwise.

64. How do inborn errors of metabolism vary in clinical and laboratory features?

Clinical Findings in Inborn Errors of Metabolism

CLINICAL MANIFESTATIONS LABORATORY FINDINGS	GENERAL TYPE OF DISORDER TO CONSIDER								
	A	B	C	D	E	F	G	H	I
Episodic nature	++	++	++	++	+	+	–	–	–
Poor feeding	++	+	++	+	+	+	+	–	–
Abnormal odor	+	+	–	+	–	–	–	–	–
Lethargy, coma	+	+	+	+	+	+	–	–	–
Seizures	+	+	+	–	+	+	+	–	+
Developmental regression	+	+	+	–	+	–	+	++	+
Hepatomegaly	+	+	+	+	+	+	+	+	+
Hepatosplenomegaly	–	–	–	–	–	–	+	+	+
Splenomegaly	–	–	–	–	–	–	–	–	+
Hypotonia	+	+	+	+	+	+	+	–	+
Cardiomyopathy	–	+	–	+	+	+	–	+	–
Coarse facies	–	–	–	–	–	–	–	++	–
Birth defects	–	+	–	–	+	–	+	–	–
Hypoglycemia	+	+	–	+	+	+	–	–	–
Acidosis	+	++	–	+	+	+	–	–	–
Hyperammonemia	+	+	++	+	+	–	–	–	–
Ketosis	+	+	+	–	–	+	–	–	–
Hypoketosis	–	–	–	+	–	–	–	–	–

A–amino acidopathies; B–organic acidopathies; C–urea-cycle defects; D–fatty-acid oxidation defects; E–mitochondrial disorders; F–carbohydrate disorders; G–peroxisomal disorders; H–mucopolysaccharidoses; I–sphingolipidoses. ++ = usually present; + = may be present; – = usually not present.
From Wappner RS: Biochemical diagnosis of genetic disease. Pediatr Ann 22:284, 1993; with permission.

65. What key urine odors are associated with inborn errors of metabolism?

Cabbage	Tyrosinemia, type I
Cat urine	3-Methylcrotonyl-CoA carboxylase deficiency
Fish	Trimethylaminuria

Hops	Oasthouse urine disease
Maple syrup	Maple syrup urine disease
Mousey or musty	Phenylketonuria
Sweaty feet or cheesy	Isovaleric acidemia; glutaric aciduria, type II

66. Which inherited metabolic disorders are commonly associated with hypoglycemia?

1. Primary errors of glucose synthesis and release, i.e., gluconeogenesis and glycogenolysis
2. Defects of fatty-acid oxidation and ketogenesis, the main sources of fuel for gluconeogenesis
3. Hyperinsulinism
4. Defects causing "metabolic poisoning" of glucose metabolism, principally the organic acidurias

67. What is the differential diagnosis for ketotic and nonketotic hypoglycemia?

Ketotic hypoglycemia
- 3-Ketoacyl-CoA thiolase deficiency (short chain)
- Acetoacetyl-CoA thiolase deficiency
- Succinyl-3-ketoacyl CoA transferase deficiency
- Glycogen storage diseases I, III, VI
- Hereditary fructose intolerance
- Respiratory chain defects and related mitochondrial defects
- Growth hormone deficiency
- Hypopituitarism
- Starvation

Nonketotic or hypoketotic hypoglycemia
- Hyperinsulinism
- Hypopituitarism
- Fatty-acid β oxidation defects and systemic carnitine deficiency
- 3-Hydroxy, 3-methyl glutaric acidemia
- Defective Ketostix or Dextrostix

68. In an acutely ill child with suspected metabolic disease, how does the liver size provide a clue to the possible diagnosis?

Generally, in patients with inborn errors of metabolism, hepatomegaly in association with acute illness is more typical of disorders of carbohydrate or fatty-acid metabolism. Less commonly, patients with urea-cycle enzyme defects or organic acidemias, such as methylmalonic acidemia, may manifest hepatomegaly. In patients without hepatomegaly, a disorder of amino acid metabolism, such as maple syrup urine disease or nonketotic hyperglycemia, is more likely.

69. What strategies are used in the chronic management of inborn errors of metabolism?

1. Dietary manipulation to avoid the substrate for deficient enzymes and precursor accumulation (e.g., give a low-phenylalanine diet in patients with phenylketonuria)
2. Augment the excretion of toxic metabolites (e.g., glycine treatment of isovaleric acidemia)
3. Supplement with an inadequately produced enzyme product (e.g., arginine therapy for urea-cycle disorders)
4. Administer additional coenzyme to increase the activity of an abnormal enzyme (e.g., vitamin B_{12} in methylmalonic acidemia)
5. Provide deficient enzyme (e.g., enzyme infusion in Gaucher disease, liver transplantation in hereditary tyrosinemia, gene replacement therapy)

Goodman SI, Greene CL: Metabolic disorders of the newborn. Pediatr Rev 15:359–365, 1994.

LIPID DISORDERS

70. How are lipoproteins categorized?

The three major lipoprotein groups are classified by their density or electrophoretic properties: very-low-density lipoproteins (VLDL or pre-β), low-density lipoproteins (LDL or β), and high-density lipoproteins (HDL or α_1). In addition, chylomicrons and an intermediate-density lipoprotein (IDL or "floating β") can be found in plasma, although their quantities are typically much less, except in children with disorders of lipid metabolism.

71. What are normal cholesterol levels for children and adolescents?

	Total Cholesterol	LDL Cholesterol
Acceptable	< 170 mg/dl	< 110 mg/dl
Borderline	170–199	110–129
High	≥ 200	≥ 130

National Cholesterol Education Program (NCEP): Report of the Expert Panel on Blood Cholesterol in Children and Adolescents. Pediatrics 89(Suppl):525–584, 1992.

72. How is LDL cholesterol calculated?

LDL cholesterol = total cholesterol – [HDL cholesterol + (total triglyceride/5)]

73. Which children should have their cholesterol measured?

This is a controversial issue with proponents and opponents of universal screening. Current recommendations, developed by the National Cholesterol Education Committee and the American Academy of Pediatrics, adopt a middle ground—to screen all children aged ≥ 2 years if there is:

1. Family history of parents or grandparents aged 55 or younger with documented premature cardiovascular disease

2. History of a parent with elevated total cholesterol (≥ 240 mg/dl)

3. Parental and/or family history is unobtainable (e.g., adoption)

Proponents of universal screening have since argued that the guidelines are not sufficiently sensitive and may miss up to 50% of children with elevated lipids.

74. Outline the six arguments against universal screening for elevated cholesterol.

1. Instrumentation for cholesterol measurement is not standardized and some children will be mislabeled.

2. If pediatric dietary recommendations (e.g., total fat < 30% of calories) are routinely followed, many children with hypercholesterolemia will achieve normal levels.

3. Serum cholesterol may not be the most sensitive indicator of future atherosclerotic heart disease.

4. Tracking (persistence of high or low levels over time) is not precise for serum cholesterol.

5. Although fatty arterial plaques occur in children, atherosclerotic events are rare before the third decade, and present evidence suggests reversibility at that age with treatment.

6. Cost of universal screening is large compared to benefits.

Committee on Nutrition: Pediatric Nutrition Handbook. Elk Grove Village, IL, American Academy of Pediatrics, 1993, p 258.

Newman TB, et al: Problems with the report of the Expert Panel on blood cholesterol levels in children and adolescents. Arch Pediatr Adolesc Med 149:241–247, 1996.

75. How are the primary genetic hyperlipidemias classified?

Frederick-son Type	Lipids Increased	Lipoproteins Increased	Prevalence	Clinical Findings
I	Triglyceride	Chylomicrons	Very rare	Eruptive xanthomas, pancreatitis, recurrent abdominal pain, lipemia retinalis, hepatosplenomegaly
IIa	Cholesterol	LDL	Common	Tendon xanthomas, PVD
IIb	Cholesterol, triglyceride	LDL + VLDL	Common	PVD, no xanthomas
III	Cholesterol, triglyceride	VLDL remnants (IDL)	Rare	PVD, yellow palm creases
IV	Triglyceride	VLDL	Uncommon	PVD, xanthomas, hyperglycemia
V	Triglyceride, cholesterol	VLDL + chylomicrons	Very rare	Pancreatitis, lipemia retinalis, xanthomas, hyperglycemia

PVD = premature vascular disease.

76. What is the most common hyperlipidemia in childhood?

Type IIa, familial hypercholesterolemia with elevated cholesterol and LDL. This condition results from a lack of functional LDL receptors on cell membranes due to various mutations. When LDL cannot attach and release cholesterol to the cell, feedback suppression of HMG-CoA reductase (the rate-limiting enzyme in cholesterol synthesis) does not occur, and cholesterol synthesis continues excessively. In the homozygous form of Type IIa, xanthomas may appear before age 10 and vascular disease before age 20. However, the homozygous form is very rare, with an incidence of 1 in 1 million births. The heterozygous variety has a much higher incidence of 1 in 500 but is less likely to produce clinical manifestations in children.

The type most likely to present in childhood is type I hyperlipoproteinemia. This disorder is characterized by an excess of chylomicron triglycerides, which typically causes recurrent abdominal pain and hepatosplenomegaly in the first 5 years of life. Although rare, it is more common than homozygous familial hypercholesterolemia (type IIa). As a rule, most of the common familial hyperlipidemias are not associated with clinical disease during childhood, but usually manifest as atherosclerotic heart disease or xanthomata in the third or later decades.

77. What are the treatments of choice for familial hypercholesterolemia?

Dietary restriction of cholesterol and fat, plus a lipid-lowering resin such as cholestyramine. Cholestyramine and the related resin, colestipol, lower plasma cholesterol by trapping bile acids in the gut and thereby causing more cholesterol to be shunted to bile acid synthesis. Other therapies include direct removal of lipoproteins by plasmapheresis, pharmacologic doses of the vitamin niacin (nicotinic acid), and orthotopic liver transplantation. Inhibitors of the rate-limiting enzyme of cholesterol synthesis, HMG-CoA reductase, are also available but are still undergoing clinical testing in children. Ex vivo gene therapy using liver cells and retroviral vectors is currently under study in adults.

78. What are causes of secondary hyperlipidemia in childhood?

General medical conditions
- Obesity
- Hypothyroidism
- Chronic renal failure
- Nephrotic syndrome
- Biliary atresia, biliary cirrhosis
- Hepatitis
- Diabetes mellitus
- Pregnancy
- Anorexia nervosa

Inborn errors of metabolism
- Glycogen storage disease (mostly type I)
- Congenital lactic acidosis
- Mitochondrial encephalomyopathies (some)
- Acute intermittent porphyria

Drugs
- β-Adrenergic blockers
- Alcohol
- Oral contraceptives
- Thiazide diuretics
- Anabolic steroids
- Corticosteroids
- Istretinoin (Accutane)

Genetic syndromes
- Werner syndrome
- Progeria
- Klinefelter syndrome
- Idiopathic hypercalcemia

79. Which is the most commonly encountered lipid-storage disorder in humans?

Gaucher disease, or glucosyl ceramide lipidosis, caused by a deficiency of β-glucocerebrosidase, is the most commonly diagnosed lipid-storage disorder. The incidence varies from 1/100,000 in non-Jewish populations to 1/2500 in Ashkenazi Jews.

80. What lipid-storage disorder should be suspected in patients with unexplained proteinuria?

Fabry disease (α-galactosidase deficiency). Proteinuria is also a characteristic of several types of sialic acid storage disease, presenting in the newborn period with nephrotic syndrome, coarse facial features, organomegaly, bony changes (dyostosis multiplex), and neurologic abnormalities.

SCREENING

81. How frequently are the various metabolic disorders detected by newborn screening?

Disorder	Frequency
Tay-Sachs disease (U.S. Jews)	1/3000
Phenylketonuria	1/10,000–25,000
Galactosemia	1/40,000–60,000
Biotinidase deficiency	1/70,000
Homocystinuria	1/50,000–150,000
Maple syrup urine disease	1/250,000–300,000

82. Which common sugar does the Clinitest screen not detect?

Sucrose. Reducing sugars, such as glucose, fructose, galactose, pentoses, and lactose, are detected, but sucrose is not a reducing sugar. The test method is straightforward. Five drops of urine and 10 drops of water are mixed, and Clinitest tablet is added. Color changes are then compared to a standard chart to determine the percentage of reducing substances. Testing for sucrose can be done by substituting hydrochloric acid for the water and boiling for a few seconds. This hydrolyzes the sucrose, and a negative test will become positive.

83. What are the common causes of false-positive tests for urine-reducing substances?
- Radiologic contrast dyes
- Stool contamination
- Antibiotics, especially ampicillin, and other drugs excreted as glucuronides
- Pentosuria from pentose-enriched fruits (true-positive but nonpathologic)
- *p*-Hydroxyphenylpyruvic acid (tyrosinemias)

84. What metabolic abnormalities can be detected with the ferric chloride test?

The ferric chloride test is one of the oldest urine metabolic tests, yet it remains a useful screen in this day of sophisticated microanalytical quantitative methods. The test is simple and quick. Two drops of 10% ferric chloride are mixed with 1 ml of fresh urine. In the presence of various organic compounds, ferric chloride will form derivatives of different colors, as below:

Disorder	Major Reactant	Metabolite Origin	Reaction
Phenylketonuria	Phenylpyruvic acid	Phenylalanine	Green
Hypertyrosinemia syndromes, severe liver disease	*p*-OH-phenylpyruvic acid	Tyrosine	Green (fades rapidly)
Histidinemia	Imidazole pyruvic acid	Histidine	Olive green
Alkaptonuria	Homogentisic acid	Tyrosine	Blue or green (fades rapidly)
Formiminotransferase deficiency	Imidazole carboxamide	Histidine	Gray
Ketoacidosis (severe)	Acetoacetate	Fatty acids, amino acids	Cherry red
Congenital lactic acidosis	Pyruvate	Amino acids, glucose	Green-gold

85. Why was the "Guthrie bacterial inhibition test" a major breakthrough?

Devised in 1961, this test permitted widespread and inexpensive screening for phenylketonuria (PKU) and then also for other inborn errors of metabolism. The guiding principle was that growth of bacteria inhibited by a toxic compound could be reversed by a physiologically similar compound (e.g., elevated metabolites). In PKU testing, a filter paper disc spotted with a newborn's blood is placed on a bacterial growth medium (agar) which contains an inhibiting substance (β-2-thienylalanine). If phenylalanine is in high concentration in the test disc, it will diffuse into the agar and permit bacterial growth. The extent of growth is proportional to the concentration of the phenylalanine. If excessive, follow-up confirmatory tests must be done.

86. In addition to PKU, what other metabolic disorders can be detected by Guthrie bacterial inhibition tests?

Compound Detected	Disorder
Phenylalanine	Phenylketonuria Hyperphenylalaninemic states
Leucine	Maple syrup urine disease
Histidine	Histidinemia
Galactose	Galactosemia
Methionine	Homocystinuria (one type, due to cystathionine synthase deficiency) Liver disease
Tyrosine	Tyrosinemia Liver disease

From Erbe RW, Boss GR: Newborn genetic screening. In Emery AEH, Rimoin DL (eds): Principles and Practice of Medical Genetics, 2nd ed. Edinburgh, Churchill Livingstone, 1990, p 1938; with permission.

87. What tests comprise a "urine metabolic screen"?
These tests vary according to individual hospital and commercial labs. In addition to the ferric chloride and reducing substances (e.g., Clinitest) testing, other liquid and chromatographic tests include:

	Principal Disorders Detected
Liquid tests	
Cyanide nitroprusside	Homocystinuria, cystinuria, tyrosinemia
Nitrosonaphthol	Tyrosinemia
2,4-Dinitrophenylhydrazine	Maple syrup urine disease, lactic acidoses
Cetylpyridinium	Mucopolysaccharidoses
Thiosulfate	Sulfate oxidase deficiency, molybdenum defects
Chromatographic tests	
Amino acid paper or column chromatography	Many amino acid disorders, renal Fanconi syndrome
Organic acid gas chromatography	Many organic acidurias and lactic acidoses
Thin-layer chromatography	Sialic acid defects, many lysosomal storage diseases (e.g., mucopolysaccharidoses)

Because pathologic metabolites may clear from the urine within hours of starting general supportive therapy, "acute" urine specimens or even just a wet diaper should be saved and sent for testing.

88. Of the disorders most often screened for in newborns, which three are potentially life-threatening in the newborn period?
• Galactosemia (increased risk of sepsis)
• Maple syrup urine disease (increased risk of cerebral edema, apnea, and seizures)
• Congenital adrenal hyperplasia (increased risk of circulatory collapse)

12. NEONATOLOGY

Philip Roth, M.D., Ph.D., Mary Catherine Harris, M.D.,
Carlos Vega-Rich, M.D., and Peter Marro, M.D.

CLINICAL ISSUES

1. Why don't preterm infants sweat?

The failure of infants born at < 30 weeks' gestation to sweat is probably due to the incomplete development and differentiation of sweat glands. In term babies, in whom more data are available, the maximal sweat response to thermal stimuli is one-third that of adults, despite a density of sweat glands which is six times higher.

2. Do infants ever shiver?

It is uncertain whether newborns shiver. In some reports, shivering was observed only at temperatures < 22–24°C. Heat generation is mainly via nonshivering thermogenesis, consisting of muscular activity and metabolism of brown fat.

3. How does brown fat keep infants warm?

Cold-stressed infants depend principally on chemical mechanisms to maintain body temperature. When placed in a cold environment, the sympathetic nervous system is activated, and norepinephrine and thyroid hormones are released. These hormones induce the lipolysis of brown fat stores, which are located primarily in the intrascapular, axillary, perirenal, mediastinal, paraspinal, and nuchal regions. Triglycerides in the brown fat deposits are broken down into fatty acids and glycerol, which enter the abundant mitochondria and generate heat. The combustion of fatty acids in brown fat is under the control of an uncoupling protein called thermogenin.

4. What are the manifestations of neonatal cold injury?

Neonatal cold injury is primarily seen in low-birthweight infants but may also be seen in full-term infants with CNS malformations. Characteristics of this syndrome include poor feeding, lethargy, and coldness to touch associated with core temperatures of ≤ 32.2°C. Despite the presence of a bright red skin color, which is secondary to decreased dissociation of oxyhemoglobin, these infants display central cyanosis. Respirations are shallow, irregular, and sometimes associated with grunting. Bradycardia as a function of the degree of temperature depression may also be seen. Other findings include CNS depression with decreased responsiveness, abdominal distention with vomiting, and edema of the skin and face which may progress to sclerema. Concomitant metabolic disturbances include metabolic acidosis, hypoglycemia, hyperkalemia, and azotemia.

5. What are the best ways to warm a hypothermic infant?

Whether rapid or slow rewarming is preferable is a much debated issue, but no good controlled studies exist to answer this question. A general approach consists of placing the infant in a heat-gaining environment to prevent further losses. This can best be achieved by warming the infant in a convectively heated incubator at 36°C with a heat shield to reduce radiant losses and increased humidity to decrease evaporative losses. Under these conditions, the air temperature is approximately equal to the environmental temperature in the incubator. Air temperature should be monitored along with skin temperature, which should not exceed rectal temperature by > 1°C. If the patient's temperature does not stabilize or increase, the incubator temperature should be increased to 37°C and the patient's temperature observed for 15 minutes. If there is still no improvement, the temperature should be increased to 38°C. If temperatures > 38°C are necessary, an overhead warmer may need to be placed over the incubator in order to warm its walls and achieve the desired effect.

6. Should an asymptomatic infant with a single umbilical artery have a screening ultrasound done for renal anomalies?

This point has been argued for years. A single umbilical artery is a rare phenomenon. In one study of nearly 35,000 infants, examination of the placenta showed that only 112 (0.32%) had a single umbilical artery. All 112 underwent renal ultrasonography, and 17% had abnormalities (45% of which persisted). Because of the rarity of the condition and the increased association of abnormalities, patients with single umbilical arteries probably should receive a screening renal ultrasound.

Bourke WG, et al: Isolated single umbilical artery: The case for routine renal screening. Arch Dis Child 68:600–601, 1993.

7. How does the handling of the umbilical cord at birth affect neonatal hemoglobin concentrations?

At the time of birth, the placental vessels may contain up to 33% of the fetal-placental blood volume. Constriction of the umbilical arteries limits blood flow from the infant, but the umbilical vein remains dilated. The extent of drainage from the placenta to the infant via the umbilical vein is very dependent on gravity. The recommendation is to keep the baby at least 20 cm below the placenta for approximately 30 seconds before clamping the cord. More elevated positioning or rapid clamping can minimize the placental transfusion and decrease red cell volume.

Oski FA: The erythrocyte and its disorders. In Nathan DG, Oski FA (eds): Hematology of Infancy and Childhood, 4th ed. Philadelphia, W.B. Saunders, 1993, pp 26–29.

8. Describe the best method of umbilical cord care in the immediate neonatal period.

No single method of cord care has been determined to be superior in preventing colonization and infections. Antimicrobial agents, such as bacitracin or triple dye, are commonly used. Alcohol accelerates drying of the cord, but it has not been shown to reduce the rates of colonization or omphalitis.

9. Which way does the umbilical cord twist?

Usually counterclockwise. Coiling of the umbilical cord occurs in approximately 95% of newborns, and most are twisted in a sinistral manner. Because this helical arrangement is absent in species in which fetuses are arranged longitudinally in a bicornuate uterus, spiraling may result from the mobility of the primate fetus. Noncoiled cords may be associated with an increased likelihood of anomalies.

Strong TH, et al: Antepartum diagnosis of noncoiled umbilical cords. Am J Obstet Gynecol 170: 1729–1733, 1994.

10. When should a parent begin to worry if an umbilical cord has not fallen off?

The umbilical cord generally dries up and sloughs by 2 weeks of life. Delayed separation can be normal up to 45 days. However, because neutrophilic and/or monocytic infiltration appears to play a major role in autodigestion, persistence of the cord beyond 30 days should prompt consideration of an underlying functional abnormality of neutrophils (leukocyte adhesion deficiency) or neutropenia.

Kemp AS, Lubitz L: Delayed cord separation in alloimmune neutropenia. Arch Dis Child 68:52–53, 1993.

11. How do you estimate the insertion distance necessary for umbilical catheters?

Measuring the distance from the umbilicus to the shoulder (lateral end of clavicle) allows an estimation of desired length.

Insertion Distance for Umbilical Catheters (cm)

SHOULDER TO UMBILICUS	AORTIC CATHETER TO DIAPHRAGM	AORTIC CATHETER TO AORTIC BIFURCATION	VENOUS CATHETER TO RIGHT ATRIUM
9	11	5	6
10	12	5	6–7
11	13	6	7
12	14	7	8
13	15	8	8–9
14	16	9	9
15	17	10	10
16	18	10–11	11
17	20	11–12	11–12

From Dunn PM: Localization of umbilical catheters by post mortem measurement. Arch Dis Child 41:69, 1966; with permission.

12. What are the risks of umbilical catheters?

Short-term risks

1. Perforation and development of retroperitoneal hemorrhage (umbilical artery [UA] catheter)
2. Decreased femoral pulses and blanching of limbs and/or buttocks (UA catheter)
3. Accidental hemorrhage (both UA and umbilical vein [UV] catheters)
4. Infection (both UA and UV catheters)

Long-term risks

1. Embolization and infarcts (both UA and UV catheters)
2. Thrombosis of hepatic vein (UV catheter)
3. Liver necrosis (UV catheter)
4. Aortic thrombi (UA catheter)
5. Renal artery thrombosis (UA catheter)
6. Infection (both UA and UV catheters)

13. What are the increased risks of twin pregnancies?

1. Premature delivery
2. Intrauterine growth retardation, including discordant growth (which may occur in up to one-third of twin pregnancies)
3. Increased perinatal mortality, especially for premature, monozygotic, and discordant twins
4. Spontaneous abortion
5. Birth asphyxia
6. Fetal malposition
7. Placental abnormalities (abruptio placentae, placenta previa)
8. Polyhydramnios

14. Why are monozygotic twins considered higher risk than dizygotic twins?

Monozygotic twins (identical twins) arise from the division of a single fertilized egg. Depending on the timing of the division of the single ovum into separate embryos, the amnionic and chorionic membranes can be either shared (if division occurs > 8 days after fertilization), separate (if < 72 hours after fertilization), or mixed (separate amnion, shared chorion if 4–8 days after fertilization). Sharing of the chorion and/or amnion is associated with potential problems of vascular anastomoses (and possible twin–twin transfusions), cord entanglements, and congenital anomalies. These problems increase the risk of intrauterine growth retardation and perinatal death. Dizygotic twins, however, result from two separately fertilized ova and, as such, usually have a separate amnion and chorion.

15. Who is at higher risk, the first- or second-born twin?
The second born twin has a 2–4-fold increased risk of developing respiratory distress syndrome and is more likely to be asphyxiated. However, the risks for sepsis and necrotizing enterocolitis may be increased in first-born twins.

16. What are the varieties of conjoined twins?
Conjoined twins are classified according to the degree and nature of their union. These are listed below in order of decreasing frequency:

Thoracopagus	Joined at the thorax
Xiphopagus	Joined at anterior abdominal wall
	Joined from the xiphoid to the umbilicus
Pygopagus	Joined at buttocks or rump
Ischiopagus	Joined at ischium
Craniopagus	Joined at head

17. Who were Cheng and Eng?
The original "Siamese twins."

18. How extensive is insensible water loss in preterm infants?
Insensible water loss is the loss of water through the lungs during respiration and from the skin by evaporation. A rough guide to the amount of insensible loss for infants in humidified isolettes is:

750–1000 gm: 65 ml/kg/day   1251–1500 gm: 40 ml/kg/day
1001–1250 gm: 55 ml/kg/day   > 1500 gm: 20 ml/kg/day

19. What factors affect insensible water loss?
Increase: prematurity, activity, fever, radiant warmer, phototherapy
Decrease: high humidity, mechanical ventilation

20. How much does phototherapy increase the fluid requirements of infants?
By 50% if no heat shield is used, or by 10–30% if a plastic heat shield is used. The increased insensible water loss is believed to result from vasodilation secondary to a direct effect of light on the precapillary arterioles in the skin.

21. When should infection with *Malassezia furfur* be suspected in the neonate?
This dermatophyte, usually found on the skin of infants without clinical disease, can cause signs and symptoms of infection in critically ill and premature infants. Infection is almost always associated with the presence of an indwelling venous catheter. The fat emulsion administered during hyperalimentation is believed to contain fatty acids required for fungal proliferation. Although treatment with amphotericin is effective, removal of the indwelling catheter appears to eliminate the infection in most cases.

22. You are informed during sign-out rounds that a newborn is suspected to have funisitis. Where should you look for that infection?
Funisitis is inflammation of the **umbilical cord vessels** and **Wharton's jelly** and has been described as either an acute exudative or subacute necrotizing process accompanying chorioamnionitis. The predominant organisms identified as etiologic agents are gram-negative bacteria, including *Escherichia coli*, *Klebsiella*, and *Pseudomonas*. Gram-positive organisms (e.g., streptococci, staphylococci) and candidal species are less commonly responsible.

23. Which infants require ophthalmologic evaluation for retinopathy of prematurity (ROP)?
The American Academy of Pediatrics recommends that an individual experienced in neonatal ophthalmology and indirect ophthalmoscopy examine the retinae of all premature neonates

(i.e., those who are delivered at < 35 weeks' gestation or who weigh < 1800 gm) who require supplemental oxygen. Infants who are less mature at birth (i.e., ≤ 30 weeks' gestation or < 1300 gm) should be examined regardless of oxygen exposure. The examination is best done prior to discharge or at 5–7 weeks of age if the infant is still hospitalized.

24. What are the stages of ROP?

Stage I: Line of demarcation separates vascular and avascular retina
Stage II: Ridging of line of demarcation secondary to scar formation
Stage III: Extraretinal fibrovascular proliferation present (In addition, in stages II and III, the term *plus disease* refers to active inflammation as manifested by tortuosity of retinal vessels, which increases the risk of progression of ROP.)
Stage IV: Subtotal retinal detachment
Stage V: Complete retinal detachment

25. What are the indications for cryotherapy or laser therapy in ROP?

In a multicenter trial by the Cryotherapy for ROP Cooperative Group, "threshold" disease, defined as a level of severity at which the risk of blindness approaches 50%, was chosen for treatment. This diagnosis required the presence of at least five contiguous or eight cumulative 30° sectors (clock hours) of stage III ROP (in zone 1 or 2) and the presence of plus disease.

26. How is vitamin E used in the prevention and treatment of ROP?

Recent trials of vitamin E therapy have *not* shown it to be effective in preventing ROP. However, because of its activity as an antioxidant, vitamin E treatment may lessen the severity of ROP. Serum vitamin E levels should be maintained at 1–2 mg/dl. Higher levels may be associated with toxicity (necrotizing enterocolitis and/or sepsis).

27. Name the conditions associated with abnormalities in maternal serum alpha-fetoprotein concentration.

Increased
- Incorrect gestational dating
- Multiple pregnancy
- Threatened abortion
- Fetomaternal hemorrhage
- Anencephaly
- Open spina bifida
- Anterior abdominal wall defects
- Congenital nephrosis
- Acardia
- Lesions of the placenta and umbilical cord
- Turner syndrome
- Cystic hygroma
- Renal agenesis
- Polycystic kidney disease
- Epidermolysis bullosa
- Hereditary persistence (AD trait)

Decreased
- Incorrect gestational dating
- Trisomy 21
- Trisomy 18
- Intrauterine growth retardation

From Taeusch W, et al (eds): Schaffer & Avery's Diseases of the Newborn, 6th ed. Philadelphia, W.B. Saunders, 1991, p 47; with permission.

28. If maternal drug abuse is suspected, which specimen from the infant is most accurate in detecting exposure?

Although urine has traditionally been tested when maternal drug abuse is a possibility, **meconium** has a greater sensitivity than urine and positive findings that persist longer. It may contain metabolites gathered over multiple weeks, compared with urine which represents more recent exposure. Of note, maternal self-reporting is notoriously inaccurate as an indicator of drug use. In addition, in some states, informed maternal consent must be given prior to drug screening of the neonate, which can hinder diagnosis and surveillance.

Ostrea EM Jr, et al: Drug screening of newborns by meconium analysis: A large-scale, prospective, epidemiologic study. Pediatrics 89:107–113, 1992.

29. What are the manifestations of drug withdrawal in the neonate?
The signs and symptoms of drug withdrawal in the neonate can be remembered by using the mnemonic "withdrawal."
W   Wakefulness
I   Irritability
T   Tremulousness, temperature variation, tachypnea
H   Hyperactivity, high-pitched persistent cry, hyperacusis, hyperreflexia, hypertonus
D   Diarrhea, diaphoresis, disorganized suck
R   Rub marks, respiratory distress, rhinorrhea
A   Apneic attacks, autonomic dysfunction
W   Weight loss or failure to gain weight
A   Alkalosis (respiratory)
L   Lacrimation
Committee on Drugs: Neonatal drug withdrawal. Pediatrics 72:896, 1983.

30. What bone is the most frequently fractured in the newborn?
The **clavicle**. This injury, which stems from excessive traction during delivery, generally results in a greenstick fracture.

31. Should palpable lymph nodes in a newborn be considered pathologic?
No. Up to 25% of newborns have palpable nodes, particularly in the inguinal and cervical regions. By 1 month of age, the prevalence is nearly 40%.
Bamji M, et al: Palpable lymph nodes in healthy newborns and infants. Pediatrics 78:573–575, 1986.

32. How loud is the noise inside an infant's isolette?
The noise usually ranges from about **50–90 db**. With the slamming of an isolette door, the level can approach 100 db. For comparison, room conversation is 60–70 db and louder rock music is 100–120 db. The American Academy of Pediatrics recommends no more than 70 db because (1) > 70 db disrupts and/or awakens sleeping infants, (2) > 70 db is associated with cardiovascular changes (e.g., increased heart rate), and (3) ototoxicity secondary to use of aminoglycoside antibiotics may be potentiated by constant loud noise.
Committee on Environmental Hazards: Noise pollution: Neonatal aspects. Pediatrics 54:483–486, 1974.

33. In infants, why is it dangerous to use an IV flush containing benzyl alcohol as a bacteriostatic agent?
In an association first recognized in 1982, IV fluids containing benzyl alcohol can result in progressive CNS depression, increasing respiratory distress with gasps (the "gasping syndrome"), severe metabolic acidosis, thrombocytopenia, hepatic and renal failure, cardiovascular collapse, and death. Benzyl alcohol may also increase the risk of kernicterus by facilitating passage of bilirubin into the CNS. It might be said, look before you flush.

34. How valuable is the footprinting of newborns for the permanent medical record?
A time-honored tradition that is, alas, of minimal benefit. Although the AAP recommended discontinuing the practice in 1983 due to the fact that in nearly 80% the quality was so poor as to render the print useless, up to 80% of U.S. hospitals continue footprinting as a means of identification. Of note, footprinting is legally mandated only in New York State.

35. What are the most common causes of fetal death?
Chromosomal abnormalities (especially in early pregnancy) and congenital malformations.

36. How long should a healthy term newborn remain hospitalized?
A controversial issue. Although some neonatal problems do not appear until several days of age, most are apparent by 6 hours of life. Nevertheless, there is an increased frequency of

hospital readmissions in patients discharged at < 48 hours and especially in those discharged at < 24 hours.

Braveman R, et al: Early discharge of newborns and mothers: A critical review of the literature. Pediatrics 96:716–726, 1995.

37. What are Spitzer's Laws of Neonatology?

1. The more stable a baby appears to be, the more likely he will "crump" that day.

2. The nicer the parents, the sicker the baby.

3. The likelihood of BPD (bronchopulmonary dysplasia) is directly proportional to the number of physicians involved in the care of that baby.

4. The longer a patient is discussed on rounds, the more certain it is that no one has the faintest idea of what's going on or what to do.

5. The sickest infant in the nursery can always be discerned by the fact that she is being cared for by the newest, most inexperienced nursing orientee.

6. The surest way to have an infant linger interminably is to inform the parents that death is imminent.

7. The more miraculous the "save," the more likely that you'll be sued for something totally inconsequential.

8. If they're not breathin', they may be seizin'.

9. Antibiotics should always be continued for _____ days. (Fill in the blank with any number from 1 to 21.)

10. If you can't figure out what's going on with a baby, call the surgeons. They won't figure it out either, but they'll sure as hell do something about it.

From Spitzer A: Spitzer's laws of neonatology. Clin Pediatr 20:733, 1981; with permission.

38. What is Throgmorton's sign?

Throgmorton's sign is the extension of the suspensory ligament of the penis prior to micturition in newborn infants. However, thousands of house officers have come to believe that this sign relates to the radiographic finding in a male in which the penis points to the side of pathology.

THE DELIVERY ROOM

39. What is the clinical significance of fetal decelerations?

The character or pattern of decelerations often seen during fetal heart rate monitoring can be a valuable indicator of fetal well-being or need for intervention.

Early decelerations: Associated with head compression. Usually of no consequence.

Variable decelerations: Observed with cord compression. May indicate fetal distress when prolonged and associated with bradycardia.

Late decelerations: Indicate uteroplacental insufficiency and the presence of fetal distress. Both variable and late decelerations may be associated with acidosis and fetal compromise.

40. How sensitive is fetal heart rate monitoring in detecting fetal asphyxia?

Abnormal decelerations have a poor positive-predictive value, with only 15–25% being associated with a significantly compromised fetus. However, normal studies have a much higher predictive value of ongoing fetal well-being.

41. What is an acceptable scalp pH in the fetus?

Fetal scalp sampling to measure blood pH is used in conjunction with electronic fetal heart rate monitoring to assess fetal well-being during labor. The range of acceptable values for fetal pH is broad. A pH ≥ 7.25 is considered normal. Values between 7.20 and 7.25 are often referred to as pre-acidotic and may be associated with an increased incidence of depression at delivery. As labor progresses, repeat testing is warranted. A pH < 7.20 may indicate significant fetal compromise.

Normal Fetal Scalp Blood Values in Labor

	EARLY FIRST STAGE	LATE FIRST STAGE	SECOND STAGE
pH	7.33 ± 0.03	7.32 ± 0.02	7.29 ± 0.04
PCO_2 (mm Hg)	44 ± 4.05	42 ± 5.1	46.3 ± 4.2
PO_2 (mm Hg)	21.8 ± 2.6	21.3 ± 2.1	16.5 ± 1.4
Bicarbonate (mmol/L)	20.1 ± 1.2	19.1 ± 2.1	17 ± 2
Base excess (mmol/L)	3.9 ± 1.9	4.1 ± 2.5	6.4 ± 1.8

From Boylan PC, Parisi VM: Fetal acid-base balance. In Creasy RK, Resnik R (eds): Maternal-Fetal Medicine, 3rd ed. Philadelphia, W. B. Saunders, 1994, p 352; with permission.

42. Is length of labor the same for male and female babies?

No. Labor length for boys is about 1 hour longer than for girls.

43. How long has meconium been present in the amniotic fluid if an infant has evidence of meconium staining?

Gross staining of the infant is a surface phenomenon proportional to the length of exposure and meconium concentration. With heavy meconium, staining of the umbilical cord begins in as little as 15 minutes, and with light meconium, after 1 hour. Yellow staining of the newborn's toenails requires 4–6 hours. Yellow staining of the vernix caseosa takes about 12–14 hours.

Miller PW, et al: Dating the time interval from meconium passage to birth. Obstet Gynecol 66:459–462, 1985.

44. Is meconium staining a good marker for neonatal asphyxia?

Because 10–20% of all deliveries have in utero passage of meconium, meconium staining alone is not a good marker for neonatal asphyxia.

45. If meconium is noted prior to or at the time of delivery, what is the recommended course of action?

Regardless of the nature of the fluid, the obstetrician should suction the infant's oro- and nasopharynx prior to delivery of the shoulders. An 8- or 10-French flexible catheter is much more effective than simple bulb syringing. The next course of action depends on the thickness of the meconium and the clinical appearance of the baby. With **thin meconium**, if the infant is crying and vigorous, visualization of the larynx and intubation is probably not necessary. With **thick meconium** in a depressed infant, the infant's pharynx should be suctioned followed by endotracheal intubation with suctioning below the vocal cords. If the infant is *vigorous*, visualization of the cords may suffice, and if no meconium is noted at that level, intubation may be deferred. However, many clinicians recommend that the trachea be suctioned whenever there is thick meconium.

46. Name the three initial steps in resuscitation.

Thermal management, clearing the airway, tactile stimulation

47. During asphyxia, how is primary apnea distinguished from secondary apnea?

A regular sequence of events occurs when an infant is asphyxiated. Initially, gasping respiratory efforts increase in depth and frequency for up to 3 minutes, followed by approximately 1 minute of **primary apnea**. If oxygen (along with stimulation) is provided during the apneic period, respiratory function spontaneously returns. If asphyxia continues, gasping then resumes for a variable period of time, terminating with the "last gasp" and followed by **secondary apnea**. During secondary apnea, the only way to restore respiratory function is with positive pressure ventilation and high concentrations of oxygen.

Thus, a linear relationship exists between the duration of asphyxia and the recovery of respiratory function following resuscitation. The longer the artificial ventilation is delayed after the "last gasp," the longer it will take to resuscitate the infant. However, clinically, the two conditions are indistinguishable.

48. How much pressure does it take to inflate the lungs of a normal infant at the moment of birth?

At the initiation of respiration shortly after birth, pressures of 40–70 cm H_2O are generated to inflate the neonatal lung.

49. How does one estimate the size of an endotracheal tube needed for resuscitation?

Endotracheal Tubes Needed for Resuscitation

TUBE SIZE (ID mm)	WEIGHT	GESTATIONAL AGE
2.5	< 1,000 gm	< 28 wks
3.0	1,001–2,000 gm	28–34 wks
3.5	2,001–3,000 gm	34–38 wks
3.5–4.0	> 3,000 gm	> 38 wks

Adapted from Bloom RS, et al: Principles of neonatal resuscitation. In Polin RA, et al: (eds): Workbook in Practical Neonatology, 2nd ed. Philadelphia, W.B. Saunders, 1993, p 12; with permission.

50. What is the "7-8-9" rule?

The "7-8-9" rule is an estimate of the length (in cm) that an oral endotracheal tube should be inserted in a 1-, 2-, or 3-kg infant, respectively. A variation of this rule is the tip-to-lip rule of adding 6 to the weight of the infant to determine the insertion distance. With good visualization, the tube should be inserted 1.0–1.5 cm below the vocal cords. Tube placement should always be verified radiographically.

51. Should infants be intubated nasally or orally?

There are studies to support both routes of intubation for newborn infants. The oral intubation school argues that since neonates are obligate nose breathers, they will demonstrate increased work of breathing as well as atelectasis following removal of nasotracheal tubes. On the other hand, the nasal intubation school suggests that orotracheal intubation results in grooving of the palate with subsequent orthodontic problems. A recent study has not confirmed the increased incidence of postextubation atelectasis in nasally intubated babies. Therefore, operator skill and institutional tradition are primary considerations in this clinical decision.

52. How is the size of the endotracheal tube related to the development of subglottic stenosis?

If the endotracheal tube size (mm)/gestational age (wks) ratio is > 0.1, there is an increased risk for development of tracheal stenosis.

53. When should epinephrine be given during a resuscitation in the delivery room?

In a depressed infant with gasping or absent respirations, 100% oxygen should be given via positive pressure ventilation (PPV). Depending on the extent of asphyxia (and depression of heart rate), cardiac compressions are usually initiated within 30 seconds. If there is no response (i.e., increased heart rate) after at least 30 seconds of PPV with 100% oxygen and chest compressions, epinephrine is indicated. Epinephrine, 1:10,000, can be given via IV, umbilical vein, or endotracheal tube at a dose of 0.1–0.3 ml/kg.

54. When is sodium bicarbonate administered in a resuscitation?

If there is no response to epinephrine in a severely asphyxiated infant (with continued apnea and a heart rate < 100), sodium bicarbonate (and/or a volume expander) should be considered. If an infant is being adequately ventilated, the partial correction of metabolic acidosis may improve pulmonary blood flow and improve oxygenation. Half-strength (4.2% solution or 0.5 mEq/l) bicarbonate is preferable, given in a dose of 2 mEq/kg slowly over 2–5 minutes.

55. Are there complications of sodium bicarbonate therapy in infants?

The relative risks of sodium bicarbonate therapy in infants are related to dosage (higher > lower), rapidity of administration (faster > slower), and osmolality (higher > lower). Physiologic complications include a transient increase in $PaCO_2$ and fall in PaO_2. The sudden expansion of blood volume and increase in cerebral blood flow may increase the risk of periventricular-intraventricular hemorrhage in preterm infants. Other potential complications include the development of hypernatremia and metabolic alkalosis.

56. If the newborn is stabilized and extent of acidosis determined by an arterial blood gas, how is the therapeutic correction calculated?

$$HCO_3 \text{ (mEq)} = \text{Base deficit (mEq/L)} \times 0.3 \text{ L/kg} \times \text{body wt (kg)}$$

Generally, it is safest to correct half the base deficit initially, and then reassess acid-base status to determine if further correction is necessary. Under optimal circumstances, sodium bicarbonate should be infused in small doses over 20–30 minutes as a dilute solution (0.5 mEq/ml).

57. What are the side effects of naloxone?

Naloxone has a history of being remarkably free of side effects, except for precipitating manifestations of sudden drug withdrawal in infants born to drug-addicted mothers. Other reported side effects relate to the sudden release of catecholamines, which can cause hypertension, sudden cardiac arrest, and cardiac dysrhythmias. It is important to remember that the half-life of naloxone is significantly shorter than that of narcotics.

58. Should umbilical arterial catheters be kept in a "low" or "high" position?

Umbilical catheters kept in a **low** position (L3–5) have a somewhat higher incidence of lower limb blanching and cyanosis compared to high lines (T6–10). However, high lines may be associated with a slightly increased risk of periventricular-intraventricular hemorrhage as well as embolization of clots to arterial vessels distal to the catheter site. No differences in the development of sepsis or necrotizing enterocolitis have been noted between infants with low or high umbilical catheters.

59. After a "traumatic" delivery, what are the commonly injured systems?

1. Cranial injuries: caput succedaneum, subconjunctival hemorrhage, cephalhematoma, skull fractures, intracranial hemorrhage, cerebral edema
2. Spinal injuries: spinal cord transection
3. Peripheral nerve injuries: brachial palsy (Erb-Duchenne paralysis, Klumpke paralysis), phrenic nerve and facial nerve paralysis
4. Visceral injuries: liver rupture or hematoma, splenic rupture, adrenal hemorrhage
5. Skeletal injuries: fractures of the clavicle, femur, and humerus

60. Who was Virginia Apgar?

Virginia Apgar, an anesthesiologist at Columbia Presbyterian Medical Center, introduced the Apgar scoring system in 1953 to assess the newborn infant's response to the stress of labor and delivery.

61. How does one remember the Apgar score?

A   Appearance (pink, mottled, or blue)
P   Pulse (> 100, < 100, or 0 bpm)
G   Grimace (response to suctioning of the nose and mouth)
A   Activity (flexed arms and legs, extended limbs, or limp)
R   Respiratory effort (crying, gasping, or no respiratory activity)

Each category is assigned a rating of 0, 1, or 2 points with a total score of 10 indicating the best possible condition. A score of < 3 at one minute implies possible asphyxia and the score at 5 minutes gauges the response to resuscitation efforts.

62. Is a low Apgar score alone sufficient to diagnose a neonate as asphyxiated?

No. It is not acceptable to label an infant as asphyxiated simply because of a low Apgar score. Asphyxiated neonates typically have a profound metabolic acidosis and demonstrate abnormalities in multiple organ systems. Signs referable to the CNS are often most prominent. The cardinal features of hypoxic-ischemic encephalopathy include seizures, alterations of consciousness, and abnormalities of tone. Disorders of reflexes, respiratory pattern, oculovestibular responses, and autonomic function are less significant components of this entity.

Committee on Fetus and Newborn: Use and abuse of the Apgar score. Pediatrics 98:141–142, 1996.

63. When should a neonatal resuscitation be stopped?

No precise answer is possible, as clinical circumstances and responses are variable. However, in one study of 58 newborns who had an Apgar score of 0 at 10 minutes despite appropriate resuscitative efforts, only 1 of 58 survived and that infant had profound cerebral palsy. Failure of response after ≥ 10 minutes should prompt consideration of cessation.

Jain L: Cardiopulmonary resuscitation of apparently stillborn infants: Survival and long-term outcome. J Pediatr 118:778–782, 1991.

DEVELOPMENT AND GROWTH

64. What is the best way to assess gestational age in the fetus?

Nägele's rule, dating pregnancy from the first day of the last menstrual period, has historically been the most reliable way to assess gestational age. However, ultrasound measurements done between 5–20 weeks of gestation can predict gestational age quite accurately. Prior to 12 weeks' gestation, crown–rump length is the measurement of choice, and beyond 12 weeks', biparietal diameter is the preferred study. In later gestation, the accuracy of fetal age determination is improved by the assessment of multiple variables (e.g., femur length, abdominal circumference, and biparietal diameter) and by serial determinations. Maternal dates should always be used as the "gold standard" unless ultrasound studies are highly discrepant. Estimates of uterine size, which approximate gestational age from 16–38 weeks, may also be clinically useful.

65. What features constitute the biophysical profile?

The biophysical profile is a scoring system that assesses fetal well-being prior to birth. Five variables are assessed: fetal breathing movements, gross body movements, fetal tone, reactive fetal heart rate, and qualitative amniotic fluid volume. Normal results equate to 2 points per variable, for a possible total of 10 points.

66. How can gestational age be determined by looking at the lens of the eye?

In fetal ocular development, a web of blood vessels on the anterior lens fades as gestation progresses. Ophthalmoscopic examination of the anterior lens allows an estimation of gestational age:

Grade 4	Grade 3	Grade 2	Grade 1
27 to 28 weeks	29 to 30 weeks	31 to 32 weeks	33 to 34 weeks

From Hittner H, et al: Assessment of gestational age by examination of the anterior capsule of the lens. J Pediatr 91:455, 1977; with permission.

67. What is the first bone in the human fetus to ossify?

The clavicle. In the long bones, the process of ossification occurs in the primary centers of ossification in the diaphysis during the embryonic period of fetal development. Although the femora are the first long bones to show traces of ossification, the clavicles, which develop initially by intramembranous ossification, begin to ossify before any other bones in the body.

68. What external characteristics are useful for estimating gestational age?

External Gestational Age Characteristics

EXTERNAL CHARACTERISTICS	GESTATIONAL AGE			
	28 WKS	32 WKS	36WKS	40 WKS
Ear cartilage	Pinna soft, remains folded	Pinna slightly harder but remains folded	Pinna harder, springs back	Pinna firm, stands erect from head
Breast tissue	None	None	1–2 mm nodule	6–7 mm nodule
External genitalia				
Male	Testes undescended, smooth scrotum	Testes in inguinal canal, few scrotal rugae	Testes high in scrotum, more scrotal rugae	Testes descended, pendulous scrotum covered with rugae
Female	Prominent clitoris, small, widely separated labia	Prominent clitoris, larger separated labia	Clitoris less prominent, labia majora cover labia minora	Clitoris covered by labia majora
Plantar surface	Smooth	1–2 anterior creases	2–3 anterior creases	Creases cover sole

From Volpe JJ: Neurology of the Newborn, 3rd ed. Philadelphia, W.B. Saunders, 1995, p 96; with permission.

69. At what gestational age does pupillary reaction to light develop?

Pupillary reaction to light may appear as early as 29 weeks' gestation but is not consistently present until approximately 32 weeks.

70. At what gestational age does a sense of smell develop?

By 32 weeks' gestation, normal premature infants respond to concentrated odor.

71. When does the fetal heart begin to contract in utero?

Contractions begin by the 22nd day of gestation. These contractions resemble peristaltic waves and begin in the sinus venosus. By the end of the 4th week, they result in unidirectional flow of blood.

72. How does fetal circulation differ from neonatal circulation?

1. Intra- and extracardiac shunts are present: placenta, ductus venosus, foramen ovale, ductus arteriosus.
2. The two ventricles work in parallel rather than in series.
3. The right ventricle pumps against a higher resistance than the left ventricle.
4. Blood flow to the lung is only a fraction of the right ventricular output.
5. The lung extracts oxygen from the blood instead of providing oxygen for it.
6. The lung continually secretes a fluid into the respiratory passages.
7. The liver is the first organ to receive maternal substances, such as oxygen, glucose, amino acids, etc.
8. The placenta is the major route of gas exchange, excretion, and acquisition of essential fetal chemicals.
9. The placenta provides a low resistance circuit.

Adams FH, Emmanouilides GC (eds): Moss' Heart Disease in Infants, Children, and Adolescents, 3rd ed. Baltimore, Williams & Wilkins, 1983, pp 11–17.

73. What changes occur in stroke volume, cardiac output, and heart rate after birth?

Both stroke volume (SV) and cardiac output (CO) increase into adolescence, whereas heart rate (HR) falls.

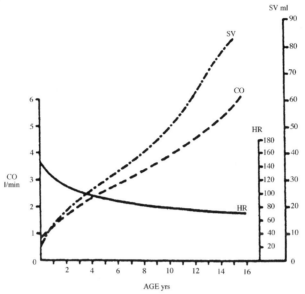

From Rudolph AM: Congenital Diseases of the Heart. Chicago, Year Book Medical Publishers, 1974; with permission.

74. Why does pulmonary vascular resistance (PVR) decline postnatally?

Within minutes after birth, the PVR drops due to rapid recruitment of peripheral arteries previously "closed." The phase of accelerated recruitment of peripheral arteries results from a combination of events, including gaseous expansion of the lung (with removal of fluid), a fall in arterial PCO_2, and a rise in arterial PO_2. PVR continues to decrease in the days following birth, principally from a gradual decrease in medial wall thickness of smaller muscular arteries (< 250 μm). Within a few months, the more proximal vessels (> 250 μm) also show a decrease in medial wall thickness. However, the specific mechanism(s) responsible for the remodeling of the pulmonary vasculature after birth are unknown.

75. How does postmaturity differ from dysmaturity?

An infant born of a postterm pregnancy (> 42 weeks' gestation) is referred to as **postmature**. The baby is **dysmature** if features of placental insufficiency are present. These include loss of subcutaneous fat and muscle mass, as well as meconium staining of the amniotic fluid, skin, and nails.

76. What is the normal rate of head growth in the preterm infant?

0.5–1.0 cm/wk during the first 2–4 months of life. An increase in the circumference of the head of ≥ 2.0 cm in 1 week should raise a suspicion of CNS pathology, such as hydrocephalus. However, some premature infants may experience rapid "catch-up" head growth following significant early stress or illness. The ratio of body length to head circumference may be used to distinguish normal from abnormal head growth. A ratio of 1.42–1.48 is reportedly normal, whereas a low ratio of 1.12–1.32 indicates relative or absolute macrocephaly.

77. How is the ponderal index used to classify growth-retarded infants?

$$\text{Ponderal index (PI)} = \frac{\text{weight (gm)}}{(\text{length [cm]})^3} \times 100$$

This index has been used to estimate the adequacy of intrauterine fetal nutrition. Values < 2.0 between 29 and 37 weeks' gestation and 2.2 beyond 37 weeks' have been associated with fetal malnutrition. Growth-retarded infants with low ponderal indices also appear to be at increased risk for the development of neonatal hypoglycemia. Maternal conditions associated with a low ponderal index (fetal malnutrition) include poor maternal weight gain, lack of prenatal care, preeclampsia, and chronic maternal illness.

78. What morbidities (short- and long-term) are known to occur more frequently in growth-retarded babies?

Short-term morbidities include perinatal asphyxia, meconium aspiration, fasting hypoglycemia, alimented hypoglycemia, polycythemia-hyperviscosity, and immunodeficiency.

Long-term morbidities include poor developmental outcome and altered postnatal growth. Most studies demonstrate normal intelligence and developmental quotients in SGA infants, although there seems to be a higher incidence of behavioral and learning problems. The presence or absence of severe perinatal asphyxia is extremely important in predicting later intellectual and neurologic function.

79. When do premature infants "catch-up" on growth charts?

Most catch-up growth takes place during the first 2 years of life, with maximal growth rates occurring between 36–40 weeks postconception. Little catch-up growth occurs after 3 years' chronologic age. Approximately 15% of infants born prematurely remain below normal weight at 3 years of age.

GASTROINTESTINAL ISSUES

80. When does the newborn infant's stomach begin to secrete acid?

The pH of gastric fluid in newborns is usually neutral or slightly acidic and decreases shortly after birth. pH values are < 3 by 6–8 hours of age and then increase again during the second week of life. Preterm infants frequently demonstrate gastric pH values > 7.

81. At what rate do the disaccharidases develop prenatally?

The disaccharidases are detectable with low activity at about 12–14 weeks of gestation, and by 24 weeks, sucrase, maltase, and isomaltase generally achieve significant levels of activity. Lactase activity lags behind and is frequently not detected until 28–30 weeks of gestation. Many preterm and term infants demonstrate lactose intolerance when measured by breath hydrogen analysis; however, the significance of subclinical lactose intolerance is controversial.

82. When is meconium usually passed after birth?

Most infants pass some meconium in the first 12 hours of life. Overall, 99% of term infants and 95% of premature infants pass meconium by 48 hours of life. However, the smallest of premature infants may have delayed passage of meconium due to relative immaturity of rectal sphincteric reflexes.

83. What differentiates meconium ileus from meconium plug syndrome?

Meconium ileus: Obstruction of the distal ileum occurs secondary to thick, tenacious concretions of inspissated meconium. A barium enema may reveal a microcolon, and 25% of cases have associated intestinal atresia due to intrauterine obstruction. Meconium ileus is a common presentation of cystic fibrosis in the newborn period.

Meconium plug syndrome: This condition presents as either delayed passage of meconium or intestinal obstruction. Barium enema usually demonstrates a normal caliber colon with multiple filling defects. Small preterm infants, infants of diabetic mothers, and infants born to mothers who received magnesium sulfate are especially likely to develop meconium plug syndrome.

There is also an increased frequency of cystic fibrosis in infants with meconium plug syndrome, although much less than with meconium ileus.

84. After an asphyxial event, how long should feeding be delayed?
During an asphyxial event, vasoconstriction of the mesenteric vessels can result in intestinal ischemia. Because of the relationship between ischemia and the incidence of necrotizing enterocolitis, feedings should be delayed for 2–3 days to allow for repair of the intestinal mucosa.

85. List the four types of congenital diaphragmatic defects.
1. Posterolateral defect, or Bochdalek hernia
2. Parasternal defect, or Morgagni hernia
3. Septum transversum defects
4. Congenitally large esophageal orifice or hiatal hernias

86. How is gastroschisis differentiated from omphalocele in the newborn infant?
Both are ventral wall defects, yet their pathogenesis and prognosis differ markedly.

	Gastroschisis	Omphalocele
Incidence	1/50,000 births	1/5,000 births
Location of defect	Right paraumbilical	Central umbilical
Umbilical cord insertion	Normal	Apex of sac
Herniation of liver	Rare	Common
Extraintestinal anomalies	Rare	Common
Chromosomal abnormalities	Rare	Common

87. Which conditions are associated with intra-abdominal calcifications?
Meconium peritonitis and **intra-abdominal tumors** are the most common disorders associated with intra-abdominal calcifications in the neonate. The calcifications of meconium peritonitis are streaky or plaque-like and occur over the abdominal surface of the diaphragm or along the flanks. Intraintestinal calcifications appear as small round densities that follow the course of the intestine and occur in association with intestinal stenoses, atresias, and aganglionosis. Intra-abdominal calcifications have also been observed in infants with adrenal hemorrhages and congenital infections.

88. How is necrotizing enterocolitis (NEC) distinguished from volvulus?

	NEC	Volvulus
Preterm infants	85–90%	30–35%
Onset by day 14 of life	85–90%	50–60%
Male:female	1:1	2:1
Associated anomalies	Rare	25–40%
Bilious emesis	Unusual	75%
Grossly bloody stools	Common	Less common
Pneumatosis intestinalis	80–90%	1–2%
Marked proximal duodenal obstruction (x-ray)	Rare	Common
Thrombocytopenia without DIC	Common	Rare

DIC, disseminated intravascular coagulation.
From Kleigman RM: Necrotizing enterocolitis: Differential diagnosis and management. In Polin RA, et al (eds): Workbook in Practical Neonatology, 2nd ed. Philadelphia, W.B. Saunders, 1993, p 456; with permission.

89. Are positive blood cultures common in babies with NEC?

Approximately 25% will have a positive blood culture at the time of diagnosis.

90. When is paracentesis indicated in a neonate with suspected NEC?

When there is a high suspicion of intestinal gangrene but no radiographic evidence of free air in the abdomen, abdominal paracentesis should be considered. A positive paracentesis, as indicated by the presence of brown fluid or bacteria on Gram stain, is diagnostic of intestinal gangrene with a specificity approaching 100%.

91. Is pneumatosis intestinalis pathognomonic for NEC?

No. Pneumatosis intestinalis can be seen in various other conditions, including Hirschsprung disease, pseudomembranous enterocolitis, neonatal ulcerative colitis, and ischemic bowel disease.

92. How long should infants with NEC be kept NPO?

Infants with true NEC (radiographic or surgical evidence) should remain NPO for a minimum of 2–3 weeks. Infants in whom the diagnosis is suspected but not proven should be treated conservatively. Many of these infants may be fed after 3–7 days.

93. Does the feeding of immunoglobulin to infants or the use of prophylactic antibotics prevent NEC?

Immunoglobulins: Preliminary studies show that formula fortified with immunoglobulins (IgA and IgG) may effectively reduce the incidence of NEC in very-low-birthweight infants. IgA may provide local mucosal protection, while IgG may neutralize toxins of ingested pathogenic bacteria. More definitive studies are needed to evaluate this promising therapy.

Antibiotics: In two small studies of high-risk, low-birthweight infants, the administration of oral kanamycin/gentamicin was effective in preventing NEC. However, study infants became colonized with organisms resistant to these antibiotics. More recent studies have failed to show a decreased incidence of NEC following prophylactic oral antibiotics. Therefore, antibiotic prophylaxis is not indicated for the prevention of NEC.

94. What is pig-bel?

Pig-bel is an NEC-like disease afflicting infants and adults in Papua, New Guinea. It is caused by ingestion of *Clostridium perfringens* type C enterotoxin.

95. How is the volume of gastric aspirate helpful in the diagnosis of intestinal obstruction in a newborn?

A large aspirate in the first 15 minutes after birth suggests obstruction. In normal term newborns, the mean gastric aspirate is about 5 ml. In newborns with obstruction (e.g., duodenal atresia, jejunal atresia, annular pancreas), the mean aspirate is approximately 60 ml. Any gastric aspirate > 20 ml should be viewed as suspicious.

Britton JR, Britton HL: Gastric aspirate volume at birth as an indication of congenital intestinal obstruction. Acta Pediatr 84:945–946, 1995.

HEMATOLOGIC ISSUES

96. When does the switchover from fetal to adult hemoglobin synthesis occur in the neonate?

The switch from production of hemoglobin F to hemoglobin A begins in a very programmed fashion in the fetus and neonate at approximately 32 weeks' gestation. At birth, approximately 50–65% of hemoglobin is type F.

97. How do the relative amounts of hemoglobin polypeptide chains vary in the fetus and infant?

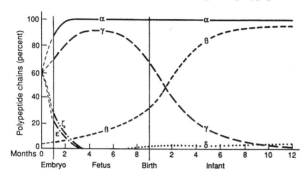

From Lane PA, et al: Hematologic disorders. In Hay WW, et al (eds): Current Pediatric Diagnosis & Treatment, 12th ed. Norwalk, CT, Appleton & Lange, 1995, p 828; with permission.

98. Does the definition of anemia vary by gestational age?

For the term infant, most authorities consider a venous blood hemoglobin of < 13.0 gm/dl or a capillary hemoglobin of < 14.5 gm/dl as consistent with anemia. In preterm infants beyond 32 weeks' gestation, hematologic values differ only minimally from those of full-term infants, and therefore the same values may be used.

99. Describe the changes in hemoglobin concentration seen during the first few days of life.

In all newborn infants, hemoglobin levels rise slightly during the first few hours of life (because of hemoconcentration) and then fall somewhat during the remainder of the first day. In healthy full-term infants, the hemoglobin concentration then stays relatively constant for the rest of the first week of life. However, appropriate-for-gestational-age infants of < 1500 gm birthweight may show a decline of 1.0–1.5 gm/day during this same period.

100. What are the indications for RBC transfusions in premature infants?

Preterm infants who are critically ill and who experience (1) large blood losses at the time of delivery, (2) repeated blood sampling, or (3) other episodes of bleeding should receive RBC transfusions to replace these losses. Anemic infants who require an inspiratory oxygen concentration ≥ 30% should be transfused to optimize oxygen-carrying capacity. In infants who are ventilator- and oxygen-dependent, maintaining the venous hematocrit > 35% should be considered. "Top-off" transfusions for clinically well infants are not generally recommended. Healthy preterm infants should be observed for the development of signs and symptoms referable to anemia (poor growth, tachycardia, apnea, bradycardia). Preterm infants with apnea and bradycardia which are unresponsive to methylxanthines may benefit from transfusion therapy. Other indications for RBC transfusions are less clear.

101. Which neonates should receive irradiated blood?

All premature infants and infants < 1500 gm should receive irradiated blood.

102. How does phlebotomy in a premature infant compare with that in an adult?

Withdrawing 1 ml of blood from a 1000-gm infant is equivalent to taking 70 ml of blood from an adult.

Blanchette VS, Ziporsky A: Assessment of anemia in newborn infants. Clin Perinatol 11:489–510, 1984.

103. Which antigens make up the Rh complex?

The Rh antigen complex is made up of six possible antigens: C, c, D, d, E, e. The vast majority of isoimmunizations causing serious neonatal disease are the result of incompatibility to the D antigen. The non-D Rh antigens (E, C, c) have been shown to cause hemolytic disease and may be associated with mild to severe hydrops fetalis.

104. How can Rh disease be prevented?

Unsensitized pregnant women who are Rh-negative should have a repeat antibody screen at approximately 28 weeks' gestation and receive 300 μg of Rh-immune globulin (RhoGAM) prophylactically. After delivery, if the infant is Rh-positive, the mother should receive an additional dose of RhoGAM. At the time of delivery, the dose of RhoGAM may be increased if the fetomaternal hemorrhage is excessively large.

105. Why is the direct Coombs' test frequently negative or weakly positive in infants with ABO incompatibility?

There are fewer A or B antigenic sites on the newborn red cell, and there is also a greater distance between antigenic sites when compared to adult red cells. There is also absorption of serum antibody by naturally occurring A and B substances scattered throughout body tissues, in foods, and gram-negative bacteria.

106. If fetomaternal hemorrhage is suspected as a cause of neonatal anemia, how is this diagnosed?

The **Kleihauer-Betke test** detects the presence of fetal cells in the maternal circulation. It involves an acid elution technique, which utilizes the property of fetal hemoglobin to resist elution in an acid medium. In a stained maternal blood smear, the fetal cells stain darkly, and the percentage of fetal red cells can be determined. One percent fetal cells in the maternal circulation indicates a bleed of 50 ml.

107. If a gastric aspirate contains blood shortly after birth, what test can determine if it is swallowed maternal blood or fetal hemorrhage?

The Apt test. This test relies on the increased sensitivity of adult hemoglobin to alkali compared with fetal hemoglobin.

Method: Mix the specimen with an equal quantity of tap water. Centrifuge or filter. Supernatant must have pink color to proceed. To 5 parts of supernatant, add 1 part of 0.25 N (1%) NaOH.

Interpretation: A pink color persisting > 2 minutes indicates fetal hemoglobin. Adult hemoglobin gives a pink color that becomes yellow in 2 minutes or less, indicating denaturation of hemoglobin.

108. How is polycythemia defined?

Polycythemia is defined by a venous hematocrit of ≥ 65%, since this exceeds the mean hematocrit found in normal newborns by 2 standard deviations. As the central venous hematocrit rises above 65%, there is a dramatic increase in viscosity. Since direct measurements of blood viscosity are not readily available in most labs, a high hematocrit is felt to be the best indicator of hyperviscosity.

109. What are the clinical manifestations of polycythemia?

In symptomatic infants, the most common presentations relate to **CNS abnormalities**, including lethargy, hypotonia, tremulousness, and irritability. With severe CNS involvement, seizures can result. **Hypoglycemia** is common. Other organ systems can be involved, including the GI tract (vomiting, distension, NEC), kidneys (renal vein thrombosis and acute renal failure), and cardiopulmonary system (respiratory distress, congestive heart failure). Peripheral manifestations can include gangrene and priapism. Of note, infants with polycythemia are often asymptomatic.

110. In what settings is polycythemia most likely to occur?

Although the most common cause is idiopathic, identifiable causes result primarily from two mechanisms:

Active (Increased Intrauterine Erythropoiesis)	Passive (Secondary to Eruthrocyte Transfusions)
Intrauterine hypoxia	Delayed cord clamping
Placental insufficiency	Intentional
SGA infants	Unassisted delivery
Postmaturity	Maternofetal transfusion
Toxemia of pregnancy	Twin-twin transfusion
Drugs (propranolol)	
Severe maternal heart disease	
Maternal smoking	
Maternal diabetes	
Neonatal hyper- or hypothyroidism	
Congenital adrenal hyperplasia	
Chromosome abnormalities	
Trisomy 13, 18, 21	
Hyperplastic visceromegaly (Beckwith syndrome)	
Decreased fetal erythrocyte deformability	

From Oski FA, Naiman JL: Hematologic Problems in the Newborn, 3rd ed. Philadelphia, W.B. Saunders, 1982; with permission.

111. Which infants with polycythemia should be treated?

Because polycythemia results from a diverse array of etiologies, it is difficult to determine whether outcome depends more on etiology or the chronic elevation of viscosity. There is controversy regarding guidelines for treatment. Many authorities recommend a partial exchange transfusion, regardless of symptoms, in infants with a central venous hematocrit ≥ 70% (due to the correlation with laboratory-measured hyperviscosity) or those with a central hematocrit ≥ 65% if there are signs and symptoms attributable to polycythemia.

112. Describe the preferred method for partial exchange transfusions in polycythemic neonates.

Partial exchange transfusions can be performed through an umbilical venous catheter, umbilical arterial catheter, or peripheral venous catheter. Aliquots equal to 5% of the estimated blood volume are withdrawn and replaced by either fresh frozen plasma, Plasmanate, 5% albumin, or normal saline. The latter two solutions may be preferable since they avoid the risks of transfusion-acquired infections associated with plasma. The amount of blood volume to be exchanged with crystalloid or colloid may be calculated using the following formula:

$$\text{Blood volume to be exchanged} = \frac{\text{Observed Hct} - \text{desired Hct (55\%)}}{\text{Observed Hct}} \times \text{Blood volume} \times \text{Body wt (kg) (85–100 ml/kg)}$$

113. What is the long-term morbidity of polycythemia in newborns?

Follow-up studies suggest that early polycythemia may be associated with mild neuropsychologic handicaps, lower school achievement, fine motor abnormalities, and more speech delay in comparison with control infants in the first years of life.

Black VD, et al: Neonatal hyperviscosity: Association with lower achievement and IQ scores at school age. Pediatrics 83:662–667, 1989.

114. What is the definition of thrombocytopenia in the neonate?

Platelet counts < 100,000 should be considered abnormal in term or preterm neonates, whereas counts in the 100,000–150,000/mm^3 range may be seen in some healthy newborns. Consequently, patients with counts in this latter category should have repeat counts as well as further studies if illness is suspected.

115. What is the differential diagnosis in a newborn with a confirmed low platelet count?

Causes of increased platelet destruction	Causes of decreased platelet production
Maternal idiopathic thrombocytopenic purpura	Congenital amegakaryocytic hypoplasia (e.g., (TAR)
Isoimmune thrombocytopenia	Bone marrow replacement
Infection	Pancytopenias (e.g., Fanconi anemia, trisomy 13 and 18)
Disseminated intravascular coagulation	
Drugs	
Extensive localized thrombosis	
Critically ill infants	**Undetermined mechanism**
Giant hemangiomas	Inborn errors of metabolism
Maternal lupus	Congenital thyrotoxicosis

From Andrew M, Kolton J: Neonatal thrombocytopenia. Clin Perinatol 11:363, 1984; with permission.

116. Describe the two main types of neonatal thrombocytopenia caused by maternal antibody.

Transplacental passage of antibody from the mother to infant can be due to (1) maternal idiopathic thrombocytopenic purpura (ITP, with the newborn a secondary target) and (2) isoimmune thrombocytopenia (with the newborn a primary target). The diseases can have a similar clinical appearance. Babies are generally well-appearing, do not have hepatosplenomegaly, and have thrombocytopenia that persists for 3–12 weeks postnatally. Differences include:

	Maternal ITP	*Isoimmune Neonatal Thrombocytopenia*
Estimated incidence	Uncertain,? 1 in 300 births	1 in 500 births
Offending antigen	Probably part of platelet membrane glycoprotein IIb–IIIa complex: on *all* platelets	PLA[1] (Zw[a]) or HLA: on father's and neonate's platelets but *not* mothers
Type of antibody	Maternal autoantibody	Maternal alloantibody (isoantibody) directed against foreign platelet antigen
Maternal platelet count	Reduced (unless previous splenectomy)	Always normal
Recurrence risk	Cannot be reliably estimated from maternal platelet count	50–85% (depending on offending antigen and zygosity of father)

From Buchanan GR: Coagulation disorders in the neonate. Pediatr Clin North Am 33:212, 1986; with permission.

117. How should women known to have a previous infant with alloimmune thrombocytopenia be evaluated during pregnancy?

Fetal thrombocytopenia can usually be detected at 20–22 weeks' gestation through percutaneous umbilical blood sampling. An additional evaluation at 37 weeks' gestation is indicated to assist in directing antepartum treatments. In utero therapy includes fetal platelet transfusions with carefully washed maternal platelets and administration of intravenous immunoglobulin to the mother.

An infant with thrombocytopenia should be delivered via cesarean section to reduce the risk of intracranial hemorrhage.

118. In the mother with new-onset thrombocytopenia during pregnancy, how can one determine the risk to the fetus?

The maternal platelet count is a poor predictor of risk of thrombocytopenia in the fetus. However, an elevated maternal titer of **circulating antiplatelet IgG** places the infant at high risk for thrombocytopenia. When maternal thrombocytopenia is limited to late pregnancy, however, the risk for developing severe neonatal thrombocytopenia is low. In mothers who have circulating antiplatelet antibody (IgG), the infant should be delivered via cesarean section, or a cordocentesis should be performed to demonstrate a normal platelet count prior to a vaginal delivery.

119. When should a thrombocytopenic infant receive a platelet transfusion?

Infants with platelet counts of $< 20,000/mm^3$, or those with clinical signs of bleeding regardless of the actual count, should receive platelet transfusions. In infants at increased risk for hemorrhage (e.g., postoperative) the platelet count should be kept $> 100,000/mm^3$.

120. How long do transfused platelets survive?

If thrombocytopenia is not the result of increased platelet destruction, the platelet count will fall approximately 10% each day and reach pretransfusion levels in approximately 1 week.

121. When do the prothrombin time and partial thromboplastin time "normalize" to adult values?

The prothrombin time reaches adult values at approximately 1 week of age, while the partial thromboplastin time does not attain adult values until 2–9 months.

122. How is disseminated intravascular coagulation (DIC) diagnosed in the neonate?

The laboratory findings in DIC include evidence of red cell fragmentation on peripheral smear; elevation of prothrombin time, partial thromboplastin time, and thrombin time; thrombocytopenia; decreased levels of factors V, VIII, and fibrinogen; and in some cases, the presence of fibrin split products.

123. How should newborn infants with DIC be managed?

Treatment should be directed primarily at the underlying disease rather than just at the coagulation defects. In many cases, treatment of the former makes specific treatment of the latter unnecessary. However, in cases in which stabilization of coagulopathy is not imminent, treatment with fresh frozen plasma and platelets is recommended. In cases where fluid overload is a major concern, exchange transfusion with fresh whole blood may be used. However, this second approach is not superior to the first with respect to resolution of DIC. The use of heparin in DIC is currently reserved for cases of thrombosis of major vessels or purpura fulminans.

124. What is the difference between early and late hemorrhagic disease of the newborn?

For evolutionary reasons that are unclear, a newborn has only about 50% of the normal vitamin-K-dependent cofactors, and unless vitamin K is given, these levels steadily decline in the first 3 days of life. In addition, breastmilk is low in vitamin K. **Early hemorrhagic disease** can be observed during the first few days of life in infants who are exclusively breastfed and who do not receive vitamin K prophylaxis at birth. They can present with bleeding from various sites (e.g., umbilical cord, circumcision). Infants born to mothers who have received medications that affect the metabolism of vitamin K (e.g., warfarin, antiepileptic medications, antituberculous drugs) are at risk to develop severe life-threatening intracranial hemorrhages at or shortly after delivery. **Late hemorrhagic disease** occurs most commonly between 1 and 3 months of life in infants who are exclusively breastfed and who develop diarrhea from a variety of causes. These infants typically did not receive vitamin K at birth or received it in an oral form. Although oral vitamin K supplementation should prevent late disease, the optimal oral dose, timing, and form of vitamin K required have not been clearly established.

Hathaway WE: Comparison of oral and parenteral vitamin K prophylaxis for prevention of late hemorrhagic disease of the newborn. J Pediatr 119:461–463, 1991.

125. Does administration of vitamin K in the newborn period increase the risk of childhood cancer?

In the early 1990s, British investigators reported an association between intramuscular vitamin K and an increased risk in childhood cancers, particularly leukemia. However, subsequent studies have refuted this claim, and perinatal use of intramuscular vitamin K is still recommended.

Klebanoff MA, et al: The risk of childhood cancer after neonatal exposure to vitamin K. N Engl J Med 329:905–908, 1993.

HYPERBILIRUBINEMIA

126. What are the normal maximum bilirubin levels for full-term healthy newborns?
The 97th percentile for bilirubin in healthy full-term infants is **12.4** mg/dl for bottlefed infants and **14.8** mg/dl for breastfed infants.

127. What maternal factors affect neonatal serum bilirubin levels?

	Increase	*Decrease*
Race	East Asian Native American Greek	Black
Maternal health issues	Primipara (?) Older mothers Diabetes Hypertension Oral contraceptive use at time of conception First trimester bleeding Decreased plasma zinc level	Smoking
Drugs administered to mother	Oxytocin Diazepam Epidural anesthesia Promethazine	Phenobarbital Meperidine Reserpine Aspirin Chloral hydrate Heroin Phenytoin Antipyrine Alcohol

From Maisels MJ: Neonatal jaundice. In Avery GB, et al (eds): Neonatology: Pathophysiology and Management of the Newborn, 4th ed. Philadelphia, J.B. Lippincott, 1994, p 639; with permission.

128. Which physiologic factors contribute to the rise in serum bilirubin in newborns?

Possible Mechanisms Involved in Physiologic Jaundice of the Newborn

Increased bilirubin load on liver cell
   ↑ RBC volume
   ↓ RBC survival
   ↑ Early-labeled bilirubin
   ↑ Enterohepatic circulation of bilirubin
Defective hepatic uptake of bilirubin from plasma
   ↓ Ligandin (Y protein)
   Binding of Y and Z proteins by other anions
   ↓ Relative hepatic uptake deficiency (phase II)
Defective bilirubin conjugation
   ↓ UDP glucuronyl transferase activity
   ↓ UDP glucose dehydrogenase activity
Defective bilirubin excretion
   Excretion impaired but not rate-limiting
Hepatic circulation
   ↓ Oxygen supply to the liver when umbilical cord clamped
   Portal blood flow bypassing liver sinusoids if ductus venosus patent

From Maisels MJ: Neonatal jaundice. In Avery GB, et al (eds): Neonatalogy: Pathophysiology and Management of the Newborn, 4th ed. Philadelphia, J.B. Lippincott, 1994, p 653; with permission.

129. Why is bilirubin toxic to the brain?

Although it is well established that unconjugated bilirubin is toxic to the CNS, the exact mechanism is not known. Bilirubin is toxic/inhibitory to a wide variety of enzymatic reactions. In vitro studies have demonstrated that bilirubin impairs water and ion exchange. Furthermore, bilirubin impairs the activation of protein kinase C, decreases phosphorylation of intermediary proteins, and decreases mitochondrial functions, substrate transport, and cell viability. Bilirubin also adversely affects the conductive properties of nerve cell membranes at both the cellular and functional level.

130. What factors suggest hemolytic disease as a cause of jaundice in the newborn?

- Family history of hemolytic disease
- Ethnicity suggestive of inherited disease (e.g., G6PD deficiency)
- Onset of jaundice before 24 hours of age
- Bilirubin rise > 0.5 mg/dl/hr
- Pallor, hepatosplenomegaly
- Failure of phototherapy to lower bilirubin level

Provisional Committee for Quality Improvement and Subcommittee on Hyperbilirubinemia: Practice parameter: Management of hyperbilirubinemia in the healthy term newborn. Pediatrics 94:558–565, 1994.

131. Which infants are "set-ups" for ABO incompatibility?

Infants who are type A or B and whose mothers are type O. In individuals with types A or B blood, naturally occurring anti-A and anti-B isoantibodies are primarily IgM and do not cross the placenta. However, in type O individuals, isoantibodies are frequently IgG. These antibodies can cross the placenta and cause hemolysis. Although approximately 12% of maternal/infant pairs qualify as "set-ups" for ABO incompatibility, < 1% of infants have significant hemolysis.

132. Should conjugated (i.e., direct-reacting) bilirubin levels be routinely obtained in children who are being evaluated for early jaundice?

The utility of a routine measurement of conjugated bilirubin in early jaundice in healthy infants is minimal. Elevated conjugated bilirubin should be suspected in infants with dark urine or urine positive for bilirubin (conjugated bilirubin is water-soluble), light-colored stools, or jaundice that persists > 3 weeks.

133. What is *vigintiphobia*?

Vigintiphobia, translated from the Latin, is "fear of 20." Traditionally, it has been common to do exchange transfusions in term infants without evidence of isoimmunization or hemolysis at bilirubin levels of 20 mg/dl to prevent kernicterus. Critics argue that this practice is without scientific evidence, and support for tolerating higher levels of bilirubin prior to intervention has grown.

Watchko JF, Oski FA: Bilirubin 20 mg/dL = vigintiphobia. Pediatrics 71:660–663, 1983.

134. When are phototherapy and exchange transfusion indicated in the term infant with hyperbilirubinemia?

This is one of the more controversial issues in pediatrics because knowledge regarding bilirubin concentration and circumstances at which CNS toxicity is likely is incomplete. Recommendations by the American Academy of Pediatrics for infants > 24 hours are as follows:

Total Serum Bilirubin (TSB) Levels (mg/dl)

AGE, HRS	CONSIDER PHO-TOTHERAPY	PHOTOTHERAPY	EXCHANGE TRANSFUSION IF INTENSIVE PHOTO-THERAPY FAILS*	EXCHANGE TRANSFUSION AND INTENSIVE PHOTO-THERAPY
25–48	≥ 12	≥ 15	≥ 20	≥ 25
49–72	≥ 15	≥ 18	≥ 25	≥ 30
> 72	≥ 17	≥ 20	≥ 25	≥ 30

* Intensive phototherapy should produce a decline of TSB of 1–2 mg/dl within 4–6 hours, and the TSB level should continue to fall and remain below the threshold level for exchange transfusion. If this does not occur, it is considered a failure of phototherapy.

From Provisional Committee for Quality Improvement and Subcommittee on Hyperbilirubinemia: Practice parameter: Management of hyperbilirubinemia in the healthy term newborn. Pediatrics 94:565, 1994; with permission.

135. What distinguishes "breast-feeding jaundice" from "breast-milk jaundice"?

Hyperbilirubinemia in breastfed infants during the first week of life is called breast-feeding jaundice and is thought to be secondary to poor caloric intake and/or dehydration. Hyperbilirubinemia in breastfed infants after the first week of life is known as breast-milk jaundice. This form of hyperbilirubinemia is believed to be caused by an increased enterohepatic circulation of bilirubin secondary to the presence of beta-glucoronidase in human milk and/or to the inhibition of the hepatic glucoronosyl transferase by a factor such as free fatty acids in some human milk samples. The incidence and duration as compared with physiologic jaundice are noted in the table.

	Physiologic Jaundice	Breast-Feeding Jaundice	Breast-Milk Jaundice
Time of onset (TSB > 7 mg/dl)	After 36 hr	2–4 days	4–7 days
Usual time of peak bilirubin	3–4 days	3–6 days	5–15 days
Peak TSB	5–12 mg/dl	> 12 mg/dl	> 10 mg/dl
Age when total bilirubin < 3 mg/dl	1–2 wk	> 3 wk	9 wk
Incidence in full-term neonates	56%	12–13%	2–4%

TSB = total serum bilirubin.
From Gourley G: Pathophysiology of breast milk jaundice. In Polin RA, Fox W (eds): Fetal and Neonatal Physiology. Philadelphia, W.B. Saunders, 1992, p 1174; with permission.

136. Why should infants at risk for breast-feeding jaundice be fed more frequently?

Breast-feeding jaundice appears to be associated with poor feeding practices. Infants breastfed on an average of > 8 times a day in the first 3 days of life have significantly lower serum bilirubin concentrations than those less frequently breastfed. Therefore, it makes sense to encourage more frequent feedings. Supplemental feedings may be of value. However, sterile water or balanced electrolyte solutions may worsen the hyperbilirubinemia associated with breast feeding and should not be used.

137. Should breast-feeding be discontinued in an infant with hyperbilirubinemia?

Only in rare metabolic disorders (e.g., galactosemia) should breast-feeding be permanently discontinued. In one study, Martinez et al. compared four interventions in breastfed newborns with a serum bilirubin concentration > 17 mg/dl. The authors concluded that most infants require no intervention. If phototherapy is used, there is no need to discontinue breast feeding.

	Intervention	Treatment Failure*
Group I	Continued breast-feeding until TSB rose to 20 mg/dl, then breast feeding stopped and phototherapy begun	24%
Group II	Breast-feeding stopped and formula substituted; phototherapy begun at TSB of 20 mg/dl	19%
Group III	Breast-feeding stopped, formula substituted, and phototherapy begun immediately	3%
Group IV	Breast-feeding continued and phototherapy begun	14%

* Total serum bilirubin (TSB) rose to 20 mg/dl.
Martinez JC, et al: Hyperbilirubinemia in the breast-fed newborn: A controlled trial of four interventions. Pediatrics 91:470–473, 1993.

138. Where does bilirubin go when you turn on the lights?

It becomes lumirubin (through structural isomerization), which is the principal pathway of bilirubin elimination. Lumirubin is rapidly excreted in bile, with a half-life of about 2 hours. Photoisomers can also be excreted in the urine.

139. What are the contraindications to phototherapy?

Infants with a significantly elevated conjugated hyperbilirubinemia or a family history of light-sensitive porphyria should not receive phototherapy.

140. What are the common adverse effects of phototherapy?

Diarrhea, increased insensible water loss, skin rashes, overheating, and the potential for burns if the lights are placed too close to the infant's skin. If direct hyperbilirubinemia is present, the bronze baby syndrome can result.

141. A newborn who develops dark skin discoloration and dark urine after beginning phototherapy likely has what condition?

The **bronze baby syndrome**. Infants who develop the syndrome typically have an elevated direct serum bilirubin concentration. The bronze baby syndrome results from retention of lumirubin that cannot be excreted in the bile. Most infants appear to recover without complications. However, in infants with significant conjugated hyperbilirubinemia, the use of phototherapy is controversial.

142. Why do babies receiving phototherapy develop diarrhea?

During phototherapy, unconjugated bilirubin is excreted into the gut in increased amounts, which enhances intestinal secretions. The diarrhea may be a consequence of the high concentrations of bilirubin within the intestinal lumen. Increased concentrations of bile salts also have been found in the gut of neonates during phototherapy and may be a factor in the pathogenesis of phototherapy-associated diarrhea. The diarrhea is not believed to be the result of a phototherapy-induced lactase deficiency.

143. How can the metallo-protoporphyrins assist in settings of hyperbilirubinemia?

Numerous studies have demonstrated that various metallo-protophorhyrins (such as zinc, tin, and chromium) can effectively inhibit heme oxygenase, which is the rate-limiting step in heme catabolism. These enzyme inhibitors can thus decrease bilirubin production. The potential toxicities remain under study and may include photosensitization and inhibition of cytochrome $p450$-drug metabolism.

Valaes T, et al: Control of jaundice in preterm newborns by an inhibitor of bilirubin production: Studies with tin-mesoporphyrin. Pediatrics 93:1–11, 1994.

144. What percentage of blood volume is removed in a one-, two-, and three-volume exchange transfusion?

Blood Volume Exchanged	Blood Volume Removed and Replaced by Exchange
1.0	63%
2.0	87%
3.0	95%

145. How quickly does the bilirubin rebound following an exchange transfusion?

Although 87% of the infant's bilirubin is removed in a two-volume exchange, the serum bilirubin concentration is only reduced to 45% of the pre-exchange level. Equilibration is complete by 30 minutes, at which time the bilirubin rises to 60% of the pre-exchange value.

146. What are the complications of exchange transfusions in the newborn?

Acute

- Hypocalcemia (secondary to binding of calcium by citrate)
- Thrombocytopenia (secondary to removal of platelets and use of stored blood that may be low in platelets)
- Hyperkalemia (secondary to higher potassium levels in stored blood)

- Hypovolemia (if blood replacement is inadequate)
- Diminished oxygen delivery (if blood stored > 5–7 days is used, the resultant loss of 2,3-DPG may have deleterious effects on oxygen delivery)

Late
- Anemia (for unknown reasons)
- Graft vs. host disease (secondary to introduction of donor lymphocytes into a relatively immunocompromised neonatal host)

147. How often does prolonged unconjugated hyperbilirubinemia occur?

About one-third of healthy breastfed infants will have persistent jaundice ≥ 14 days. In formula-fed infants, this prolonged jaundice occurs in < 1% of neonates.

148. What are the pathologic causes of prolonged unconjugated hyperbilirubinemia?

1. Hemolytic disorders
   Isoimmunization
   Inherited defects of red cell metabolism
   Acquired hemolytic disorders secondary to infections, drugs, and micro-angiopathies
2. Extravasation of blood: petechiae; hematomas; pulmonary, cerebral, or retroperitoneal hemorrhages; cephalhematomas
3. Swallowed blood
4. Increased enterohepatic circulation of bilirubin
   Intestinal obstruction
   Pyloric stenosis
   Meconium ileus
   Paralytic ileus, drug-induced ileus
   Hirschsprung disease
5. Hypothyroidism
6. Hypopituitarism
7. Familial nonhemolytic jaundice:
   Types 1 and 2
   Gilbert disease
8. Lucey-Driscoll syndrome
9. Mixed disturbances in which both unconjugated and conjugated hyperbilirubinemia may be present
   Galactosemia
   Tyrosinosis
   Hypermethioninemia
   Cystic fibrosis

From Oski FA: Unconjugated hyperbilirubinemia.In Taeusch HW, et al (eds): Diseases of the Newborn, 6th ed. Philadelphia, W.B. Saunders, 1991, p 758; with permission.

149. How much potential bilirubin is there in meconium?

Analysis of meconium stools from preterm and term infants indicates that there is 1 mg bilirubin/gm wet weight and that 50% is unconjugated. At birth, the amount of meconium in the gut is estimated to be between 100–200 gm.

150. What is delta bilirubin?

When bilirubin is measured by high pressure lipid chromatography (HPLC), the total bilirubin includes the unconjugated fraction, conjugated fraction, and a fraction that is covalently bound to albumin—the delta bilirubin fraction. It was named delta because it is the fourth bilirubin peak on the HPLC elution curve. Most laboratories utilize the diazonium test which results in delta bilirubin being included in the conjugated fraction. At present, there is no clear clinical significance for delta bilirubin.

151. What is the relationship between delayed neonatal jaundice and urinary tract infection (UTI)?

Unexplained jaundice developing between 10–60 days of age can be associated with a UTI in infants. The typical patient is usually afebrile (in two-thirds of cases) with hepatomegaly and often minimal systemic symptoms. Hyperbilirubinemia is usually conjugated, and liver transaminases may be normal or mildly elevated. Treatment of the UTI (usually caused by *Escherichia coli*) results in reversal of the jaundice, which is felt to be caused by liver dysfunction secondary to endotoxins. Sepsis with bacterial hepatitis usually presents earlier with a more sick infant.

152. Who was Sister Ward?

In the early 1950s, Sister Ward was the nurse in charge of the unit for premature infants at Rochford General Hospital in Essex, England. On warm summer days, Sister Ward would take her infants to the courtyard to give them a little fresh air and sunshine. It was following such an afternoon of sunshine that Sister Ward observed that sunlight was able to "bleach" the skin of jaundiced neonates. The account of her discovery, as recorded by R.H. Dobbs, follows:

> One particularly fine summer's day in 1956, during a ward routine, Sister Ward diffidently showed us a premature baby, carefully undressed and with fully exposed abdomen. The infant was pale yellow except for a strongly demarcated triangle of skin very much yellower than the rest of the body. I asked her, "Sister, what did you paint it with—iodine or flavine—and why?" But she replied that she thought it must have been the sun. "What do you mean Sister? Suntan takes days to develop after the erythema has faded." Sister Ward looked increasingly uncomfortable, and explained that she thought it was a jaundiced baby, much darker where a corner of the sheet had covered the area. "It's the rest of the body that seems to have faded." We left it at that, and as the infant did well and went home, fresh air treatment of prematurity continued.

METABOLIC ISSUES

153. Define neonatal hypoglycemia.

Although there is no universally accepted definition, neonatal hypoglycemia is commonly defined as a serum glucose of < 35 mg/dl in a term infant and < 25 mg/dl in a preterm or low-birthweight infant during the first 3 days of life. However, because the fetal glucose level is typically ≥ 40 mg/dl and older children can be symptomatic with glucose levels ≤ 40 mg/dl, any glucose level < 40 mg/dl should be viewed as abnormal and treated.

154. When is hypoglycemia most likely to occur in a neonate?

During gestation, glucose is freely transferred across the placenta by the process of facilitated diffusion. However, after birth, the infant must adjust to the sudden withdrawal of this transplacental supply. In all infants, there is a nadir in blood sugar between 1–3 hours of life. This fall is accentuated in preterm infants, infants of diabetic mothers, infants with erythroblastosis fetalis, asphyxiated infants, and infants who are small or large for gestational age.

155. How should hypoglycemia be treated?

Both symptomatic and asymptomatic hypoglycemia should be treated. If an asymptomatic infant can take oral feedings, these may suffice initially. Otherwise, the infant should receive therapy based on the response:

- Initially, the infant is given a bolus of IV glucose (200 mg/kg or 2 ml/kg of $D_{10}W$), followed by a glucose infusion of 6–8 mg/kg/min (0.36–0.48 ml/kg/hr of $D_{10}W$) with frequent glucose monitoring and increases in infusion rates and concentrations as needed.
- Glucagon, 1 mg IM, can be given as an anti-insulin measure until an IV is established, but glucagon is not as helpful in the low-birthweight infant.
- If $\geq 15–20$ mg/kg/min is required, glucocorticoids (hydrocortisone, 5 mg/kg/day, or prednisone, 2 mg/kg/day) can enhance gluconeogenesis. Diazoxide (10–15 mg/kg/day) can suppress insulin secretion.

156. In a newborn requiring a glucose infusion of ≥ 15 mg/kg/min, what condition should be suspected?

A marked hyperinsulinemic state. This can be seen in a variety of conditions: nesidioblastosis (primary hyperplasia of the islets of Langerhans), islet cell adenomas, maternal diabetes mellitus, Rh incompatibility, maternal drug use (e.g., thiazide diuretics or tocolytics), or Beckwith-Wiedemann syndrome. The absence of ketone bodies in an infant with increased insulin levels, a high glucose requirement, and a low serum glucose level makes one of the islet cell disorders likely. All but the first two diagnoses are discernible by history and/or exam.

157. A large-for-gestational-age newborn is noted to have a large tongue, a large umbilical hernia, ear creases, and hypoglycemia. What diagnosis should be suspected?

Beckwith-Wiedemann syndrome. This genetic overgrowth syndrome occurs in about 1 in 14,000 deliveries. Although most cases are sporadic, parentally transmitted cytogenetic abnormalities can occur on chromosome 11. In addition to the features mentioned above, other common findings include other abdominal wall defects (e.g., omphalocele, diastasis recti), infraorbital creases, visceromegaly, and GI malrotation. In the delivery room, associated features including a large and thickened placenta, polyhydramnios, and long umbilical cord may be noted.

Weng EY, et al: Beckwith-Wiedemann syndrome. Clin Pediatr 34:317–326, 1995.

158. Discuss the mechanism of neonatal hypoglycemia after administration of tocolytic drugs to mothers.

Beta-agonists used as tocolytics may cause beta-cell hyperplasia in the fetal pancreas, leading to elevated fetal insulin levels and hypoglycemia in the immediate postnatal period. The risk of hypoglycemia seems to be associated with long-term use of the beta-agonists, especially if therapy is discontinued < 2 days prior to delivery.

159. Describe the manifestations of hypocalcemia in the neonate.

The major manifestations are **jitteriness** and **seizures**. Additional signs such as high-pitched cry, laryngospasm, Chvostek's sign (facial muscle twitching on tapping), and Trousseau's sign (carpopedal spasm) may be present, but more commonly these are absent during the neonatal period.

160. What is the differential diagnosis of hypocalcemia in the neonate?

Early neonatal hypocalcemia (first 3 days of life)
1. Premature infants
2. Infants with birth asphyxia
3. Infants of diabetic mothers

Late neonatal hypocalcemia (after end of first week)
1. High-phosphate cow's milk formula
2. Intestinal malabsorption
3. Postdiarrheal acidosis
4. Hypomagnesemia
5. Neonatal hypoparathyroidism
6. Rickets

Decreased ionized fraction of calcium
1. Citrate (exchange transfusion)
2. Increased free fatty acid (Intralipid)
3. Alkalosis

161. When should hypocalcemia be treated in the neonate?

Hypocalcemia should be treated when it is associated with signs or symptoms or when the serum calcium level is < 7.0 mg/dl. The first line of therapy generally consists of increasing the amount of calcium in the IV infusion to achieve 75 mg of elemental Ca/kg/day and following serum levels every 6–8 hours. Infusion of bolus IV calcium (10% calcium gluconate, 2 ml/kg) over 10 minutes should be reserved for the infant with seizures. In the asymptomatic infant, hypocalcemia most frequently resolves spontaneously without need for further therapy.

162. When should the serum magnesium concentration be measured in a neonate?

It should be measured in any hypocalcemic infant not responding to calcium therapy, hypotonic infants born to mothers who received magnesium sulfate therapy prior to delivery, and infants with seizures of unknown etiology.

163. How is hypomagnesemia treated?

Hypomagnesemic infants should be treated with 0.25 ml/kg of a 50% solution (100 mg of elemental Mg/ml) given intramuscularly. Magnesium levels are followed and the dosage repeated if necessary.

NEONATAL SEPSIS

164. Describe the common clinical presentations of evolving neonatal sepsis.

Symptoms and signs of sepsis may be minimal and nonspecific. As the rap goes, "In the newborn, anything can be a sign of anything." Temperature instability (both hyper- and hypothermia), respiratory distress, apnea, cyanosis, GI changes (vomiting, distention, diarrhea, anorexia), and CNS features (irritability, lethargy, weak suck) can all be early presentations of sepsis. Of course, these can also overlap with many noninfectious processes, making the diagnosis difficult. Risk factors for sepsis (e.g., prematurity, prolonged rupture of membranes, chorioamnionitis) should increase the urgency for more detailed evaluations. While the search for the definitive screening lab test continues, cultures remain the only certain method of verifying infection.

165. Can sepsis be distinguished from other causes of respiratory distress in the neonate?

Not reliably. Diagnosis is confirmed only by a positive blood, urine, or CSF culture.

166. In a newborn with suspected sepsis, is a normal total WBC count reassuring?

It shouldn't be. Total WBC counts are of limited value in the diagnosis of bacterial sepsis in the newborn. In one-third of infants with proven bacterial disease, total WBC counts are normal, particularly early in the course of infection.

167. Which neutrophil indices are of value as a screen for sepsis?

The most sensitive neutrophil index for identifying septic infants is the **immature to total (I:T) neutrophil ratio**. An I:T ratio of > 0.2 has been considered abnormal, although some studies have suggested a ratio as high as 0.27 may be seen in healthy term newborns. **Neutropenia** (total WBC < 5000/mm³ or absolute neutrophil count < 1750/mm³) is the most specific indicator. The least sensitive neutrophil index is the absolute band count (normal < 2000/mm³). Generally, abnormal neutrophil indices have low positive-predictive values (about 40%) and therefore are not helpful in clearly identifying which infants are infected. However, they have a much higher negative-predictive value, particularly if repeated 12 hours after birth, and thus can be very helpful in determining which infants do *not* have infection.

168. How helpful is a gastric aspirate in evaluation of infection?

Examination of gastric aspirates for leukocytes and bacteria was previously thought to be useful in identifying infants at risk for sepsis. However, the leukocytes are of maternal origin, and the bacteria represent organisms colonizing or infecting the amniotic cavity. They do not necessarily indicate fetal or neonatal infection.

169. Should a urine culture be done as part of the sepsis evaluation in the neonate?

A urine culture can be excluded as part of a sepsis evaluation in the first days of life. Urine cultures are very infrequently positive in infants < 72 hours of age, except when associated with renal anomalies.

170. Should a lumbar puncture (LP) be done on all newborns as part of the sepsis evaluation?

The need for LP in the sepsis evaluation of a newborn is controversial, with some authors suggesting its omission in asymptomatic infants. However, in symptomatic infants, an LP should be strongly considered because (1) bacterial meningitis can be present in newborns without CNS symptoms, (2) a significant number (15–30%) can have meningitis without bacteremia, and (3) meningitis can coexist in premature infants with suspected respiratory distress syndrome. The procedure should be postponed in an infant with cardiorespiratory instability or significant thrombocytopenia.

Wiswell TE, et al: No lumbar puncture in the evaluation for early neonatal sepsis: Will meningitis be missed? Pediatrics 95:803–806, 1995.

171. What is the ideal position for an infant to receive a lumbar puncture?

Infants who undergo LP in an upright position (with head support and spina flexion) exhibit less hypoxia and hypercarbia. If a lateral recumbent position is used, partial neck extension helps to minimize the respiratory stresses.

172. Are skin surface cultures helpful in the evaluation of suspected neonatal sepsis?

The theoretic value of these cultures is that they might help to identify the possible etiologic agents and thus guide therapy. However, an analysis of nearly 25,000 cultures in > 3,300 patients revealed that surface cultures correlated with urine, blood, or CSF cultures in only about 50% of cases. Most agree that surface cultures in this setting have little clinical value.

Evans ME, et al: Sensitivity, specificity, and predictive value of body surface cultures in a neonatal intensive care unit. JAMA 259:248–252, 1988.

Fulginiti VA, Ray CG: Body surface cultures in the newborn infant: An exercise in futility, wastefulness, and inappropriate practice. Am J Dis Child 142:19–20, 1988.

173. If a mother has received intrapartum antibiotics, how should an asymptomatic infant be managed?

The administration of antibiotics to a mother during labor invalidates cultures taken from the infant (unless positive) and often creates some clinical soul-searching. Some suggest the use of a sepsis screen, with a positive screen defined as two or more abnormal values. Particularly in infants < 37 weeks' gestation, a positive screen warrants a full course of antibiotics.

Sepsis screen	Abnormal value
• WBC count	≤ 5000 or ≥ 30,000/mm³
• Absolute neutrophil count	< 1750/mm³
• Immature-to-total neutrophil ratio	≥ 0.2
• C-reactive protein	≥ 0.8 mg/dl
• Micro-erythrocyte rate (ESR)	≥ 15 mm/hr

Polin RA, St. Geme JW III: Neonatal sepsis. Adv Pediatr Infect Dis 7:25–61, 1992.

174. Discuss the pathogenesis of early-onset bacterial infection.

Blanc has designated the sequence of events leading to early-onset bacterial infection as the "ascending amniotic infection syndrome." Infection begins with colonization of the maternal genital tract. Pathogenic bacteria then spread upward through the cervix and into the amniotic cavity, resulting in chorioamnionitis. Susceptible infants either inhale or swallow infected amniotic fluid and develop generalized sepsis. Although chorioamnionitis increases the risk of both fetal and neonatal infection, < 5% of mothers with this condition deliver infected infants.

Blanc WA: Pathways of fetal and early neonatal infection. J Pediatr 59:473–496, 1961.

175. What are the most common pathogens responsible for sepsis in the neonate?

Gram-negative bacteria (particularly *Escherichia coli*) and **group B streptococci**. Of note is the emergence of coagulase-negative staphylococci as the most common organisms responsible for nosocomial infections in most newborn intensive care units.

176. Compare early-onset and late-onset group B streptococcal sepsis.

Comparison of Early- and Late-Onset Group B Streptococcal Sepsis

FEATURE	EARLY ONSET (< 7 DAYS)	LATE ONSET (≥ 7 DAYS)
Median age at onset	1 hr	27 days
Incidence of prematurity	Increased	Not increased
Maternal obstetric complications	Frequent (70%)	Uncommon
Common manifestations	Septicemia (25–40%)	Meningitis (30–40%)
	Meningitis (5–15%)	Bacteremia without focus
	Pneumonia (35–55%)	(40–50%)
		Osteoarthritis (5–10%)
Serotypes isolated	Ia, Ib/c, Ia/c (30%)	III (93%)
	II (30%)	
	III (40% nonmeningeal; 80% meningeal isolates)	
Mortality rate	10–15%	2–6%

From Baker C: Group B streptococcal infections. In Remington JS, Klein JO (eds): Infectious Diseases of the Fetus and Newborn Infant, 4th ed. Philadelphia, W.B. Saunders, 1995, p 1010; with permission.

177. Which maternal carriers of group B streptococci (GBS) warrant prophylactic antibiotics?

Up to 40% of pregnant women are positive for GBS on anorectal or vaginal cultures. Since neonatal prophylaxis is not sufficiently effective (> 60% of infants with infection are symptomatic at or shortly after birth), selective maternal chemoprophylaxis has been proposed as a means to decrease vertical transmission of the organism. If maternal cultures are positive for GBS, risk factors that warrant intrapartum antibiotics include:

1. Preterm labor at < 37 weeks' gestation
2. Premature rupture of membranes at < 37 weeks' gestation
3. Prolonged rupture of membranes at any gestation
4. Fever during labor
5. Multiple births
6. Previous delivery of a sibling with invasive GBS disease

Committee on Infectious Diseases, Committee on the Fetus and Newborn: Guidelines for prevention of group B streptococcal (GBS) infection by chemoprophylaxis. Pediatrics 90:775–778, 1992.

178. In cultures positive for coagulase-negative staphylococci, what distinguishes contamination from "true" infection?

To help in differentiating a "true" coagulase-negative staphylococcal infection from blood culture contamination (especially in infants with central catheters), blood cultures should be obtained from two different sites. In infants with infections, both cultures should grow coagulase-negative staphylococci with identical sensitivity patterns. If only a single blood culture is obtained, some authors have suggested that a colony count of ≥ 50 cfu/ml is suggestive evidence of "true" bacteremia. In clinical practice, however, that number of cfus has a relatively poor predictive accuracy.

179. How is systemic candidiasis diagnosed in the neonate?

By cultures of blood, urine, and CSF or other body fluids that are generally sterile. Since cultures are only intermittently positive, multiple systemic cultures should be obtained. A urinalysis demonstrating budding yeasts or hyphae should raise suspicion of systemic infection. Gram stains of buffy coat smears may also demonstrate organisms. An ophthalmologic exam may indicate the presence of candidal endophthalmitis.

180. What is the preferred treatment of candidal sepsis and meningitis?

Systemic candidiasis is treated with amphotericin B intravenously for 4 weeks. Treatment is started at 0.1 mg/kg in a single daily dose infused over 4–6 hours. The dose is gradually increased over several days until a maximum daily dosage of 0.5–1.0 mg/kg is achieved. 5-Flucytosine (50–150 mg/kg/day) should be used to supplement amphotericin B if the infection is severe, the organism is resistant to amphotericin, or the CNS is involved.

181. Is prophylactic use of intravenous immunoglobulin (IVIG) indicated in newborns?

Although the data are conflicting, no clearcut proof indicates that routine administration of IVIG is effective in preventing nosocomial sepsis or decreasing mortality.

Hill HR: Intravenous immunoglobulin use in the neonate: Role in prophylaxis and therapy of infection. Pediatr Infect Dis J 12:549–559, 1993.

182. When is immunoglobulin therapy indicated in the acutely infected infant?

Although most studies have focused on the use of IVIG for prophylaxis, a few studies have examined its role as an adjunct to antibiotics in the acute treatment of sepsis. There appears to be a modest improvement in survival, but the numbers of patients remain too small to warrant any conclusions.

183. What is the role of fibronectin in neonatal sepsis?

Fibronectins are large-molecular-weight glycoproteins, present on most cell surfaces, that have vital roles in cell migration, proliferation, inflammation, hemostasis, and wound healing. In bacterial sepsis, fibronectin levels are decreased, which may contribute to dysfunction of the neonatal reticuloendothelial function. Clinical trials will determine if purified preparations of fibronectin are an effective immunotherapeutic agent.

Polin RA: Role of fibronectin in diseases of newborn infants and children. Rev Infect Dis 12:5428–5435, 1990.

NEUROLOGIC ISSUES

184. Give the normal CSF values for healthy neonates.

In the CSF examination of a group of high-risk neonates who did not have infection, the values (mean and range) were:

	Term	Preterm
WBC count (cells/mm³)	8.2 (0–32)	9.0 (0–29)
Protein (mg/dl)	90 (20–170)	115 (65–150)
Glucose (mg/dl)	52 (34–119)	50 (24–63)
CSF/blood glucose (%)	81 (44–248)	74 (55–105)

Adapted from Sarff LD, et al: Cerebrospinal fluid evaluation in neonates: Comparison of high risk infants with and without meningitis. J Pediatr 88:473, 1976; with permission.

185. Following a difficult delivery, what three major forms of extracranial hemorrhage can occur?

Caput succedaneum, cephalhematoma, and subgaleal hemorrhage.

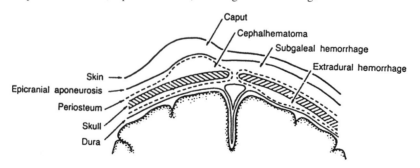

Major Varieties of Traumatic Extracranial Hemorrhage

LESION	FEATURES OF EX-TERNAL SWELLING	INCREASES AFTER BIRTH	CROSSES SUTURE LINES	MARKED ACUTE BLOOD LOSS
Caput succedaneum	Soft, pitting	No	Yes	No
Subgaleal hemorrhage	Firm, fluctuant	Yes	Yes	Yes
Cephalhematoma	Firm, tense	Yes	No	No

From Volpe JJ (ed): Neurology of the Newborn, 3rd ed. Philadelphia, W.B. Saunders, 1995, p 770; with permission.

186. If a cephalhematoma is suspected, should a skull x-ray be done to evaluate for fracture?

Cephalhematomas occur in up to 2.5% of livebirths. The incidence of associated fractures ranges from 5–25% in studies. These fractures are almost always linear and nondepressed and do not require treatment. Thus, in an asymptomatic infant with a cephalhematoma over the convexity of the skull and without suspicion of a depressed fracture, x-ray is not necessary. If the exam suggests cranial depression or neurologic signs are present, radiographic imaging is warranted.

187. Should all preterm infants by examined by cranial ultrasound?

Because of the relative noninvasiveness of ultrasound, most neonatologists recommend that a single cranial ultrasonogram be obtained in the first week of life in infants born at < 35 weeks' gestational age.

188. In screening for intraventricular hemorrhage (IVH), when is the best time to perform an ultrasound?

In series of infants studied by ultrasonography, approximately 50% had the onset of hemorrhage in the first day of life, 25% on the second day, and 15% on the third day. Thus, a single scan on the fourth day of life would be expected to detect > 90% of IVHs. However, approximately 20–40% of hemorrhages show evidence of extension within 3–5 days after initial diagnosis, and thus a second scan is indicated after about 5 days after the first to determine the maximal extent of hemorrhage.

189. Describe the three clinical presentations of IVH.

1. A **catastrophic deterioration** characterized by an inexorable evolution in minutes to hours. Major features include stupor or coma, respiratory disturbances including apnea, generalized tonic seizures, decerebrate posturing, flaccid quadriparesis, fixed pupils, and absent "doll's eyes." Associated features include falling hematocrit, bulging anterior fontanel, hypotension, bradycardia, temperature instability, metabolic acidosis, and abnormal water homeostasis (SIADH or diabetes insipidus).

2. A **saltatory deterioration** that follows a stuttering evolution over hours to days. Important features include altered level of consciousness, decreased motility, decreased tone, abnormal eye movements (e.g., downward vertical drift, skew deviation), and an abnormally tight popliteal angle (< 130° for premature infants and < 110° for term infants).

3. A **clinically silent syndrome** often associated with an unexplained fall in hematocrit or failure of hematocrit to rise after transfusion.

190. How are IVHs classified?

Most traditional systems of classification include a grading system according to increasing severity:

Grade I   Germinal matrix hemorrhage only
Grade II   IVH without ventricular dilatation
Grade III IVH with ventricular dilatation
Grade IV   Grade III hemorrhage plus intraparenchymal involvement

Some authorities have abandoned the grade IV classification in favor of "periventricular hemorrhagic infarction" to emphasize that these lesions have a different pathophysiology and are not simply extensions of matrix or IVH into parenchymal tissue. As such, the extent of parenchymal involvement rather than the grade of hemorrhage is more important in determining prognosis.

191. What is the cause of hydrocephalus following an intracranial hemorrhage?

The acute hydrocephalus is believed to be secondary to impairment of CSF absorption by the arachnoid membrane caused by the particulate blood clot. In subacute/chronic hydrocephalus, ventricular enlargement is due to an obliterative arachnoiditis (likely a chemical inflammatory response from the continued presence of blood) which usually causes a communicating hydrocephalus. Less commonly, obstruction of the aqueduct of Sylvius can lead to a noncommunicating hydrocephalus.

192. How common is progressive posthemorrhagic ventricular enlargement?

The likelihood of this phenomenon depends on the extent of the initial hemorrhage, ranging from only about a 5% likelihood in Grade I IVH to 80% in Grade IV IVH.

193. Can serial lumbar punctures prevent posthemorrhagic hydrocephalus?

No. Although LPs are useful in lowering increased intracranial pressure and in treating hydrocephalus once it has developed, they are of no benefit in preventing the onset. Infants with slowly progressive ventricular dilation and increasing head circumference who do not show signs of spontaneous arrest and improvement within 4 weeks should undergo a trial of serial LPs. Their effectiveness should be assessed with ultrasound. If there is no benefit, the placement of a ventriculoperitoneal shunt is necessary.

194. How much fluid should be removed by lumbar puncture in an infant with ventriculomegaly?

Because the volume of CSF in the dilated ventricles of infants with posthemorrhagic hydrocephalus is large, the removal of a significant amount (10–15 ml/kg) is usually required.

195. What causes subarachnoid hemorrhage (SAH) in the newborn?

SAH in the neonate is believed to result from traumatic or hypoxic events that increase traction on, or flow through, small fragile vascular channels, which are the remnants of anastomoses present between the leptomeningeal arteries during brain development.

196. What are the three clinical presentations of SAH?

1. **Asymptomatic**. In most cases, only small amounts of hemorrhage have occurred, and minimal or no clinical signs are present.

2. **Well baby with seizures**. In patients without significant hypoxic-ischemic encephalopathy, seizures secondary to SAH have their onset on the second day of life. In the interictal period, these babies appear well.

3. **Catastrophic deterioration**. In rare instances, newborn infants with large SAHs follow a rapidly fatal course characterized by coma, respiratory disturbance, seizures, loss of brainstem reflexes, and flaccidity.

197. Which areas of the CNS are injured by hypoxia and ischemia?

Full-term infants: Asphyxia produces injury in the peripheral and dorsal aspects of the cerebral cortex. Lesions involve gyri at the depths of the sulci as well as the neuronal nuclei of the basal ganglia.

Premature infants: Injury is localized to the germinal matrix and the periventricular region, while the cortex is relatively spared.

198. What are the five major neuropathological varieties of neonatal hypoxic-ischemic encephalopathy?

1. Selective neuronal necrosis: usually occurs in a characteristic, although possibly widespread, region.

2. Status marmoratus: following neuronal loss, the development of gliosis and hypermyelination, often in the basal ganglia and thalamus

3. Parasagittal cerebral injury: "watershed infarcts" due to ischemia

4. Periventricular leukomalacia: loss of white matter in characteristic patterns due to ischemia, particularly in premature infants

5. Focal and multifocal ischemic brain necrosis: infarction due to ischemia, with large areas of necrosis in the distribution of major vessels

199. How does Erb palsy differ from Klumpke palsy?

Neonatal *brachial plexus injuries* occur in < 0.5% of deliveries and are often associated with shoulder dystocia and breech or forceps delivery. Of the two, Erb palsy is more common.

Erb palsy	Klumpke palsy
• Involves upper plexus (C5, C6, and, in 50% of cases, C7)	• Involves lower plexus (C8, T1)
• Arm held adducted, internally rotated, and pronated with wrist flexed and fingers flexed ("waiter's tip" position)	• Small muscles of hand and wrist affected ("claw hand")
• Biceps reflex absent, Moro reflex with hand movement but no shoulder abduction, palmar grasp present	• Up to one-third have associated Horner syndrome
• 5% have ipsilateral diaphragmatic involvement	

200. How is brachial plexus injury treated?

Therapy must be aimed at preventing contractures. For the first 7–10 days, the arm is gently immobilized against the abdomen to minimize further hemorrhage and/or swelling. Following this initial period, passive range of motion exercises at the shoulder, elbow, wrist, and hand are performed. In addition, wrist splints to stabilize the fingers and avoid contractures should be used.

201. What is the outcome of neonatal brachial plexus palsy?

Approximately 90% of patients have normal examinations by 12 months of age. Onset of recovery within 2 weeks and involvement of only the proximal upper extremity are both favorable prognostic signs.

202. In newborns with facial paralysis, how is peripheral nerve involvement distinguished from central nerve involvement?

Peripheral: Usually results from compression of the peripheral portion of the nerve by prolonged pressure from the maternal sacral promontory. The use of forceps alone is not thought to be an important causative factor. Peripheral paralysis is unilateral. The forehead is smooth on the affected side, and the eye is persistently open.

Central: Often results from contralateral CNS injury (temporal bone fracture and/or posterior fossa hemorrhage or tissue destruction). It involves only the lower half or two-thirds of the face. The forehead and eyelids are not affected.

In both forms of paralysis, the mouth is drawn to the normal side when crying, and the nasolabial fold is obliterated on the affected side.

203. Is ankle clonus normal in the newborn infant?

Bilateral ankle clonus of 5–10 beats may be a normal finding, especially in infants who are crying, hungry, or jittery. This is particularly true if the clonus is unaccompanied by other signs of upper motor neuron dysfunction.

204. Do newborns prefer to turn their heads to the right or left?

Healthy neonates prefer to turn their heads to the right, which may reflect the normal asymmetry of cerebral function at this age. This preference has been observed as early as 28 weeks' gestation. By 39 weeks' gestation, 90% of newborn infants spend ≥ 80% of the time with their head turned to the right side.

NUTRITION

205. How many calories are required daily for growth in a healthy, growing, preterm infant?
Preterm infants need approximately **120 cal/kg/day**. About 45% of the caloric intake should be carbohydrate, 45% fat, and 10% protein. Infants who expend increased calories (e.g., those with chronic lung disease, fever, cold stress, etc.) may need up to 150 cal/kg/day.

206. What is the rationale for starting with dilute formula for feeding the preterm infant?
The preterm infant is often started on formula feeds that are one-quarter or one-half strength. Although there are no data to support this clinical practice, many neonatologists believe that starting with dilute formula lessens the likelihood of feeding intolerance and possibly avoids serious complications such as necrotizing enterocolitis. The osmolality of the formula used may be a key determinant of the rapidity of gastric emptying.

207. What are the nutritional advantages of formulas designed for preterm babies?

Feeding Component	*Advantage*
Protein 60/40 whey casein	Improved digestion; increased amounts of cystine, taurine
Carbohydrate glucose polymers + lactose	Glucose polymers are better absorbed than lactose because of decreased production of intestinal lactase in the preterm infant
Fats: medium chain triglycerides (MCTs), corn/coconut	MCTs are absorbed directly into portal vein and are less dependent on bile salts for emulsification and micelle formation
Minerals: increased calcium, phosphorus	Improved bone mineralization
Calories: 24 cal/oz	Increased growth

208. How quickly can feedings be increased in preterm infants?
Feedings must be tailored to the premature infant based on the level of immaturity and current level of illness. While the average physiologic gastric capacity increases from 2 to 27 ml/kg over a course of 10 days, it is suggested that enteral feeds be advanced slowly (< 20 ml/kg/day) to decrease the risk of necrotizing enterocolitis.

209. What are the documented medical benefits of breast-feeding?
Proven benefits
1. Fewer episodes of otitis media and respiratory and GI illness occur in breastfed infants.
2. Human milk facilitates the growth of beneficial, nonpathogenic flora, compared with pathogenic anaerobes and coliforms that predominate in infants fed formula.
3. Formula-fed infants have reduced quantities of host defense proteins in the GI tract (e.g., lactoferrin and secretory IgA).
Suggested but unproven benefits
1. Decreased incidence of neonatal sepsis and necrotizing enterocolitis in preterm infants
2. Enhancement of subsequent intelligence
3. Reduction in incidence of atherosclerosis
4. Reduction in incidence of diabetes mellitus

210. How does maternal breast milk differ for a full-term versus premature baby?
The composition of human milk for preterm infants differs from that for term infants in a number of ways. Per 100 ml, it is higher in calories (67–72 kcal vs 62–68), higher in protein

(1.7–2.1 gm vs 1.2–1.7 gm), higher in lipid (3.4–4.4 gm vs 3.0–4.0 gm), lower in carbohydrates, higher in multiple minerals and trace elements (especially Na, Cl, Fe, Zn, Cu), and higher in vitamins (especially vitamins A and E).

Van Aerde J: Nutrition and metabolism in the high risk neonate. In Fanaroff AA, Martin RJ (eds): Neonatal-Perinatal Medicine, 5th ed. St. Louis, Mosby, 1992, pp 492–495.

211. How does colostrum differ from mature human breast milk?

Colostrum is the thick yellowish mammary secretion that is characteristic in the first postpartum week. It is higher in phospholipids, cholesterol, and protein concentration and lower in lactose and total fat composition than mature breast milk. Colostrum is particularly rich in immunoglobulins, especially secretory IgA.

212. In breast-feeding, how do fore milk and hind milk differ?

The caloric density of human milk increases in a nonlinear fashion while the infant is breast-feeding. Hind milk (produced at the end of the feeding) can have a fat content that is 50% higher than fore milk.

213. What are contraindications to breast-feeding?

Inborn errors of metabolism: galactosemia, phenylketonuria, urea-cycle defects

Infections: HIV, tuberculosis, hepatitis B, HTLV-I, cytomegalovirus, herpes simplex (when lesions are present on breast)

Medications: sulfonamides, tetracycline, metronidazole, radioactive medicines, chemotherapeutic agents (alkylating agents), antithyroid medications

214. Should breast-feeding be discontinued if the mother is on antibiotics?

In general, no. Sulfonamides have the potential to displace bilirubin from albumin and should be avoided during the first week of life. Tetracycline, which can cause tooth discoloration and enamel hypoplasia, should not be taken by lactating women. Most authorities also suggest that chloramphenicol not be administered to nursing mothers, although drug levels are unlikely to become high enough to produce the "gray baby" syndrome. Although no adverse effects have been seen in metronidazole-exposed infants, this drug is potentially mutagenic and carcinogenic. Therefore, breast-feeding should be discontinued while a mother is receiving metronidazole (Flagyl) and for a minimum of 12 hours after it has been stopped.

215. Should breastfed babies be supplemented with water?

Although a common practice, there is no basis for the supplementation of breast-feeding with water. Babies with water supplementation do not have any lesser degree of physiologic jaundice, may have more weight loss than nonsupplemented babies, and are less likely to be breastfed at 3 months than those nonsupplemented.

216. How long should infants be breastfed per feeding?

Infants nurse between 4–20 minutes per breast. Although the majority of milk volume is consumed during the first 4 minutes of nursing, the caloric density is greater during the later phase of breast feeding. If > 25 minutes is needed by an infant to empty a breast, one should suspect either poor milk production, an abnormal "let-down" response, or ineffective "latch-on."

217. What are the signs of inadequate intake in a breastfed infant?

- Irregular or nonsustained sucking at breast
- < 5 large, seedy, yellow stools each day during first month
- Failure to have a wet diaper with each feeding
- Nursing < 10 minutes/breast at each feeding
- Failure to demand to nurse at least 8 times daily
- Taking only 1 breast at each feeding

• Crying, fussing, and appearing hungry after most feedings
• Gaining < 1 oz/day

Neifert MR, Seacat JM: A guide to successful breast-feeding. Contemp Pediatr 3:32, 1986.

218. Do breast milk and cow's milk vary in lactose content?

Breast milk is 7% lactose, compared with whole or skim milk which is 4.8%.

219. What advice should be given to a mother who plans to express and save breast milk for later feedings?

Ideally, she should collect the milk as cleanly as possible and then store it rapidly at 3°–4°C or less. The milk should be used within 48 hours. If prolonged storage is necessary, the milk should be kept frozen at a temperature of at least –20°C. Once the milk has thawed, it should not be refrozen.

220. Should mothers with silicone breast implants breast-feed their infants?

Concerns have been raised that women with silicone implants have an increased incidence of associated rheumatologic illnesses, particularly scleroderma, and that breast-fed infants of mothers with implants are more likely to develop severe distal esophageal dysmotility (scleroderma-like). Until there is scientific clarification (and tort reform), prudence warrants advising such mothers of the potential risk of breast-feeding.

Levine JJ, et al: Scleroderma-like esophageal disease in children breast-fed by mothers with silicone breast implants. JAMA 271:213–216, 1994.

221. What are the advantages of a 60/40 whey/casein ratio in infant formulas?

The term 60/40 refers to the percentage of whey (lactalbumin) and casein in human milk or cow's milk formulas. This ratio makes for small curds and therefore easy digestibility by the infant. The 60/40 ratio is of particular advantage in the preterm infant because it is associated with lower levels of serum ammonia and a decreased incidence of metabolic acidosis. Only human milk or formulas that supply protein in this ratio provide adequate amounts of the amino acids cystine and taurine, which may be essential for the preterm infant.

222. How much formula should an average infant drink per day?

A healthy term newborn in the first 1–2 days of life may drink only 0.5–1 oz every 3–4 hours. Once feedings are well established, infants may ingest 200 ml/kg/day or more.

223. Must infant formulas be sterilized?

As a rule, no. The terminal sterilization of prepared formula by boiling the bottle for 25 minutes offers no advantage over simple cleansing of the bottles and nipples in hot, soapy water and the subsequent use of unsterilized tap water in formula preparation. If bacteriologically safe tap water is used, no differences in rates of gastroenteritis occur.

Gerber MA, et al: Sterilization of infant formula. Clin Pediatr 22:344–349, 1983.

224. Among infant formulas, is low-iron or regular iron-fortified better?

Generally, low-iron formula has 1.5 mg of elemental Fe/l, while regular iron-fortified formula has 12 mg/l. Infants who are not breastfed should be placed on regular iron-fortified formula.

Although a greater percentage of iron is absorbed from the ingested low-iron formula, the quantity may not be sufficient to protect against the development of iron-deficiency anemia. In addition, despite anecdotal experiences, the incidence of colic, constipation, vomiting, and fussiness does not vary between infants fed the two formulas. If a breastfed baby is to receive an occasional supplement, the low-iron formula is preferable because it is less likely to saturate lactoferrin, which is present in breast milk and important in suppressing the growth of *Escherichia coli*.

225. May milk be heated in a microwave oven?

No. Microwave heating produces uneven temperatures. Also, human milk is easily damaged by high temperatures.

226. Why are newborns who drink cow's milk at risk for development of hypocalcemia?

Cow's milk contains six times as much phosphorus as human milk (950 mg/l vs 162 mg/l). The neonatal kidney is unable to excrete this excessive phosphorus load, and hyperphosphatemia results. Since serum calcium and phosphorus concentrations are inversely correlated, the initial impact is increased deposition of calcium in bone and a decreased calcitriol (1,25-dihydroxyvitamin D) synthesis, which ultimately lead to hypocalcemia.

227. Is vitamin supplementation necessary in exclusively breastfed term infants?

Vitamin deficiencies are rare in breastfed infants, and as a rule, supplementation is not necessary. Exceptions include:

1. Vitamin D supplementation in black or darkly-pigmented babies or in settings where maternal and infant sunlight exposure is minimal. Breast milk is low in vitamin D (approx. 22 IU/l).

2. Malnourished mothers.

3. Mothers who are strict vegetarians. The concentration of B vitamins in their breast milk can be low.

Committee on Nutrition: Pediatric Nutrition Handbook, 3rd ed. Elk Grove Village, IL, American Academy of Pediatrics, 1993, pp 36–37.

228. Can infants with umbilical arterial catheters be fed safely?

The adequacy of GI perfusion and the risk of necrotizing enterocolitis have been major concerns in feeding infants with umbilical arterial catheters. However, no definite evidence exists that these catheters, by themselves, increase the risk of NEC when they are in place during feedings.

229. What is the mechanism of hyperalimentation-induced cholestasis?

The mechanism remains uncertain, although amino acid toxicity has been frequently implicated. Dextrose infusions may also be hepatotoxic, but Intralipid administration is probably not causative in this syndrome. Infants fed a high-protein regimen (3–6 gm/kg/day) develop a higher level of direct bilirubin at an earlier time than infants receiving a lower protein load. Other possible etiologies include (1) decreased bile flow and gut motility secondary to the lack of oral alimentation and immaturity of the enterohepatic circulation; (2) cholestasis secondary to absorption of bacterial toxins from the gut during bowel stasis; or (3) amino acid deficiency in hyperalimentation mixtures.

230. How can hyperalimentation-induced cholestasis be prevented?

Cholestasis secondary to intravenous hyperalimentation is a multifactorial disease. Newer balanced mixtures of amino acids, which include taurine, may help reduce the incidence of cholestasis. The development of cholestasis can only be prevented by establishing enteral feeds. Even minimal enteral feeds may be helpful in reducing the incidence of hyperalimentation-induced cholestasis.

231. What is the treatment for hyperalimentation-induced cholestasis?

The preferred treatment is to stop IV hyperalimentation and begin enteral feedings. If IV hyperalimentation cannot be discontinued, the amount of protein infused should be reduced to 2 gm/kg/day and the cal/N ratio kept below 200. In most infants, the condition is transient and resolves without further therapy. In infants with severe intrahepatic cholestasis, phenobarbital has been shown to stimulate bile secretion and lower serum bilirubin levels. Recent studies have also suggested that ursodeoxycholic acid, a choleretic and predominant bile acid in the polar bear, may alleviate hyperalimentation-induced cholestasis.

232. How should lipid infusions be monitored?

Intralipid infusions should be monitored by measuring weekly triglyceride and cholesterol levels. Visible clearing from the serum may also be measured through a capillary tube, but this technique is probably much less reliable. Glucose levels should also be followed, as lipids cause enhanced gluconeogenesis secondary to increased fatty acid oxidation.

233. Should Intralipid usage be curtailed in the infant with hyperbilirubinemia or respiratory distress?

During lipid hydrolysis, free fatty acids are generated which may compete with bilirubin for binding to albumin. However, to date, no studies suggest a higher incidence of kernicterus in infants receiving Intralipid. Lipid deposits have been noted at autopsy in alveolar macrophages and capillaries following Intralipid administration. These adverse effects of Intralipid on pulmonary function and bilirubin binding are related both to the dose and rate of Infusion. A lipid dose of 1 gm/kg administered over 15 hours is safe for any size newborn infant. Therefore, hyperbilirubinemia and respiratory distress are not contraindications to the use of Intralipid. In an infant nearing the point of exchange transfusion or receiving 100% oxygen, lipid emulsions should be used with caution.

234. If alimentation is being administered through a peripheral vein, is heparinization necessary?

The administration of heparin to premature infants in a concentration of 1 U/ml has been shown to improve the clearance of lipids. Therefore, heparin should be used whenever fats are being administered intravenously.

235. What is nonnutritive sucking?

Nonnutritive sucking is a mode of sucking unique to humans and is characterized by a highly regular, burst-pause pattern. Nonnutritive sucking occurs in all sleep and awake states, although less often during quiet sleep and crying. It assumes a recognizable rhythmic pattern after 33 weeks' gestation.

236. How do protein requirements vary with mode of nutrient delivery (intravenous vs enteral)?

Whether delivered intravenously or enterally, the protein requirements needed to achieve in utero accretion rates are similar. Preterm infants have slightly higher protein requirements (3.0–3.5 gm/kg/day) than term infants (2.0–2.5 gm/kg/day).

237. Which amino acids are essential for the preterm infant?

Essential	Conditionally Essential
• Leucine	• Cysteine
• Isoleucine	• Taurine
• Valine	• Tyrosine
• Threonine	• Arginine
• Methionine	• Glutamine
• Phenylalanine	
• Tryptophan	
• Lysine	

238. Which fatty acids are essential for the neonate?

Linoleic acid and **linolenic acid**. In infants weighing < 1750 gm who experience delay or difficulty in maintaining full enteral feedings, arachidonic and docosahexaenoic fatty acids may also be essential. These fatty acids are vital for normal brain development, myelination, cell proliferation, and retinal function. Fatty acids in human milk are composed of 12–15% linoleic acid.

239. What are the manifestations of essential-fatty-acid deficiency?

Scaly dermatitis, alopecia, thrombocytopenia (and platelet dysfunction), failure to thrive, and increased susceptibility to recurrent infection. To prevent and treat fatty-acid deficiency, 4–5% of caloric intake should be provided as linoleic acid and 1% as linolenic acid. This requirement can be met by 0.5–1.0 gm/kg/day of intravenous lipids.

240. Why are nucleotides being added to a number of infant formulas?

Dietary nucleotides may play a role in early neonatal life in the desaturation and elongation of essential fatty acids which are necessary for brain and retinal development. The addition of nucleotides to formula, simulating the composition in breast milk, may be especially important during early development. Nucleotides are present in relatively large amounts in human milk, and several studies have suggested an important role for nucleotides in immune function, GI function, and lipoprotein metabolism.

241. What causes osteopenia of prematurity?

During the period of rapid growth, many preterm infants exhibit undermineralization of bone (rickets of prematurity). This condition results primarily from an insufficient intake of calcium and phosporus, although vitamin D insufficiency, aluminum toxicity, or liver disease can be contributing factors.

242. What tests make up a "rickets screen"?

Serum calcium, phosporus, and **alkaline phosphatase**. Infants with osteopenia of prematurity (i.e., rickets) can maintain a normal serum calcium and phosporus until late in the disease, and so increased alkaline phosphatase is usually seen first. Routine radiographs can demonstrate generalized osteopenia with widening, cupping, and fraying of the metaphyses and fractures. In research settings, adequacy of mineral status can also be followed by serial serum concentrations of osteocalcin and calciotropic hormones and by bone photon densitometry.

243. How is osteopenia of prematurity prevented?

Calcium and phosporus should be supplied in amounts that approximate the intrauterine accretion rates (120–140 mg/kg/day for calcium and 65–75 mg/kg/day for phosphorus). Since only 65% of calcium and 85% of phosporus is absorbed when preterm infants are fed enterally, the amounts must be readjusted upward in infants receiving formula.

244. Describe the manifestations of vitamin E deficiency in the neonate.

Hemolytic anemia (with reticulocytosis), **peripheral edema**, and **thrombocytosis**. Vitamin E is important in stabilizing the red cell membrane, and a deficiency can result in a mild hemolytic anemia. The American Academy of Pediatrics recommends that 0.7 IU of vitamin E/100 kcal be present in feedings for preterm infants.

245. What are the manifestations of zinc and copper deficiency in the neonate?

Zinc deficiency: dry skin, growth retardation, hepatosplenomegaly, impaired wound healing, hair loss, perioral and perianal rashes, decreased resistance to infection.

Copper deficiency: hypochromic microcytic anemia, neutropenia, bony abnormalities.

RESPIRATORY ISSUES

246. What causes infants to grunt?

Infants with respiratory disease tend to expire through closed or partially closed vocal cords in order to elevate transpulmonary pressure and therefore increase lung volume. The latter effect results in an improved ventilation/perfusion ratio with better gas exchange. It is during the last part of expiration when gas is expelled through the partially closed vocal cords that the audible grunt is produced.

247. What do hyperpnea and tachypnea signify in the neonate?

Hyperpnea refers to deep relatively unlabored respirations at mildly increased rates. It is typical of situations in which there is reduced pulmonary blood flow (e.g., pulmonary atresia) and results from ventilation of underperfused alveoli. **Tachypnea** refers to shallow, rapid, and somewhat labored respirations and is seen in the setting of low lung compliance (e.g., primary lung disease and pulmonary edema).

248. Why do newborn infants breathe faster than adults?

The total work of breathing, which is the sum of elastic and resistance work, varies with ventilatory pattern (tidal volume and rate). The respiratory centers attempt to achieve a given minute ventilation with a pattern that minimizes work. This minimum energy expenditure is achieved at higher respiratory rates in infants than in adults (35–40 breaths/min vs. 16 breaths/min).

249. Until what age are infants obligate nose breathers?

Although 30% of newborn infants breathe through their mouth and nose or both, the remaining 70% are obligate nose breathers until the third to sixth week of life.

250. Discuss the effects of severe hypercarbia ($PCO_2 \geq 100$ mm Hg) if there is no associated hypoxia.

There are few data in human newborns on the effects of isolated severe hypercarbia in the absence of hypoxia. However, results from animal studies and limited clinical observations in humans suggest that this condition can lead to a pressure-passive cerebral circulation and an increased risk of intraventricular hemorrhage. In addition, the high $PaCO_2$ may disrupt the blood–brain barrier and enhance the deposition of molecules such as bilirubin in the CNS, leading to kernicterus. Finally, on a more cellular level, data in animal model systems demonstrate alterations in brain cell membrane lipid peroxidation as well as Na^+–K^+ ATPase activity. The significance of these latter findings remains undetermined.

251. How do blood oxygen content, oxygen saturation, and PO_2 differ?

PO_2 is the partial pressure of oxygen in equilibrium with blood. The percentage of hemoglobin that is bound with oxygen at a given PO_2 is the **oxygen saturation**. The **oxygen content**, which is measured in vol %, is the total volume of oxygen bound to hemoglobin plus the volume dissolved in blood, the latter of which is generally negligible at normal values of PO_2. The oxygen content can be calculated as follows:

$$1.34 \text{ ml } O_2/\text{gm hemoglobin} \times \text{hemoglobin (gm/dl)} \times \text{oxygen saturation}$$

252. What is mean airway pressure? Which settings on the ventilator affect mean airway pressure?

Mean airway pressure (P̄aw) is a measure of the average pressure to which the lungs are exposed during the respiratory cycle and can be calculated by dividing the area under the airway pressure curve by the duration of the cycle. P̄aw is affected by changes in inspiratory flow, peak inspiratory pressure (PIP), positive end-expiratory pressure (PEEP), and ratio of inspiratory to expiratory time (I/E ratio).

253. In an infant receiving mechanical ventilation, what is an acceptable range for pH, PCO_2, and PO_2?

The goal of mechanical ventilation is to maintain the arterial PO_2 in the range of 50–80 mm Hg and arterial pH between 7.30–7.41. Earlier recommendations advocated maintenance of PCO_2 between 35–45 mm Hg. Some neonatologists now recommend that the PCO_2 be allowed to rise to levels as high as 55–60 mm Hg in order to minimize barotrauma. It is still controversial whether sustained hypercarbia has adverse side effects.

254. What mechanical ventilator settings are likely to affect PO_2 and PCO_2?

Since many ventilatory changes may affect both oxygenation and ventilation to some degree, the following table is an oversimplified but, nevertheless, useful guide:

Ventilator Setting	PO_2	PCO_2
PIP	↑	↓
PEEP	↑	↑
Frequency	↑ or NE*	↓
I:E	↑	NE†
FiO_2	↑	NE
Flow rate	↑	NE

NE = no consistent effect; PIP = positive inspiratory pressure; PEEP = positive end-expiratory pressure; I:E = ratio of inspiratory to expiratory time.

* At very high respiratory rates, inspiratory time may be so short as to compromise oxygenation. Furthermore, at a very high frequency, there is an increase in inadvertent PEEP which can result in CO_2 accumulation.

† CO_2 elimination may be affected at extremely low expiratory times.

255. What are the physiologic effects of positive end-expiratory pressure (PEEP)?

PEEP can prevent alveolar collapse, maintain lung volume at end expiration, and improve ventilation-perfusion mismatch. However, an increase in PEEP may decrease tidal volume and impede CO_2 elimination. Elevations in PEEP to nonphysiologic values may decrease lung compliance, impair venous return, decrease cardiac output, and reduce tissue oxygen delivery.

256. How is the optimal PEEP determined?

The "optimal PEEP" is the end-expiratory pressure at which oxygenation is maximal with minimum effect on cardiovascular function. The best way to determine optimal PEEP is controversial. In practice, the PEEP setting is generally maintained at a level equal to 10% of the inspired oxygen concentration. For example, if the inspired oxygen concentration is 60%, the PEEP should be kept in the 5–7 range; if 40%, the 4–5 range, etc.

257. When is intermittent continuous positive airway pressure (CPAP) indicated in the nonventilated infant?

Intermittent CPAP, delivered by mask, is used in nonventilated infants to reduce the incidence of segmental or lobar atelectasis following prolonged endotracheal intubation.

258. In infants with chronic lung disease receiving supplemental oxygen, what is the approximate FiO_2 delivered by nasal cannula at various flow rates?

The FiO_2 delivered by nasal cannula in an infant is dependent on the respiratory rate and minute ventilation, positioning of the cannula, and the extent of nasal versus oral breathing. Smaller infants (with lower minute ventilation) entrain less room air and thus receive more oxygen for a given flow rate. As a general rule, for infants < 3500 gm, the delivery of 100% O_2 by nasal cannula at a flow rate of 0.125 l/min corresponds to an FiO_2 of 28–30%, and at 0.5 l/min, to an FiO_2 of approximately 35%. For infants > 3500 gm, 0.5 l/min corresponds to an FiO_2 of 28 and 2.0 l/min to 35%.

Fan LL, Voyles JB: Determination of inspired oxygen delivered by nasal cannula in infants with chronic lung disease. J Pediatr 106:923–925, 1983.

259. Should newborn infants receiving mechanical ventilation be pharmacologically paralyzed?

Neuromuscular paralysis is not recommended as routine treatment for mechanically ventilated infants. However, in specific instances, such as persistence of fetal circulation, neuromuscular paralysis may benefit infants whose activity/agitation may increase right-to-left shunting and decrease oxygenation. Paralysis may also reduce the incidence of pneumothorax and intraventricular hemorrhage in infants with respiratory distress.

260. How do high-frequency oscillatory ventilation (HFOV) and high-frequency jet ventilation (HFJV) differ?

	HFOV	*HFJV*
Frequency	10–30 Hz	10–40 Hz
Total volume	Determined by oscillator	Increased by gas entrainment
I:E ratio	Constant*	Variable
Expiratory phase	Active	Passive
	Less risk of gas trapping	More risk of gas trapping
Airway damage	Similar to IPPV	Necrotizing tracheobronchitis[†]
May be used in combination with IPPV	Yes	Yes

* Some oscillators have adjustable I:E ratios.
† May be no different from conventional ventilation. IPPV = intermittent positive pressure ventilation.

In general, HFJV has been used more commonly in infants with severe pulmonary interstitial emphysema, while HFOV has been of greater value in preventing "air-leak syndrome" in infants requiring "high" settings. Neither ventilator has been proven superior to conventional ventilation in the management of infants with uncomplicated respiratory distress syndrome (RDS). Furthermore, it is controversial if either form of high-frequency ventilation lessens the incidence of bronchopulmonary dysplasia (BPD).

From Bancalari E, Goldberg RN: High-frequency ventilation in the neonate. Clin Perinatol 14:581, 1987; with permission.

261. What is the preferred method of suctioning in premature infants?

Two varieties of endotracheal tube (ETT) suctioning are used in premature infants:

1. **"Shallow" suctioning**, in which the catheter is introduced 0.5–1 cm below the tip of the ETT.

2. **"Deep" suctioning**, in which the catheter is introduced until resistance is felt, and then withdrawn 1 cm before suction is applied.

Shallow suctioning may be the preferred method for premature infants because of a lesser risk of traumatic injury. It should be done with a catheter no larger than two-thirds of the inner diameter of the ETT and with a negative pressure no greater than 60–100 mm Hg. Suctioning should be performed as often as necessary to maintain ETT patency, with a minimum of once every several hours. Suctioning increases intracranial pressure, slows the heart rate, and decreases lung volumes. Infants who are being suctioned commonly become hypoxemic, which may worsen ongoing pulmonary hypertension.

262. How successful are operative procedures to reverse subglottic stenosis?

Cricoid split and endoscopic excision of a subglottic lesion have been used to treat subglottic stenosis with success rates of > 75%.

263. What tests can be done to estimate lung maturity prenatally?

Most prenatal tests for lung maturity are designed to detect the presence of surfactant. The following tests are those most commonly used:

Lecithin/sphingomyelin (L/S) ratio: Since lecithin is a major component of surfactant, and sphingomyelin concentration is relatively constant during gestation, the L/S ratio can be used as a measure of lung maturity. An L/S of ≥ 2.0 carries a low risk of RDS and is generally attained at 34–35 weeks' gestation. While ratios of 1.5–2.0 carry a 40% risk of RDS, values of < 1.5 carry a risk of 75%. The L/S ratio is *not* reliable in pregnancies with Rh disease or maternal diabetes. Furthermore, the test cannot be performed on fluid contaminated with blood or meconium.

Phosphatidylglycerol: This surface-acting, stabilizing factor is present at > 35 weeks' gestation. Thus, its presence is indicative of lung maturity, but its absence offers no definitive help in management. The measurement can be performed on blood- or meconium-contaminated fluid and is available as a standardized latex agglutination assay. Many clinicians quantitate both the L/S ratio and phosphatidylglycerol as part of a lung profile.

Foam stability or shake test: These tests depend on the ability of surfactant-rich fluid to form stable bubbles when mixed or shaken with ethanol. The foam stability index has been developed as a standardized test using constant amounts of ethanol with different dilutions of amniotic fluid. Stable bubbles at ≥ 0.48 dilution are suggestive of mature lungs. The test is, however, limited by a high incidence of false-negative results.

Fluorescence polarimetry: This test may be used to measure microviscosity of amniotic fluid, which decreases as lung matures. This method involves expensive equipment and is not routinely available.

Optical density (OD): The OD of phospholipids in amniotic fluid peaks at 650 nm. This test is rapid and routinely available, but it may not be as reliable as other tests.

264. What is the function of surfactant?

Surfactant is a surface-active material comprised of a mixture rich in phosphatidylcholine (64%), phosphatidylglycerol (8%), and lesser amounts of proteins and other lipids. Surfactant acts as an anti-atelectasis factor in the alveolar lining by lowering surface tension at diminished lung volumes and increasing it at high volumes. This allows for maintenance of functional residual capacity, which acts as a reservoir to prevent wide fluctuation in arterial PO_2 and PCO_2 during respiration. In patients with RDS, surfactants have been shown to decrease the need for supplemental oxygen therapy, lower mortality rates, and decrease the incidence of air-leak syndromes. The incidence of BPD has also been reduced in some studies.

265. Do the kinds of surfactant used to treat infants with RDS differ in effectiveness?

Two general classes of surfactant are available for replacement therapy: natural surfactants prepared from mammalian lungs (e.g., Survanta, Infasurf, Curosurf) and synthetic surfactants (e.g., Exosurf, ALEC). Although natural surfactant extracts seem to have a better immediate effect (less supplemental oxygen required, fewer pneumothoraces), long-term clinical outcomes (e.g., chronic lung disease, death) with synthetic surfactants are comparable.

The Vermont-Oxford Neonatal Network: Comparison of surfactants in respiratory distress syndrome. Pediatrics 97:1–6, 1996.

266. In surfactant therapy, is prophylaxis or "rescue" treatment better?

When and to whom surfactant should be administered remains a heavily studied topic. Ideally, it is administered to surfactant-deficient infants as soon as possible. However, while some institutions routinely administer surfactant to all infants less than a set gestational age (e.g., 31 weeks) as soon as possible after birth, others wait for clinical signs of RDS before initiating therapy. Until precise measures are available to rapidly assess the extent of surfactant sufficiency in an infant, the debate will continue. Early administration of surfactant is more important for the very-low-birth-weight infant, in whom it has been shown to reduce mortality and lower the incidence of BPD.

267. What are the adverse effects of prophylactically administering surfactant in the delivery room?

- 20–60% of healthy infants whose gestational age is ≤ 30 weeks will be treated unnecessarily.
- It imposes extra risks and unwarranted expenses.
- Use of surfactant may lead to a transient decrease in oxygen saturation.
- It delays resuscitation efforts and stabilization.
- In comparison with rescue treatment, the use of prophylactic surfactant may worsen neurodevelopmental outcome and increase the incidence of chronic lung disease (controversial).

268. When should infants with RDS be mechanically ventilated?

Mechanical ventilation is initiated when the diagnosis of respiratory failure is made.

Laboratory criteria for respiratory failure

1. Respiratory acidosis with pH < 7.20 and PCO_2 > 60 mmHg

2. Severe hypoxemia with $PaO_2 < 50$–60 mm Hg despite an FiO_2 of 0.7–1.0 and an adequate trial of continuous positive airway pressure

Clinical criteria for respiratory failure
1. Severe retractions
2. Cyanosis
3. Intractable apnea

269. How is pulmonary interstitial emphysema (PIE) treated?

PIE is an air-leak syndrome that is usually a complication of mechanical ventilation. Thus, therapy for PIE is usually aimed at reduction of the peak inflating pressure (through jet ventilation if necessary). In cases of localized PIE, dependent positioning of the involved lung as well as selective mainstem bronchial intubation and ventilation of the uninvolved lung are beneficial. When medical management of localized PIE fails, surgical lobectomy may be considered.

270. Is the meconium aspiration syndrome a function of meconium aspirated in utero or at birth?

The meconium aspiration syndrome is commonly defined as respiratory distress in a meconium-stained newborn with scattered infiltrates on x-ray, no alternative explanation for the clinical findings, and a high incidence of pulmonary vasoconstriction which leads to persistent pulmonary hypertension of the newborn. Some argue that in utero gasping of meconium leads to pulmonary vascular hypertrophy demonstrable by early biopsy, while others argue that aspiration after birth with an evolving syndrome is more likely since a high proportion of infants (up to 60%) are healthy and vigorous at birth. The likely answer is that both are involved and that this syndrome is a spectrum of diseases.

Wiswell TE, Bent RC: Meconium staining and the meconium aspiration syndrome. Pediatr Clin North Am 40:955–981, 1993.

271. Where is the proper location for a chest tube?

Chest tubes should be placed in the fourth intercostal space at the midaxillary line. For evacuation of a pneumothorax, they should then be directed anteriorly toward the apex of the thorax and advanced to the midclavicular line.

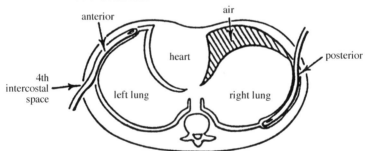

Anterior versus posterior position of the chest tube for drainage of air or fluid. Since air usually collects anteromedially in the supine neonate, the posterior tip is less appropriate. (From Fletcher MA, et al: Atlas of Procedures in Neonatology. Philadelphia, J.B. Lippincott, 1983, p 265; with permission.)

272. What is the pathophysiology of pulmonary hemorrhage in the neonate?

Pulmonary hemorrhage has been associated with a number of clinical conditions, including prematurity, asphyxia, sepsis, aspiration, intrauterine growth retardation, congenital heart disease, patent ductus arteriosus, and coagulopathies. Studies have indicated that lung effluents in these patients actually represent hemorrhagic pulmonary edema and not whole blood. The unifying feature in this disorder is an elevation in pulmonary capillary pressure which results either from acute left ventricular failure or conditions favoring increased filtration of fluid, such as hypoproteinemia, hypervolemia, and lung injury.

273. Which infants benefit most from extracorporeal membrane oxygenation (ECMO)?

ECMO is prolonged cardiopulmonary bypass used as a therapy in neonates. Newborn infants (< 1 week old) with reversible pulmonary disease complicated by persistent pulmonary hypertension are most likely to benefit from ECMO therapy. The most common associated diagnoses include meconium aspiration syndrome, respiratory distress syndrome, sepsis/pneumonia, and congenital diaphragmatic hernia.

274. What are the indications for instituting ECMO therapy?

ECMO therapy is usually indicated when an infant fails to oxygenate adequately (despite maximal ventilatory support with 100% oxygen) or shows acute deterioration. Most ECMO centers use one or more of the following formulas to identify candidates with an expected mortality $\geq 80\%$.

1. Alveolar/arterial oxygen gradient ($AaDO_2$) > 605 for 8–12 hours.

$AaDO_2$ (approximately) = $713 - (PaO_2 + PaCO_2)$ when the FiO_2 is 1.0 (100% inspired oxygen).

2. Oxygen index (OI) ≥ 40 on three of five consecutive arterial blood gases obtained 30–60 minutes apart.

$$OI = \text{mean airway pressure} \times FiO_2/PaO_2 \times 100.$$

3. PaO_2 < 50 mm Hg for 4 hours.

Other criteria include:
- Gestational age ≥ 34 weeks
- Birthweight > 2000 gm
- No evidence of bleeding or intraventricular hemorrhage
- Reversible lung disease

275. What percentage of infants are normal after receiving ECMO?

The overall survival of infants placed on ECMO is > 80%. The short-term outcome data suggest that approximately two-thirds of infants are normal following ECMO. It is difficult to determine if moderate to severe neurologic deficits seen in some survivors after ECMO are secondary to the infant's condition prior to bypass or to the risks of ECMO therapy.

276. What are the risks of and contraindications to ECMO?

The risk of thrombosis is an ever-present threat during ECMO therapy. Therefore, all infants on ECMO are heparinized. However, heparinization creates an increased risk for systemic bleeding and/or intracranial hemorrhage. Long-term morbidities are generally referable to the CNS.

Contraindications to ECMO include uncontrolled bleeding, grade II or greater intraventricular hemorrhage, irreversible pulmonary disease, and significant prematurity (birthweight < 2000 gm, gestational age < 34 weeks).

277. What characterizes the diagnosis of bronchopulmonary dysplasia (BPD)?

Since BPD was first reported in 1967, the clinical definition and diagnosis have evolved to include all patients who, after mechanical ventilation, remain oxygen-dependent for > 28 days and have persistent changes on chest radiographs. The pathologic diagnosis remains unchanged and is characterized by areas of emphysema and collapse with interstitial edema and fibrosis. The airway epithelium demonstrates hyperplasia and squamous metaplasia and the smooth muscle in the airways and vasculature frequently demonstrates hyperplasia.

278. Why is combination diuretic therapy used in infants with BPD?

Chlorothiazide/spironolactone and furosemide are used in infants with chronic lung disease to improve pulmonary compliance and decrease resistance by eliminating excess sodium and water. Furosemide produces an increase in venous capacitance and may have the added benefit of reducing right ventricular preload. Spironolactone and chlorothiazide are commonly used in combination with furosemide to minimize calcium wasting and decrease the incidence of nephrocalcinosis. In clinical practice, however, infants receiving combination therapy still waste calcium.

279. Is there a long-term benefit to diuretic therapy in BPD?

Long-term diuretic therapy in infants with BPD improves pulmonary function, decreases airway resistance, increases pulmonary compliance, and allows weaning of supplemental oxygen. However, the duration of supplemental oxygen may not be shortened. Furthermore, the long-term effect on infant mortality is not entirely clear. Diuretic therapy is not without side effects, including electrolyte imbalance, nephrocalcinosis, bone demineralization, and ototoxicity.

Kao LC, et al: Randomized trial of long-term diuretic therapy for infants with oxygen-dependent bronchopulmonary dysplasia. J Pediatr 124:772–781, 1994.

280. What is the role of vitamin A supplementation in preventing or reducing the severity of BPD?

Because vitamin A is involved in the proliferation and differentiation of epithelial cells, it is thought to play an important role in the repair process in the lung following barotrauma and oxygen exposure. In fact, vitamin A deficiency has been associated with the development of BPD. However, studies examining the effects of vitamin A supplementation on the incidence of BPD have not been conclusive.

281. When should steroids be initiated in neonates with BPD?

Infants between 2–4 weeks of age who are infection-free, are ventilator- and oxygen-dependent, and have early radiographic signs of BPD may benefit from treatment with steroids. It remains unclear if earlier administration is beneficial. Dexamethasone clearly improves lung function and compliance in infants with BPD within 72 hours after initiation. In turn, larger numbers of infants can be weaned from assisted ventilation and extubated. The impact is less clear with regard to the duration of supplemental oxygen required, length of hospital stay, and infant mortality. Side effects can include adrenal suppression, gastroduodenal perforation, hypertension, and hyperglycemia.

Ng PC: The effectiveness and side effects of dexamethasone in preterm infants with bronchopulmonary dysplasia. Arch Dis Child 68:330–337, 1993.

282. What is a BPD spell?

BPD spells have not been well characterized. In many infants the spell is clearly due to bronchial constriction. Most of these infants are believed to have airway smooth muscle hypertrophy. Other causes of BPD spells include cor pulmonale, tracheomalacia, aspiration, and atelectasis. The frequency of spells can generally be minimized by administering bronchodilators, diuretics, and oxygen. Some infants may require increased levels of end-expiratory pressure as a treatment for tracheomalacia or the use of sedatives to decrease agitation.

283. Why are infants with BPD at increased risk for poor neurodevelopmental outcome?

1. Recurrent episodes of hypoxia secondary to chronic lung disease and BPD spells
2. BPD is associated with intraventricular hemorrhage and periventricular leukomalacia.
3. Poor nutrition during periods of critical brain growth
4. Prolonged illness and hospitalization preclude normal stimulation and parent-infant interaction

Gerdes JS: Bronchopulmonary dysplasia. In Polin RA, et al (eds): Workbook in Practical Neonatology, 2nd ed. Philadelphia, W.B. Saunders, 1993, pp 189–206.

284. What is the difference between apnea and periodic breathing?

Apnea is defined as periods of cessation of respiration for > 10–15 seconds with or without cyanosis, pallor, hypotonia, and/or bradycardia, or for < 10 seconds accompanied by bradycardia. **Periodic breathing**, which is commonly seen in preterm infants, is defined as recurrent sequences of respiratory pauses of 5–10 seconds followed by 10–15 seconds of rapid respirations. Periodic breathing is not associated with bradycardia. Both apnea and periodic breathing reflect lack of maturation of respiratory control centers in the preterm infant.

285. When should apnea be treated?

In all cases of apnea, an underlying cause should be sought and treated if found. In idiopathic apnea, therapy should be initiated when episodes do not resolve with gentle tactile stimulation and require vigorous stimulation, or when patients have a frequency of > 2 episodes/8 hours.

286. What is the impact of apnea and bradycardia on cerebral blood flow in the preterm newborn?

Episodes of apnea associated with a decrease in heart rate to < 80 bpm can result in hypotension. Furthermore, these events may be accompanied by decreased diastolic and systolic cerebral blood flow velocities.

287. What methods are effective for treating apnea of prematurity?

1. Use of oscillating waterbeds
2. Administration of continuous positive airway pressure (CPAP) (especially helpful in apnea with an obstructive component)
3. Provision of supplemental oxygen (with or without CPAP)
4. Administration of respiratory stimulants (methylxanthines or doxapram).

If supplemental oxygen is used, the PaO_2 must be carefully monitored either directly by arterial blood gases or indirectly by noninvasive oxygen monitoring devices (e.g., pulse oximetry).

288. Is caffeine or theophylline more effective in lessening apnea of prematurity?

There is no evidence to date that one methylxanthine is more effective than the other in reducing the frequency of apnea in premature infants. Caffeine, however, has become the preferred medication for several reasons: it is excreted more slowly, can be given once daily, achieves a more stable plasma level, and has fewer GI and CNS side effects.

289. When is doxapram indicated in treating apnea of prematurity?

Doxapram is a potent respiratory stimulant with predominantly peripheral chemoreceptor effects. It does not appear to be any more effective than the methylxanthines in the treatment of apnea of prematurity and has a potentially greater toxicity. However, doxapram may be helpful when used in addition to methylxanthines to avoid positive pressure therapies (i.e., CPAP or mechanical ventilation).

Brion LP, et al: Low dose doxapram for apnea unresponsive to aminophylline in VLBW infants. J Perinatol 11:359–364, 1991.

290. What are the criteria for discontinuing the use of an apnea monitor or methylxanthines?

Methylxanthines are usually discontinued after an apnea-free period of 4–8 weeks. The apnea monitor is then discontinued 4–8 weeks later if there is no recurrence of symptomatic apnea. A home pneumogram should be recorded before monitor discontinuance.

291. Do home apnea monitors help prevent SIDS?

The use of monitors generates considerable controversy in pediatric and neonatal circles. Infants who are usually considered for monitoring include siblings of SIDS victims, infants who have had apparent life-threatening events, infants with abnormal "predictive" studies (e.g., abnormal pneumograms, spectral cry analyses, or brainstem auditory evoked responses), or infants with apnea of prematurity. Opponents of monitors argue that no controlled studies have been done to indicate home monitoring is effective in SIDS prevention. Furthermore, monitoring is often expensive and may be anxiety-provoking (due to the false alarms). Proponents cite anecdotal data demonstrating a lower incidence of SIDS with home monitoring and a reduction in parental anxiety and stress.

Burnell RH, Beal SM: Monitoring and sudden infant death. J Paediatr Child Health 30:461–462, 1994.

13. NEPHROLOGY

John W. Foreman, M.D.

ACID-BASE AND ELECTROLYTE DISORDERS

1. What nonrenal factors affect potassium balance?

Increased Potassium Release by Cells	**Increased Potassium Uptake by Cells**
• Acidosis	• Alkalosis
• α-Adrenergic agonists	• Insulin
• Exercise (rise in serum potassium depends on intensity of exercise)	• β-Adrenergic agonists
• Increased plasma osmolality	

Aldosterone promotes potassium excretion by the kidney. Diet has little effect on serum potassium values, except with extremes of intake.

2. How does serum potassium concentration change with alterations in serum pH?

In patients with alkalosis, potassium moves into cells as hydrogen moves out of cells in an effort to diminish the alkalinity. The opposite occurs in conditions of acidosis. For every 0.1 unit rise or fall in pH, there is a corresponding change in the potassium concentration between 0.4 and 0.6 mEq/L. In organic acidosis, the change in potassium concentration is less.

3. What are the clinical and physiologic consequences of hypokalemia?

- Causes muscle weakness and paralysis, which can lead to hypoventilation and apnea
- Leads to constipation and ileus
- Increases susceptibility for ventricular ectopic rhythms and fibrillation, especially in children receiving digitalis
- Interferes with the ability of the kidney to concentrate urine, leading to polyuria

4. List the common causes of hypokalemia.

- Diuretics, occasionally laxatives
- Metabolic alkalosis—especially in patients with pyloric stenosis
- Diabetic ketoacidosis
- Diarrhea
- Renal tubular acidosis, types 1 and 2
- Fanconi syndrome
- Bartter syndrome
- Hyperreninemic hypertension—usually due to renal artery stenosis
- Hyperaldosteronism—usually secondary to cirrhosis or congestive heart failure

5. What should be the maximum rate and concentration of potassium infusions?

Ideally, if potassium supplementation or replacement is needed, the concentration of potassium in the intravenous fluids should *not* exceed 40 mEq/L if given by a peripheral vein or 80 mEq/L if given by a central vein. Infusion rates should not be > 0.3 mEq K^+/kg/hr. Faster delivery can lead to local irritation of the veins, paresthesias and/or weakness, and cardiac arrest because of changes in transmembrane potentials. For life-threatening conditions due to hypokalemia, such as cardiac dysrhythmias or respiratory paralysis in a patient without alkalosis or acidosis, the rate may be increased up to 1 mEq K^+/kg/hr given centrally by an infusion pump. A continuous EKG monitor should be in place.

Cronan KM, Norman ME: Renal and electrolyte emergencies. In Fleisher GR, Ludwig S (eds): Textbook of Pediatric Emergency Medicine, 3rd ed. Baltimore, Williams & Wilkins, 1993, pp 677–682.

6. Which foods are high in potassium?

Food	Portion	Potassium (mg)
Raisins	2/3 cup	751
Baked potato	1 medium	503
Cocoa	1 cup	480
Orange juice	8 oz	474
Banana	1 medium	451
French fries	3/5 cup	364
Carrot	1 raw	341

7. List the causes of hyperkalemia in children.

Increased intake
- Oral including salt substitutes
- Intravenous
- Exchange transfusion, use of aged packed RBCs

Transcellular outward movement
- Metabolic and acute respiratory acidosis
- Insulin deficiency and hyperglycemia in uncontrolled diabetes mellitus
- Increased tissue catabolism—trauma, chemotherapy, hemolysis, rhabdo-myolysis
- Exercise
- Medication related—digoxin, β-blockers, succinylcholine, arginine
- Familial hyperkalemic periodic paralysis

Decreased renal excretion
- Acute oliguric renal failure—acute glomerulo-nephritis or acute tubular necrosis
- Oliguric end-stage renal failure
- Hypovolemia
- Hypoaldosteronism
- Medications—potassium-sparing diuretics, ACE inhibitors
- Distal renal tubular acidosis, type IV
- Renal defect in potassium excretion—familial or obstructive

Pseudohyperkalemia (laboratory artifact)
- Thrombocytosis, leukocytosis, hemolysis
- Abnormal leaky RBC membrane

From McDonald RA: Disorders of potassium balance. Pediatr Ann 24:36, 1995; with permission.

8. In what situations can a child be hyponatremic but not hypotonic?

1. *Elevated plasma lipids and plasma proteins.* Both increase plasma volume and tonicity but decrease the relative amount of plasma water. In general, measurements of serum Na^+ are expressed per plasma volume and not plasma water. Therefore, the Na^+ concentration can be artifactually low ("pseudohyponatremia") in hypertriglyceride states such as diabetic ketoacidosis. On average, an increase in triglyceride concentration of 1 g/dl will decrease serum Na^+ concentrations by 2 mEq/L.

2. *Increased extracellular osmotically active solutes.* When glucose, mannitol, glycerol, or another osmotically active substance is added to or increased in the extracellular space, the osmotic gradient pulls water from the cells and dilutes the serum Na^+. Hyponatremia can result, although the serum osmolality remains normal or elevated. This situation is most commonly encountered in diabetic ketoacidosis, and as a rule, for each 100-mg/dl increase in serum glucose, the Na^+ is decreased by 1.6 mEq/L.

9. How is the cause of hyponatremia established?

Artifactual causes of hyponatremia should be ruled out. Furthermore, if the urine specific gravity is < 1.003, causes of water intoxication (e.g., administration of inappropriate IV fluids, use of low-solute formulas or plain water in infants, excessive use of tap water enemas or pathologic drinking behavior in psychiatric patients) should be sought by history. If none of these causes are likely, clinical evaluation based on the patient's volume status and urinary sodium concentration will help categorize the disorder.

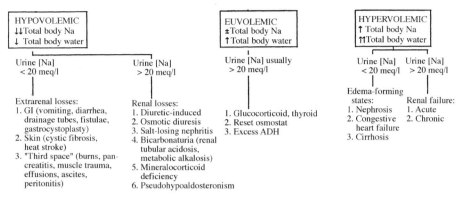

From Avner ED: Clinical disorders of water metabolism: hyponatremia and hypernatremia. Pediatr Ann 24:26, 1995; with permission.

10. What is the emergency treatment of symptomatic hyponatremia?

Symptoms of hyponatremia usually do not occur until the plasma $[Na^+]$ is < 120 mEq/L, but they may occur at higher concentrations if the change has been sudden. Symptoms can range from GI complaints (anorexia, nausea, vomiting) to mental status changes (headaches, irritability, disorientation, cloudy sensorium) and may ultimately lead to seizures, coma, and death. Patients with CNS symptoms should receive urgent treatment with hypertonic saline (3%). One ml/kg raises the serum [Na] approximately 1 mEq/L. It is relatively safe to infuse hypertonic saline at a rate of 3 ml/kg every 10–20 minutes until symptoms remit. Further treatment can be more gradual, with normal saline or fluid restriction based on whether the hyponatremia is due to Na loss or water excess.

11. How is the cause of hypernatremia established?

A combination of history, clinical assessment of the patient's volume status, and a urine sodium concentration measurement is helpful in establishing the diagnostic categories.

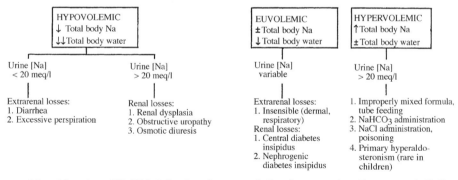

Adapted from Avner ED: Clinical disorders of water metabolism: hyponatremia and hypernatremia. Pediatr Ann 24:28, 1995.

12. Why is the treatment of hypernatremic dehydration so precarious?

In hypernatremic dehydration, the increased extracellular tonicity draws fluid from the intracellular compartment until the tonicity is balanced on each side of the membrane. However, the brain can generate "idiogenic osmoles" to minimize the loss of fluids. These idiogenic osmoles are principally amino acids and other organic solutes. With rehydration, the loss of these idiogenic osmoles occurs slowly. Therefore, if the correction is too rapid and the serum sodium concentration falls quickly, water flows from the extracellular compartment into the cerebral intracellular compartments, causing cerebral edema. This can lead to seizures, cerebral hemorrhage, and even death. To prevent this situation, the serum [Na] should not be allowed to fall faster than 0.5 mEq/L/hr and ideally not more than 15 mEq/L in 24 hours.

13. What is the normal anion gap from infancy to adulthood?

The anion gap or delta is the difference between the serum [Na] and the sum of the serum [Cl⁻] plus serum bicarbonate, usually measured as total CO_2. This difference represents the unmeasured anions, such as organic acids, sulfate, and phosphate. The mean anion gap in children from age 9 months to 19 years is 8 ± 2 mEq/L if the blood is assayed immediately; however, if the blood is analyzed 4 hours later, the mean is closer to 11 mEq/L, which is similar to that of adults (12 ± 2 mEq/L). An elevated anion gap, in practice, occurs when this difference is > 15–16 mEq/L.

14. What are the causes of an elevated anion gap acidosis?

The mnemonic **MUDPILES** is commonly used to recall these acidoses, which occur in a variety of clinical scenarios, including certain ingestions.

Methanol
Uremia (renal failure)
Diabetic ketoacidosis, diarrhea of infancy
Paraldehyde, phenformin
Iron, isoniazid, inborn errors of metabolism
Lactic acidosis (seen in clinical situations associated with hypoxia, severe cardiorespiratory
   depression, shock, prolonged seizures)
Ethanol, ethylene glycol
Salicylates

15. What is the urinary anion gap?

This indirect estimate of urinary ammonium excretion (and thus acid excretion) is calculated by subtracting the urinary chloride concentration from the sum of sodium and potassium concentrations:

$$\text{Anion gap} = Na^+ + K^+ - Cl^-$$

If the anion gap is negative, it suggests a large chloride excretion and adequate ammonium excretion. The urinary anion gap is negative in hyperchloremic metabolic acidosis secondary to diarrhea, untreated proximal renal tubular acidosis, or prior administration of an acid load. If the anion gap is positive, it suggests a distal acidification effect, as in distal renal tubular acidosis. Its results are not reliable if there are large amounts of unmeasured anions such as ketoacids, penicillin, or salicylates.

16. How limited is the respiratory response to metabolic alkalosis?

Metabolic alkalosis occurs when a net gain of alkali or loss of acid leads to a rise in the serum bicarbonate concentration and pH. In metabolic alkalosis, as in metabolic acidosis, there is a measure of respiratory compensation in response to the change in pH. This response, accomplished by alveolar hypoventilation, is limited by the overriding need to maintain an adequate blood oxygen concentration. Usually the PCO_2 will not rise above 50–55 mmHg despite severe alkalosis.

17. Discuss the differential diagnosis for a child presenting with primary metabolic alkalosis.

Metabolic alkalosis (MA) can be divided into two major categories based on the urinary Cl⁻ concentration and the response to volume expansion with a saline infusion. The **saline-responsive** metabolic alkaloses usually have a urine Cl⁻ concentration that is < 10 mEq/L and significant volume depletion. The classic example is pyloric stenosis. The **saline-resistant** alkaloses are associated with a high urine Cl⁻ and often hypertension. In most cases, mineralocorticoid excess plays the central role in the generation of the acid-base disturbance.

Causes of Saline-responsive MA	Causes of Saline-resistant MA
• Pyloric stenosis	• Primary hyperaldosteronism (extremely rare
• Vomiting	in pediatrics)
• Excessive upper GI suctioning	• Hyperreninemic hypertension
• Congenital chloride diarrhea	• Renal artery stenosis

- Laxative abuse
- Diuretic abuse
- Cystic fibrosis
- Chloride-deficient formulas in infants
- Posthypercapnia syndrome
- Poorly reabsorbable anion administration
- Post-treatment of organic acidemias

- Heritable block in steroid hormone synthesis
  17α-OH deficiency
  11β-OH deficiency
- Licorice
- Liddle syndrome
- Bartter syndrome
- Severe potassium deficiency

18. What is the pathophysiologic basis for "contraction alkalosis"?

Strictly speaking, contraction alkalosis refers to the loss of total body water with little or no loss of total body bicarbonate. This leads to an increase in the serum bicarbonate concentration and therefore alkalosis. However, this condition is most often seen in a setting of loss of gastric contents, such as pyloric stenosis, which leads to both volume and NaCl loss as well as hydrogen ion loss in the gastric secretions. The NaCl losses increase proximal absorption of sodium bicarbonate, maintaining the alkalosis and the release of aldosterone. Aldosterone facilitates the exchange of sodium for potassium. It also augments hydrogen ion secretion for sodium in the distal nephron, giving rise to the paradoxical aciduria often seen in the face of systemic alkalosis.

19. How does the "4-2-1" rule for maintenance fluid therapy work?

Infants weighing 3–10 kg have a maintenance fluid requirement of 100 ml/kg/day. For patients weighing 11–20 kg, the maintenance fluids are 1000 ml/day plus 50 ml/day for each kg of weight between 11 and 20 kg. For children weighing > 20 kg, the maintenance fluids are 1500 ml/day plus 20 ml/day for each kg of weight above 20 kg. If this daily requirement triad of 100-50-20 is divided by 24 hours to obtain an hourly rate of fluid requirements, then a rough estimate of 4-2-1 results. For example, the daily fluid requirement for a 24-kg child would be 1580 ml, or an hourly flow rate of $(10 \text{ kg} \times 4) + (10 \text{ kg} \times 2) + (4 \text{ kg} \times 1) = 64$ ml/hr. This rule is applicable up to about 80 kg.

CLINICAL ISSUES

20. How common is asymptomatic microhematuria?

Approximately 2–3% of school-aged children have a positive reaction for blood on repeated urinalyses, but this rate drops to 0.5% after 6 months of follow-up studies.

21. What distinguishes lower from upper tract bleeding?

This differentiation can be difficult. Red cells from upper tract (i.e., glomerular) bleeding are small and dysmorphic with blurs and blebs, while those from the lower tract are normal in size and shape or slightly crenated. This difference is best observed with phase contrast microscopy. The presence of red cell casts indicates upper tract bleeding. The presence of 1+ or more protein suggests renal pathology. Direct visualization by cytoscopy and ureteroscopy can often distinguish between upper and lower bleeding.

22. How does the "three glass test" localize the site of hematuria?

The three glass test involves having the patient void initially into one glass, then into a second glass, and then into a third glass. Hematuria found only in the first glass suggests a lesion in the urethra. Blood in the third glass supposedly indicates bladder neck and trigone pathology. Blood in all three glasses suggests that the bleeding is from the bladder, ureter, or kidney. Usually, getting a child to void in one cup (let alone three) is a major accomplishment. Needless to say, this test has not been particularly useful in pediatrics.

23. What historical and laboratory features are important in the evaluation of persistent hematuria?

History

- Family history of renal disease, hematuria, hearing loss, hemoglobinopathies, bleeding disorders, stone disease

• Drug use (e.g., anticoagulants, aspirin, sulfonamides)
• Trauma
• Abdominal, suprapubic, flank pain, or dysuria
• Recent illnesses

Laboratory
• Urine culture
• Urine calcium excretion
• Complete blood count
• Electrolytes, BUN, creatinine
• C3 and C4 levels
• Serologic evidence of recent streptococcal infection
• Hemoglobin electrophoresis (if sickle cell trait or disease is suspected)
• Renal ultrasound
Fitzwater DS, Wyatt RJ: Hematuria. Pediatr Rev 15:102–108, 1994.

24. How common is hypercalciuria as a cause of hematuria?

Nearly one-third of children with isolated hematuria have hypercalciuria as the cause. About 5% of healthy white children in the United States have this condition. The mechanism of hematuria is unclear but may involve irritation of the renal tubules by calcium-containing crystals. Treatment includes limited dietary restriction of a calcium, increased fluid intake, and thiazide diuretics if there is a history of nephrolithiasis or nephrocalcinosis.

25. What causes benign familial hematuria?

In this diagnosis of exclusion, multiple family members have microscopic (and occasionally gross) hematuria without significant proteinuria, abnormal renal function, or identifiable cause (e.g., hypercalciuria). Family history is not suggestive of any other serious renal problems, including deafness (Alport disease). Although renal biopsies are not usually done, the likely culprit is a thin glomerular basement membrane, especially the lamina densa.

26. At what age do most children achieve urinary continence?

Daytime: 50% by age 2½, 95% by age 4
Nighttime: 65% by age 3, 75% by age 4, 90% by age 8, and 98% by ages 12–14 years

27. What are the causes of nocturnal enuresis?

97% of the causes are nonpathologic, and only 3% are due to disease states. Suspicious symptoms include intermittent daytime wetness, polydipsia, polyuria, history of CNS trauma, constipation, or encopresis. Potentially treatable surgical conditions should be suspected if there is constant dampness, a dribbling urinary stream, abnormalities in gait, or loud nighttime snoring with apnea.

Nondisease states (97%)
• Small functional bladder capacity
• Inability to delay micturition urge
• Nighttime polyuria secondary to relatively low antidiuretic hormone levels
• Nighttime polyuria because of excessive evening fluid intake
• Nonarousing when bladder is full ("deep sleepers")

Disease states (3%)

Medically treatable	Surgically treatable
• Urinary tract infection (UTI)	• Ectopic ureter
• Diabetes mellitus	• Lower UTI
• Diabetes insipidus	• Neurogenic bladder
• Fecal impaction	• Bladder calculus or foreign body
• Constipation	• Obstructive sleep apnea secondary to adenoidal enlargement

Schmitt BD: Nocturnal enuresis: Finding the treatment that fits the child. Contemp Pediatr 7:72, 1990.

28. How effective are the various treatments for nocturnal enuresis?
No treatment: 15% spontaneous cure rate annually
Conditioning alarms: remission, 55–90%; relapse, 40%
Imipramine: remission, 50%; relapse, 75%
Desmopressin (DDAVP): remission, 25%; relapse, 95%

29. How is diurnal enuresis defined?
Daytime wetting (diurnal enuresis) is defined as a lack of bladder control during waking hours in a child old enough to maintain control. In otherwise normal children, diurnal enuresis is not considered a problem until age $2\frac{1}{2}$–3 years. During the first several years after toilet training, many children wet themselves when they postpone voiding because they are so engrossed in current activities. This is probably normal if it occurs less than twice a week.

30. What are the causes of diurnal enuresis?
1. **Organic causes** account for < 5% of cases. Of these, urinary tract infections are probably the most common. An ectopic ureter should be suspected if dampness is constantly present; most children with diurnal enuresis have intermittent wetness. Rarely, a neurogenic bladder can cause this problem. Severe lower urinary tract obstruction can lead to bladder distention with overflow incontinence. Finally, pelvic masses, such as presacral teratoma, hydrocolpos, or fecal impaction, which press on the bladder, can lead to stress incontinence with running, coughing, or lifting.
2. **Physiologic types** of daytime wetting include vaginal reflux of urine, giggle incontinence, and urgency incontinence. Reflux of urine into the vagina during micturition occurs frequently; after normal voiding, when the girl stands up and walks, the urine seeps out of the vagina and wets the underpants. Giggle incontinence is a sudden, involuntary, uncontrollable, and complete emptying of the bladder when giggling or laughing. Tickling or excitement may also lead to this problem. Urgency incontinence can be defined as an attack of intense bladder spasms that leads to abrupt voiding and wetting.
3. **Psychogenic causes** may be stress-related. Wetting can occur in any child who is significantly frightened. Chronic stress, such as the loss of a close relative, marital discord, or hospitalization, can also lead to this kind of daytime wetting. The resistant child is one who is about $2\frac{1}{2}$ years of age and refuses to be toilet trained. Seventy percent are males who are predominantly or totally wet. Often, this situation has occurred because of high-pressured attempts at toilet training. Most children with daytime wetness and nighttime dryness have a behavioral basis for the problem.

31. What simple exercises may help a child with daytime incontinence?
Kegel exercises are exercises of the pelvic muscles. The pelvic muscles can be stimulated in children by instructing them to void, then starting and stopping the urinary stream two or three times by means of pelvic contractions. These maneuvers can then be done at other times without voiding. Voluntary contracture of the pelvic floor muscles is reflexively accompanied by relaxation of the detrusor muscle. These exercises may be helpful in children with daytime incontinence.

Schneider MS, et al: Kegel exercises and childhood incontinence: A new role for an old treatment? J Pediatr 124:91–92, 1994.

32. What is the normal bladder capacity of children?
In ounces, child's age plus 2. Normal adult bladder capacity is 12–16 oz.

Berger RM, et al: Bladder capacity (ounces) equals age (years) plus 2 predicts normal bladder capacity and aids in diagnosis of abnormal voiding patterns. J Urol 129:347, 1983.

33. What physical findings should prompt a search for an underlying renal abnormality?
- Abdominal mass
- High imperforate anus
- Neonatal ascites
- Oligohydramnios

- Perineal hypospadias
- Exstrophy of the bladder
- Ambiguous genitalia
- Prune belly abdomen

- Anuria-oliguria (especially in neonate)
- Aniridia, hemihypertrophy (Wilms tumor)
- Poor urinary stream
- Persistent wetness

34. A newborn male with a distended, flabby, and wrinkled abdomen and with a greatly diminished urinary output likely has what condition?

Prune belly syndrome, or congenital absence of the abdominal musculature (also called Eagle-Barrett syndrome). Occurring predominantly in males, this condition has no known familial or genetic basis. It is associated with multiple other congenital malformations, especially urinary tract dilation with a greatly enlarged bladder and dilated and tortuous ureters. Bilateral cryptorchidism is common. Renal involvement is quite variable, ranging from complete agenesis to no involvement. It also may be unilateral. Chronic UTIs are common.

35. Which entities are known to cause renal papillary necrosis?

Diabetes, analgesic abuse, sickle cell trait and disease, pyelonephritis, urinary tract obstruction, and hypotension (usually in neonates).

36. In what settings does renal vein thrombosis occur?

Renal vein thrombosis usually occurs in the sick infant, especially in the first month of life. Dehydration, shock, septicemia, asphyxia, and cyanotic congenital heart disease (especially following angiography) are predisposing factors. The usual presenting features are a sudden change in the infant's clinical condition associated with hematuria, oliguria, proteinuria, and a flank mass. Thrombocytopenia is common, but hypertension is not. An intravenous pyelogram is often not helpful since the kidney with the thrombosis usually does not visualize. An ultrasound study, demonstrating the renal vein clot and an enlarged kidney, or a radionuclide study is usually more useful. The differential diagnoses include acute tubular or cortical necrosis, multicystic dysplasia, renal arterial thrombosis, adrenal hemorrhage, renal trauma, hydronephrosis, neuroblastoma, nephroblastomatosis, and Wilms tumor.

37. What is the differential diagnosis of an abdominal mass in the neonate?

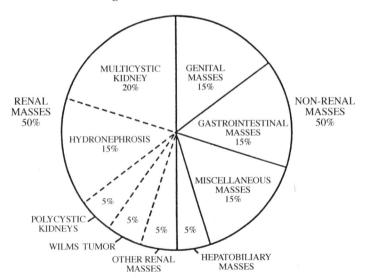

From Sunshine, et al: In Fanaroff AA, Martin RF (eds): Behrman's Neonatal–Perinatal Medicine: Diseases of the Fetus and Infant. St. Louis, Mosby, 1983, p 531; with permission.

38. What is acceptable urine output in a newborn?

The minimum and maximum volumes of urine output are determined by the amount of solute to be excreted and the maximal renal diluting and concentrating ability (which are 30–50 mOsm/L and 700–800 mOsm/L, respectively). Most clinicians find a urine output of at least 2 ml/kg/hr acceptable. This value, however, is a calculated one based on an average solute intake and knowledge about the concentrating and diluting capacities of the neonatal kidney. Infants with high solute intakes may need more urine output, and those with low intakes may need less.

39. How does relative renal blood flow differ in infants and adults?

In adults, about 20–25% of cardiac output is directed toward the kidney. In full-term infants, only about 6% is directed toward the kidney; this increases to 8–10% by the end of the first week.

40. How do you treat labial adhesions?

Labial adhesions are a relatively common gynecologic finding in girls between 4 months and 6 years of age. They may be complete or partial and are felt to be secondary to local inflammation in a low-estrogen setting with resulting skin agglutination. Treatment consists of eliminating the underlying inflammation if caused by an infection, sitz baths twice daily, maintenance of good perineal hygiene, and topical application of a 1% conjugated estrogen cream over the entire adhesion at bedtime for 3 weeks. The use of estrogen has an 80–90% cure rate and may be followed by application of a petroleum jelly for 1–2 months nightly. It should be noted that the natural history of untreated asymptomatic labial adhesions is self-resolution: 50% resolve within 6 months and nearly 100% by 18 months. Surgical correction is almost never needed.

Prasad SM: Labial adhesions. Pediatr Rev 15:87–88, 1994.

GLOMERULONEPHRITIS

41. In an evaluation of a patient with hematuria, what features suggest glomerulonephritis?

Three presentations can occur:

1. **Acute glomerulonephritis:** Edema, proteinuria of 1+ or greater, hypertension, oliguria, dysmorphic RBCs (small, misshapen RBC with blebs) on urinalysis, red cells casts on urinalysis; if rapidly progressive glomerulonephritis, may progress to anuria and uremia

2. **Chronic glomerulonephritis:** Minimal acute symptoms; may present with chronic fatigue, failure to thrive, or unexplained anemia with features of chronic renal failure, hypertension, abnormal urinalysis, azotemia

3. **Nephrotic syndrome:** Proteinuria > 40 mg/m^2/hr, edema, hypoproteinemia, hyperlipidemia

42. If glomerulonephritis is suspected, what lab tests should be considered?

- Urinalysis
- Serum C3 (possibly C4)
- Streptococcal serologies
- Throat culture; skin culture if lesions present
- Serum albumin
- Fluorescent antinuclear antibody (if systemic lupus erythematosus is suspected)
- Hepatitis B serology (if suspected)
- Antinuclear cytoplasmic antibody (if rapidly progressive glomerulonephritis or vasculitis present)

43. Which glomerulonephritides are associated with hypocomplementemia?

- Poststreptococcal
- Other postinfectious causes (may have normal complement)
- Subacute bacterial endocarditis
- Shunt nephritis
- Systemic lupus erythematosus
- Membranoproliferative

44. Which diseases present with nephritis and nephrosis in children?

Hematuria (Gross or Microscopic)	Acute Glomerulonephritis	Nephrotic Syndrome
IgA nephropathy (Berger disease)	Acute proliferative	Minimal change disease
Benign recurrent hematuria	Poststreptococcal	Focal glomerulosclerosis
Alport syndrome	Subacute bacterial endocarditis	Membranous nephropathy
Henoch-Schönlein purpura	IgA nephropathy (Berger disease)	Membranoproliferative glomerulonephritis
	Rapidly progressive	Mesangial proliferative
	Membranoproliferative	Systemic lupus erythematosus
	Hemolytic-uremic syndrome	Congenital nephrotic syndrome
	Henoch-Schönlein purpura	AIDS
	Systemic lupus erythematosus	

45. What is the usual time course for poststreptococcal glomerulonephritis?

Approximately 7–14 days following a pharyngitis and 14–21 days following a pyoderma with group A β-hemolytic streptococci, children present typically with tea-colored urine and edema. The acute phase (e.g., hypertension and gross hematuria) can last up to 3 weeks. Serum complement levels usually remain depressed for up to 8 weeks, and persistence beyond this point suggests another diagnosis. Chronic microscopic hematuria can persist up to 18 months. Complete recovery occurs in 95–98% of patients.

46. Does treatment of streptococcal skin or pharyngeal infections prevent poststreptococcal glomerulonephritis?

No study has ever demonstrated that treatment of impetigo or pharyngitis prevents renal complications in the index case. Clearly, acute rheumatic fever does not occur following the skin infections, and glomerulonephritis is limited to infections with a few serotypes, especially 49, 55, 57, and 60, which appear to be less prevalent in recent years. However, treatment lessens the likelihood of contagious spread to hosts who may be susceptible to renal complications. Serum antistreptolysin titers, which are elevated in pharyngeal infections, are usually not elevated following skin infections. Therefore, to confirm the diagnosis of an antecedent skin infection, anti-hyaluronidase and anti-DNase B titers should be obtained.

47. What is the Streptozyme test?

This commonly used screening test for recent streptococcal infection utilizes a patient's serum to agglutinate RBCs coated with a variety of streptococcal antigens. It is usually positive about 7–10 days after the onset of an infection, as compared with 3–6 weeks for anti-streptolysin 0 titers and 6–8 weeks for anti-DNase B titers. Difficulties with standardization of the reagents have limited its clinical utility.

48. A 9-year-old boy with intermittent episodes of gross hematuria associated with febrile upper respiratory infections likely has what type of glomerular disease?

IgA nephropathy (Berger disease). It is the most common cause of chronic glomerulonephritis in persons of European or Asian descent. In children, IgA nephropathy typically causes asymptomatic microscopic hematuria with periods of gross hematuria during febrile infections unrelated to the urinary tract. Most children are normotensive with minimal edema during exacerbations. However, about 25% go on to develop chronic renal insufficiency, especially those with hypertension and persistent proteinuria. The etiology is unclear, and diagnosis is established by renal biopsy with demonstration of IgA in the mesangium of the glomerulus.

Wyatt RJ, et al: IgA nephropathy: Long-term prognosis for pediatric patients. J Pediatr 127:913–919, 1995.

49. In children with the classic Alport syndrome, when does deafness develop?

Primarily inherited in an X-linked dominant fashion, Alport syndrome is a variety of disorders characterized by chronic glomerulonephritis and deafness. In the classic syndrome, high-frequency nerve deafness usually develops following the onset of renal disease. The abnormality may not be noted initially because conversational hearing can be be normal and deficits are detected only by audiometry. Most patients with deafness will present before age 15.

50. What are the causes of chronic glomerulonephritis?
- Membranoproliferative glomerulonephritis
- Membranous glomerulopathy
- Alport syndrome
- Systemic lupus erythematosus
- Focal glomerulosclerosis
- Diffuse proliferative glomerulonephritis
- Henoch-Schönlein purpura
- Crescentic glomerulonephritis (rapidly progressive GN)
- IgA nephropathy (Berger disease)

These are the main causes of chronic glomerulonephritis. Strictly speaking, membranous glomerulopathy and focal glomerulosclerosis are not inflammatory diseases, so they are not glomerulonephritides. Hemolytic-uremic syndrome is another important cause of chronic renal failure but is not a chronic glomerulonephritis.

51. Which chronic infections are associated with membranous glomerulonephritis?
The most common infection associated with membranous nephropathy is **hepatitis B**. In most children, the liver function studies are entirely normal. HBsAg should be looked for in otherwise normal patients with membranous nephropathy. This lesion has also been observed in congenital and secondary **syphilis** and **malaria**.

HYPERTENSION

52. How do you determine the appropriate cuff size in measuring blood pressure for a given patient?
Cuff size depends on limb diameter. The inflatable bag of the cuff should be about 20% wider than the diameter of the arm or leg. As a rule of thumb, a cuff that is approximately two-thirds the width of the upper extremity is adequate for measurement. The cuff must also be long enough to encircle the limb fully. One that is too small can produce falsely elevated blood pressure readings, and one that is too large can produce falsely low blood pressure readings, although the latter is more unusual.

53. Which Korotkoff sound should be used for determining the blood pressure?
The Korotkoff sounds are produced by the flow of blood as the constricting blood pressure cuff is gradually released. There are five phases of Korotkoff sounds. The first appearance of a clear, tapping sound is called **phase I** and represents the systolic pressure. As the cuff continues to be released, soft murmurs can be auscultated—**phase II**. These are followed by louder murmurs during **phase III**, as the volume of blood passing through the constricted artery increases. The sounds become abruptly muffled in **phase IV** and disappear in **phase V**, which is usually within 10 mmHg of phase IV. Diastolic pressure measured through an intrarterial catheter corresponds most closely to phase V. When the difference between phases IV and V is > 10 mmHg, both pressures should be recorded. In many children, disappearance of the sounds never occurs, and the sound are heard all the way to zero. Again, both levels should be recorded.

54. What constitutes significant and severe hypertension?
The Second Task Force on Blood Pressure Control in Children devised numerical classifications of significant and severe hypertension. Other factors, such as the rapidity of onset and association of end-organ damage or dysfunction, are important issues that must be considered in addition to simple numerical elevation.

Age	Significant Hypertension (mmHg)	Severe Hypertension (mmHg)
7 days	SBP ≥ 96	SBP ≥ 106
8–30 days	SBP ≥ 104	SBP ≥ 110
< 2 yr	SBP ≥ 112	SBP ≥ 118
	DBP ≥ 74	DBP ≥ 82
3–5 yr	SBP ≥ 116	SBP ≥ 124
	DBP ≥ 76	DBP ≥ 84
6–9 yr	SBP ≥122	SBP ≥130
	DBP ≥ 78	DBP ≥ 86
10–12 yr	SBP ≥ 126	SBP ≥ 134
	DBP ≥ 82	DBP ≥ 90
13–15 yr	SBP ≥ 136	SBP ≥ 144
	DBP ≥ 86	DBP ≥ 92
16–18 yr	SBP ≥ 142	SBP ≥ 150
	DBP ≥ 92	DBP ≥ 98

SBP = systolic blood pressure; DBP = diastolic blood pressure.
Task Force on Blood Pressure Control in Children: Report of the Second Task Force on Blood Pressure Control in Children—1987. Pediatrics 79:1–25, 1987.

55. What is the natural history of essential hypertension in children?

Approximately 30–40% of children who are hypertensive become hypertensive adults. This is especially true for black males.

Gillman MW, et al: Identifying children at high risk for the development of essential hypertension. J Pediatr 122:837–845, 1993.

56. How does normal blood pressure vary according to the size of a newborn?

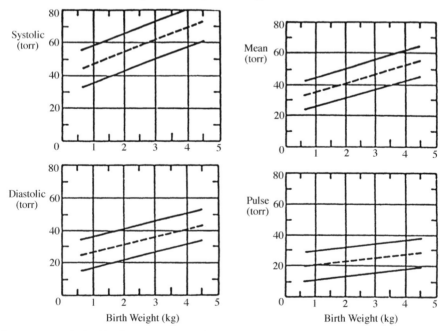

Pressures were obtained by direct measurement through an umbilical artery catheter in healthy newborn infants of various weights during first 12 hours of life. Broken lines represent linear regressions; solid lines represent 95% confidence limits. Shown are systolic and diastolic pressures, mean aortic pressure, and pulse pressure (systolic-diastolic pressure amplitude). From Vesmold HT, et al: Aortic blood pressure during the first 12 hours of life in infants with birth weight 610 to 4220 grams. Pediatrics 67:611, 1981; with permission.

57. When should hypertension be treated in the neonate?

Hypertension is defined as a blood pressure > 90/60 mmHg in term neonates and > 80/45 in preterm infants. A sustained systolic blood pressure > 100 mmHg in the neonate should be investigated and treated.

58. What workup is indicated in an adolescent with hypertension?

The need for a workup is to exclude surgically correctable causes or underlying renal disease. Clearly, the first step is a careful history and physical examination, which will aid in the selection of additional tests. A strong family history of essential hypertension suggests that an extensive workup will not be fruitful. The minimum evaluation should include a urinalysis and serum creatinine or blood urea nitrogen (BUN) to exclude intrinsic renal disease. An ultrasound also would be prudent to exclude structural renal disease. An arteriogram is indicated for children with severe hypertension (diastolic pressure > 120 mmHg) after excluding other renal causes.

59. List the causes of secondary hypertension in children and adolescents.

Cause	Acute Hypertension	Chronic Hypertension	
Renal	Acute glomerulonephritis Acute renal failure Hemolytic-uremic syndrome	Congenital defects Chronic pyelonephritis Hydronephrosis	Tumors of the kidney Hypoplastic kidney Collagen vascular disease
Endocrine	—	Pheochromocytoma Hyperthyroidism (systolic)	Primary aldosteronism Neuroblastoma
Vascular	Renovascular trauma	Coarctation of the aorta Renal artery stenosis Takayasu arteritis	Renal arteriovenous fistula Neurofibromatosis Tuberous sclerosis
Neurogenic	Increased intracranial pressure Guillain-Barré syndrome	Dysautonomia	—
Metabolic	Hypercalcemia Hypernatremia	—	—
Drugs	Cocaine Phencyclidine (PCP) Amphetamines	Nonsteroidal antiinflammatory drugs Oral contraceptives	Anabolic steroids Corticosteroids Alcohol
Miscellaneous	Burns Leg traction	Heavy metal poisons	—

Adapted from Daniels SR, Loggie JM: Essential hypertension. Adolesc Med State Art Rev 2:555, 1991; with permission.

60. What historical information suggests a secondary cause of hypertension?

History	Suggests
Known UTI; recurrent abdominal or flank pain with frequency, urgency, dysuria; secondary enuresis	Renal disease
Joint pains, rash, fever, edema	Renal disease, vasculitis
Complicated neonatal course, umbilical artery catheter	Renal artery stenosis
Renal trauma	Renal artery stenosis
Drug use (e.g., sympathomimetics, anabolic steroids, oral contraceptives, illicit drugs)	Drug-induced hypertension
Aberrant course or timing of secondary sexual characteristics; virilization	Adrenal disorder
Muscle cramping, constipation, weakness	Hyperaldosteronism (primary or secondary)
Excessive sweating, episodes of pallor and flushing	Pheochromocytoma

Adapted from Hiner LB, Falkner B: Renovascular hypertension in children. Pediatr Clin North Am 40:128–129, 1993; with permission.

61. List the features on physical exam that suggest a secondary cause of hypertension.

Physical Finding	Possible Secondary Cause
Blood pressure	
> 140/100 at any age	Multiple secondary causes
Leg BP < arm BP	Coarctation of the aorta
Poor growth	Chronic renal disease
Short stature, features of Turner syndrome	Coarctation of the aorta
Multiple café-au-lait spots or neurofibromas	Renal artery stenosis, pheochromocytoma
Decreased or delayed pulse in leg	Coarctation of the aorta
Vascular bruits	
Over large vessels	Arteritis
Over upper abdomen, flank	Renal artery stenosis
Flank or upper quadrant mass	Renal malformation, renal or adrenal tumor
Excessive virilization or secondary sex characteristics inappropriate for age	Adrenal disorder
Extremities	
Edema	Renal disease
Excessive sweating	Pheochromocytoma

Adapted from Hiner LB, Falkner B: Renovascular hypertension in children. Pediatr Clin North Am 40:128–129, 1993; with permission.

62. How is the "captopril challenge" test done?

The captopril challenge test is designed to screen for renovascular hypertension. In patients with significant unilateral renal artery stenosis, perfusion of the kidney downstream from the renal artery stenosis is dependent on angiotensin II; the effect is blocked by captopril. In the captopril test, standard nuclear medicine scanning of the kidneys is performed, and the radioactivity observed in each kidney is compared before and after administering captopril. With significant renal artery stenosis, there is a sharp reduction in the radioactivity in the kidney ipsilateral to the stenosis after captopril administration. This test may be falsely negative if there is bilateral renal artery stenosis.

63. What are the mechanisms of action and side effects of furosemide?

Furosemide acts principally in the medullary diluting segment of the ascending limb of the loop of Henle by inhibiting sodium, potassium, and chloride cotransport, thereby causing their increased excretion. It also inhibits calcium and magnesium reabsorption in the loop such that up to 30–35% of the filtered load can be lost. The onset of action occurs 5 minutes after intravenous injection and 1 hour after oral ingestion. The peak effect occurs at 2 hours, and the duration of action is 6–8 hours.

The usual side effects of furosemide result from its diuretic action, i.e., volume contraction, hyponatremia, hypokalemia and metabolic acidosis. Because of the hypercalciuric effect, prolonged administration has been linked to renal stone formation, especially in neonates. Ototoxicity has been observed in patients with reduced renal function after large intravenous doses. Furosemide is a sulfonamide, and patients with sulfonamide sensitivity may develop an allergic reaction.

64. How do thiazide diuretics differ from furosemide?

Compared to furosemide, hydrochlorothiazide and chlorothiazide directly inhibit sodium and chloride reabsorption in the early portion of the distal tubule (rather than loop of Henle). Onset (1–2 hours), peak (4–6 hours), and duration (12–24 hours) are more delayed than with furosemide. Thiazides are less potent than furosemide in treating edema, but they are more potent in treating hypertension. They are also useful in the treatment of hypercalciuria, nephrogenic diabetes insipidus, and proximal renal tubular acidosis. As with furosemide, they may cause volume contraction and hypokalemia, but they are also associated with the development of hyperuricemia and hyperglycemia (rarely).

65. Which medications are useful in hypertensive emergencies?

- Sublingual nifedipine (calcium channel blocker)
- IV labetalol (α/β-receptor blockade)
- IV sodium nitroprusside (direct arteriolar and venous dilator)
- IV diazoxide (direct arterial vasodilator)
- IV hydralazine (direct arterial vasodilator)
- IV esmolol (β-blocker)
- IV enalaprilat (ACE inhibitor)

• Emergency treatment of hypertension in children is indicated if signs or symptoms of CNS dysfunction are present (e.g., headache, confusion, lethargy, visual problems, papilledema, seizures). The drug of choice and optimal rate of blood pressure decline are uncertain. Traditionally, IV diazoxide and hydralazine have been the primary agents, but some argue that the magnitude of the effects may be difficult to predict and lead to an excessively rapid fall in blood pressure with sequelae of cortical blindness, stroke, and renal failure. Other medications, particularly labetalol and nitroprusside, have been touted as safer, particularly if used in incremental dosing to lower the excessive blood pressure by about one-third over the first 6 hours of treatment and the remaining two-thirds over the ensuing 36–48 hours.

Deal J, et al: Management of hypertensive emergencies. Arch Dis Child 67:1089, 1992.

66. Why shouldn't patients with hypertension and/or using diuretics eat licorice?

True licorice contains glycyrrhizic acid, which has mineralocorticoid (e.g., sodium-retaining) properties. However, most American licorice contains only licorice flavoring and thus has no mineralocorticoid properties. Some chewing tobacco also contains licorice and has been associated with an excess mineralocorticoid syndrome. Think of this if you are called to evaluate an edematous Philadelphia Phillies batboy.

PROTEINURIA/NEPHROTIC SYNDROME

67. On a routine urinalysis, an asymptomatic 7-year-old boy has 1+ protein noted on dipstick. How should this child be evaluated?

If he has no overt signs, symptoms, or other abnormalities on urinalysis to suggest nephritis, then the initial step is to determine if the proteinuria is transient or persistent. This is done by rechecking the urine at least two times over a 2–4-week period. If persistent, the presence or absence of orthostatic proteinuria must be determined and the amount of protein quantified.

1. **Transient** (and intermittent) proteinuria occurs during febrile episodes, vigorous exertion, cold exposure, dehydration, stress, and seizures.

2. **Orthostatic** proteinuria refers to abnormal protein excretion observed only when the patient is upright. A definitive diagnosis can be made by collecting a timed urine specimen while the patient is recumbent and comparing the result with a specimen collected while the patient is upright. Both results are extrapolated to 24 hours and compared to normal values. The recumbent excretion must be within the range for normal age-matched peers, while the upright excretion can, and usually does, exceed the normal range. A dipstick value of trace or negative protein in the recumbent specimen is probably adequate, especially if the specific gravity exceeds 1.018. Orthostatic proteinuria is most commonly observed in teenagers. A complete 24-hour urine protein collection should not exceed 1 gm.

3. **Persistent** proteinuria is more worrisome and must be quantitated. A timed urine collection demonstrating > 4 mg/m^2/day of protein is significant and requires evaluation for potential renal disease. Indicated tests can include serum electrolytes, BUN, creatinine, cholesterol, antinuclear antibodies screen, complement levels, renal ultrasound, and renal biopsy.

68. What is the natural history of orthostatic proteinuria?

Few prospective data exist on the long-term outcome of children and adolescents, but followup data on young adults up to 50 years after diagnosis demonstrate a benign clinical course. Most agree that the prognosis is excellent, although the etiology remains unclear. Since some significant glomerular diseases can present with orthostatic proteinuria, it is advisable to monitor protein quantification, urinalysis, and renal function once or twice a year, particularly in the first years after diagnosis. If hypertension, hematuria, decreased renal function, or increased protein-uria develop, then additional evaluation and referral to a nephrologist should be considered.

Glassock R: Postural proteinuria: No cause for concern. N Engl J Med 305:639–641, 1981.

69. What level constitutes "significant" proteinuria?

Protein excretion of > 4 mg/m²/hr on a timed urine collection. Children with nephrosis ex-crete > 40 mg/m²/hr. The upper limit of protein excretion in adults is 150 mg/day. A urine pro-tein/urine creatinine ratio of > 0.5 in children under 2 years of age and > 0.2 in older children is considered excessive.

24-Hour Urine Protein Excretion at Different Ages

AGE	PROTEIN CONCENTRATION (mg/L)	TOTAL PROTEIN IN 24 HRS (mg)*	PROTEIN/M² BSA/24 HRS (mg)*
Premature (5–30 days)	88–845	29 (14–60)	182 (88–377)
Full-term	94–455	32 (15–68)	145 (68–309)
2–12 mos	70–315	38 (17–85)	109 (48–244)
2–4 yrs	45–217	49 (20–121)	91 (37–223)
4–10 yrs	50–223	71 (26–194)	85 (31–234)
10–16 yrs	45–391	83 (29–238)	63 (22–181)

BSA = body surface area.
* Data expressed as mean and, in parentheses, 95% confidence limits calculated from log transformed data.
Modified from Miltényi M: Urinary protein excretion in healthy children. Clin Nephrol 12:216, 1979; with permission.

70. In the presence of gross hematuria, what amount of protein excretion is considered abnormal?

> 500 mg/m²/day

71. What constellation of clinical findings defines nephrotic syndrome?

The nephrotic syndrome consists of heavy proteinuria (> 40 mg/m²/hr), hypoalbuminemia, edema, and hyperlipidemia. The most common cause, especially in toddlers, and preschoolers, is minimal change disease.

72. How is a spot urine test helpful in the determination of the nephrotic syndrome?

A standard 24-hour urine collection for protein can be cumbersome, and the spot urine test has been shown to have good correlation. The protein (mg/dl) and creatinine (mg/dl) concentra-tions are measured in a single urine specimen and the protein/creatinine ratio calculated. A result > 0.2 is considered abnormal for excessive proteinuria, > 1.0 is suspicious for nephrotic syn-drome, and > 2.5 is diagnostic for proteinuria in the nephrotic range. If the diagnosis remains un-clear, a 24-hour collection should be obtained.

Kelsch RC, Sedman AD: Nephrotic syndrome. Pediatr Rev 14:30–38, 1993.

73. At what level of albumin do children usually start to develop edema?

When the serum level of albumin falls below 2.7 gm/dl, edema usually begins to develop. Below 1.8 gm/dl, edema is almost always present.

74. Is urinary protein electrophoresis helpful in evaluating children with persistent proteinuria?

It is rarely useful, but results showing predominantly albumin indicate selective excretion and are suggestive of mild glomerular disease, such as minimal change disease. A wide range of proteins indicates nonselective excretion and is suggestive of more severe glomerular disease (if large molecular-weight globulins, such as immunoglobulins) or tubular disease (if small molecu-lar-weight globulins).

75. What portion of the kidney produces Tamm-Horsfall protein?

Tamm-Horsfall protein is a large mucoprotein secreted into the urine by cells of the thick ascending limb of the loop of Henle. It is the matrix of a cast.

76. Describe the clinical features of minimal change nephrotic syndrome.

Also called minimal lesion nephrotic syndrome because of the normal light-microscopic findings and reversible glomerular foot process alterations on electron microscopy, this entity is most common in children aged 1–7, in whom it causes 80% of cases of nephrotic syndrome. Edema is present but blood pressure is usually normal, gross hematuria is absent, urinalysis is usually normal except for proteinuria (20% have microhematuria but no RBC casts), screening labs (e.g., creatinine, serum complement, antinuclear antibodies) are normal, and there is no evidence of systemic disease. Empiric corticosteroid treatment without the need for renal biopsy is commonly advised.

77. What are the recommended primary and secondary therapies for idiopathic nephrosis?

The **primary** treatment of idiopathic nephrotic syndrome is steroids, usually prednisone. Various doses have been recommended, ranging from 2–60 mg/m^2/day with a maximum dose of 60 mg/day. Alternate-day steroids are not particularly effective in inducing remission. Multiple doses throughout the day are more effective than a single daily dose. Daily steroids are continued until the urine is free of protein or for a complete month, regardless of protein excretion. The daily prednisone is then followed by a course of alternate-day therapy for 1–3 months. A mistake often made is to stop the steroids too quickly. One approach is to treat the initial episode of nephrosis with 2 mg/kg/day of prednisone for 1 month, then give that same dose every other morning as a single dose, and begin tapering the steroids over the next 2 months. Relapses are treated similarly, except the switch to alternate-day steroids is done when the urine dipstick shows a negative or trace reaction for protein for several days.

Secondary therapies for idiopathic nephrotic syndrome include cytotoxic drugs (cyclophosphamide and chlorambucil), prostaglandin inhibitors, and diuretics. Cytotoxic drugs are considered in the child in whom the steroids have become more harmful than helpful. Indications include significant growth failure, aseptic necrosis of bone, severe hypertension, gross obesity, and cataracts. Some children who were initially responsive to steroids but later become resistant may again become responsive after a course of cytotoxic drugs.

78. When are furosemide and albumin therapy indicated in nephrotic syndrome?

Intravenous albumin, followed by a potent diuretic such as furosemide, is used to induce diuresis in a child with nephrotic syndrome. This measure is only temporary, since the rise in albumin will lead to increased protein excretion, returning the serum level to the previous steady-state value. However, it is useful in a child with incapacitating **anasarca** in conjunction with other measures such as sodium restriction and steroids. Furosemide and albumin are also used in children with **cellulitis** and **skin breakdown** due to edema and in those with **respiratory embarrassment** from pleural effusions. In more acute situations, the pleural space should be drained with a needle. Albumin alone is useful in the child with a **rising BUN** secondary to decreased renal perfusion, a situation most often seen after vigorous diuretic therapy. Albumin alone is also indicated in the nephrotic child with **shock** from hypovolemia to promote transfer of interstitial water into the intravascular compartment. The usual course of action is to give 0.5–1 gm/kg of 25% albumin intravenously over 1–2 hours followed by 1–4 mg/kg of furosemide (euphemistically called the "albumin-Lasix sandwich"). Respiratory rate and blood pressure should be monitored during treatment, and the diuretic administered earlier if the blood pressure rises significantly or if there is difficulty with respiration.

79. How quickly do patients with minimal change nephrotic syndrome respond to steroid therapy?

In patients who are placed on prednisone for their initial episode, up to 95% will respond in the first month, with the mean time being 10–13 days. Response is indicated by normalization of urinary protein excretion and diuresis.

80. What is the mechanism of hyperlipidemia associated with severe proteinuria?

Elevations in the plasma concentrations of cholesterol and triglycerides are characteristically seen in children with nephrotic syndrome. Low-density lipoproteins (LDL) and very-low-density lipoproteins (VLDL) are also increased, but high-density lipoproteins (HDL) may be high, normal, or low. The mechanisms underlying these lipid alterations include both enhanced hepatic production of VLDL and decreased peripheral catabolism/utilization of VLDL. With very low plasma oncotic pressure, conversion of VLDL to LDL may be impaired. HDL may be lost in the urine in severely proteinuric states. Although total cholesterol rises in most nephrotics, the ratio of LDL to HDL cholesterol may actually be low. It is this ratio which is more predictive of the risk of atherosclerosis, and it varies from patient to patient. Lowering of plasma lipids with an infusion of albumin suggests that the oncotic pressure or possibly the plasma viscosity is an important determinant of these abnormalities. Normalization of the plasma lipids, however, is usually the last feature of the nephrotic syndrome to resolve.

81. What is the mechanism of hypercoagulability associated with nephrotic syndrome?

Many factors seem to be involved in the hypercoagulable state. Blood viscosity (in part due to hyperlipidemia) is increased. Platelet adhesiveness is increased. Nearly all coagulation factors and clotting inhibitors are altered, such as lower levels of antithrombin III, protein C, and protein S. The overall tendency favors increased coagulation and decreased fibrinolysis.

82. List the infectious causes of nephrotic syndrome in children.

Bacterial: post-streptococcal, infective endocarditis, shunt nephritis, leprosy, syphilis
Viral: hepatitis B virus, HIV, hepatitis C virus, and rarely other viruses
Protozoal: malaria, toxoplasmosis
Parasitic: schistosomiasis

83. Which organisms are responsible for peritonitis in children with nephrotic syndrome?

Pneumococcus remains an important cause, although gram-negative organisms, especially *Escherichia coli*, account for 25–50% of cases.

84. Which causes of nephrotic syndrome are likely to progress to renal impairment?

Cause	% Progressing
Minimal change	2–3
Focal segmental sclerosis	30–50
Membranoproliferative (untreated)	90
Membranous	10–30
Systemic lupus erythematosus	30–40
Henoch-Schönlein purpura	40
Diabetes mellitus	100
AIDS nephropathy	100

These outcomes do not reflect the change in outcome with treatment of membranoproliferative glomerulonephritis, in which only a very small percentage of cases may progress. Only 1–5% of all patients with Henoch-Schönlein purpura will develop chronic renal impairment, with the percent shown reflecting those with nephrotic syndrome. Again, only a fraction of patients with diabetes mellitus develop nephrotic syndrome, but those who do almost universally develop evidence of chronic renal impairment.

85. Discuss the prognostic factors in children with nephrotic syndrome.

Age is one of the best prognostic factors. Children initially presenting before age 6 have an 85–90% chance of minimal change disease. Children 6–12 years old have a 50% chance. For teenagers, the probability of minimal change disease drops to 25%. Complete resolution of the nephrotic syndrome with steroid therapy is also associated with a 90–95% chance of minimal change disease. A **low serum complement** level and **raised BUN** or **creatinine** (not responsive to volume) are also poor prognostic signs, since minimal change disease is very unlikely with these laboratory abnormalities. Finally, **nephrotic syndrome** in a child with glomerulonephritis usually indicates a more severe disease and a poorer prognosis.

86. When should renal biopsy be performed in a child with nephrosis?

A renal biopsy is not necessary in most children with nephrosis. Biopsy is reasonable to consider in children with idiopathic nephrotic syndrome under age 1 year or over age 10–12 years since the incidence of minimal change disease in such children is much less. Children with hypocomplementemia, azotemia not responsive to volume and albumin, gross hematuria, and red cell casts on urinalysis should also have a biopsy to aid in the decision whether to treat with steroids. Several studies have pointed out that the response to prednisone is nearly as good as a biopsy in predicting whether the pathology is minimal change or not. Complete remission of the proteinuria indicates a high (80–90%) likelihood of minimal change disease, and no response indicates a 95% chance of another diagnosis. Children who have no response or only some reduction in their proteinuria after a month of therapy should be biopsied. A more difficult issue is when to biopsy children with frequent relapses, and this usually is a matter of nephrologic style. One approach is to biopsy them when the consideration of adding a cytotoxic agent is raised or when they become steroid-resistant.

RENAL FAILURE

87. Which is a more sensitive index of altered glomerular filtration: BUN or creatinine?

Both have drawbacks. Changes in BUN tend to be more sensitive to alterations in diet and extracellular volume compared to the serum creatinine. Conversely, a reduced muscle mass can lower the serum creatinine concentration, masking mild renal insufficiency. In general, a rise in BUN is evident earlier than a rise in serum creatinine in mild renal insufficiency. Incremental increase in creatinine can have major significance, with an increase from 0.5 mg/dl to 1.0 mg/dl representing a 50% decrease in glomerular filtration.

88. What is the Schwartz formula for estimating creatinine clearance?

$$\text{Creatinine clearance (ml/1.73 m}^2\text{/min)} = \frac{\text{height (cm)} \times (0.55)}{\text{Serum creatinine (mg/dl)}}$$

This formula was derived from measurements in children aged 0.5–20 years. It is best applied to children > 2 years when glomerular filtration rate bears a constant relationship to body surface area. For children < 1 year of age, the constant (0.55) changes to 0.45.

Schwartz GJ, et al: A simple estimate of glomerular filtration rate in children derived from body length and plasma creatinine. Pediatrics 58:259–263, 1976.

89. How do you distinguish prerenal azotemia from established renal failure?

Prerenal Azotemia vs. Renal Failure

PARAMETERS	PRERENAL	RENAL
Urine osmolality	> 500	< 350
Urine/plasma osmolality	> 1.3	< 1.1
Urine/plasma urea	> 8	< 3
Urine/plasma creatinine	> 40	< 20
FE_{Na}*	< 1%	> 2%
RFI[†]	< 1%	> 2%

* FE_{Na} = fractional excretion of Na = $\dfrac{U_{Na} \cdot P_{Cr}}{P_{Na} \cdot U_{Cr}} \times 100$

[†] RFI = renal failure index = $\dfrac{U_{Na} \cdot P_{Cr}}{U_{Cr}}$

The FE_{Na} and RFI can be done on an untimed "spot" urine. These tests are useful only in patients with hypovolemia in whom one is trying to distinguish prerenal oliguria from established acute tubular necrosis (ATN). Patients with postrenal causes (obstruction) tend to have values similar to those in ATN patients, while patients with acute glomerulonephritis have values similar to those in prerenal patients. Diuretics, especially potent loop diuretics, invalidate all of these indices.

90. What is the most common cause of acute renal failure in children in the United States?
Hemolytic-uremic syndrome (HUS). HUS is classified as either diarrhea-associated or non-diarrhea-associated. The diarrhea-associated type usually follows an episode of infection with verotoxin-producing *Escherichia coli* (especially O157:H7) or *Shigella dysenteriae* type 1.

91. What is the classic triad of clinical findings in HUS?
• Microangiopathic hemolytic anemia (blood smear showing RBC fragments and schistocytes)
• Azotemia
• Thrombocytopenia (not always present)

92. Which diseases should be considered in the differential diagnosis of HUS?
HUS in a young child is not generally confused with other disorders.
1. **Acute autoimmune hemolytic anemia** can occasionally be confused with HUS, especially if hemoglobinuria has caused renal injury. The blood smear in this disorder is quite different from that in HUS, and the Coombs' test is positive in the anemia and negative in HUS.
2. In the older child and teenager, distinguishing **thrombotic thrombocytopenia purpura** (TTP) from HUS can be difficult. However, TTP is rare in children and tends to have marked CNS involvement and less renal disease.
3. **Systemic vasculitis**, such as systemic lupus erythematosus, can cause microangiopathic hemolytic anemia, thrombocytopenia, and azotemia. These disorders, however, usually involve many organs and are associated with a number of abnormal laboratory tests, such as hypocomplementemia, antinuclear antibodies, and circulating immune complexes, which easily distinguish them from HUS.
4. **Shock**, especially with septicemia, can lead to disseminated intravascular coagulopathy, which causes thrombocytopenia and a microangiopathic anemia. Many such children also develop acute renal failure. Shock is the dominant problem in these children, which is not typically a part of HUS. Further, these children have marked abnormalities of the clotting system (in addition to thrombocytopenia), which is not typical for HUS.

93. List the poor prognostic indicators in HUS.
• Non-diarrhea-associated HUS (recurrent, hereditary)
• Age < 1 year
• Prolonged period of anuria
• Severe hypertension
• CNS findings (e.g., hemiparesis, stroke, seizure, coma)
• Elevated WBC count (> 20,000/mm³)
Stewart CL, Tina LU: Hemolytic-uremic syndrome. Pediatr Rev 14:218–224, 1993.

94. What biomedical data suggest myoglobinuria as the etiology of acute renal failure?
Myoglobinuria or hemoglobinuria should be considered whenever the urine dipstick indicates *significant blood but few or no RBCs are observed* in the sediment from fresh urine. One should remember, however, that RBCs will lyse if allowed to stand at room temperature for a long time, especially if the urine is alkaline or dilute. Adding ammonium sulfate (2.8 gm to 5 ml of urine) will precipitate hemoglobin and clear the urine of the brown or red color secondary to this pigment. The dipstick test should also become negative. Since ammonium sulfate does not precipitate myoglobin, no effect will be seen. In children with myoglobinuria, there is often evidence of rhabdomyolysis, myalgia, and weakness, and muscle enzymes are elevated. If renal failure occurs, the creatinine rises very quickly secondary to the loss of creatine from muscle. The

BUN/serum creatinine ratio will often be < 10 (normally, in renal failure it is ≥ 20:1). Hemoglobinuria is caused by massive hemolysis, which can be suspected by a pink to red discoloration of the serum.

95. Give the indications for peritoneal dialysis or hemodialysis in the child with acute renal failure.

Peritoneal dialysis or hemodialysis should be instituted when other more conservative medical interventions have failed to control the problems associated with renal failure. Specific indications for dialysis include:

1. Hyperkalemia unresponsive to potassium restriction and Kayexalate administration
2. Hypertension, congestive failure, or edema secondary to volume overload that is unresponsive to volume restriction and diuretics
3. Significant acidosis that cannot be treated with sodium bicarbonate because of volume overload
4. Signs of uremia such as stupor or coma, seizures, GI bleeding, and pericarditis
5. Elevated BUN concentration (?). (Dialysis is usually instituted when the BUN reaches 100 mg/dl, although it may be started sooner or later in individual patients depending on whether they are recovering from or just developing renal failure.)
6. Drug overdose or intoxication

96. How does acidosis develop in chronic renal failure?

The most common mechanism of acidosis in chronic renal failure is the retention of nonvolatile acids produced from the catabolism of protein. This acidosis is associated with an elevated anion gap and usually appears when the GFR drops below 30% of normal. Interestingly, it tends to be nonprogressive. The serum bicarbonate concentration is maintained in the 12–18-mEq/L range because bone salts are used to buffer the acid at the expense of further renal osteodystrophy. Hyperchloremic, "non-delta" acidosis can also be seen in chronic renal failure. This usually occurs with diabetic nephropathy and obstructive uropathy. The mechanism of this acidosis presumably is from decreased aldosterone production or decreased tubular sensitivity to aldosterone, which results in diminished distal tubular acidification.

97. What electrolyte disturbances occur in children with chronic renal failure?

Just about anything can happen and usually will. The earliest abnormalities are **hyperphosphatemia** and **acidosis**, which appear with a GFR < 30% of normal. With progression of renal disease, **hypocalcemia** and **hypermagnesemia** appear. Hyperkalemia is usually not observed until the GFR is < 10% of normal. Similarly, hyponatremia secondary to water overload usually is not noted until the GFR is quite low.

98. "Renal rickets" refers to what condition?

Renal osteodystrophy. This manifestation of chronic renal disease is characterized clinically by poor linear growth, bowing of the long bones, slipped capital femoral epiphyses, and osteonecrosis of the femoral head. It is due to the effects of hyperparathyroidism, low calcitriol levels, and poor bone mineralization.

99. How should the diet be altered in a child with chronic renal failure?

1. Ensure an adequate caloric intake, especially in an infant with CRF. Inadequate caloric intake can occur even when the GFR is > 50% of normal.
2. Reduce phosphate intake to 700–1200 mg/day to control hyperparathyroidism. This usually means almost eliminating dairy products and providing calcium supplements. Calcium supplements also prevent hyperphosphatemia by binding dietary phosphate and preventing its absorption.
3. Protein restriction to 1–1.5 gm/kg/day in the older child and 1.5–2 gm/kg/day in infants is recommended to minimize uremic symptoms when the BUN exceeds 70 mg/dl. Earlier restriction of protein has been proposed to slow the progression of renal failure, but appears not to alter the progression significantly.

4. Potassium restriction is necessary when hyperkalemia is present, and sodium restriction is necessary in the presence of edema and/or hypertension.

SURGICAL ISSUES

100. What are the risks of circumcision?

The most common complications are bleeding and infection. With poor technique, injury or amputation of the glans can occur. Meatal stenosis as a consequence of meatal ulceration is another complication.

101. Is circumcision now medically indicated?

The debate continues. Data support that newborn circumcision protects males against UTIs in infancy and adulthood. Circumcision may decrease the transmission of certain sexually transmitted diseases (syphilis, chancroid, herpes simplex, human papillomavirus, HIV), but these data are not as substantial. Other benefits can include improved lifetime genital hygiene, elimination of phimosis and local foreskin infections, and a lower incidence of penile cancer. The decision at present, however, still rests primarily on nonmedical issues.

Schoen EJ: Circumcision updated—indicated? Pediatrics 92:860–861, 1993.

102. Describe the proper method of anesthesia for neonatal circumcision.

Up to 85% of infant males in the U.S. undergo circumcision, and worldwide it remains the most commonly performed operation. Until recently, it was usually performed by most without anesthesia or analgesia. Although pacifiers, topical agents (30% lidocaine, EMLA cream), and parenteral analgesics (e.g, acetaminophen) help alleviate some discomfort, the most effective means of minimizing pain is a dorsal penile nerve block. This consists of injecting 0.3–0.4 ml of 1% lidocaine *without* epinephrine in both sides of the dorsal penile base. The safety record of this method, when properly performed, is excellent.

Strauss SG, et al: Progress in pain control for very young infants. Contemp Pediatr 12:80–100, 1995.

103. How are the degrees of hypospadias classified?

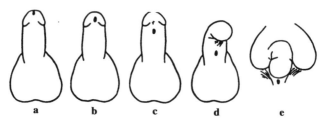

a   b   c   d   e

Degrees of hypospadias are classified according to the site of urethral opening: (a) normal meatus, (b) coronal or glandular, (c) distal shaft, (d) proximal shaft, and (e) perineal with bifid scrotum and penoscrotal transposition. Penoscrotal hypospadias not depicted.

From Perlmutter AD: Hypospadias. In Edelmann CM Jr (ed): Pediatric Kidney Disease. Boston, Little, Brown and Co., Boston, 1978, p 1235; with permission.

104. What are the implications of hypospadias?

Hypospadias occurs in 1–2/1000 livebirths and results from failure or delay in midline fusion of the urethral folds. It is often associated with a ventral band of fibrous tissue (chordee) that causes ventral curvature of the penis, especially with an erection, making intercourse difficult or impossible. In assessing hypospadias, it is useful to describe where the urethral meatus appears—glandular, distal shaft, proximal shaft, or perineal—and also the degree and location of chordee.

A number of associated genitourinary abnormalities have been described with hypospadias including meatal stenosis, inguinal hernias, undescended testes, and enlarged utricle masculinus (vestigial vagina). The incidence of these abnormalities rises sharply with the more severe degrees of hypospadias. In the mild forms, which account for most cases, radiography or endoscopy of the urinary tract is unnecessary. The treatment of hypospadias is surgical repair, usually as a one-step procedure. With the advent of microsurgical techniques, the optimal time for repair appears to be 6–12 months of age.

105. What distinguishes phimosis and paraphimosis?

Phimosis is the narrowing of the distal foreskin, preventing its retraction over the glans of the penis. In newborns, retraction is difficult due to normal adhesions which gradually self-resolve. Chronic inflammation or scarring can cause true phimosis with persistent narrowing and may require circumcision.

Paraphimosis is the incarceration of a retracted foreskin behind the glans. It occurs when the retracted foreskin is not repositioned. Progressive edema results, which, if uncorrected, can lead to ischemic breakdown. Local anesthesia, ice, and manual reduction usually correct the problem, but if these are unsuccessful, surgical reduction is necessary.

106. How should urethral prolapse be managed in young girls?

Urethral prolapse is an uncommon problem, occurring mainly in young black girls. They present with an anterior, bleeding introital mass, perineal discomfort, and mild dysuria. Many options have been tried, from sitz baths alone to aggressive surgical fixation of the bladder neck. The recommended therapy is primary surgical excision on an outpatient basis.

107. What is the natural history of hydroceles?

Small hydroceles in infancy are benign and spontaneously resolve by 9–12 months of age. Large hydroceles rarely resolve and may cause vascular compromise and testicular atrophy; these should be resected. A communicating hydrocele (which changes in size) indicates a completely patent processus vaginalis and has the potential for hernia formation. This variety also should be repaired.

108. When should undescended testicles be repaired?

The optimal time for surgery on an undescended testes is 12 months of age or shortly thereafter. Cryptorchidism usually resolves without intervention. Seventy-five percent of full-term infants and 90% of premature cryptorchid newborns will have full testicular descent by age 9 months. Spontaneous testis descent after 9 months is unlikely. In the second year of life, ultrastructural changes in the seminiferous tubules of the undescended testes begin to appear, which may be halted by orchipexy.

Section on Urology: Timing of elective surgery on the genitalia of male children with particular reference to the risks, benefits, and psychological effects of surgery and anesthesia. Pediatrics 97:590–594, 1996.

109. How young can a child be for consideration for renal transplantation?

Newborns have been successfully transplanted, so size and age are not absolute barriers. However, most centers are reluctant to transplant a child under 8–10 kg because the rate of graft loss secondary to technical factors is high. The success rate improves markedly above age 2.

110. Which primary kidney diseases recur in the transplanted patient?

The most common recurrent disease is focal segmental sclerosis, but membranoproliferative glomerulonephritis (especially type II), hemolytic-uremic syndrome, and oxalosis (unless a liver transplant is also done) also recur. With the exception of oxalosis, however, rejection remains by far the most common cause for graft failure.

111. How closely must the kidney donor and recipient be genetically matched to ensure graft survival?

As with blood transfusions, ABO blood groups must match in the donor and recipient. Furthermore, it is routine to crossmatch the recipient's sera against donor T lymphocytes (testing for preformed antibodies) to ensure there is no reaction. Some increase in overall graft survival is seen with fewer genetic mismatches between recipient and donor, especially at the HLA-B and DR loci, but long-term graft survival has occurred in patients with complete mismatch at all HLA loci.

112. How successful are cadaveric renal transplants?

60% of cadaveric renal transplants are functioning after 3 years compared to 80% from live-related donors.

113. What are the long-term risks of azathioprine and cyclosporine in renal transplant patients?

Azathioprine	Cyclosporine	
• Infections	• Infections	• Hepatotoxicity
• Neutropenia	• Hypertension	• Tremors, convulsions
• Lymphomas	• Lymphomas	• Hypertrichosis
• Cholestasis	• Nephrotoxicity	• Gum hyperplasia
	• Hyperlipidemia	

114. What are the manifestations of allograft rejection?

1. **Hyperacute rejection**, in which the kidney immediately becomes blue, pale, and poorly perfused, occurs as soon as recipient blood flows into the kidney. It is caused by preformed antibodies to the donor kidney and is a rare event because of current cross-matching techniques.

2. **Acute rejection** can be associated with fever, graft tenderness and swelling, oliguria, rising BUN and creatinine, hypertension, and edema. With the use of cyclosporine, fever and graft tenderness are unusual. A rising BUN and creatinine and worsening hypertension are more commonly noted. In small children receiving adult kidneys, worsening hypertension can be the earliest sign of rejection, with a rise in the serum creatinine concentration occurring much later.

3. **Chronic rejection** is insidious, with slowly worsening renal function as the only sign.

TUBULAR DISORDERS

115. Name the four main types of renal tubular acidosis (RTA).

Type 1—impairment in distal acidification
Type 2—impairment in bicarbonate reclamation
Type 3—combination of types 1 and 2
Type 4—secondary to a lack of, or insensitivity to, aldosterone

All four types are associated with a hyperchloremic, normal anion gap acidosis.

116. Describe the clinical and laboratory manifestations of the various RTAs.

	Type 1 (Classic, distal)	Type 2 (Proximal)	Type 3 (Hybrid)	Type 4 (Aldosterone deficiency)
Growth failure	+++	++	++	+++
Hypokalemic muscle weakness	++	+	+	Hyperkalemia
Nephrocalcinosis	Frequent	Rare	±	Rare
Low citrate excretion	+++	±	±	±
FE of filtered HCO_3 at normal serum HCO_3 levels	< 5%	> 15%	5–15%	< 15%
Daily alkali treatment (mEq/kg)	1–10	5–20	1–10	1–5
Daily potassium requirement	Decreases with correction	Increases with correction	±	
Urine pH	> 5.5	< 5.5	> 5.5	< 5.5
Presence of other tubular defects	Rare	Common	Rare	Rare
Metabolic bone disease	Rare	Common	Rare	Rare
Urine anion gap	Positive	Negative	Positive	Positive

+, Present; ++, common; +++, very common; ±, variable. FE = fractional excretion.
Adapted from Chan JCM: Renal tubular acidosis. J Pediatr 103:327, 1983; and Zelikovic I: Renal tubular acidosis. Pediatr Ann 24:53, 1995; with permission.

Types 1, 2, and 3 RTA are associated with hypokalemia, whereas type 4 is characterized by hyperkalemia in addition to hyperchloremic acidosis. Hypercalciuria is typical of type 1 RTA and, in conjunction with hypocitraturia, often leads to nephrocalcinosis and renal calculi. Type 2 is often part of a more global defect of proximal tubule function, the **Fanconi syndrome**, characterized by aminoaciduria, hypophosphatemia, glycosuria, and rickets. Type 4 RTA is most commonly observed in patients with obstructive uropathy, congenital adrenal hyperplasia, and adrenal insufficiency. Other symptoms and signs that are common with all forms of RTA are growth failure, polyuria, polydipsia, recurrent dehydration, and vomiting.

117. What are the causes of classic type 2 RTA?
  Isolated: transient, sporadic, hereditary
  Fanconi syndrome: idiopathic, hereditary, cystinosis, tyrosinemia, galactosemia, glycogen storage disease, Lowe syndrome, Wilson disease, cytochrome *c* oxidase deficiency, lead, mercury, cadmium poisoning
    Drugs: outdated tetracycline, acetazolamide, sulfanilamide
    Disorders of calcium metabolism: hyperparathyroidism, vitamin D deficiency
    CNS degenerative: metachromatic leukodystrophy, Leigh encephalopathy
    Renal: medullary cystic disease, transplant rejection

118. How is the diagnosis of proximal RTA established?
Because the primary problem is a defect in the reabsorption of filtered bicarbonate in the proximal tubule, the key is to normalize the body's serum HCO_3 level and then demonstrate an increased spillage of HCO_3 in the urine as the tubule's lower threshold is reached. Two methods are commonly used:

One method involves giving oral or intravenous bicarbonate until the urine pH increases to 6.0 and then measuring serum HCO_3 levels. This pH change occurs when the serum HCO_3 is > 21 mEq/L in infants and > 22–23 mEq/L in older children. In proximal RTA, this pH change occurs at lower levels, such as 16–19 mEq/L.

The simpler method is to measure the fractional excretion (FE) of bicarbonate, as the serum bicarbonate level is raised toward normal:

$$FE_{HCO_3} = ([U_{HCO_3} \times P_{Cr}] \times 100)/[P_{HCO_3} \times U_{Cr}])$$

where U indicates urinary values, P is plasma values, and Cr is creatinine. In normal children, the FE_{HCO_3} is < 5%, while in children with proximal RTA it is > 15%.

119. What disorders are associated with classic type 1 distal RTA?
  Primary
    Sporadic, hereditary
  Secondary
    Disorders associated with nephrocalcinosis: idiopathic hypercalciuria, hyperthyroidism, hyperparathyroidism, vitamin D intoxication, Wilson disease, Fabry disease, hereditary fructose intolerance
    Autoimmune disorders: systemic lupus erythematosus, Sjögren's syndrome, hypergammaglobulinemia
    Renal disorders: chronic pyelonephritis, hydronephrosis, medullary cystic disease
    Various genetic disorders: sickle cell anemia, Ehlers-Danlos syndrome, carbonic anhydrase B deficiency, Marfan syndrome
    Drugs: amphotericin B, lithium

120. How is the diagnosis of classic distal RTA established?
Because the primary problem is an inability to acidify the urine properly, the key to diagnosis is demonstrating an inability to lower the urine pH to < 5.5 in the setting of metabolic acidemia. Most distal RTA patients have low serum HCO_3 levels, making direct urine testing possible.

However, in some patients, provocative acidifying challenges with ammonium chloride or argi-nine hydrochloride are necessary. Alternatively, furosemide can be used to stimulate the distal tubule to secrete hydrogen ions. In patients with distal RTA, measured net acid secretion is also diminished.

Another test of hydrogen ion secretion involves loading the patient with bicarbonate. Normally, distally secreted hydrogen ions combine with bicarbonate to form carbonic acid, which is catalyzed to water and CO_2. In patients with distal RTA, less carbonic acid (and thus CO_2) is produced. When the difference between the urine and blood CO_2 concentration is < 20 mmHg, distal RTA is likely.

121. An 8-month-old with failure to thrive, hypokalemic metabolic alkalosis, and hyper-plasia of the juxtaglomerular apparatus on renal biopsy is admitted to your service. What is the most likely diagnosis?

Bartter syndrome. This disorder of the renal tubules is of unclear etiology but is believed to be a defect in chloride reabsorption. It leads to volume contraction, increased aldosterone se-cretion, and profound hypokalemia. In the state of volume contraction, plasma renin levels are high, but patients remain normotensive and relatively unresponsive to the pressor effects of an-giotensin II and norepinephrine. A variety of urinary abnormalities exist, including excessive chloride, sodium, magnesium, and potassium excretion. These mineral and electrolyte abnor-malities can lead to symptoms of fatigue, muscle cramps, weakness, excessive thirst, and exces-sive urination.

URINALYSIS

122. How do glucosuria and proteinuria affect urine specific gravity?

Specific gravity is the ratio of the weight of a volume of urine to a similar volume of water. It is affected by the number and weight of particles in the urine. Because of their weight, glucose and protein can affect the specific gravity. For each 1 gm/dl of protein, the specific gravity in-creases by 0.003, and for each 1 gm/dl of glucose, by 0.004. In practice, this usually does not affect the clinical interpretation as to whether the urine is concentrated or not.

123. Which substances give a positive urine Clinitest?

Glucose, fructose, galactose, pentose, lactose, cephalosporins, large amounts of ascorbic acid.

124. What causes black urine?

Black or dark brown urine is observed in children with **alkaptonuria** due to the excretion of homogentisic acid. The urine does not turn black immediately, but only after exposure to air. Black urine can also be seen in **melanotic sarcoma** from melanin excretion. Brown urine is also observed in glomerulonephritis.

125. What causes milky urine?

The precipitation of calcium phosphate or urates can turn the urine milky, especially when the specimen is stored in the refrigerator. Warming the urine to body temperature causes these precipitated salts to return to solution, removing the milky appearance. Purulent material associ-ated with infections of the bladder and urethra may also cause the urine to appear milky. Lymph can also cause a milky urine as a result from lymphatic obstruction (rare cause of milky urine).

126. What causes red urine without hematuria?

Red urine can be caused by porphyrins, beets, blackberries, vegetable dyes, drugs such as phenolphthalein (used in laxatives), and urates (especially in neonates). Hemoglobinuria and myoglobinuria usually cause a brown color. *Serratia marcescens* can produce a red pigment, making the diaper red.

127. What causes pneumaturia?

Pneumaturia is the passage of gas bubbles in the urine. It can occur as a result of a fistula between the bladder and bowel or vagina. Fistulae can be congenital abnormalities or result from infection, neoplasms, inflammatory bowel disease, or instrumentation of the bladder. Rarely, UTIs with gas-producing bacteria can lead to pneumaturia. This condition is most often observed in diabetics.

128. What is the significance of red cell casts in the urine?

Finding red cell casts on urinalysis almost always indicates the presence of **glomerulonephritis**. Casts have, however, been observed after strenuous exercise and renal trauma (including renal biopsy).

129. What is the significance of white cell casts in the urine?

White cell casts are found in a variety of renal disorders. They are noted in patients with acute glomerulonephritis (especially post-streptococcal), although red cell casts are more common. White cell casts are the typical casts in **interstitial nephritis** and **pyelonephritis**. Indeed, the presence of white cell casts in a child with a UTI indicates pyelonephritis.

130. How do dipstick tests for pyuria work?

Most dipsticks provide an indirect measurement of urinary specific gravity and pH and assess the presence of protein, glucose, blood, nitrites, and leukocyte esterase. The leukocyte esterase test detects esterases released from WBCs that have broken down and is an indirect test for the presence of WBCs in urine. The nitrite test detects nitrites, which can be produced by most gram-negative urinary bacteria by the reduction of dietary nitrates. Most gram-positive organisms cannot do this reduction. The organisms must reside in the presence of dietary nitrates for hours before the reduction can take place, and thus nitrite testing has its greatest value in the analysis of a first morning specimen.

Lohr JHA: Use of routine urinalysis in making a presumptive diagnosis of urinary tract infection in children. Pediatr Infect Dis J 10:646–650, 1991.

131. Should screening urinalyses be done on asymptomatic children?

A continuing area of debate. The American Academy of Pediatrics recommends a urinalysis in infancy (age < 1 yr), the preschool age group (ages 1–4 yrs), late childhood (ages 5–12), and adolescence. However, the likelihood of detecting conditions that will benefit from early diagnosis and treatment is exceedingly low. Nearly all cases of microscopic hematuria, intermittent proteinuria, and bacteriuria in asymptomatic patients appear to have no significant long-term morbidity. Many authorities question the routine urinalysis as fraught with uncertainty and unlikely cost-effectiveness.

Hoekelman RA: Is screening urinalysis worthwhile in asymptomatic pediatric patients? Pediatr Ann 23:459–460, 1994.

132. Should all children have a routine urinalysis on hospital admission?

In patients without signs or symptoms attributable to the urinary tract, the value of routine urinalysis on admission is debatable. At present local custom prevails.
- **Arguments against:**
  1. The low likelihood of significant pathology if microhematuria, proteinuria, glycosuria and/or pyuria are detected, particularly in older children
  2. Inconsistency of followup of abnormalities on urinalysis done in an inpatient setting
  3. Excessive cost
- **Arguments for:**
  1. Difficulties in identifying high-risk patients by history or exam alone
  2. Lack of primary care in many patients
  3. Detection of even a few preventable cases of chronic renal failure justifies its use

Mitchell N, Stapleton FB: Routine admission urinalysis examination in pediatric patients: A poor value. Pediatrics 86:345–349, 1990.

URINARY TRACT INFECTIONS

133. How sensitive is pyuria as an indicator for bacteriuria?

About 80% of children with a UTI will have > 10 WBC/high-power field (hpf). About 20% of normal children will also have pyuria. This finding is helpful but cannot be relied on alone to make or exclude a UTI diagnosis. In older children, in whom UTI symptoms are more reliable indicators of infection, a negative nitrite test, negative leukocyte esterase test, and absence of UTI symptoms are highly correlated with the absence of infection. However, babies require a culture to exclude UTI.

Kramer MS, et al: Urine testing in young febrile children: A risk-benefit analysis. J Pediatr 125:6–13, 1995.

Shaw KN, et al: Clinical evaluation of a rapid screening test for urinary tract infections. J Pediatr 118:733–735, 1991.

134. Should children be screened for asymptomatic bacteriuria?

Although 1–2% of girls older than age 5 have persistent bacteriuria, mass screening at present is not recommended for the following reasons:

- In girls with radiologically demonstrable anatomic abnormalities (0.2–0.5%), most renal injury appears to occur before age 5 and may not progress.
- Older girls with asymptomatic bacteriuria and normal anatomy are unlikely to have sequelae if untreated.

Screening of infants and toddlers is technically more difficult, and the merits of screening are unclear. Infants and children at high risk should be considered for screening.

135. Which children are at increased risk for bacteriuria or a symptomatic UTI?

Premature infants discharged from neonatal intensive care units

Children with:

- Immunodeficiencies or underlying systemic disease
- Urinary tract abnormalities
- Renal calculi
- Neurogenic bladder or voiding dysfunction
- Chronic severe constipation
- Family history of UTI, renal anomalies, or reflux

Girls < 5 years of age with a history of UTI

136. How common are UTIs in febrile infants < 2 months of age?

In one study of 442 such infants, 7.5% had UTIs. In a subgroup of infants in whom the utility of urinalysis in predicting a positive urine culture was being evaluated, 40% with UTI demonstrated by catheterization or suprapubic aspiration had no pyuria and no bacteria detectable on smears of an unspun sample.

Crain EF, Gershel JC: Urinary tract infections in febrile infants younger than eight weeks of age. Pediatrics 86:363–367, 1990.

137. Why should urine specimens be refrigerated if they cannot be immediately processed?

The storage of urine specimens at room temperature is one of the most common causes of false-positive results. When left at room temperature, enteric organisms in specimens have a growth-doubling time of 30 minutes, and thus colony counts become an unreliable gauge. If a urine specimen cannot be processed within 15 minutes, it should be refrigerated at < 4°C.

138. What amounts constitute a positive urine culture?

By definition, significant bacteriuria is present in clean-catch samples if > 100,000 organisms of a single species/ml is cultured. Colony counts between 10,000–100,000 are suspicious and require reculturing, and < 10,000 organisms usually indicates contamination. If the specimen is obtained by catheterization, colony counts > 10,000 indicate infection. If the specimen is obtained by suprapubic aspiration, the presence of any bacteria indicates infection.

139. What are the characteristics of complicated UTIs?

Complicated UTIs imply the presence of either an anatomic abnormality, such as obstruction or vesicoureteral reflux, or a functional abnormality, such as a neurogenic bladder, indwelling catheter, or voiding dysfunction. Patients with complicated UTIs are more likely to have fever, flank pain, and a toxic appearance and tend to relapse after treatment.

140. Which organism should be suspected when a patient presents with UTI symptoms and a very alkaline urine?

Proteus mainly, also *Pseudomonas*, and occasionally *Escherichia coli*.

141. What is the cause of an elevated blood ammonia concentration in a child with a UTI due to *Proteus*?

Proteus produces the enzyme urease, which hydrolyzes urea to ammonia. This results in a highly alkaline urine with a significant fraction of the generated ammonia as NH_3. NH_3 can diffuse easily into the bloodstream, where it is ionized to NH_4^+ and is trapped. Thus a *Proteus* UTI has the potential of causing hyperammonemia, which can be further aggravated in children who have urinary stasis.

Samtoy B: Ammonia encephalopathy secondary to urinary tract infection with *Proteus mirabilis*. Pediatrics 65:294–297, 1980.

142. How is cystitis distinguished clinically from pyelonephritis?

Often with difficulty. Pyelonephritis tends to have more constitutional symptoms, such as fever, rigors, and flank and back pain, while cystitis has more bladder symptoms, such as wetting, dysuria, frequency, and urgency. The presence of white cell casts or impaired urinary concentrating ability is more indicative of pyelonephritis. Pyelonephritis tends to be associated with more elevations in sedimentation rate and C-reactive protein, but there is enough overlap with cystitis to make the distinction difficult in the individual patient. Detection of antibody-coated bacteria (a sign of upper tract disease in the adult) is not helpful in the pediatric age group. Renal DMSA cortical scintigraphy has a much greater sensitivity than voiding cystourethrography, intravenous pyelography, and renal ultrasonography in confirming the diagnosis.

143. How should a child with a UTI be evaluated?

Younger children and those with more severe symptoms warrant a more thorough evaluation for possible anatomic abnormalities and reflux. As a rule, boys at any age, girls < age 5, older girls with recurrent UTIs, and any child with pyelonephritis warrant evaluation with a renal ultrasound and voiding cystourethrogram (VCUG) or radionuclide cystogram. Many authorities also advise a renal cortical scan with DMSA (dimercaptosuccinic acid) for the diagnosis of acute pyelonephritis and permanent focal scars. The need for and extent of evaluation for patients with asymptomatic bacteriuria remain controversial.

Lerner GR: Urinary tract infections in children. Pediatr Ann 23:463–473, 1994.

144. When are prophylactic antibiotics indicated in a child with recurrent UTIs?

1. Maintenance therapy in an infant or child with a first-time UTI following acute treatment until appropriate imaging studies can be done
2. Grade II or higher vesicoureteral reflux until resolution
3. Infants with various forms of obstructive uropathy (such as posterior urethral valves) until surgical correction is achieved
4. For 6–12 months in children and adolescents with recurrent UTIs and normal urinary tract anatomy; if infection develops during an antibiotic-free trial period, therapy is resumed.

145. Which antibiotics are used for prophylaxis?

Nitrofurantoin (1–2 mg/kg) or trimethoprim-sulfamethoxazole (1–2 mg/kg of the trimethoprim component) is used as a single daily therapy. At these doses (less than therapeutic), urine concentrations result in adequate inhibitory activity, coverage is wide-ranging, and development of resistant flora is minimal.

UROLITHIASIS

146. What is the composition of calculi causing kidney stones in children?

Stone Composition	North America (n = 340)	Europe (n = 315)
Calcium	58%	37%
Struvite	25%	54%
Cystine	6%	3%
Uric acid/urate	9%	2%
Others	2%	4%

Modified from Polinsky MS, et al: Urolithiasis in childhood. Pediatr Clin North Am 34:683–710, 1987.

147. What disorders of childhood are known to cause calcium urolithiasis?
  A. Normocalcemic hypercalciuria
    1. Idiopathic hypercalciuria (absorptive, renal)
    2. Distal renal tubular acidosis
    3. Drug-induced (furosemide)
  B. Hypercalcemic hypercalciuria
    1. Immobilization
    2. Idiopathic hypercalcemia of infancy
    3. Hypervitaminosis D
    4. Adrenocorticosteroid excess (Cushing syndrome, exogenous)
    5. Primary hyperparathyroidism
    6. Hyperthyroidism
    7. Adrenal insufficiency
    8. Milk-alkali syndrome
  C. Hyperoxaluria
    1. Enteric hyperoxaluria
    2. Hereditary hyperoxaluria (types I and II)
    3. Pyridoxine deficiency
  D. Other causes
    1. Idiopathic calcium urolithiasis
    2. Hyperuricosuria
    3. Hypocitraturia
Nakano M, et al: Renal calculi. In Barakat AY (ed): Renal Disease in Children. Berlin, Springer-Verlag, 1990, p 373.

148. Which disorders cause urate stones?
  • Leukemia, lymphoma
  • Lesch-Nyhan syndrome
  • Glycogen storage disease (type I)
  • Polycythemia
  • Chronic volume depletion

149. How does manipulation of urine pH affect renal calculi?
  Calcium oxalate stones, the most common type of renal calculi, are unaffected by the urine pH. These stones can be treated with thiazides diuretics, which increase renal calcium reabsorption. **Calcium phosphate** stones, which occur in distal renal tubular acidosis, respond to treatment with alkali. **Uric acid** stones form in acid urine and also respond to alkalinization.

Additional therapy includes a reduction in purine intake and allopurinol to block the formation of uric acid. Urine alkalinization, in combination with penicillamine and a large fluid intake, helps to prevent formation of **cystine stones**. **Struvite** or **infection stones** form in extremely alkaline urine. Urine acidification along with antibiotics are the cornerstones of treatment for these stones.

150. How is hypercalciuria defined in the infant and child?

The strict definition of hypercalciuria in the child is > 4 mg of urinary calcium/kg/24 hr. A fasting urine calcium/creatinine ratio > 0.2 or nonfasting ratio > 0.25 is suggestive of hypercalciuria in the child > 6 years old. For children aged 1½–6 years, this ratio is < 0.4; for children from 7–18 months, it is < 0.6; and for infants < 7 months, it is < 0.86.

Sargent, et al: Normal values for random urinary calcium to creatinine ratios in infancy. J Pediatr 123:393–397, 1993.

151. When is lithotripsy or surgery indicated in children with kidney stones?

Most children with stones will spontaneously pass them. Lithotripsy is useful in children with large pelvic or bladder stones that are radiopaque in which fluoroscopy can be used to focus the shock waves. Surgery is reserved for children with stones causing urinary obstruction and for staghorn calculi that cannot be dissolved medically or fragmented by lithotripsy. Cystine stones also cannot be fragmented by lithotripsy.

Cohen TD, et al: Pediatric urolithiasis: Medical and surgical management. Urology 47:292–303, 1996.

VESICOURETERAL REFLUX

152. How is vesicoureteral reflux graded?

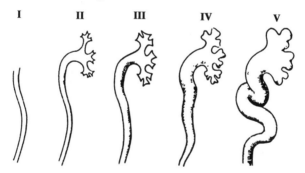

| I | II | III | IV | V |

Grade I	Ureter only
Grade II	Ureter, pelvis, and calices; no dilation, normal caliceal fornices
Grade III	Mild dilation and/or tortuosity of the ureter and mild dilation of the renal pelvis; minor blunting of the fornices
Grade IV	Moderate dilation and/or tortuosity of the ureter and moderate dilation of the renal pelvis and calices; maintenance of the papillary impressions in most calices
Grade V	Significant blunting of most fornices; papillary impressions are no longer visible in most of the calices; gross dilation and tortuosity of the ureter; gross dilation of the renal pelvis and calices

From Duckett JD, Bellinger MF: A plea for standardized grading of vesicoureteral reflux. Eur Urol 8:74–77, 1982; with permission.

153. In addition to reflux, what other pathologic bladder findings may be noted on a voiding cystourethrogram?

Diverticula may be seen, especially in the presence of outflow obstruction. A posterior urethral valve or urethral stricture can be detected during the voiding phase of the study. A ureterocele may be seen and appears as a filling defect in the bladder. Other features to note are the capacity of the bladder, whether the wall is thickened from muscular hypertrophy or is smooth, and the residual volume after voiding.

154. What is the natural history of vesicoureteral reflux?

Overall, reflux spontaneously resolves in 20–30% of patients every 2 years for a long-term disappearance of up to 80%. The extent of disappearance, however, varies by the grade of reflux on initial diagnosis. Nondilating grades of reflux (grades I–III) spontaneously resolve in 85% of patients as they get older, but more severe, dilating grades (grades IV–V) resolve in only 40%.

Edwards D, et al: Disappearance of vesicoureteral reflux during long-term prophylaxis of urinary tract infection in children. BMJ 2:285–288, 1977.

155. How should urinary reflux be managed?

Grade I reflux does not extend into the kidney and has been rarely associated with renal injury. In virtually all these children, the reflux resolves with time. Approximately 75% of children with **grades II or III** reflux will improve in time at a rate of 10% per year. Nightly administration of nitrofurantoin or trimethoprim/sulfamethoxazole is usually effective in preventing further infections in these children. Urine culture should be obtained every 3 months or whenever symptoms of an infection are present. Reevaluation of a child for presence of reflux, renal growth, and extent of scarring should be done at least every 2 years until the reflux resolves.

Children with **grade V** reflux should probably have surgical correction because the risk of renal damage is high, especially in infants, and the chance of spontaneous resolution is low. The chance of **grade IV** reflux spontaneously resolving is less than that in lower grades of reflux, but still, a significant percentage will spontaneously stop refluxing. These children could be managed medically for several years and then considered for surgical correction if the reflux persists, especially if it remains as a high grade of reflux. Another management option is to do cystoscopy and then surgically correct the reflux if it appears that the intravesical tunnel is short. This decision should be individualized in consultation with a pediatric urologist or nephrologist.

156. How does the radiation exposure differ between radionuclide cystography (RNC) and voiding cystourethrography (VCUG)?

RNC has approximately 100 times less the absorbed radiation dose compared with a single x-ray VCUG. RNC is felt to be as sensitive as VCUG in detecting vesicoureteral reflux and is recommended as the initial study in examining the female child with a UTI, screening of siblings with reflux, evaluating the child with myelomeningocele, and for ongoing followup of significant reflux.

Conway JJ, Cohn RA: Evolving role of nuclear medicine for the diagnosis and management of urinary tract infection. J Pediatr 124:87–90, 1994.

157. Should asymptomatic siblings of a patient with vesicoureteral reflux have urologic imaging done as a screen for reflux?

The incidence of vesicoureteral reflux is thought to be < 1% in normal children, but it may be as high as 45% in siblings of patients with reflux. Consequently, many recommend screening of siblings early in life.

14. NEUROLOGY

Peter Bingham, M.D., and Robert R. Clancy, M.D.

ANTIEPILEPTIC DRUGS

1. Which antiepileptic drugs (AEDs) are recommended for idiopathic generalized tonic-clonic seizures in children?

The "traditional" AEDs (phenobarbital, primidone, phenytoin) are no longer considered the drugs of choice for grand mal seizures for many age groups, although **phenobarbital** remains the drug of choice for neonatal seizures. Studies have shown that most of the major anticonvulsants are comparable in reducing or eliminating seizure recurrences. However, because many children with seizures require treatment for years, the impact of chronic use of anticonvulsant drugs on the body and brain is a concern. For example, the long-term use of phenytoin may be associated with coarsened facial features, hirsutism, cerebellar atrophy, and gingival hyperplasia. Perhaps more importantly, there is a growing awareness of the neurologic side effects affecting behavior, mood, cognitive processing, memory, and attention provoked by phenobarbital and phenytoin. For these reasons, **carbamazepine** and **valproate** have emerged as the current drugs of choice for grand mal seizures.

2. What is the AED of choice for petit mal epilepsy?

Ethosuximide (Zarontin). Most patients with petit mal epilepsy have only absence attacks during which there is some disturbance of consciousness, alertness, or reactivity while the EEG shows the classic pattern of generalized 3/second spike and slow-wave discharges. Ethosuximide is currently the drug of choice for several reasons:

1. It works well for many patients. It not only stops the clinical attacks of absence but it often normalizes the EEG by "erasing" the 3/second spike-wave discharges.

2. It is well tolerated by most patients. Although rare cases of serious bone marrow, liver, or dermatologic disorders have occurred, routine or frequent blood tests are not considered obligatory by most physicians.

3. It has a relatively long serum half-life (40 hrs). Thus once or twice a day dosing is appropriate and represents a real convenience to the patient.

4. It is relatively inexpensive.

3. What is the drug of choice for coexisting petit mal and grand mal seizures?

Divalproex sodium (Depakote). Its broad spectrum of activity provides excellent coverage for both seizure types. Most patients with absence seizures are > 2 years, at which time there is little risk of hepatotoxicity from valproic acid. Despite the relatively short elimination half-life (6–10 hrs), twice a day dosing may be used. Divalproex acid is considered to have a very low risk of unwanted cognitive side effects.

4. What idiosyncratic drug reactions are associated with antiepileptic medications?

Carbamazepine:	leukopenia, aplastic anemia, thrombocytopenia, hepatic dysfunction, rashes
Ethosuximide:	leukopenia, pancytopenia, rashes
Phenobarbital:	rashes, Stevens-Johnson syndrome, hepatic dysfunction
Phenytoin:	hepatic dysfunction, lymphadenopathy, movement disorder, Stevens-Johnson syndrome, fulminant hepatic failure
Valproic acid:	fulminant hepatic failure, hyperammonemia, pancreatitis, thrombocytopenia, rash, stupor

Freeman JM, Holmes GL: Should uncomplicated seizures be treated? Curr Probl Pediatr 24:143, 1994.

5. Give the suggested dosing and therapeutic ranges for AEDs.

Guidelines for Doses of Established Antiepileptic Drugs in Children

AED	STANDARD MAINTENANCE DOSE (RANGE) (mg/kg/day)	NO. OF DOSES/DAY	TARGET PLASMA DRUG CONCENTRATION (RANGE) (µg/ml)	STEADY STATE REACHED (days)
Carbamazepine	10–25	2–4	4–12	3–6
Clonazepam	0.025–0.1	2–4	40–80 ng/ml	5–10
Ethosuximide	15–30	1–2	40–100	5–6
Phenobarbital	4–8	1–2	15–40	10–21
Phenytoin	5–15	1–3	10–20	3–10
Primidone	20–30	1–3	5–12	1–5
Valproic acid	15–40	1–3	50–120	2–4

Note that therapeutic ranges are somewhat arbitrary. Levels above "normal" may be maintained to control seizures if side effects do not occur.

Adapted from Brodie MJ, Dichter MA: Antiepileptic drugs. N Engl J Med 334:171, 1996; with permission.

6. What are the common side effects of phenytoin?

Phenytoin (Dilantin) promotes connective tissue growth that is ultimately manifest as gum hyperplasia, coarsening facial features, hypertrophic (keloid) scar formation, and sometimes Dupuytren contractures. Facial and body hair growth is also stimulated. Lymphoidal hypertrophy may appear as tonsillar enlargement. Lowered serum folate levels may eventually produce a megaloblastic anemia or mild peripheral neuropathy. The use of phenytoin may accelerate the hepatic elimination of vitamin D, resulting in rickets.

The neurologic side effects include subtle mood, behavioral, or cognitive effects, even within the normal therapeutic range. Signals of overmedication include nystagmus (blood level > 20 µg/µl), ataxia (> 30 µg/ml), and somnolence (> 40 µg/ml). Irreversible ataxia and cerebellar atrophy from Purkinje cell loss may follow chronic phenytoin use.

7. What are the risks of felbamate?

In 1993, felbamate was approved for treatment of partial and generalized seizures associated with the Lennox-Gastaut syndrome in children and for various other epilepsies in adults. Subsequent case reports identified rare associations with aplastic anemia and acute liver failure in adults. The FDA subsequently recommended its use for severe and uncontrollable epilepsy when potential benefits might outweigh possible risks. The risks and benefits of felbamate should be thoroughly discussed with the family before treatment is begun.

Dichter MA, Brodie MJ: Drug therapy: New antiepileptic drugs. N Engl J Med 334:1583–1590, 1996.

8. Which AEDs can be given rectally for acute management of seizures?

If intravenous or intraosseous routes are unavailable, options for rectal administration include:

Diazepam	0.2–0.5 mg/kg of parenteral solution
	Onset of action in 2–10 min and peak concentration in 2–30 min
Lorazepam	0.05–0.1 mg/kg of parenteral solution
	Peak concentration in 30–120 min
Paraldehyde	0.3 ml/kg of oral solution diluted in equal volume of mineral oil
	Effect in 20 min; peak concentration in 150 min
	Glass syringe needed for administration (if plastic used, plunger may bond to syringe barrel)

Of note, numerous AEDs (e.g., carbamazepine, valproic acid) do not have parenteral formulations because of their poor water solubility. However, when an oral route is not feasible (e.g., due to acute gastritis) and seizures are uncontrolled, rectal administration may also be considered.

Graves NM, Kriel RL: Rectal administration of AEDs in children. Pediatr Neurol 3:321–326, 1987.

9. After what period can AEDs be safely discontinued?

A trial of AED withdrawal may be considered if the child has remained completely seizure-free for 2 years. The highest remission rate is in those who are otherwise neurologically normal and in whom the EEG at the time of discontinuation lacks specific epileptiform features and displays a normal background. The highest relapse rate occurs in those who also have other neurologic abnormalities (e.g., mental retardation, cerebral palsy) and whose EEG at the time of discontinuation displays clear spikes or sharp waves with background slowing.

Shinnar S, et al: Discontinuing antiepileptic drugs in children with epilepsy: A prospective study. Ann neurol 35:534–538, 1994.

10. When the decision is made to discontinue AEDs, should the taper period be long or short?

In practice, all AEDs are gradually tapered rather than abruptly discontinued, even though there is no actual withdrawal state produced by a "cold turkey" reduction of most AEDs (phenytoin, carbamazepine, valproate, ethosuximide). In contrast, a **withdrawal syndrome** of agitation, signs of autonomic overactivity, and seizures follow the sudden elimination of habitually consumed diazepam or short-acting barbiturates (such as secobarbital). The long elimination half-life of phenobarbital lessens the risk of withdrawal symptoms following abrupt discontinuation.

In a study of over 100 children who had been seizure-free for either 2 or 4 years, the risk of seizure recurrence during tapering and after discontinuation of the AED was no different if the period of taper was 6 weeks or 9 months. Rapid tapering appears to be an acceptable means of discontinuation.

Tennison M, et al: Discontinuing antiepileptic drugs in children with epilepsy: A comparison of a six-week and a nine-month taper period. N Engl J Med 330:1407–1410, 1994.

CEREBRAL PALSY

11. How is cerebral palsy (CP) defined?

CP constitutes a heterogeneous group of nonprogressive disorders of movement and posture manifest early in life attributed to various known (e.g., central nervous system anomalies, hypoxic insults) and unknown etiologies involving the immature brain. While the disorder is defined as static, clinical manifestations often change over time as the central nervous system matures.

12. How is cerebral palsy classified?

Clinical classification is based on the nature of the movement disorder, muscle tone, and anatomic distribution. A single patient may have more than one type.

1. **Spastic CP** (65%): characterized by neurologic signs of upper motor neuron damage with increased "clasp knife" muscle tone, increased deep tendon reflexes, pathologic reflexes, and spastic weakness. Spastic CP is subclassified based on distribution:
   - **Hemiplegia** (30%): primarily unilateral involvement, arm usually more than leg
   - **Quadriplegia** (5%): all limbs involved, with legs often more involved than arms
   - **Diplegia** (30%): legs much more involved than arms, which may show no or only minimal impairment

2. **Dyskinetic CP** (20%): characterized by prominent involuntary movements and/or fluctuating muscle tone with choreoathetosis the most common subtype. Distribution is usually symmetric among the four limbs.

3. **Ataxic CP** (15%)

Palmer FB, Hoon AH: Cerebral palsy. In Parker S, Zuckerman B (ed): Behavioral and Developmental Pediatrics. Boston, Little, Brown & Co., 1995, pp 88–94.

13. What proportion of cerebral palsy is related to birth asphyxia?

Contrary to popular perception, large longitudinal studies indicate that perinatal asphyxia is an important, but relatively minor, cause. Estimates range from a low of 3% to a high of 21%.

Nelson KB: What proportion of cerebral palsy is related to birth asphyxia? J Pediatr 112:572–574, 1988.

14. Why is CP difficult to diagnose clinically in the first year of life?

1. Hypotonia is more common than hypertonia and spasticity in the first year, making prediction of CP difficult.

2. Early abundance of primitive reflexes (with variable persistence) may confuse clinical picture.

3. Infant has a limited variety of volitional movements for evaluation.

4. Substantial myelination takes months to evolve and may delay the clinical picture of abnormal tone and increased deep tendon reflexes.

5. Most infants who develop CP do not have identifiable risk factors. Most cases are not related to labor and delivery events.

Shapiro BK, Capute AJ: Cerebral palsy. In Oski FA (ed): Principles and Practice of Pediatrics, 2nd ed. Philadelphia, J.B. Lippincott, 1994, pp 679–686.

15. How well do Apgar scores correlate with the development of CP?

In a large study of 49,000 infants, a low Apgar score correlated poorly with the development of CP. Of term infants with scores of 0–3 at 1 or 5 minutes, 95% did not develop CP. Of those with scores of 0–3 at 10 minutes, 84% did not develop CP. If the 10-minute Apgar improved to 4 or more, the rate for CP was < 1%. A low Apgar score (0–3) at 20 minutes, however, had an observed CP rate of nearly 60%. Conversely, nearly 75% of patients with CP had 5-minute Apgar scores of 7–10.

Nelson KB, Ellenberg JH: Apgar scores as predictors of chronic neurologic disability. Pediatrics 68:36–44, 1981.

16. What problems are commonly associated with cerebral palsy?

- Mental retardation: two-thirds of total patients; most commonly observed in children with spastic quadriplegia
- Learning disabilities
- Ophthalmologic abnormalities (strabismus, amblyopia, nystagmus, refractive errors)
- Hearing deficits
- Communication disorders
- Seizures: one-third of total patients; most commonly observed in children with spastic hemiplegia
- Failure to thrive
- Feeding problems
- Gastroesophageal reflux
- Behavioral and emotional problems (especially attention deficit hyperactivity disorder, depression)

Eicher PS, Batshaw ML: Cerebral palsy. Pediatric Clin North Am 40:537–551, 1993.

17. What features in an infant suggest a progressive CNS disorder rather than CP as the cause of a motor deficit?

1. Abnormally increasing head circumference (possible hydrocephalus, tumor)

2. Eye anomalies such as cataracts, retinal pigmentary degeneration, optic atrophy (possible neurodegenerative disease)

3. Skin abnormalities such as vitiligo, café-au-lait spots, nevus flammeus (possible Sturge-Weber disease, neurofibromatosis)

4. Hepatomegaly and/or splenomegaly (possible storage disease)

5. Decreased or absent deep tendon reflexes

6. Sensory abnormalities (loss of diminished sense of pain, position, vibration, or light touch)

Taft LT: Cerebral palsy. Pediatr Rev 6:41, 1984.

18. How effective is selective dorsal rhizotomy in the treatment of spasticity in CP?

Selective dorsal rhizotomy involves the cutting of lumbar spinal laminae and dura, isolating the dorsal nerve roots, and cutting selected fibers. Studies have shown benefits in reducing spasticity and improving range of motion, but the precise effects of the surgery are difficult to predict. Questions remain about which patients will benefit, which fibers should be cut, and what are the long-term complications of lumbar laminotomy.

Boscarino LF, et al: Effects of selective dorsal rhizotomy on gait in children with cerebral palsy. J Pediatr Orthop 13:174–179, 1993.

CEREBROSPINAL FLUID DYNAMICS

19. What is normal CSF pressure?

CSF pressure, as measured during a lumbar puncture, varies with age, positional technique and combativeness of the patient. Normal CSF opening pressure, as measured with the patient in the *recumbent lateral* position, is up to 50 mm H_2O in neonates, up to 85–110 mm H_2O in young infants, and up to 150 mm H_2O in older children. As measured with the patient in the *flexed lateral* position, CSF pressure is higher, ranging from 100–280 mm H_2O in children. With the patient in the sitting position, average pressures are even higher.

Ellis RW: Lumbar cerebrospinal fluid opening pressure measured in a flexed lateral decubitus position in children. Pediatrics 93:622–623, 1994.

Bonadio WA: The cerebrospinal fluid: Physiologic aspects and alterations associated with bacterial meningitis. Pediatr Infect Dis J 11:423–432, 1992.

20. How can CSF pressure be measured without a manometer?

Ellis et al. have devised a method of estimating pressure by counting drops of CSF. For example, if a 22-gauge 1.5-in spinal needle is used, the number of drops counted in 21 seconds equals the pressure in *cm* of H_2O.

Ellis RW, et al: A simple method of estimating cerebrospinal fluid pressure during lumbar puncture. Pediatrics 89:895–897, 1992..

21. What is the normal CSF volume in an infant, child, and adolescent?

Estimates of normal are 40 ml in a term newborn, increasing to 70 ml for a 7-year-old, and to 150 ml for a teenager and adult. Of note, approximately 15% of the total volume of CSF is replaced hourly.

Cutler RWP, Spertell RB: Cerebrospinal fluid: A selective review. Ann Neurol 11:1, 1982.

22. What are the common causes of an elevated CSF protein?

Elevated CSF protein is a nonspecific finding encountered in various neurologic disorders. Several common etiologies should be considered.

1. **Infection:** tuberculous meningitis, acute bacterial meningitis (pneumococcal, meningococcal, *Haemophilus influenzae*), syphilitic or viral meningitis, or encephalitis

2. **Inflammation:** Guillain-Barré syndrome, multiple sclerosis, peripheral neuropathy, or postinfectious encephalopathy

3. **Tumor** of the cerebral hemispheres or spinal cord

4. **Vascular accidents**, such as cerebral hemorrhage (including subarachnoid hemorrhage, subdural hemorrhage, intracerebral hemorrhages) or stroke due to cranial arteritis, diabetes mellitus, or hypertension

5. **Degenerative disorders** involving white matter disease (e.g., Krabbe disease).

6. **Metabolic disorders** such as uremia

7. **Toxins** such as lead

23. As tests of meningeal irritation, what constitutes a positive Kernig sign or Brudzinski sign?

Kernig sign: The straight-leg-raising sign. It consists of flexing the hip to 90° and attempting to extend the knee. Limitation of knee extension due to painful resistance is a positive sign.

Brudzinski sign: A positive sign is present if a reflex flexion of thighs occurs when a patient's neck is passively flexed.

24. What are the physical signs of meningeal irritation in the neonate?

In neonates, the physical signs of meningeal irritation may be overshadowed by systemic dysfunction, such as poor feeding, respiratory distress, or jaundice. Perhaps this is because meningitis commonly follows seeding of the meninges by systemic sepsis. Only a few patients present predominantly with frank neurologic signs, such as coma, seizures, or abnormal posture. Pure nuchal rigidity is rare in the newborn. More commonly, there is widespread increase of extensor tone in the neck, trunk, and limb musculature. Meningismus is not seen in every patient of any age, even with advanced purulent meningitis, and should not be considered a *sine qua non* for the diagnosis.

25. How does meningismus differ from meningism?

The term **meningismus** has various meanings. It is most commonly used to refer to the signs and symptoms of meningeal irritation associated with meningitis (abnormal CSF profile), including headache, nuchal rigidity, and positive Kernig and Brudzinski signs. Some also use this term to describe headache or stiff neck seen without meningitis, as in intracranial hypertension.

Meningism was commonly used in the older medical literature to denote the sudden onset of headache and mild meningeal signs without meningitis in the setting of an acute febrile illness. These symptoms can occur in the setting of acute systemic viral or bacterial infections, such as streptococcal pharyngitis or roseola infantum. The CSF profile is normal except for mildly increased CSF pressure.

26. How do the manifestations of increased intracranial pressure differ in an infant compared to an older child?

Infant: bulging fontanelle, failure to thrive, macrocephaly, setting sun sign, shrill cry
Child: headache, nausea, vomiting, mental changes, diplopia, papilledema
Fenichel GM: Clinical Pediatric Neurology, 2nd ed. Philadelphia, W.B. Saunders, 1993, p 89.

27. What comprises Cushing's triad?

Cushing's triad consists of the development of slow or irregular respirations, slow pulse, and elevated blood pressure resulting from an increase in intracranial pressure (ICP). Cushing's triad may be observed in children with increased ICP or compression of the posterior fossa, which houses the medullary circulatory control center.

28. Describe the characteristic features of pseudotumor cerebri.

Pseudotumor cerebri consists of an increased ICP in the absence of a demonstrable mass lesion and with a normal CSF formula. Characteristic features include:
1. Headache, fatigue, vomiting, anorexia, stiff neck, and diplopia from increased ICP
2. Normal neurologic examination except for papilledema or a third or sixth nerve palsy
3. Normal CT scan except sometimes for small ventricles
4. Normal CSF profile with the exception of an elevated opening pressure

29. What causes pseudotumor cerebri?

Although there are multiple possible causes, over 90% of cases are idiopathic. Among the reported causes are:
1. Drugs: tetracycline, nalidixic acid, nitrofurantoin, corticosteroids, excess vitamin A.
2. Endocrine disorders: hyperthyroidism, Cushing's syndrome, hypoparathyroidism.
3. Thrombosis of the dural venous sinuses due to head trauma, otitis media, mastoiditis, or obstruction of jugular veins in the superior vena cava syndrome.

30. What morbidity is associated with pseudotumor cerebri?

Visual loss. All patients with this disorder should have periodic formal testing of visual fields. Patients with well-developed papilledema may complain of fleeting visual loss (obscurations) that may be accentuated by the Valsalva maneuver or by standing up. This sign is believed to represent reduction of optic nerve blood flow due to arterial compression. Visual obscurations do not necessarily imply imminent "stroke" of the optic nerves.

31. What treatment is recommended for severe cases of pseudotumor cerebri?

Patients with sustained visual field loss or severe refractory headache are candidates for treatment. Specific treatment depends on the presence of an identifiable precipitant, which should be removed when possible. For example, the cessation of the offending medication, such as tetracycline, or weight reduction in obese patients is recommended. Nonspecific treatment includes the administration of acetazolamide, furosemide, or hydrochlorothiazide and sometimes corticosteroids. In severe cases surgical intervention is available in the form of the installation of a lumboperitoneal shunt or optic nerve sheath decompression.

32. Can anything be done to minimize the chance of a post-lumbar puncture headache?

The risk of headache may be decreased by:
1. Avoiding a head-up posture during the procedure, and
2. Using the smallest possible needle (22 gauge or smaller) and advancing the bevel "up" with the patient in the decubitus position.

There is debate over whether maintenance of a prone position several hours following the procedure can prevent the headache.

33. Why may it be dangerous to do a lumbar puncture using a needle with the stylette removed?

The (unproven) theory is that the stylette may prevent nerve roots of the cauda equina from becoming entrapped in the needle and may cause less disruption of the dural sac. Another concern is that without the stylette, skin cells may enter the core of the needle, where they can be introduced into the subarachnoid space and form an epidermoid tumor.

CLINICAL ISSUES

34. How does the presentation of stroke differ between infants and older children?

Infants present usually with a seizure, whereas older children present with acute hemiplegia.

35. What is the differential diagnosis of stroke in children?

Cerebrovascular disease, or stroke, can be due to primary vascular disease, bleeding disorder (hemorrhagic stroke), or a variety of secondary problems that lead to thrombotic or embolic occlusions (most commonly the middle cerebral artery). Diagnostic possibilities include:

Cardioembolic: cyanotic congenital heart disease, atrial myxoma, endocarditis, rheumatic or other valvular heart disease

Hematologic: hemoglobinopathies (especially sickle cell disease), hypercoagulable states (antithrombin III deficiency, protein C or S deficiency), hyperviscosity (leukemia, hyperproteinemia, thrombocytosis), coagulation disorders (lupus-associated antibodies, hemophilia, thrombocytopenia, factor V abnormalities, hyperhomocysteinemia)

Circulatory: vasculitis (infectious or inflammatory), occlusive (homocystinuria, arteriosclerosis, fibromuscular dysplasia of the internal carotid artery, post-traumatic carotid scarring), carotid or vertebral artery dissection, moyamoya disease, atrioventricular malformation with steal syndrome, anomalous circulation, post-traumatic air embolism, arterial aneurysm, hemiplegic migraine

Metabolic: mitochondrial disease

36. What is the derivation of "moyamoya" in moyamoya disease?

Moyamoya, Japanese for "puff of smoke," refers to the cerebral angiographic appearance in patients with this primary vascular disease which results in stenosis of the internal carotid artery. It also occurs in a wide variety of conditions, such as neurofibromatosis type 1, sickle cell disease, Down syndrome, and tuberous sclerosis, in addition to the idiopathic condition that is endemic in Japan. Because it is a chronic condition, fine vascular collaterals can develop, and it is these collaterals that create the "puff of smoke" appearance on angiography.

37. Describe the clinical findings seen in cavernous sinus thrombosis?

Within the confined space of the cavernous sinus lie all three cranial nerves which move the eye (oculomotor, trochlear, and abducent nerves) and the upper two divisions of the trigeminal nerve (ophthalmic V_1 and maxillary V_2). The venous drainage of the orbit exits via the cavernous sinus. Orbital infections thus quickly spread to these contiguous venous structures and result in an acute thrombophlebitis. Thrombosis of the venous channels of the cavernous sinus results in desperate systemic illness with fulminant constitutional signs such as fever, headache, prostration, and local signs of proptosis, prominent redness, swelling, and edema of the eyelid and bulbar conjunctiva (chemosis), visual loss, papilledema, ophthalmoplegia (due to dysfunction of cranial nerves III, IV, and VI) and paraesthesias, numbness, or local pain in the distribution of V_1.

38. What are the acceptable criteria for pronouncing a patient brain dead?

Brain death is said to have occurred when all brain functions are irreversibly lost. Spinal cord, peripheral nerve, or reflex muscular activity may persist despite brain death. The clinical hallmark of brain death is deep, unremitting, unresponsive coma. Consciousness requires the presence of (1) an intact brainstem, which contains the "on and off" switch of vigilance—the ascending reticular activating system; and (2) the cerebral hemispheres, which house the content of consciousness such as memories, thoughts, and skillful motor control. Patients with suspected brain death should be observed over 12–24 hours for:

1. Unresponsive coma and absence of eye opening, extraocular movements, vocalizations, or other cerebral-generated activity.

2. Absent brainstem reflexes such as the pupillary light reflex, reflex extraocular movements (elicited by irrigation of the ears with cold water or doll's eyes reflex), eye blink generated by hand clap, spontaneous respirations, gag reflex, coughing, or sucking.

3. Absent cerebral cortical activity as evidenced by a properly recorded "flat," "isoelectric," or ECS (electrocerebral silence) EEG, the absence of blood flow to the hemispheres by cerebral arteriography, or the presence of ICP that exceeds mean blood pressure for several hours.

The most difficult patients in whom to diagnose brain death are the neonate and infants < 2 months of age. For this age group, more stringent criteria are recommended: (1) the diagnosis of brain death should be deferred until the infant is at least 1 week old; and (2) the patient should be observed in the "brain dead state" for at least 48 hours before the declaration of brain death and the termination of life support.

Task Force on Brain Death in Children: Guidelines for the determination of brain death in children. Pediatrics 80:298, 1987.

39. What is the differential diagnosis of an intracranial bruit?

An intracranial bruit can be found in up to 50% of normal children. Disorders that may be associated with an intracranial bruit include:

• Fever	• Cerebral angioma	• Intracerebral tumors
• Thyrotoxicosis	• Cerebral aneurysm	• Any cause of increased ICP
• Anemia	• Cerebral arteriovenous	• Meningitis
• Cardiac murmurs	malformations	

Mace JW, et al: Cranial bruits in purulent meningitis in children. N Engl J Med 278:1420, 1968.

40. In a previously normal child who develops acute ataxia, what are the two most common diagnoses?

1. Drug ingestion, especially antiepileptic drugs and antihistamines

2. Acute postinfectious cerebellitis, most commonly following varicella. This is a diagnosis of exclusion if a drug screen, CT or MRI, CSF evaluation, and other testing is negative.

41. What clinical features help to distinguish peripheral from central vertigo?

Peripheral vertigo implies dysfunction of the labyrinth or vestibular nerve, while central vertigo is associated with abnormalities of the brainstem or temporal lobe.

Peripheral

1. Hearing loss, tinnitus, and otalgia may be associated.
2. Past pointing and falling in direction of unilateral disease occur.
3. In bilateral disease, ataxia occurs with eyes closed.
4. Vestibular and positional nystagmus are present.

Central

1. Cerebellar and cranial nerve dysfunction frequently associated.
2. No hearing loss.
3. Alteration of consciousness may be associated.

Fenichel GM: Clinical Pediatric Neurology. Philadelphia, W.B. Saunders, 1993, pp 354–359.

42. How is the Nylen-Barany maneuver performed?

Also called the Hallpike-Barany or Hallpike-Dix, this maneuver is used in the evaluation of vertigo when vestibular disease is suspected; it is a method to elicit paroxysmal positional nystagmus. A seated patient is asked to lie supine with his or her head hanging off the examining table with a 45° rotation. The patient's eyes are observed for the direction and duration of nystagmus. The maneuver is repeated to the opposite side and once again with the head in midline. If the patient does not exhibit nystagmus or symptoms during the maneuver, then a vestibular problem is unlikely as the cause of vertigo.

43. Define "persistent vegetative state."

This is "a form of eyes-open permanent unconsciousness in which the patient has periods of wakefulness and physiological sleep/wake cycles, but at no time is the patient aware of himself or herself or the environment." If this state persists for > 3 months in children, the long-term outlook is grim.

American Academy of Neurology: Position of the American Academy of Neurology on certain aspects of the care and management of the persistent vegetative state patient. Neurology 39:125, 1989.

44. What are the causes of toe-walking?

- Cerebral palsy (spastic diplegia)
- Spinal dysraphism
- Intraspinal and filum terminale tumors
- Isolated congenital shortening of the Achilles tendon
- Muscular dystrophy
- Hereditary or acquired polyneuropathies
- Equinovarus deformity
- Variation of normal in early stages of walking
- Normal development pattern in some toddlers

45. In what settings is hyperacusis noted?

Hyperacusis, or increased sensitivity to sound, is found in patients with injury to the facial nerve (VII), which innervates the stapedius muscle, or injury to the trigeminal nerve (V), which innervates the tensor tympani muscle. Exaggerated startle response to sound or vibration occurs in lysosomal storage diseases (e.g., sphingolipidoses such as Tay-Sachs disease, GM_1 gangliosidosis, Sandhoff disease), Williams syndrome, hyperkalemia, tetanus, and strychnine poisoning.

46. What is the most common cause of "asymmetric crying facies"?

In this entity, one side of the lower lip depresses on crying (the normal side) and the other does not. Often misdiagnosed as a facial nerve palsy secondary to forceps delivery, the most common cause is **congenital absence of the depressor anguli oris muscle** of the lower lip. Its occasional association with heart defects warrants electrocardiography and chest x-ray in these patients.

47. In which condition is "risus sardonicus" seen?

The sardonic smile is seen in patients with **tetanus** and is due to the spasm of facial muscles.

48. Discuss the common causes of peripheral seventh nerve palsy.

Facial weakness due to lesion of the facial nerve (cranial nerve VII) is common. The facial weakness involves both the upper and lower face and affects both emotional and volitional facial movements. Any part of the nerve can be disturbed: the nucleus itself, the axon as it passes through the pons, or the peripheral portion of the nerve. Common etiologies include:

1. Trauma
2. Developmental hypoplasia or aplasia including the Möbius anomalad
3. Bell's palsy (usually idiopathic but may follow nonspecific viral infections)
4. Infections including the Ramsay Hunt syndrome (herpes zoster invasion of the geniculate ganglion producing herpetic vesicles behind the ear and painful paralysis of facial nerve); Lyme disease; local invasion from suppurative mastoiditis or otitis media; mumps, varicella, or enterovirus neuritis; sequelae of bacterial meningitis; and parotid gland infection, inflammation, or tumor
5. Guillain-Barré syndrome
6. Tumor of brainstem or cerebellar pontine angle tumors
7. Inflammatory disorders such as sarcoidosis

49. During recovery from a Bell's palsy, why do the eyes water at mealtime?

These are crocodile tears. The facial nerve supplies autonomic motor function to the lacrimal and salivary glands. Because of aberrant reinnervation in the course of healing from a facial nerve palsy, tasting a meal can trigger tearing rather than salivation. Folklore has it that crocodiles feel compassion for their victims and weep while munching.

50. What is the significance of the Babinski reflex?

The Babinski reflex is the extension of the great toe in response to stroking the lateral outer sole of the foot. Most healthy children beyond the newborn period have a flexor response of the toe. The presence of extension may indicate an abnormality of the corticospinal tracts.

51. When is the Chaddock maneuver helpful?

The Chaddock maneuver is another means of eliciting an extensor toe response. It involves stroking the outer edge of the dorsum of the foot. It is useful in those patients in whom plantar stimulation results in reflex grasping (e.g., newborns) or withdrawal.

52. How is the Hoffman reflex test performed?

Like the Babinski reflex, the Hoffman reflex is a test for corticospinal tract abnormalities. In a patient with such pathology, downward flicking of the nail (on the second or third finger) by the examiner results in flexion of the distal phalanx of the thumb. Ordinarily, there is no response or one very muted.

Swaiman KF: Neurologic exam of the older child. In Swaiman KF (ed): Pediatric Neurology, 2nd ed. St. Louis, Mosby-Year Book, 1994, p 21.

FEBRILE SEIZURES

53. What features make a febrile seizure complex rather than simple?

A **simple** febrile seizure is a generalized convulsion that is relatively brief (< 15 min) and occurs as a solitary event (1 attack/24 hrs) in the setting of fever not due to CNS infection. **Complex** (also called atypical or complicated) febrile seizures may be focal, extended in duration, or repetitive. They suggest a more serious problem. For example, a focal seizure raises concern of a localized or lateralized functional disturbance of the CNS. An unusually long seizure (> 15 min) also raises the suspicion of primary CNS infectious, structural, or metabolic disease. Repeated seizures within a 24-hour period likewise imply a potentially more serious disorder or impending status epilepticus.

54. What ancillary testing should be considered in a patient with a complex febrile seizure?

Most children with their first atypical febrile seizure should undergo a **CSF exam** to rule out intracranial infection. Children with focal motor seizures or postictal lateralized deficits (motor paresis, unilateral sensory or visual loss, sustained eye deviation, or aphasia) require a **CT scan** to check for a structural abnormality. The immediate performance of an **EEG** offers limited insight into the patient's disease. Prominent generalized postictal slowing is not unexpected. Definite focal slowing suggests a possible structural abnormality. For a *simple* febrile seizure, an EEG is *not* indicated as it is not predictive of either the risk of recurrence of febrile seizures or the development of epilepsy.

Provisional Committee on Quality Improvement: Practice parameter: The neurodiagnostic evaluation of the child with a first simple febrile seizure. Pediatrics 97:769–775, 1996.

55. What does a definite epileptiform abnormality on EEG in the setting of febrile seizure represent?

1. An inherited EEG trait if a close relative has genuine epilepsy (children may inherit an "abnormal EEG" from an epileptic parent without actually inheriting clinical epilepsy).

2. A sporadic, unrelated, epileptic EEG abnormality (about 2–3% of healthy children with no family history of epilepsy have an incidental unexpected epileptiform EEG abnormality but do not develop clinical seizures).

3. A "lowered seizure threshold" with the implication that the febrile seizure may have been an early expression of genuine epilepsy precipitated by the stress of fever and threatens to recur without the provocation of fever.

56. How dangerous are febrile seizures?

In a previously normal child, the risk of death, neurologic damage, or persistent cognitive impairment from a single febrile seizure is near zero. These potential complications are more likely with complex febrile seizures, but the risk is still exceedingly low. Impaired cognition in the latter group is more likely if afebrile seizures subsequently develop.

57. How frequently do febrile seizures recur?

Febrile seizures affect 2–5% of children under 6 years of age. About 30% have a recurrence. The risk increases to 50% if the patient's first seizure occurred before the first birthday. In this age group, there is also a 30% chance of multiple recurrences, compared to an 11% risk of multiple recurrences if the first seizure occurred after age 1 year.

58. What is the risk of epilepsy following a febrile seizure?

The risk depends on several variables. In otherwise normal children with a simple febrile seizure, the risk of later epilepsy is only 1%. The risk of epilepsy is higher if:

1. There is a close family history of nonfebrile seizures.
2. Prior neurologic or developmental abnormalities existed.
3. The patient had an atypical or complex febrile seizure, defined as focal seizures, seizures lasting 15 minutes, and/or multiple attacks within 24 hours.

If all three risk factors are present, the likelihood of later epilepsy increases to 5–10%.

59. Following a febrile seizure, should a child be treated with prophylactic antiepileptics?

For most children, a simple febrile seizure is an unwanted but transient disruption of their health, and treatment is not necessary. Treatment may be considered in the very young child if febrile seizures recur and in those with preexisting neurologic abnormalities or with complex febrile seizures. Long-term prophylaxis does not improve the prognosis in terms of subsequent epilepsy, motor or cognitive ability.

Knudson FU, et al: Long term outcome of prophylaxis for febrile convulsions. Arch Dis Child 74:13–18, 1996.

60. Discuss the antiepileptic regimens used prophylactically in children with histories of complex febrile seizures.

1. Continuous daily prophylactic administration of **phenobarbital** to produce a minimum serum level of 15 μg/ml. The daily use of primidone is effective, but the side effect profile is similar and it probably has little advantage over phenobarbital. Comparable protection against febrile

seizures may be achieved with **valproic acid**, but its use is not recommended for children under age 2 because of the risk of hepatotoxicity. Neither carbamazepine nor phenytoin appears effective in preventing the recurrence of febrile seizures.

2. **Oral diazepam** (0.33 mg/kg) given every 8 hours during a febrile illness reduces the risk of febrile seizures by nearly 50%. However, the side effects may obscure the clinical picture, especially in meningitis; nearly half of the children using this regimen develop ataxia, lethargy, or irritability.

3. **Rectal diazepam** or **lorazepam** for administration by parents either prophylactically or in the event of a prolonged febrile seizure.

Rosman NP, et al: A controlled trial of diazepam administered during febrile illness to prevent recurrence of febrile seizures. N Engl J Med 329:79–84, 1993.

HEADACHE

61. What are the emergency priorities in evaluating a child with a severe headache?

As with all common presenting symptoms, the main priority is to rule out diagnostic possibilities that may be life-threatening:
- Malignant hypertension
- Increased intracranial pressure (e.g., mass lesion and/or acute hydrocephalus)
- Intracranial infections (e.g., meningitis, encephalitis)
- Subarachnoid hemorrhage
- Stroke

Acute angle closure glaucoma may present as headache but is rare in children.

62. When should neuroimaging be considered in a child with headache?

- Abnormal neurologic signs
- Headache increasing in frequency and severity
- Headache occurring in early morning or awakening child from sleep
- Headache made worse by straining or by sneezing or coughing
  (may be a sign of increased ICP)
- Headache associated with severe vomiting without nausea
- Headache worsened or helped significantly by a change in position
- Fall-off in linear growth rate
- Recent school failure or significant behavioral changes
- New-onset seizures, especially if seizure has a focal onset
- Migraine headache and seizure occurring in the same episode, with vascular symptoms
  preceding the seizure (20–50% risk of tumor or arteriovenous malformation)
- Cluster headaches in any child or teenager

Halsam RHA: Migraine headaches. In Behrman RE, et al (ed): Nelson textbook of Pediatrics, 15th ed. Philadelphia, W.B. Saunders, 1992, p 1507.

63. What is the origin of the word "migraine"?

Ancient Greek physicians recognized a specific type of recurring head pain that was unilateral. The modern word *migraine* is a French modification of the archaic term *hemikrania*.

64. Give the diagnostic criteria for common migraine.

Common migraine is also called migraine without aura. Diagnostic criteria from the International Headache Society include:
- 5 attacks
- Duration of 4–72 hours
- Characteristics (two out of four):
    1. Unilateral   2. Pulsating   3. Moderate or severe   4. Aggravated by physical activity
- Concomitant features (one out of two):
    1. Nausea and/or vomiting   2. Photophobia/phonophobia

Singer HS: Migraine headaches in children. Pediatr Rev 15:94, 1994.

65. Which physical findings are important in the initial evaluation of possible migraine headache?

1. Height and weight should be normal for age. Pituitary tumor, craniopharyngioma, or partial ornithine transcarbamylase deficiency may all result in growth failure and mimic migraine headache. Head circumference should be normal, ruling out hydrocephalus.

2. Skin should be checked for abnormalities. Throbbing headaches are common in neurofibromatosis and systemic lupus erythymatosus, both of which have easily recognizable skin manifestations.

3. Blood pressure should be normal.

4. Check for sinus tenderness or pain with head movement (implying cervical spine disease). The patient should be examined for carious teeth, misaligned bite, or disordered chewing and jaw opening (temporomandibular joint dysfunction).

5. Auscultation should reveal no cranial bruits (if present, suggest possible arteriovenous malformation, or mass lesion).

6. The neurologic examination should be normal.

66. When do children begin to have migraine headaches?

About 20% suffer their first headache before age 10 years.

67. Which foods have been associated with the development of migraine headaches?

Tyramine-rich foods (cheese, red wine), foods with monosodium glutamate (Chinese and Mexican food), nitrate-rich foods (smoked meats, salami), marinated foods, alcoholic beverages, caffeinated beverages, chocolate, citrus fruits, beans.

68. What is the most common form of complex migraine in children?

Complex migraines are those migraine headaches accompanied by transient neurologic signs or symptoms. These include hemiplegic migraine, ophthalmoplegic migraine (orbital pain with third nerve palsy), acute confusional state, and the Alice-in-Wonderland syndrome (hallucinations and distortion of object size). The most common form is **basilar artery migraine**, which has a variety of symptoms including blurred vision, vertigo, ataxia, dysarthria, and loss of consciousness.

69. What nonpharmacologic therapy is available for the treatment of migraine?

• Migraine elimination diet
• Normalization of sleep habits
• Discontinuance of possible triggering medications
  (e.g., analgesic overuse, bronchodilators, oral contraceptives)
• Biofeedback
• Relaxation therapy
• Family counseling (if family stress is a trigger)

70. Are biofeedback and self-hypnosis useful in the management of juvenile migraine headaches?

These nonpharmacological approaches have their advocates, with reported response rates comparable to those of drug therapy. Disadvantages include limited availability, expense, time commitment, and variability in the quality of instruction and the subject's motivation. For similar reasons, the efficacy of these approaches is hard to document.

Barowsky E: The use of biofeedback in the treatment of disorders of childhood. Ann NY Acad Sci 602:221, 1990.

71. What are the best medications to abort a severe migraine attack that has not responded to acetaminophen or nonsteroidal antiinflammatory drugs?

• Ergotamines
• Midrin (isometheptene mucate, dichloralphenazone, acetaminophen)
• Sumatriptan

72. Who should be started on prophylactic medication for migraine headaches?

There are no precise criteria, but generally prophylactic treatment should be considered if:

1. Headaches with aura occur frequently
2. Headaches with aura are poorly responsive to abortive medication
3. School attendance is significantly affected
4. Headaches, though infrequent, last for several days

73. What medications are used in children for prevention of migraine headaches?

- Beta-blockers (especially propranolol)
- Calcium channel blockers (especially verapamil)
- Nonsteroidal antiinflammatory medications (especially naproxen)
- Tricyclic antidepressants (especially amitriptyline)
- Antiepileptics (especially divalproex sodium)
- Cyproheptadine

Igarashi M, et al: Pharmacologic treatment of childhood migraine. J Pediatr 120:653–657, 1992.

74. How long are the prophylactic medications continued?

The optimal duration of therapy remains unclear, but many authorities suggest a treatment duration of 4–6 months followed by an attempt at weaning. Less than 50% will require reinitiation of medication.

75. Why are migraine headaches and epilepsy thought to be linked?

1. Both are familial, paroxysmal and associated with transitory neurologic disturbances.
2. There is an increased incidence of epilepsy in migraineurs and migraine in epileptics.
3. Headache can be a seizure manifestation.
4. Abnormal EEGs occur in both disorders (asymptomatic central spikes occur in 9% of children with migraine vs 2% of healthy children).

Fenichel GM: Clinical Pediatric Neurology, 2nd ed. Philadelphia, W.B. Saunders, 1993, p 26.

MOVEMENT DISORDERS

76. Name the various types of pathologic hyperkinetic movements.

Tremors:	Rhythmic oscillatory movements, both supination-pronation and flexion-extension, seen in resting state or with activity
Chorea:	Slow, writhing movements
Athetosis:	Slow, distal writhing movements
Stereotypy:	Repetitive, purposeless motions (e.g., body rocking, head rolling) that resemble voluntary movements often associated with akathisia (sensory and motor restlessness)
Dystonia:	Involuntary, twisting, sustained movements; may result in abnormal postures and progress to contractures
Ballismus:	Abrupt, random, violent, flinging movements, often proximal and unilateral
Myoclonus:	Abrupt, brief, jerklike contractions of one or more muscles, often stimulus-sensitive
Tics:	Rapid, sudden, repetitive movements or vocalizations

Jankovic J: Basal ganglia and neurotransmitter disorders. In Oski FA, et al (eds): Principles and Practice of Pediatrics, 2nd ed. Philadelphia, J.B. Lippincott, 1994, pp 2113–2125.

77. What disorders are commonly associated with the various hyperkinetic movements?

Tremors, resting:	Primary juvenile Parkinson disease, secondary Parkinson disease
Tremors, kinetic:	Essential (familial) tremor, cerebellar disorders, brainstem tumors, hyperthyroidism, Wilson disease, electrolyte disturbance (e.g., glucose, calcium, magnesium), heavy metal intoxication (e.g., lead, mercury), multiple sclerosis

Chorea:	Sydenham chorea (associated with rheumatic fever), Huntington disease, hyperthyroidism, infectious mononucleosis, pregnancy, anticonvulsants, neuroleptic drugs, closed head injury, systemic lupus erythematosus
Athetosis:	Cerebral palsy, other static encephalopathies, Lesch-Nyhan syndrome, kernicterus
Stereotypy:	Autism, Rett syndrome, neuroleptic drugs (i.e., tardive dyskinesia), schizophrenia
Dystonia:	Idiopathic primary dystonias (e.g., torsion dystonia), Sandifer syndrome, spasmus nutans, neuroleptic drugs, static encephalopathy, perinatal asphyxia, familial dystonia (sometimes dopa-responsive)
Ballismus:	Encephalitis, closed-head injury
Myoclonus:	Sleep myoclonus, benign myoclonus of infancy, post-anoxic encephalopathy, uremic encephalopathy, hyperthyroidism, urea-cycle defects, side effects of tricyclic therapy, slow virus infections, Wilson disease, myoclonus-opsoclonus, neuroblastoma, epileptic encephalopathies, mitochondrial disease, prion disease, Tay-Sachs, startle disease, sialidosis

78. What constitutes a tic?

Tics are brief, sudden, repetitive, stereotyped, involuntary, and purposeless movements or vocalizations. They most commonly involve muscles of the head, neck, and respiratory tract. Their frequency can be increased by anxiety, stress, excitement, and fatigue and is decreased during sleep and relaxation, activities involving high concentration, and at times, through voluntary action. In some cases, premonitory feelings (e.g., irritation, tickle, temperature change) can precipitate the motor or vocal response.

79. What is the range of clinical tics?

Tics can be motor or vocal, simple or complex, clonic or dystonic.

Motor (simple clonic):	Eye blinking, eye jerking, head twitching, shoulder shrugging
Motor (simple dystonic):	Bruxism, abdominal tensing, shoulder rotation
Motor (complex):	Grunting , barking, sniffing, snorting, throat clearing
Vocal (complex):	Coprolalia (obscene words), echolalia (repeating another's words), palilalia (rapidly repeating one's own words)

80. What makes a tic tick?

Transient and chronic tic disorders usually do not have an identifiable cause. However, dyskinesias such as tics can be found in association with a number of other conditions:

Chromosomal abnormalities:	Down syndrome, fragile X syndrome
Developmental syndromes:	Autism, pervasive developmental disorder, Rett syndrome
Drugs:	Anticonvulsants, stimulants (e.g., amphetamines, cocaine, methylphenidate, pemoline)
Infections:	Encephalitis, post-rubella syndrome

81. How should simple tics be treated?

Simple tics generally do not require pharmacologic intervention and can be treated expectantly by developing relaxation techniques, by minimizing stresses that exacerbate the problem, by avoidance of punishment for tics, and by decreasing fixation on the problem. Most simple tics self-resolve in 2–12 months.

82. When do tics warrant pharmacologic intervention?

Tics that have a significant disabling impact on a child's educational, social or psychological well-being (particularly if they have been present for > 1 year) may require intervention. When the complexity of tics increases or the diagnosis of Tourette syndrome is suspected, pharmacotherapy should also be considered. Most theories point to a hyperdopaminergic state of the basal ganglia as the most likely etiology for unregulated movements. Pharmacologic manage-ment includes administration of dopamine blockers (e.g., fluphenazine, haloperidol) or clonidine (method and site of action unclear) or cessation of any stimulant drugs (which can cause dopamine release). Because of the high associated incidence of obsessive-compulsive disorder and attention deficit hyperactivity disorder (ADHD), other medications may be needed, and con-sultation with a pediatric psychiatrist or neurologist is often warranted.

83. What are the diagnostic criteria for Tourette syndrome?

Gilles de la Tourette syndrome is a condition of vocal and motor tics with varying severity characterized by:

1. Multiple motor tics
2. One or more vocal tics
3. Onset before age 21
4. Waxing and waning course
5. Presence of tics for > 1 year
6. No identifiable medical etiology

84. What percentage of patients with Tourette syndrome demonstrate coprolalia?

Coprolalia is an irresistible urge to utter profanities, occurring as a phonic tic. Only 20–40% of patients with Tourette syndrome have this phenomenon, and it is not essential for the diagnosis.

85. What behavioral problems are associated with Tourette syndrome?

Obsessive-compulsive disorder (30–70%)

Attention deficit hyperactivity disorder (50–60%)

Learning disabilities

Sleep abnormalities

86. Why is the diagnosis of Tourette syndrome commonly delayed?

1. Tendency to associate unusual symptoms with attention-getting or psychologic problems
2. Incorrect belief that all children with Tourette syndrome must have severe tics
3. Attributing vocal tics to upper respiratory infections, allergies, sinus or bronchial problems
4. Diagnosing eye blinking or ocular tics as ophthalmologic problems
5. Mistaken belief that coprolalia (shouting of obscenities) is an essential diagnostic feature

Singer HS: Tic disorders. Pediatric Ann 22:22–29, 1993.

87. What is the cause of tardive dyskinesia?

Tardive dyskinesia is a hyperkinetic disorder of abnormal movements, most commonly in-volving the face (e.g., lip smacking or pursing, chewing, grimacing, tongue protruding). Tardive dyskinesia occurs during treatment with neuroleptics (e.g., chlorpromazine, haloperidol, meto-clopramide) or within 6 months of their discontinuance. This disorder is felt to be secondary to dopaminergic dysfunction of the basal ganglia, as these drugs act as dopamine receptor blockers.

88. For a patient on neuroleptic medication, how long must therapy last before symptoms of tardive dyskinesia can develop?

About 3 months of continuous or intermittent treatment with neuroleptics is needed before the risk of tardive dyskinesia increases.

89. Which movement disorder in children presents with "dancing eyes and dancing feet"?

Opsoclonus-myoclonus (infantile polymyoclonus syndrome or acute myoclonic encepha-lopathy of infants) is a rare but distinctive movement disorder. Opsoclonus is characterized by wild, chaotic, fluttering, irregular, rapid, conjugate bursts of eye movements (saccadomania). Myo-clonus is sudden, shock-like muscular twitches of the face, limbs, or trunk. The anatomic site of pathology is the cerebellar outflow tracts, including the dentato-rubro-thalamo-cortical networks. The etiology may be direct viral invasion, postinfectious encephalopathy, or neuroblastoma.

90. A 10-month old child with head tilt, head nodding and nystagmus is likely to have what condition?

Spasmus nutans is a rare, acquired movement disorder of unknown etiology beginning be-tween ages 4 and 14 months. The full triad consists of head tilt (torticollis), head nodding, and nystagmus. The condition often presents first with the head nodding, which is out of synchrony with the speed, direction, and tempo of the nystagmus. The condition lasts several months to years and usually fades by age 5 years. The nystagmus is present in the primary position (with the patient looking straight ahead) but is characteristically unilateral or markedly asymmetrical. The nystagmus has a pendular quality. (A pendulum arm sweeps arcs of equal magnitude and velocity). The direction of the nystagmus can be horizontal, vertical, or rotatory and may vary with the direction of gaze. Spasmus nutans has occasionally been associated with developmental abnormalities or optic chiasmal gliomas. Congenital or sensory nystagmus should also be considered. Therefore, a CT scan should be obtained before reassuring the parents of the benign nature and favorable outcome of the disorder.

NEONATAL SEIZURES

91. How are neonatal seizures classified clinically?
Although there is no universally accepted standard classification system, one based on clinical criteria is commonly used. It divides neonatal seizures into four types:

Subtle   **Tonic** (focal or generalized)
Clonic (focal or multifocal)   **Myoclonic** (focal, multifocal, or generalized)

All seizure types are recognized as paroxysmal alterations in behavioral, motor, or autonomic function. Not all clinically observed phenomena, however, are accompanied by associated epileptic surface-EEG activity.

92. In premature and full-term infants, how do the causes of seizures vary in relative frequency and time of onset?

Variance in Relative Frequency and Time of Onset of Causes of Seizures

	POSTNATAL TIME OF ONSET		RELATIVE FREQUENCY	
ETIOLOGY	0-3 DAYS	> 3 DAYS	PREMATURE	FULL-TERM
Hypoxic-ischemic	+		+++	+++
Intracranial hemorrhage*	+	+	++	+
Hypoglycemia	+		+	+
Hypocalcemia	+	+	+	+
Intracranial infection†	+	+	++	+
Developmental defects	+	+	++	++
Drug withdrawal	+	+	+	+

* Hemorrhages are principally germinal matrix-intraventricular in the premature infant and subarachnoid or subdural in the term infant.
† Early seizures occur usually after intrauterine nonbacterial infections (e.g., toxoplasmosis, CMV infection), and later seizures usually occur with herpes simplex encephalitis or bacterial meningitis.
From Volpe JJ (ed): Neurology of the Newborn, 3rd ed. Philadelphia, W.B. Saunders, 1995, p 184; with permission.

93. Why are focal seizures in the neonate not necessarily indicative of a focal brain abnormality?
The immature CNS cannot sustain a synchronized, well-orchestrated, generalized seizure. The anatomic basis for this observation is the paucity of myelination in the newborn brain. More extensive myelination is required for conduction of discharges throughout the brain in generalized seizures. Focal seizures in newborns often arise from diffuse, toxic, or metabolic conditions, whose epileptogenic influence affects those cortical areas of the brain mature enough to produce a seizure. On the other hand, stroke, localized hemorrhage, and trauma do occur in infants and should be included in the differential diagnosis of seizures in this age group.
Painter MJ, Gaus RN: Neonatal seizures: Diagnosis and treatment. J Child Neurol 6:101–108, 1991.

94. What is the most common type of clinical seizure in the neonatal period?

The so-called **subtle seizure**. Rather than arising as an abrupt dramatic "convulsion" with obvious forceful twitching or posturing of the muscles, the subtle seizure appears as an unnatural, repetitive, stereotyped choreography, featuring oral-buccal-lingual movements, eye blinking, nystagmus, lip smacking, or complex integrated limb movements (swimming, pedaling, or rowing) and other fragments of activity drawn from the limited repertoire of normal infant activity.

95. What behavioral states may be confused with seizures in neonates?

A variety of "seizure-like" behaviors, which show no evidence of simultaneous EEG discharges consistent with seizures, are believed to originate in the brainstem and spinal cord without superimposed inhibitory cortical influences. These include jitteriness, movements during REM sleep, "rowing:" and "bicycling" movements, decorticate and decerebrate posturing, and autonomic dysfunctions.

96. What is an acceptable workup in a newborn with seizures?

The workup should include a careful prenatal and natal history as well as a complete physical examination. Laboratory studies should include blood for glucose, electrolytes, calcium, phosphorus, and magnesium. A lumbar puncture should be performed to rule out meningitis, and and ultrasound, CT scan, or MRI should be obtained when intracranial hemorrhage or a developmental defect is suspected. Additional studies, where warranted, include a blood ammonia level, and blood and urine studies for organic and amino acid analysis.

97. How are seizures differentiated from tremors in the neonate?

Clinical Feature	Jitteriness	Seizure
Abnormality of gaze or eye movement	0	+
Movements exquisitely stimulus-sensitive	+	0
Predominant movement	Tremor	Clonic jerking
Movements cease with passive flexion	+	0
Autonomic changes	0	+

From Volpe JJ: Neurology of the Newborn, 3rd ed. Philadelphia, W.S. Saunders, 1995, p 182; with permission.

98. Does tonic posturing require treatment?

Generalized tonic posturing and subtle clinical phenomena not associated with concurrent autonomic disturbance or EEG seizure activity are nonepileptic events which should not be treated with anticonvulsant medication. Such events rarely affect ventilatory or cardiovascular function and require high levels of anticonvulsant drug therapy for suppression.

99. How should an infant with seizures be treated?

Due to the potential deleterious effects of seizures on the CNS, initiation of therapy is urgent. Therapies should be administered only after ventilation and perfusion are adequately established.

Hypoglycemia	Glucose, 10% solution: 2 ml/kg IV
No hypoglycemia	Phenobarbital: 20 mg/kg IV (10–15 min)
	If necessary—
	Additional phenobarbital: 5 mg/kg (10–15 min) to a maximum of 20 mg/kg (consider omission of this additional phenobarbital if infant is severely "asphyxiated")
	Phenytoin: 20 mg/kg IV (1 mg/kg/min)
	Lorazepam: 0.05–0.10 mg/kg IV
Other (as indicated)	Calcium gluconate, 5% solution: 4 ml/kg IV
	Magnesium sulfate, 50% solution: 0.2 ml/kg IM
	Pyridoxine: 50–100 mg IV

From Volpe JJ: Neurology of the Newborn, 3rd ed. Philadelphia, W.B. Saunders, 1995, p 196; with permission.

100. What is the treatment for refractory seizures in the neonate?

Frequent and recurrent seizures are not uncommon in newborns and are especially common in the setting of asphyxia. If seizures are refractory to a full 40-mg/kg initial dose of phenobarbital, phenytoin up to 20 mg/kg is administered. If seizures still persist, addition of drugs in the benzodiazepine family (e.g., diazepam, lorazepam) or paraldehyde is generally effective. It is important to ensure that no underling biochemical disturbance is present before the serum levels of anticonvulsants are raised to maximal concentrations. Although pyridoxine-dependent seizures are rare, a trial dose of pyridoxine should be administered intravenously to infants with recurrent seizures of uncertain etiology. If possible, simultaneous EEG recording should be performed to document the cessation of seizure activity and the normalization of the EEG within minutes of pyridoxine treatment.

101. After an infant has recovered from a seizure, how long should medication be continued?

Maintenance therapy typically involves the use of phenobarbital, because it is difficult to achieve therapeutic levels of phenytoin with oral administration in infancy and other medications are (e.g., carbamazepine) are less well-studied. Although phenobarbital is generally well tolerated, it may have deleterious effects on behavior, attention span, and possibly brain development. It does not prevent the later development of epilepsy. Many authorities recommend discontinuing therapy if the neurologic exam has normalized. In addition, if the neurologic exam is abnormal but an EEG by age 3 months reveals no seizure activity, consideration can also be given to stopping phenobarbital.

102. Are seizures without concurrent hypoxia or acidosis harmful in a neonate?

Although the hypoxemia and hypercarbia that accompany seizures may result in brain injury, CNS damage can be produced by other associated events as well:

1. Increased cerebral blood flow accompanying seizures may result in hemorrhagic infarction of vulnerable vascular beds (e.g., the germinal matrix in premature infants).

2. Changes in the concentrations of critical high-energy phosphate compounds (e.g., ATP, phosphocreatinine) may lead to irreparable injury.

3. Depletion of brain substrates such as glucose despite increased cerebral blood flow.

4. Excessive release of synaptic excitatory amino acids, such as glutamate, which exert a toxic effect at sites where they would otherwise serve as neurotransmitters (experimental animal data).

103. In neonatal seizures, how does the cause affect the prognosis?

Relationship Between Cause and Prognosis of Neonatal Seizure

ETIOLOGY	FAVORABLE OUTCOME*	MIXED OUTCOME	UNFAVORABLE OUTCOME*
Toxic-metabolic	Simple late-onset hypocalcemia Hypomagnesemia Hyponatremia Mepivacaine toxicity	Hypoglycemia Early-onset complicated hypocalcemia Pyridoxine dependency	Some aminoacidurias
Asphyxia	–	Mild hypoxic-ischemic encephalopathy	Severe hypoxic-ischemic encephalopathy
Hemorrhage	Uncomplicated subarachnoid hemorrhage	Subdural hematoma Intraventricular hemorrhage (grades I and II)	Intraventricular hemorrhage (grades III and IV)
Infection	—	Aseptic meningoencephalitis; some bacterial meningitides	Herpes simplex encephalitis; some bacterial meningitides
Structural		Simple traumatic contusion	Malformations of CNS

* Favorable prognosis implies at least an 85–90% chance of survival and subsequent normal development. Unfavorable prognosis implies a high likelihood (85–90%) of death or serious handicap in survivors.
From Clancy RR: Neonatal seizures. In Polin RA, et al (eds): Workbook in Practical Neonatology, 2nd ed. Philadelphia, W.B. Saunders, 1993, p 359; with permission.

104. Of what prognostic value is the interictal EEG in a neonate with seizures?

It can have significant prognostic value. Severe interictal EEG abnormalities (e.g., burst-suppression, marked voltage suppression, flat or isoelectric) are highly predictive (90%) of a fatal outcome or severe neurologic sequelae. Conversely, a normal interictal EEG in a term infant with seizures confers a very low (10%) likelihood of significant neurologic impairment. Moderate abnormalities (e.g., voltage asymmetries, immature patterns) have a mixed outcome.

NEUROCUTANEOUS SYNDROMES

105. What are the three most common neurocutaneous syndromes?
• Neurofibromatosis
• Tuberous sclerosis
• Sturge-Weber syndrome

106. Describe the inheritance patterns of the various neurocutaneous syndromes.

Neurofibromatosis	Autosomal dominant
Tuberous sclerosis	Autosomal dominant
Von Hippel-Lindau syndrome	Autosomal dominant
Incontinentia pigmenti	X-linked dominant
Sturge-Weber syndrome	Sporadic
Klippel-Trenaunay-Weber syndrome	Sporadic

107. What is the derivation of the term *phakomatosis*?

The term *phakomatosis* is derived from the Greek *phakos*, meaning spot, and refers to patchy, circumscribed dermatologic lesions that are the hallmark of this group of disorders. In addition to dermatologic features, these syndromes have hamartomatous involvement of multiple tissues, especially the CNS and eye. More commonly, the term neurocutaneous syndrome is used.

108. What are the diagnostic criteria for neurofibromatosis-1 (NF1)?

Two or more of the following:
• Café-au-lait spots (6 or more > 5 mm in diameter before puberty; 6 or more > 15 mm in diameter after puberty)
• Skinfold freckling (axillary or inguinal region)
• Neurofibromas (2 or more) of any type or 1 plexiform neurofibroma
• Optic glioma
• Lisch nodules (2 or more)
• Characteristic bony lesion (i.e., sphenoid dysplasia, thinning of cortex of long bones, with or without pseudoarthrosis)
• First-degree relative with NF1

109. How does NF1 differ from NF2?

NF1, classic von Recklinghausen disease, is much more common (1:3000–4000 births) and accounts for up to 90% of cases of neurofibromatosis. NF2 (1:50,000 births) is characterized by bilateral acoustic neuromas, intracranial and intraspinal tumors, and affected first-degree relatives. NF1 has been linked to alterations on chromosome 17, while NF2 is linked to alterations on chromosome 22. Dermatologic findings and peripheral neuromas are rare in NF2. Other rarer subtypes of neurofibromatoses (e.g., segmental distribution) have been described.

110. How common are café-au-lait spots at birth?

Up to 2% of black infants will have three café-au-lait spots at birth, while even one café-au-lait spot occurs in only 0.3% of white infants. White infants with multiple café-au-lait spots at birth are more likely than black infants to develop neurofibromatosis. In older children, a single café-au-lait spot > 5 mm can be found in 10% of white and 25% of black children.

Hurwitz S: Neurofibromatosis. In Clinical Pediatric Dermatology, 2nd ed. Philadelphia, W.B. Saunders, 1993, pp 624–629.

111. If a 2-year-old has 7 café-au-lait spots > 5 mm in diameter, what is the likelihood that neurofibromatosis will develop?

Up to 75% of these children, if followed sequentially, will develop one of the varieties of neurofibromatosis, most commonly type 1. Yearly follow-up should include a careful skin examination, ophthalmologic evaluation, and blood pressure measurement.

Korf BR: Diagnostic outcome in children with multiple café-au-lait spots. Pediatrics 90:924–927, 1992.

112. How common is a positive family history in cases of NF1?

Because of the high spontaneous mutation rate for this autosomal dominant disease, only about 50% of newly diagnosed cases are associated with a positive family history.

113. What are Lisch nodules?

Pigmented iris hamartomas. Of note, while these are not usually present at birth in patients with NF1, up to 90% will develop multiple Lisch nodules by age 6.

114. Give the primary diagnostic features of tuberous sclerosis.

- Facial angiofibromas
- Subungual or periungual fibromas
- Cortical tubers
- Subependymal nodules or giant cell astrocytomas (histologic confirmation)
- Multiple calcified subependymal nodules protruding into the ventricle (radiographic confirmation)
- Multiple retinal astrocytomas

Roach ES: Neurocutaneous syndromes. Pediatr Clin North Am 39:597, 1992.

115. What is the most common presenting symptom of tuberous sclerosis?

Seizures. Up to 90% of patients with tuberous sclerosis develop seizures of varying types. Tuberous sclerosis is the cause of 5–10% of cases of infantile spasms. Up to 60% of patients have varying degrees of mental retardation.

116. What are skin findings in tuberous sclerosis?

Skin Findings in Tuberous Sclerosis

AGE AT ONSET	SKIN FINDINGS	INCIDENCE
Birth or later	Hypopigmented macules	80%
2–5 years	Angiofibromas	70%
2–5 years	Shagreen patches	35%
Puberty	Periungual and gingival fibromas	20–50%
Birth or later	Café-au-lait spots	25%

117. Why is the term *adenoma sebaceum* a misnomer when used to describe patients with tuberous sclerosis?

On biopsy, these papules are actually angiofibromas; they have no connection to sebaceous units or adenomas. This rash occurs in about 75% of patients with tuberous sclerosis, usually developing on the nose and face between ages 5 and 13 years. It is red, papular, and monomorphous and is often mistaken for acne.

118. What is the "tuber" of tuberous sclerosis?

These 1–2-cm lesions consist of small stellate neurons and astroglial elements felt to be primitive cell lines resulting from abnormal differentiation. They may be located in various cortical regions. They are firm to the touch, like a small potato or tuber.

119. What is the tissue type of a shagreen patch?

A shagreen patch is an area of cutaneous thickening with a pebbled surface that, on biopsy, is a connective tissue nevus. The term *shagreen* derives from a type of leather that is embossed by knobs in the course of processing.

120. Which types of facial port-wine stains are most strongly associated with ophthalmic or CNS complications?

Port-wine stains can occur as isolated cutaneous birthmarks or, particularly in the areas under-lying the birthmark, in association with structural abnormalities in (1) choroidal vessels of the eye leading to glaucoma, (2) leptomeningeal vessels in the the the brain leading to seizures (Sturge-Weber syndrome), and (3) hemangiomas in the spinal cord (Cobb syndrome). In a study by Tallman et al., glaucoma and/or seizures were most associated with port-wine stains in children demonstrating:

1. Involvement of the eyelids
2. Bilateral distribution of the birthmark
3. Unilateral involvement of all three branches (V_1, V_2, V_3) of the trigeminal nerve.

Ophthalmologic assessment and radiologic studies (CT or MRI) are indicated for children exhibiting these findings.

Tallman B, et al: Location of port-wine stains and the likelihood of ophthalmic and/or central nervous system complications. Pediatrics 87:323–327, 1991.

121. What are the three stages of incontinentia pigmenti?

Incontinentia pigmenti is an X-linked dominant disorder associated with seizures and mental retardation. The condition is presumed lethal to males *in utero* because nearly 100% of cases are female.

Stage 1:   Vesicular stage—lines of blisters on the trunk and extremities in the newborn which disappear in weeks or months. They may resemble herpetic vesicles. Microscopic examination of the vesicular fluid demonstrates eosinophils.

Stage 2:   Verrucous stage—lesions develop around age 3–7 months that are brown and hyperkeratotic, resembling warts. These disappear over 1–2 years.

Stage 3:   Pigmented stage—whorled, swirling (marble cake-like) macular hyperpigmented lines develop. These may fade over time, leaving only remnant hypopigmentation in late adolescence or adulthood (which is sometimes considered a fourth stage).

NEUROMUSCULAR DISORDERS

122. What constitutes the motor unit?

The anatomic unit of histologic organization of striated skeletal muscle is the fiber, micro-scopically visible as a long cylindrical cell with numerous nuclei dispersed along its length. Numerous parallel fibers are grouped together into fascicles, visible to the naked eye. The func-tional unit of organization of skeletal muscle is the motor unit which includes (1) the anterior horn cell or alpha motor neuron, whose cell body lies in the ventral gray mass of the spinal cord; (2) its axon, which leaves the cord in the ventral root and courses in the peripheral nerve wrapped in its myelin sheath; and (3) several target muscle fibers within the same fascicle. Thus, the smallest natural amount of muscle activity is the firing of one motor neuron, producing contrac-tion of its multiple target fibers.

123. How do muscle fibrillation and fasciculation differ?

A **fibrillation** is the spontaneous contraction of an *individual muscle fiber*. It produces no shortening of the muscle and cannot be observed through the skin but may rarely be visible in the tongue. Fibrillations are detected by an electromyographic (EMG) examination and recognized as ir-regular, asynchronous, brief (1–5 msec), low-voltage (20–300 μV), electrical discharges of the muscle fiber that recur with a frequency of 1–30/second. They usually arise in the setting of denerva-tion from injury to the cell body or axon but may also occur in primary disorders such as myopathy.

A **fasciculation** is the spontaneous, relatively synchronous contraction of *numerous fibers within a fascicle* which belong to the same motor unit. The contraction may produce a visible movement of the muscle and can be seen through the skin. On EMG examination, the electrical discharge of the fasciculation is distinctly longer (8–20 msec) and has a higher voltage (2–6 mV) than the fibrillation potential. Fasciculations recur at irregular intervals with a frequency of 1–50/minute. Benign fasciculations in the calf and small muscles of the hands or feet can be seen in some healthy people. Fasciculations are not characteristic of primary muscle diseases. They are usually associated with denervation of any cause but are especially prominent in disorders of anterior horn cells such as Werdnig-Hoffman disease.

124. How can the anatomic site responsible for muscle weakness be determined clinically?

Clinical Determination of Anatomic Site Responsible for Muscle Weakness

	UPPER MOTOR NEURON	ANTERIOR HORN CELL	NEUROMUSCULAR JUNCTION	PERIPHERAL NERVE	MUSCLE
Tone	Increased (may be decreased acutely)	Decreased	Normal, variable	Decreased	Decreased
Distribution	Pattern (hemiparesis, paraparesis, etc.) Distal > proximal	Variable, asymmetric	Fluctuating, cranial nerve involvement	Nerve distribution	Proximal > distal
Reflexes	Increased (may be decreased early)	Decreased to absent	Normal (unless severely involved)	Decreased to absent	Decreased
Babinski	Extensor	Flexor	Flexor	Flexor	Flexor
Other	Cognitive dysfunction, atrophy only very late	Fasciculations, atrophy, no sensory involvement	Fluctuating course	Sensory nerve involvement, atrophy, rare fasciculations	No sensory deficits; may be tenderness and signs of inflammation

From Packer RJ, Berman PH: Neurologic emergencies. In Fleisher GR, Ludwig S (eds): Textbook of Pediatric Emergency Medicine, 3rd ed. Baltimore, Williams & Wilkins, 1993, p 584; with permission.

125. What are the causes of acute generalized weakness?

Infectious/postinfectious: acute infectious myositis, Guillain-Barré syndrome, enteroviral infection

Metabolic disorders: acute intermittent porphyria, hereditary tyrosinemia

Neuromuscular blockade: botulism, tick paralysis

Periodic paralysis: familial (hyperkalemic, hypokalemic, normokalemic)

Fenichel GM: Clinical Pediatric Neurology, 2nd ed. Philadelphia, W.B. Saunders, 1993, p 187.

126. If a child presents with weakness, what aspects of history and physical exam suggest a myopathic process?

History
- Onset gradual rather than sudden
- Proximal weakness predominates (e.g., climbing stairs, running) rather than distal weakness (more characteristic of neuropathy)
- Absence of sensory abnormalities, such as "pins-and-needles" sensations
- No bowel and bladder abnormalities

Physical exam
- Proximal weakness > distal weakness (except in myotonic dystrophy)\
- Positive Gower's sign (patient arises from sitting position by pushing the trunk erect by bracing arms against anterior thigh, due to weakness of the pelvic girdle and lower extremities)
- Neck flexion weaker than neck extension
- In early stages, reflexes normal or only slightly decreased
- Normal sensory exam
- Muscle wasting, but no fasciculations
- Muscle hypertrophy seen in some dystrophies

Weiner HL, Urion DK, Levitt LP: Pediatric Neurology for the House Officer. Baltimore, William & Wilkins, 1988, pp 136–147.

127. How does EMG help differentiate between myopathic and neurogenic disorders?

EMG measures the electrical activity of resting and voluntary muscle activity. Normally, the action potentials are of standardized duration and amplitude with 2–4 distinguishable phases. In **myopathic** conditions, the durations and amplitudes are shorter than expected. In **neuropathies**, they are longer. In both conditions, extra phases (i.e., polyphasic units) are usually noted.

128. How is pseudoparalysis distinguished from true neuromuscular disease?

Pseudoparalysis (hysterical paralysis) or weakness may be seen in conversion reactions (i.e., emotional conflicts presenting as symptoms). In conversion reactions, sensation, deep tendon reflexes, and the Babinski response are normal. Movement may also be noted during sleep. The Hoover test is helpful in unilateral paralysis. With the patient lying supine on the table, the examiner places a hand under the heel of the unaffected limb and asks the patient to raise the plegic limb. In pseudoparalysis, no pressure is felt under the heel on the unaffected side.

129. Describe the differential diagnoses of hypotonia.

Hypotonia is a common but nonspecific sign in neonates and young infants.

1. It may represent a nonspecific sign in any acute serious medical illness, such as sepsis, shock, dehydration, or hypoglycemia.

2. It may be encountered in the context of chromosomal abnormalities such as Down syndrome.

3. It may represent a disturbance of connective tissue, producing excessive joint laxity.

4. It is commonly encountered in metabolic encephalopathies, such as hypothyroidism, Lowe syndrome, or Canavan disease.

5. It may indicate the presence of a CNS disorder, such as cerebellar dysfunction, acute spinal cord disease, neuromuscular disorder, hypotonic cerebral palsy, or benign congenital hypotonia.

In the absence of an acute encephalopathy the differential diagnosis of hypotonia is best approached by asking the question: Does the patient have normal strength despite the hypotonia, or is the patient weak and hypotonic? The combination of weakness and hypotonia usually points to an abnormality of the anterior horn cell or the peripheral neuromuscular apparatus, whereas hypotonia with normal strength is more characteristic of brain or spinal cord disturbances.

130. How can you detect myotonia clinically?

Myotonia is the painless tonic spasm of delayed muscle relaxation following a contraction. It can be elicited by grip (e.g., handshake), forced eyelid closure (or delayed eye opening in crying infants), lid lag after upward gaze, or by percussion over various sites (e.g., thenar eminence or tongue).

131. In a newborn with weakness and hypotonia, what obstetric and delivery features suggest a diagnosis of myotonic dystrophy?

History of spontaneous abortions, polyhydramnios, decreased fetal movements, delays in second-stage labor, retained placenta, and postpartum hemorrhage all raise the concern for

congenital myotonic dystrophy. Because the mother is nearly always affected in congenital myotonic dystrophy, a careful clinical and EMG evaluation of the mother is essential.

132. Why is myotonic dystrophy an example of the phenomenon of "anticipation"?

Genetic studies have shown that the defect in myotonic dystrophy is an expansion of a trinucleotide (CTG) in a gene on the long arm of chromosome 19 that codes for a protein kinase. In
successive generations, this repeating sequence has a tendency to increase, sometimes into the
thousands (normal is < 40 CTG repeats), and the extent of repetition correlates with the severity
of the disease. Thus, each succeeding generation is likely to get more extensive manifestations
and earlier presentations of the disease (i.e., the phenomenon of "anticipation").

133. How does the pathophysiology of infant botulism differ from that of food-borne botulism?

Infant botulism results from the ingestion of *Clostridium botulinum* spores which germinate,
multiply, and produce toxin in the infant's intestine. The source of the spores is often unknown, but
it has been linked to honey in some cases, and spores have been found in corn syrups. Therefore,
these foods are not advised for infants < 1 year of age. In **food-borne botulism**, preformed toxin is
already present in the food. Improper canning and anaerobic storage permits spore germination,
growth, and toxin formation which results in symptoms if the toxin is not destroyed by proper heating. **Wound botulism**, which is rare, occurs if spores enter a deep wound and germinate.

134. What is the earliest indication for intubation in an infant with botulism?

Loss of protective airway reflexes. This occurs before respiratory compromise or failure
because diaphragmatic function is not impaired until 90–95% of the synaptic receptors are occupied.
Indeed, an infant with hypercarbia or hypoxia is at very high risk for imminent respiratory failure.
Schreiner MS, et al: Infant botulism: A review of 12 years' experience at the Children's Hospital of
Philadelphia. Pediatrics 87:159–165, 1991.

135. Why are antibiotics and antitoxins not used in cases of infant botulism?

• By the time the diagnosis is made, most patients are usually stable or improving.
• Antibiotics may result in bacterial death with the the potential release of additional toxin.
• Risk of serum sickness and anaphylaxis.
• Circulating unbound toxin is not found in ongoing disease.
• Previously bound toxin is irreversibly bound (recovery based on growth of new nerve
  sprouts).
• Excellent prognosis with aggressive supportive care alone.
Finegold SM, Arnon SS: Clostridial intoxication and infection. In Feigin RD, Cherry JD (eds):
Textbook of Pediatric Infectious Diseases, 2nd ed. Philadelphia, W.B. Saunders, 1987, p 1121.

136. In an infant with severe weakness and suspected botulism, why is the use of aminogly-cosides relatively contraindicated?

The botulism toxin acts by irreversibly blocking acetylcholine release from the presynaptic
nerve terminals. Aminoglycosides, as well as tetracyclines, clindamycin, and trimethoprim, also
interfere with acetylcholine release. Therefore, they have the potential to act synergistically with
the botulinum toxin to worsen or prolong neuromuscular paralysis.

137. Why does botulism occur more commonly in mountain locales?

Most cases of food-borne botulism result from ingestion of improperly canned or cooked
food. Usually, boiling for 10 minutes destroys the botulinum toxin if it is present in food.
However, in the higher altitudes of mountainous areas, water boils at a lower temperature, which
may be insufficient for exotoxin destruction.

138. How is neonatal myasthenia gravis differentiated from infant botulism?

Very few cases of **botulism** have been reported in neonates. Symptoms have always occurred after discharge from the neonatal nursery. Botulism is usually heralded by constipation,

followed by early facial and pharyngeal weakness, ptosis, and *dilated, sluggishly reactive pupils* with *diminished deep tendon reflexes*. The injection of edrophonium does not improve muscle strength. EMG examination demonstrates distinctive abnormalities such as brief small-amplitude polyphasic potentials (BSAPs) and an incremental response in the amplitude of evoked muscle potentials to repetitive nerve stimulation. Stool cultures may be positive for the toxin or clostridia organism.

Myasthenia gravis usually presents at birth or within the first few days of life. There may be a family history of myasthenia in the mother or siblings. The distribution of weakness depends on the specific subtype of myasthenia, but *pupils and deep tendon reflexes are spared*. The EMG examination shows a distinctive progressive decline in the amplitude of compound motor action potentials with repetitive stimulation of the nerve. Edrophonium temporarily improves the patient's clinical strength and abolishes the pathologic EMG response to repetitive stimulation.

139. What are the risks to a neonate born to a mother with myasthenia gravis?

Passively acquired neonatal myasthenia develops in about 10% of infants born to myasthenic mothers due to the transplacental transfer of antibody directed against acetylcholine receptors (AChR) in striated muscle. Signs and symptoms of weakness typically arise within the first hours or days of life. Pathologic muscle fatigability commonly causes feeding difficulty, generalized weakness, hypotonia and respiratory depression. Ptosis and impaired eye movements occur in only 15% of cases. The weakness virtually always resolves as the body burden of anti-AChR immunoglobulin diminishes. Symptoms typically persist about 2 weeks but may require several months to disappear entirely. General supportive treatment is usually adequate, but oral or intramuscular neostigmine may help to diminish symptoms.

140. How does the pathophysiology differ in juvenile versus congenital myasthenia gravis?

Juvenile (and adult) myasthenia gravis is caused by circulating antibodies to the acetylcholine receptor of the postsynaptic neuromuscular junction. Congenital myasthenia gravis does not have an autoimmune basis. It is caused by morphologic or physiologic features affecting the pre- and postsynaptic junctions, including defects in ACh synthesis, endplate acetylcholinesterase deficiency, and endplate AChR deficiency.

141. How is the edrophonium (Tensilon) test done?

Edrophonium is a rapid-acting anticholinesterase drug of short duration that improves symptoms of myasthenia gravis by inhibiting the breakdown of ACh and increasing its concentration in the neuromuscular junction. A test dose of 0.015 mg/kg is given intravenously, and if tolerated, the full dose of 0.15 mg/kg (up to 10 mg) is given. If measurable improvement in ocular muscle or extremity strength occurs, myasthenia gravis is likely. Because edrophonium may precipitate a cholinergic crisis (e.g., bradycardia, hypotension, vomiting, bronchospasm), atropine and resuscitation equipment should be available.

142. Does a negative antibody test exclude the diagnosis of juvenile myasthenia gravis?

No. Up to 90% of children with juvenile myasthenia have measurable anti-AChR antibodies, but in the other 10%, continued clinical suspicion is necessary because their symptoms are usually milder (e.g., ocular muscle weakness or minimal generalized weakness). In these children, other tests (e.g., edrophonium, electrophysiologic studies, single-fiber EMG) may be needed to make the diagnosis.

143. What are the four characteristic features of damage to the anterior horn cells?

Weakness, fasciculations, atrophy, and hyporeflexia.

144. What processes can damage the anterior horn cells?

1. Degenerative (spinal muscular atrophy): Werdnig-Hoffman, Kugelberg-Welander, Pena-Shokeir, and Manden-Walker syndromes

2. Metabolic: Tay-Sachs disease (hexosaminidase deficiency), Pompe disease, Batten disease (ceroid-lipofuscinosis), hyperglycinemia, neonatal adrenoleukodystrophy

3. Infections: poliovirus, coxsackievirus, ECHO viruses

145. How are the inherited progressive spinal muscular atrophies distinguished?

Recessive spinal muscular atrophy (SMA) of both early (type 1) and late (type 3) onset have been linked to the same region chromosome 5. A diagnostic test using PCR that has high sensitivity and specificity is available.

Progressive Spinal Muscular Atrophies

DISORDER	INHERITANCE	AGE OF ONSET	CLINICAL FEATURES
Acute infantile SMA (Werdnig-Hoffmann disease, SMA type 1)	Autosomal recessive	In utero–6 mos	Frog-leg posture; areflexia; tongue atrophy and fasciculations; progressive swallowing and respiratory problems; survival < 4 yrs
Intermediate SMA (chronic Werdnig-Hoffmann disease, SMA type 2)	Autosomal recessive; rarely autosomal dominant	3 mos–15 yrs	Proximal weakness; most sit unsupported; decreased or absent reflexes; high incidence of scoliosis, contractures; survival may be up to 30 years
Kugelberg-Welander disease (SMA type 3)	Autosomal recessive; rarely autosomal dominant	5 yrs–15 yrs	May be part of spectrum of SMA 2; hip girdle weakness; calf hypertrophy; decreased or absent reflexes; may be ambulatory until fourth decade

Adapted from Parke JT: Disorders of the anterior horn cell. In Oski FA, et al (eds): Principles and Practice of Pediatrics, 2nd ed. Philadelphia, J.B. Lippincott, 1994, p 2068; with permission.

146. What is the clinical importance of dystrophin?

Dystrophin is a muscle protein that is presumed to be involved in anchoring the contractile apparatus of striated and cardiac muscle to the cell membrane. Due to a gene mutation, this protein is completely missing in patients with Duchenne muscular dystrophy. On the other hand, muscle tissue from patients with Becker muscular dystrophy contains reduced amounts of dystrophin or, occasionally, a protein of abnormal size.

147. How are Duchenne and Becker muscular dystrophy distinguished?
Duchenne Muscular Dystrophy

Genetics: X-linked; several different deletions/point mutations in dystrophin gene result in a completely nonfunctional protein. New mutations occur. Carrier females may have mild weakness or cardiomyopathy.

Diagnosis: whole blood DNA may reveal a deletion in ~ 65%. Otherwise, EMG and muscle biopsy are definitive.

Manifestations: regular, stereotyped course of progressive, proximal weakness, calf hypertrophy, loss of ambulation by 11 years, worsening scoliosis and contractures, eventual dilated cardiomyopathy and/or respiratory failure.

Becker Muscular Dystrophy

Genetics: X-linked; various mutations in dystrophin gene result in reduced amount or partially functional protein.

Diagnosis: as for Duchenne; a more benign course and the reduced dystrophin levels in muscle cells (by immunostaining) distinguish the two diseases.

Neurology

Manifestations: milder, slower course compared to Duchenne; calf hypertrophy, ambulatory until 14–15 years or beyond.

Bieber FR, Hoffman EP: Duchenne and Becker muscular dystrophies: Genetics, prenatal diagnosis, and future prospects. Clin Perinatol 17:845–865, 1990.

148. Is prednisone effective in Duchenne muscular dystrophy?

At least four studies from several major centers have documented an improvement in strength with an optimal dose of 0.75 mg/kg/day. The strengthening effect lasts for up to 3 years while the steroid is continued. Appropriate timing and duration of treatment have not been established, and side effects (weight gain and increased susceptibility to infection) may outweigh the benefits in many cases.

Fenichel GM, et al: Longterm benefit from prednisone treatment in Duchenne's muscular dystrophy. Neurology 41:1874–1877, 1991.

149. In an individual infected with poliovirus, how likely is the development of paralysis?

In immunocompetent hosts, up to 95% of poliovirus infections in susceptible individuals are asymptomatic. About 4–8% experience a minor illness of low-grade fever, sore throat, and malaise. Less than 1–2% experience CNS involvement, which can include aseptic meningitis (nonparalytic poliomyelitis) and paralytic poliomyelitis. Only 0.1% of total infections result in residual paralysis.

150. What are the hereditary neuropathies?

Some disorders of the peripheral nerve result from an inherited molecular or biochemical disturbance. Although relatively uncommon, they collectively account for a substantial percentage of neuropathies that are supposedly "idiopathic." Inheritance is most commonly dominant (e.g., Type 1 or demyelinating Charcot-Marie-Tooth disease) but may be recessive or X-linked. They present as a chronic, slowly progressive, noninflammatory degeneration of the nerve cell body, peripheral axon, or Schwann cells (myelin). The neurologic consequences may be predominantly sensory (e.g., congenital insensitivity to pain), or mixed motor and sensory abnormalities (e.g., Charcot-Marie-Tooth). Deafness, optic neuropathy, and autonomic neuropathy are occasionally associated.

151. What is the principal neuropathology in Guillain-Barré syndrome (GBS)?

GBS (more properly called Landry-Guillain-Barré syndrome) is an acute idiopathic polyradiculoneuritis. It is the most common acute or subacute polyneuropathy encountered in clinical practice. The disease is characterized by the presence of multifocal areas of inflammatory demyelination of nerve roots and peripheral nerves. As a result of the loss of the healthy myelin covering, the conduction of nerve impulses (action potentials) may be blocked or dispersed. The resulting clinical effects are predominantly motor—the evolution of flaccid, areflexic paralysis. There is a variable degree of motor weakness. Some individuals have mild brief weakness, whereas fulminant paralysis occurs in others. Autonomic signs (e.g., tachycardia, hypertension) or sensory symptoms such as painful dysesthesias are not uncommon but are overshadowed by the motor signs.

152. What CSF findings are characteristic of GBS?

The classic CSF finding is the **albuminocytologic dissociation**. Most common infections or inflammatory processes generate an elevation of white blood cell count *and* protein. The CSF profile in GBS includes a normal cell count with elevated protein, usually in the range of 50–100 mg/dl, but at the onset of disease, the CSF protein concentration may be normal.

153. Outline the management of acute Guillain-Barré syndrome.

Early clinical monitoring is focused on the development of bulbar or respiratory insufficiency. Bulbar weakness manifests as unilateral or bilateral facial weakness, diplopia, hoarseness, drooling, depressed gag reflex, or dysphagia. Frank respiratory insufficiency may be preceded by air hunger, dyspnea, or a soft muffled voice (hypophonia). The autonomic nervous system is occasionally involved, as signified by the presence of labile blood pressure and body temperature. The contemporary management of GBS includes the following:

1. Observation in an intensive care unit with frequent monitoring of vital signs.

2. The early institution of plasmapheresis where available. Intravenous gamma globulin may also be helpful in this setting, although randomized trials comparing this therapy with plasmapheresis in children have not yet been done.

3. If bulbar signs are present, the patient is placed NPO and the mouth is suctioned frequently. Hydration is maintained intravenously and nutritional support provided by NG feedings.

4. The vital capacity (VC) is measured frequently. In children, the normal VC may be calculated as VC = 200 ml × age (in yrs). If the VC falls < 25% of normal, endotracheal intubation is done. Careful pulmonary toilet is conducted to minimize atelectasis, aspiration, and pneumonia.

5. Meticulous nursing care includes careful patient positioning to prevent pressure sores, compression of peripheral nerves, and venous thrombosis.

6. Physical therapy is conducted to prevent the development of contractures by passive range of movement exercises and splinting to maintain physiologic hand and limb postures until muscle strength returns.

154. What is the prognosis for children with GBS?

Children seem to recover quicker and better than adults. Fewer than 10% have significant residual deficits. In rare cases, the neuropathy recurs as "chronic inflammatory demyelinating polyneuropathy."

Bradshaw DY, Jones HR Jr: Guillain-Barre in children: Clinical course, electrodiagnosis, and prognosis. Muscle Nerve 15:500–506, 1992.

155. How does multiple sclerosis (MS) present in childhood?

MS is extremely rare in childhood (0.2–2.0% of all cases). Studies of affected children demonstrate a variable predominance of boys in early childhood and females during adolescence. Transient visual or sensory symptoms are relatively common presentations. CSF examination may demonstrate mild (< 25 cells/mm^3) mononuclear pleocytosis with an increasing probability of oligoclonal bands with each recurrence. MRI is the single most useful diagnostic test: the presence of multiple, periventricular white matter plaques (bright areas on T_2 images) confirms the diagnosis.

Duquette P, et al: Clinical profiles of 125 children with multiple sclerosis. J Pediatr 111:359, 1987.

156. When are "doll's eyes" movements considered normal or abnormal?

The oculovestibular reflex (also called oculocephalic, proprioceptive head-turning reflex, or doll's eyes reflex) is used most commonly as a test of brainstem function. The patient's eyelids are held open while the head is briskly rotated from side-to-side. A positive response is contraversive conjugate eye deviation (i.e., as the head rotates to the right, both eyes deviate to the left). Doll's eyes movements are interpreted as follows:

1. In healthy awake newborn infants (who cannot inhibit or override the reflex with willful eye movements), the reflex is easy to elicit and is a normal finding. It can be used to test the range of extraocular movements of infants in the first weeks of life.

2. In healthy, awake, mature individuals, normal vision overrides the reflex, which is thus normally absent, and so the eyes follow the head-turning.

3. In coma with preserved brainstem function, the depressed cortex does not override the reflex, and doll's eyes movements occur in rapid head rotation. Indeed, the purpose of eliciting this reflex in the comatose patient is to demonstrate that the brainstem still functions normally.

4. In coma with brainstem damage, the neural circuits that carry out the reflex are impaired and the reflex is abolished.

157. How are "cold calorics" done?

As a test of brainstem function in an obtunded or comatose individual, 5 ml of ice cold water is placed in the external ear canal (after ensuring integrity of the tympanic membrane) with the head elevated at 30°. A normal response occurs with deviation of the eyes to the side in which the water was placed. No response indicates severe dysfunction of the brainstem and the medial longitudinal fasciculus.

158. What causes pinpoint pupils?

Pupillary size represents a dynamic balance between the constricting influence of the third nerve (representing the parasympathetic autonomic nervous system) and the dilating influence of the ciliary nerve (which conducts fibers of the sympathetic nervous system). Pinpoint pupils imply that the constricting influence of the third cranial nerve is not balanced by opposing sympathetic dilation. This could result from a *structural lesion in the pons* through which descend the sympathetic pathways. Small, reactive pupils also accompany some metabolic disorders. Opiates such as heroin or morphine produce pinpoint pupils that resemble those seen in pontine lesions. Various other agents also produce constriction of the pupils including propoxyphene, organophosphates, carbamate insecticides, barbiturates, clonidine, meprobamate, and pilocarpine eye drops, as well as mushroom or nutmeg poisoning.

159. What is the differential diagnosis of ptosis?

Ptosis is the downward displacement of the upper eyelid due to dysfunction of the muscles that elevate the eyelid. A drooping eyelid may represent "pseudoptosis"due to swelling of the eyelid caused by local edema or active blepharospasm. True ptosis results from weakness of the eyelid muscles or interruption of its nerve supply. Primary muscular etiologies include congenital ptosis, which may occur alone or in the setting of Turner or Smith-Lemli-Opitz syndrome, myasthenia gravis, botulism, and some muscular dystrophies. Neurologic causes include Horner syndrome, which results from the interruption of the sympathetic supply to Muller's smooth eyelid muscle, and third nerve palsy, which innervates the levator palpebral muscle.

160. What is the significance of the Marcus Gunn pupil?

The pupils are normally equal in size (except for patients with physiologic anisocoria) due to the consensual light reflex: light entering either eye produces the same strength "signal" for constriction of both the stimulated and nonstimulated pupil. Some diseases of the maculae or optic nerves affect one side more than the other. For example, a meningioma may develop on one optic nerve sheath. As a result of unilateral or asymmetrical optic nerve dysfunction, a Marcus Gunn pupil (afferent pupillary defect) may result. See question 161 for method of testing.

161. How is the "swinging flashlight test" done?

This tests for the Marcus Gunn pupil.

1. The patient is examined in a dim room, and fixation is directed to a distant target (this permits maximal pupillary dilation due to lack of direct light and accommodation reflexes).

2. Light presented to the "good" eye produces equal constriction of both pupils. The flashlight is swung briskly over the bridge of the nose to the eye with the "defective" optic nerve. The abnormal pupil remains momentarily constricted from the lingering effects of the consensual light response. However, the impaired eye with its reduced pupillomotor signal soon escapes the consensual reflex and actually dilates despite being directly stimulated with light. The pupil that paradoxically dilates to direct light stimulation displays the **afferent defect**.

162. A child whose eyelids elevate rather than close with yawning has what condition?

The **Marcus Gunn reflex**, also known as the jaw-winking phenomenon, presumably arises from a congenital "miswiring" of the oculomotor and trigeminal nerves. In this anomaly, ptosis follows jaw closure and eyelid elevation follows jaw opening.

163. What are the causes of optic atrophy in children?

Optic atrophy is characterized by disc pallor and attenuated vasculature on fundoscopy. Severe atrophy may also produce an abnormal pupillary light reflex and deficit of either acuity, visual field, or color vision. It should be distinguished from optic nerve hypoplasia, in which fundoscopy shows a nerve head of diminished circumference but normal color and vasculature.

The causes of optic atrophy include structural (spenoid sinus mucocele, neuroblastoma, chronic elevation of intracranial pressure, or other orbital/chiasmatic neoplasms), metabolic-toxic (hyperthyroidism, vitamin B deficiency, Leber optic atrophy, various leukodystrophies, mitochondrial diseases, methanol, chloroquine, or amiodarone exposure), and various recessive syndromes with other variable neurologic signs (mental retardation, paraparesis), and demyelinating (optic neuritis, multiple sclerosis) diseases.

SEIZURE DISORDERS

164. How often are EEGs abnormal in healthy children?

Approximately 10% of "normal" children have mild, nonspecific abnormalities in background activity. About 2–3% of healthy children have unexpected incidental epileptiform (i.e., spikes or sharp wave) patterns. Some may have heritable, familial EEG abnormalities without a clinical seizure disorder.

165. Which disorders may commonly mimic epilepsy?

Many conditions are characterized by the sudden onset of abnormal consciousness, awareness, reactivity, behavior, posture, tone, sensation, or autonomic function. Syncope, breath-holding spells, migraine, hypoglycemia, narcolepsy, cataplexy, sleep apnea, gastroesophageal reflux, and parasomnias (night terrors, sleep walking, sleep talking, nocturnal enuresis) feature an abrupt or "paroxysmal" alteration of brain function and suggest the possibility of epilepsy. Perhaps one of the most difficult attacks to distinguish is the "pseudoseizure," also called a pseudoepileptic seizure or hysterical seizure. These attacks are outwardly modeled after the patient's subconscious or conscious perception of a seizure and occur without abnormal electrical discharges of neurons in the CNS.

166. How are seizures in children classified?

Seizures are broadly classified by their clinical and EEG characteristics.

• **Generalized** seizures entail simultaneous, synchronous EEG discharges in both hemispheres. There may be complete loss of consciousness from the onset. **Primary** generalized seizures include some of the familial and sporadic epilepsy syndromes such as childhood absence (formerly termed petit mal) seizures, while **secondarily** generalized seizures arise from localized lesions of the cortex. Generalized seizures of both types may involve a variety of motor patterns: tonic-clonic (formerly termed grand mal), myoclonic, atonic, clonic, and tonic.

• **Partial** seizures (formerly termed focal) are divided into simple and complex types. **Complex** partial (formerly termed psychomotor) seizures produce an alteration of consciousness. **Simple** partial seizures occur in the presence of a normal level of consciousness.

167. If a previously normal child has an afebrile, generalized tonic-clonic seizure, what should parents be told about the risk of recurrence?

Studies indicate that the recurrence rate is between 25 and 50%. The EEG is an important predictor of recurrence. A subsequent normal EEG reduces the risk to 25%. Occurrence of the seizure during sleep increases the risk to 50%. The child's age at the time of first seizure or the duration of the seizure do not affect the recurrence risk.

Shinnar S, et al: Risk of seizure recurrence following unprovoked seizure in childhood: A prospective study. Pediatrics 85:1076–1085, 1990.

Shinnar S, et al: Sleep state and the risk of seizure recurrence following a first unprovoked seizure in childhood. Neurology 43:701–706, 1993.

168. Name the four most common inherited seizure syndromes.

1. Febrile convulsions
2. Benign childhood partial (rolandic) seizures
3. Absence seizures
4. Juvenile myoclonic epilepsy (of Janz)

169. Should all children with a new-onset afebrile generalized seizure have a CT or MRI evaluation?

While most adults with new-onset seizures should have a head imaging study (preferably MRI), the relatively high frequency of idiopathic seizure disorders in children often obviates a

scan in those with generalized seizures, nonfocal EEGs, and normal neurologic exams. Consider obtaining a cranial imaging study for:
1. Any seizure with focal components (other than mere eye deviation)
2. Newborns and young infants with seizures
3. Status epilepticus at any age
4. Focal slowing or focal paroxysmal activity on EEG

170. What characterizes hypsarrhythmic EEG patterns?

The term figuratively means "mountainous slowing." It describes the classic interictal EEG of infantile spasms and is characterized by extremely high-voltage, slowed, disorganized brain waves with multifocal spike activity. Hypsarrhythmia may either precede or follow the onset of infantile spasms. This EEG configuration may appear first or most obviously in non-REM sleep and confirms the clinical diagnosis of infantile spasms.

171. Name the proposed three main types of infantile spasms.

Infantile spasms are a unique epileptic syndrome of infancy and childhood characterized by clusters of spasms, usually beginning between 3 and 9 months of age. Traditionally classified as a myoclonic epilepsy, a phenomenologic division of infantile spasms into **flexor**, **extensor**, and **mixed-type** spasms has been proposed on the basis of detailed video-EEG monitoring. However, such a division has no etiologic or prognostic significance. Idiopathic infantile spasms, which present in previously neurologically normal infants, should be distinguished from the more ominous symptomatic spasms, which occur with serious and diffuse CNS disturbances (e.g., perinatal hypoxic-ischemic encephalopathy, tuberous sclerosis, congenital CMV infection, structural brain anomalies).

Commission on Pediatric Epilepsy, International League Against Epilepsy: Workshop on infantile spasms. Epilepsia 33:195, 1992.

172. How commonly is a cause identified in infantile spasms?

A cause can be identified in up to 75% of children with infantile spasms, usually in those symptomatic at the time of the initial seizure. Of identifiable causes, three-fourths are prenatal/perinatal and one-fourth are postnatal.

Prenatal/perinatal: hypoxic-ischemic encephalopathy, tuberous sclerosis, intrauterine infection (e.g., cytomegalovirus), brain malformations (e.g., lissencephaly), inborn metabolic errors (e.g., nonketotic hyperglycinemia)

Postnatal: infectious (e.g., herpes encephalitis), hypoxic-ischemic encephalopathy, head trauma

Papazian O: Common epileptic syndromes in children. Pediatr Ann 20:15–24, 1991.

173. What is the prognosis for infants with infantile spasms?

Prognosis in large part depends on the clinical state at the time of the first seizure. In the cryptogenic or idiopathic group (10–25% of total), development and the neurologic exam and studies are normal at the onset. With ACTH treatment, 40–65% will have a complete or near-complete recovery. In the symptomatic group (85–90% of total), neurologic deficits and/or cranial abnormalities are present before the first seizure. In this group, complete or near-complete recovery is achieved by only 5–15%.

174. What is the rationale for administering ACTH or corticosteroids to children with infantile spasms?

In children with infantile spasms, there is believed to be a disturbance in the cortical-brain-stem-adrenal axis, resulting in elevated levels of an endogenous epileptogenic substance (i.e., corticotropin-releasing factor, CRF). Although the precise method of action is unclear, the administration of ACTH or steroids may serve as a negative feedback inhibitor of CRF. Studies suggest that ACTH therapy of even short-term duration may be more efficacious than corticosteroids and is particularly useful in cryptogenic infantile spasms of recent onset.

Baram TZ, et al: High-dose corticosteroids (ACTH) versus prednisone for infantile spasms: A prospective, randomized, blinded study. Pediatrics 97:375–378, 1996.

175. What are the diagnostic criteria for rolandic epilepsy?

Rolandic epilepsy (benign focal epilepsy of childhood) is a common epilepsy syndrome that has received little recognition in the United States. The following criteria establish the diagnosis:

1. It begins during school age in otherwise healthy and neurologically normal children.
2. The seizures are idiopathic or familial (rolandic epilepsy may be inherited in an autosomal dominant fashion).
3. The clinical seizures may be simple or complex, partial or generalized. The simple partial seizure may begin during the daytime as a sensory disturbance on the tongue or focal clonic facial twitching. During sleep, generalized seizures seem to predominate.
4. The EEG shows a distinctive type of sharp-slow wave discharges localized to the rolandic (central, midtemporal, central-temporal, or sylvian) regions.
5. Ancillary neurodiagnostic tests are normal.

Rolandic epilepsy is often referred to as a benign syndrome because (1) the individual is otherwise normal; (2) the seizures are usually easily controlled with low doses of a single anticonvulsant; and (3) the seizures virtually always abate after puberty.

176. A teenager, like his father, develops brief, bilateral, intermittent jerking of his arms. What seizure disorder is he likely to have?

Myoclonic epilepsy of Janz or juvenile myoclonic epilepsy (JME) is a familial form of primary generalized epilepsy typically showing "fast" 3–5-Hz spike and wave discharges on EEG and autosomal dominant inheritance. Absence or tonic-clonic seizures may precede the characteristic myoclonic jerks, which usually begin in adolescence. The myoclonus may be asymmetric and consciousness is preserved. Divalproex sodium is the drug of choice. The probability of lifelong remission is small.

177. What is the clinical triad of the Lennox-Gastaut syndrome?

Disorganized **slow spike and wave activity** on an EEG, **mental retardation**, and **seizures** of various types. The most common seizure type is an axial, tonic seizure during sleep, but myoclonic, focal, clonic, akinetic, tonic-clonic, and atypical absence spells occur regularly. Seizures usually begin between ages 1.5–8 years and are notoriously difficult to control. They occasionally respond to divalproex sodium or a ketogenic diet. There is a high rate of associated neurologic abnormalities, including cerebral palsy. The Lennox-Gastaut syndrome may follow infantile spasms as the infant matures.

178. List the varieties of partial epilepsy of childhood.

Simple partial seizures (without alteration in consciousness):
• Motor (e.g., clonic jerking of facial muscles)
• Somatosensory (e.g., numbness of a leg)
• Special sensory (e.g., visual or auditory sensations)
• Autonomic (e.g., piloerection, sweating, pupillary dilatation)
• Combinations of the above

Complex partial seizures: any signs included in simple partial seizures but involving alteration or loss of consciousness.

In addition, all seizures are categorized by etiology as either idiopathic or symptomatic, the latter occurring in association with some other brain abnormality.

179. Describe the types of absence seizures.

Typical Absence
EEG: 3-Hz spike and wave
Observations: Abrupt onset and ending
Simple—unresponsiveness with no other associated feature
Complex—unresponsiveness with mild atonic, myoclonic, or tonic features or automatisms

Atypical Absence (most common in Lennox-Gastaut syndrome)
EEG: 2-Hz (or slower) spike and wave
Observations: gradual onset and ending; unresponsive with more prolonged
and pronounced atonic, tonic, myoclonic, or tonic activity

180. In a child suspected of having absence seizures, how can a seizure be elicited during an exam?

Hyperventilation for at least 3 minutes is a useful provocative maneuver to precipitate an absence seizure. Young patients may be coaxed into overbreathing by making a game of it. Hold a tissue paper in front of the child's mouth. Instruct the patient to keep breathing fast enough to keep the tissue aloft.

181. What percentage of patients with absence seizures also have occasional grand mal seizures?

About 30%.

182. How is status epilepticus defined?

1. More than 30 minutes of continuous seizure activity
2. Recurrent seizures without full recovery of consciousness between seizures

183. What are the most common precipitants of status epilepticus in children?

Fever/infection	36%	CNS infection	5%
Medication change	20%	Trauma	4%
Unknown	9%	Cerebrovascular	3%
Metabolic	8%	Ethanol/drug-related	2%
Congenital	7%	Tumor	1%
Anoxia	5%		

Dodson WE, et al: Treatment of convulsive status epilepticus: Recommendations of the Epilepsy Foundation of America's Working Group on Status Epilepticus. JAMA 270:855, 1993.

184. How should a child who presents with status epilepticus be managed?

0–5 minutes: Maintain airway by head positioning or oropharyngeal airway. Administer nasal oxygen. Suction as needed. Obtain and frequently monitor vital signs. Observe and examine the patient. Establish an intravenous line. If a rapid reagent strip for glucose testing is not available, administer 2 ml/kg of $D_{25}W$. In an infant with no known seizure disorder, give pyridoxine, 100 mg IV.

6–9 minutes: Obtain venous blood for laboratory determinations (e.g., glucose, serum chemistries, hematology studies, toxicology screen, culture, anticonvulsant levels if known epileptic). Obtain a periodic arterial blood gas and/or monitor oxygenation by pulse oximetry.

10–20 minutes: Administer (1) lorazepam, 0.1 mg/kg (up to 4 mg) at 2 mg/min IV, *or* (2) diazepam, 0.2 mg/kg (up to 10 mg) at 5 mg/min IV. May repeat diazepam in 5 minutes if seizure persists.

21–60 minutes: If seizures persist, administer phenytoin (20 mg/kg) at 1–2 mg/kg/min IV while monitoring heart rate and/or ECG. The infusion should be slowed if dysrhythmia or QT-interval widening develops.

> 60 minutes: If seizures persist for 15 minutes after use of phenytoin, give phenobarbital (20 mg/kg) IV. With use of phenobarbital following benzodiazepines, the risk of respiratory depression is increased and the likely need for intubation increases. If phenobarbital fails to stop the seizure, other measures, such as general anesthesia, are usually necessary.

Dodson WE, et al: Treatment of convulsive status epilepticus: Recommendations of the Epilepsy Foundation of America's Working Group on Status Epilepticus. JAMA 270:854–859, 1993.

185. What is the significance of a burst-suppression pattern in an EEG?

Burst-suppression refers to a very abnormal EEG pattern observed in a variety of serious diffuse acute encephalopathies, such as meningitis, encephalitis, head injury, or hypoxic-ischemic injury. The ongoing EEG activity is no longer continuous but rather appears as a sudden "burst" of abnormal electrical patterns followed by an abnormal "suppression" of brain waves. This EEG pattern originates from the cerebral cortex, which is no longer operating under the influence or guidance of the midbrain and thalami due to disruption of their connecting fibers. Burst-suppression is not specific from an etiologic viewpoint. Many neurologic illnesses can produce it if they are diffuse and sufficiently severe.

A burst-suppression EEG indicates an important acute, severe disturbance of brain functioning. This pattern is often considered an ominous EEG prognostic sign because many with this abnormality die and survivors are at high risk for permanent neurologic sequelae. Bursts-suppression can sometimes appear briefly as an immediate postictal finding that quickly evolves into a less abnormal state. This does not necessarily indicate an unfavorable outcome. The intravenous administration of benzodiazepines to stop status epilepticus can also result in a transient burst-suppression background. Similarly, large doses of barbiturates or general anesthesia may cause a reversible burst-suppression EEG with an expected return to normalcy after the drug is discontinued. Finally, some children with infantile spasms and a hypsarrhythmic EEG display a burst-suppression EEG pattern only during sleep.

186. When is surgical treatment indicated in partial seizures?

1. The seizures significantly disrupt the quality of life.

2. The seizures are refractory to concerted trials of the major groups of anticonvulsants pushed to the patient's tolerance.

3. EEG monitoring uncovers a focal, reproducible focus from which seizure discharges uniformly correlate with the "target" seizure.

4. The cortex identified by monitoring is from an expendable portion of the brain.

Spencer SS, Katz A: Arriving at the surgical options for intractable seizures. Semin Neurol 10:422–420, 1990.

Engel J Jr: Surgery for seizures. N Engl J Med 334:647–652, 1996.

SPINAL CORD DISORDERS

187. Which spinal segments do each of the common reflexes test?

Localizations of Reflexes

DEEP TENDON REFLEX	SUPERFICIAL REFLEX	PERIPHERAL NERVE	SEGMENTAL ORGANIZATION
	Pupillary	Optic/oculomotor	CN II–III
Jaw jerk		Trigeminal	CN V
	Corneal	Trigeminal/facial	CN V–VII
	Gag	Glossopharyngeal/vagal	CN IX–X
Biceps		Musculocutaneous	C5–6
Brachioradialis		Radial	C5–6
Triceps		Radial	C6–8
Finger flexion		Median/ulnar	C7–T1
Abdominal reflex		Thoracic	T8–12
	Umbilical	Thoracic	T8–12
	Cremasteric	Genitofemoral	L1–2
Adductor		Femoral/obturator	L2–4
Quadriceps		Femoral	L2–4
	Plantar reflex	Sciatic	S1–2
	Anal wink	Pudendal	S3–5

188. What are "early" signs of spinal cord compression?

Early spinal cord compression may be easily overlooked before flagrant motor or sensory signs are prominent. Some early clinical clues that may be helpful in detecting this compression promptly include:

1. Scoliosis producing sustained poor posture.
2. Back pain or abdominal pain that begins abruptly or paroxysmally during sleep.
3. Increased sensitivity of the spinal column to local pressure or percussion.
4. In extramedullary tumors that compress the cord, prodromal pains of radicular distribution are common because such tumors often arise from the posterior nerve roots themselves.
5. Bowel or bladder dysfunction may be a presenting feature of sacral or conus medullaris compression.
6. Since the somatotopic organization of sensory fibers places the sacral and lumbar dermatomes nearest to the cord surface, extrinsic compression commonly results first in diminished sensation in the anogenital region and lower limbs.

189. How common are asymptomatic spinal anomalies in normal children?

Up to 5% of children have spina bifida occulta, an incomplete fusion of the posterior vertebral arches, usually noted as a radiographic incidental finding. The defect most commonly involves the lower lumbar lamina of L5 and S1.

190. When should an occult spinal dysraphism be suspected?

Occult spinal dysraphism should be suspected in children who have the following dorsal midline features:

1. An abnormal collection of hair
2. Cutaneous abnormalities (e.g., hemangioma or pigmented nevi)
3. Cutaneous dimples or tracts or a subcutaneous mass on the lower back

In 80–90% of cases, there is an associated vertebral abnormality. The diagnosis should also be suspected in patients with symptoms of progressive lower extremity weakness or sensory loss, gait abnormalities, foot deformities, or neurogenic bowel and bladder problems.

191. What is the full anatomic expression of myelomeningocele?

Children with myelomeningocele have a complex, multifaceted, congenital disorder of structure which represents a dysraphic state—a defective closure of the embryonic neural groove. In its full expression, it is typified anatomically by:

1. The presence of unfused or excessively separated vertebral arches of the bony spine (spina bifida).
2. Cystic dilation of the meninges which surround the spinal cord (meningocele).
3. Cystic dilation of the spinal cord itself (myelocele).
4. Hydrocephalus and spectrum of congenital cerebral abnormalities.

192. If the diagnosis of myelomeningocele is made prenatally, should delivery be done by cesarean section?

In one study infants delivered by cesarean section prior to the onset of labor had significantly less paralysis at age 2 years than did infants with comparable lesions who were delivered vaginally following a period of labor.

Luthy DA, et al: Cesarean section before the onset of labor and subsequent motor function in infants with meningocele diagnosed antenatally. N Engl J Med 324:662–666, 1991.

193. Which congenital cerebral disorders are associated with myelomeningocele?

1. A type II **Arnold-Chiari malformation** may occur in which the hindbrain is abnormal and enclosed in a small posterior fossa. The medulla oblongata and the "tonsils" of the cerebellum are displaced or herniated downward to occupy the normal position of the upper cervical cord. The impaired egress of CSF caused by aqueductal stenosis commonly results in

hydrocephalus. Arnold-Chiari malformations sometimes coexist with other abnormalities of the cerebral cortex.

2. More severe **cerebral malformations** may occur in the maximal expression of the dysraphic state. Incomplete closure of the cranial bones results in cranium bifidum. Protrusion of abnormal brain tissue through the defective skull bone results in an encephalocele. Gross failure of neural groove fusion results in craniorachischisis or, in its maximal form, anencephaly.

3. **Hydrocephalus** is seen in 95% of children with thoracic or high lumbar myelomeningocele. The incidence decreases progressively with more caudal spinal defects to a minimum of 60% if the myelomeningocele is located in the sacrum.

194. What is the usual cause of stridor in a child with myelomeningocele?

The stridor is usually due to **dysfunction of the vagus nerve**, which innervates the muscles of the vocal cords. In their *resting* position, the edges of the cords meet in the midline; in speech, they move apart. Hence, in bilateral vagal nerve palsies, the free edges of the vocal cords are closely opposed and obstruct air flow, resulting in stridor. In symptomatic patients the motor nucleus of the vagus nerve may be congenitally hypoplastic or aplastic. More commonly, the vagal dysfunction is believed to arise from a mechanical traction injury secondary to hydrocephalus, which produces progressive herniation and inferior displacement of the abnormal hindbrain. Shunting the hydrocephalus may alleviate the traction and improve the stridor. Sometimes, the later recurrence of stridor indicates reaccumulation of hydrocephalus due to ventriculoperitoneal shunt failure.

195. What are the four principal options for managing urinary incontinence in patients with myelomeningocele?

About 80% of patients have a neurogenic bladder, most commonly a small, poorly compliant bladder and an open and fixed sphincter. Options include:

1. Clean intermittent catheterization which results in more complete emptying than simple Credé maneuvers
2. Artificial urinary sphincter to increase outlet resistance
3. Surgical urinary diversion (e.g., cutaneous vesicostomy), which is uncommonly used
4. Augmentation cystoplasty to increase bladder capacity in combination with the use of oxybutynin (a smooth muscle antispasmodic)

Blum RW, Pfaffinger K: Myelodysplasia in childhood and adolescence. Pediatr Rev 15:480–488, 1994.

196. How frequently is myelomeningocele associated with mental retardation?

Only 15–20% of patients have associated mental retardation. Hydrocephalus per se does not cause the mental retardation associated with this syndrome. (Recall that children with appropriately treated congenital hydrocephalus due to simple aqueductal stenosis usually have normal psychomotor development). Lower intellectual function is more commonly seen in patients with higher cord lesions, hydrocephalus, ventriculoperitoneal shunts, and a history of intracranial bleeding or infections. Mental retardation is usually attributed to acquired secondary CNS infection or subtle microscopic anomalies of neuronal migration and differentiation, which may coexist with the macroscopically visible malformation of the hindbrain.

197. In an infant born with myelomeningocele, how does the initial evaluation predict long-term ambulation potential?

Thoracic: No hip flexion is noted; almost no younger children will ambulate, and only about a third of adolescents will ambulate with the aid of extensive braces and crutches.

High lumbar (L1, L2): Able to flex hips but no knee extension; about a third of children and adolescents will ambulate, but with extensive assistive devices

Mid lumbar (L3):   Able to flex hips and extend knee; percentage of ambulators midway between those with high and low lumbar lesions.

Low lumbar (L4, L5):   Able to flex knee and dorsiflex ankle; nearly half of younger children and nearly all adolescents will ambulate with varying degrees of braces or crutches.

Sacral (S1–S4):   Able to plantarflex ankles and move toes; nearly all children and adolescents will ambulate with minimal or no assistive devices.

15. ONCOLOGY

Wayne Rackoff, M.D., and Beverly J. Lange, M.D.

CHEMOTHERAPY/RADIATION

1. How do various anticancer drugs exert their effects?

1. Interruption of DNA synthesis through inhibition of nucleotide synthesis (methotrexate), substitution of nonfunctional nucleotides in the DNA strand (cytarabine), strand breaks and cross-linking (cyclophosphamide), and intercalation (doxorubicin).
2. Interruption of cell division as a result of interruption of the mitotic spindle (vincristine)
3. Interference with RNA synthesis (dactinomycin)
4. Interference with protein synthesis (L-asparaginase)
5. Promotion of cell differentiation (retinoic acid)
6. Direct damage to cell membrane (corticosteroids)

2. Why does drug resistance develop during the course of chemotherapy?

Resistance to chemotherapeutic agents probably has several mechanisms, only a few of which are understood. The *MDR* (multiple drug resistance) gene is associated with resistance to chemotherapy in a number of tumors. The protein product of the *MDR* gene, P-glycoprotein, is responsible for pumping toxic substances out of cells. It may be responsible for resistance to vinca alkaloids, epipodophyllotoxins, and antitumor antibiotics, all of which can be actively excluded from cells by the MDR protein. Presumably, the gene is induced by exposure to chemotherapy.

Resistance to methotrexate occurs by a different mechanism. Exposure to methotrexate results in the amplification of genes that encode enzymes which circumvent the block in hydrofolate reductase activity caused by the drug.

3. What types of chemotherapy can cause diabetes mellitus?

Patients receiving chemotherapy for acute lymphoblastic leukemia may develop diabetes mellitus as a result of **prednisone** therapy. Patients who develop steroid-induced diabetes often have some family history of diabetes. Steroid-induced diabetes is almost always self-limited. Patients may also develop diabetes as a sequela of hemorrhagic pancreatitis caused by **L-asparaginase**. The pancreatitis may completely destroy the islet cells. This form of diabetes requires lifelong insulin therapy.

4. What acute or subacute CNS complications can result from chemotherapy for leukemia?

Corticosteroids: psychosis
Cytarabine: cerebellar dysfunction, nystagmus
Methotrexate (intrathecal): chemical arachnoiditis, myelopathy
L-Asparaginase: hemorrhage, thrombosis
Radiotherapy: somnolence syndrome (approx 5–8 wks after therapy)
Berg SL, Poplack DG: Complications of leukemia. Pediatr Rev 12:313–318, 1991.

5. In what setting is MESNA used?

MESNA (sodium 2-mercaptoethane sulfonate) is a synthetic sulfhydryl compound used to prevent hemorrhagic cystitis after treatment with cyclophosphamide or ifosfamide. MESNA protects the bladder by detoxifying the acrolein byproducts excreted after treatment with these drugs.

6. How should you monitor the cardiotoxicity associated with chemotherapy?

Cardiac toxicity is usually associated with the anthracyclines, doxorubicin, and daunorubicin. It is most important not to exceed doses known to be associated with cardiomyopathy and to estimate a one-third increase in "effective cardiotoxic dose" if the heart has been irradiated. Reduction in shortening fraction in the face of an adequate preload suggests early damage. It is generally recommended to perform an echocardiogram before anthracycline is begun, at 200 mg/m^2, 300 mg/m^2, 400 mg/m^2, and at each 50 mg/m^2 thereafter, and then 1 year after therapy stops. There is no formula for predicting when heart failure will occur in a given individual. It may occur many years after the completion of therapy; therefore, every-other-year echocardiography and EKG should be continued indefinitely. The risk of clinical cardiomyopathy is about 5% at 450–500 mg/m^2. Prolonged infusion therapy rather than bolus therapy may increase the tolerance to high doses.

7. Should children receiving chemotherapy be given routine immunizations?

Children who are receiving chemotherapy can be given routine diphtheria/tetanus/pertussis (DTP) immunization when they have discontinued the intensive part of treatment. They should not be given live-virus vaccines (measles, mumps, rubella, polio). They can receive the Salk vaccine for polio protection, but the response may be suboptimal. Patients with severe pulmonary disease secondary to malignancy or cancer treatment should receive influenza immunization. They can receive pneumococcal, Hib, and DTP/DTaP vaccines if clinically indicated. The response is likely to be suboptimal, particularly if treatment includes steroid, cyclophosphamide, or radiation therapy. However, there is no evidence that tolerance is induced with immunization.

8. Which antiemetic drugs are most effective in controlling the nausea and vomiting associated with chemotherapy?

Ondansetron (Zofran) and **granisetron** (Kytril), serotonin receptor antagonists, are the most effective drugs available for controlling chemotherapy-associated emesis. They do not cause sedation or extrapyramidal reactions but have been associated with headaches and flushing in some patients. The efficacy of these drugs may be enhanced by the addition of dexamethasone. They are not effective for delayed emesis, which begins 3–5 days after the start of chemotherapy. Combinations of phenothiazines/antihistamines and metaclopramide/antihistamines (with or without dexamethasone) are effective for early-onset and delayed emesis but have more side effects than ondansetron or granisetron.

9. What are the short-term toxicities of radiation therapy?

The toxicities associated with radiotherapy depend on the location of radiation fields and the dose. These toxicities may be worsened by the use of radiomimetic drugs, such as d-actinomycin. Common short-term problems include nausea, vomiting, mucositis, and skin erythema and desquamation. Myelosuppression may occur when large fields are used. Acute nephritis is possible when the kidneys are in the radiation field.

10. What are the late complications of cranial irradiation and chemotherapy?

Endocrinologic: growth hormone deficiency, hypothyroidism, hypogonadism, impaired fertility, premature ovarian failure

Neuropsychologic: attention/memory deficits, IQ deficits, leukoencephalopathy

Other: second malignancy

11. How is body surface area calculated in children?

Body surface area (BSA) is most commonly used in chemotherapy calculations and is usually derived from nomograms after height and weight are measured. A rapid (and reasonably reliable) estimate is as follows:

$$\text{BSA (m}^2) = (\text{weight [lbs]}/60) + 0.1$$

Barton DH: Quick calculation for body surface area in children. Consultant 34:907, 1994.

CLINICAL ISSUES

12. Does "reverse isolation" help prevent infection in neutropenic patients?

Reverse isolation is the placement of a patient in a single room with all medical staff and visitors wearing gowns, masks, and gloves. It is ineffective in preventing illness in neutropenic patients because most infections arise from the patient's endogenous microbial flora. Other measures that have been shown to have little value are (1) the patient's wearing of a surgical mask outside his or her room and (2) avoidance of fresh fruits and vegetables to minimize acquisition of bacteria, particularly gram-negative organisms.

13. In patients undergoing chemotherapy, how is "fever and neutropenia" defined?

If a patient has < 500 total combined polymorphonuclear leukocytes and band cells per cubic millimeter and develops an oral temperature > 38.5°C or more than three successive readings of > 38°C in a 24-hour period, fever and neutropenia are present. Empiric broad-spectrum antibiotic therapy should be initiated.

14. How should cancer patients with fever and neutropenia be managed?

Patients with neutropenia are at high risk for bacterial sepsis, and prolonged neutropenia may be associated with systemic mycotic infection. Therefore, fever in the neutropenic patient demands an immediate physical exam to identify a possible source of infection, cultures of urine, peripheral blood, and blood from any central venous access device, and the initiation of broad-spectrum antibiotics. The choice of antibiotics should include coverage of *Pseudomonas* species and staphylococci. Vancomycin should be considered if the patient has a central venous catheter or ventriculoperitoneal shunt, which increase the likelihood of a coagulase-negative staphylococcal infection.

Pizzo PA, et al: The child with cancer and infection: I. Empiric therapy for fever and neutropenia and preventive strategies. J Pediatr 119:679–694, 1991.

15. What are the indications for modifying a standard empiric antibiotic regimen in a patient with fever and neutropenia?

Event	Recommendation
Bacteremia	Gram-positive isolate, add vancomycin
	Gram-negative isolate, modify regimen if indicated by antibiotic susceptibility tests
Catheter-related infection	Add vancomycin if gram-positive isolate
	Consider catheter removal if cultures remain positive for ≥ 72 hrs or if a tunnel infection occurs
Severe mucositis	Add anaerobic coverage with clindamycin or metronidazole
	If vesicular lesions are present, culture for herpes virus and consider acyclovir
Interstitial or progressive pneumonitis	Consider bronchoalveolar lavage or biopsy
	Add TMP-SMX (20 mg/kg/day) and erythromycin
Perirectal pain or cellulitis	Add anaerobic coverage with clindamycin or metronidazole
Suspected typhlitis	Add anaerobic coverage with clindamycin or metronidazole
	Early empiric use of amphotericin B (fever ≥ 3 days)
Suspected esophagitis	Esophagoscopy
	Consider antifungal therapy with ketoconazole or fluconazole
Persistent fever and granulo-cytopenia for ≥ 7 days	Patient reevaluation
	Add empiric amphotericin B

TMP-SMX: trimethoprim-sulfamethoxazole.
From Katz JA, Mustafa MM: Management of fever in granulocytopenic children with cancer. Pediatr Infect Dis J 12:333, 1993; with permission.

16. When are granulocyte transfusions indicated in the infected granulocytopenic cancer patient?

The only established indication for granulocyte transfusion in the febrile neutropenic cancer patient is a blood culture persistently positive for gram-negative bacteria in a patient receiving appropriate antibiotics. The benefit of granulocytes in typhlitis, abscesses, pneumonitis, fungemia, or persistent fever is not established.

17. What is the triad of tumor lysis syndrome?

Hyperuricemia, **hyperkalemia**, and **hyperphosphatemia**. These metabolic complications occur as a result of the rapid lysis of a large tumor burden, especially in Burkitt lymphoma and in T-cell leukemia/lymphoma. Secondary renal failure and symptomatic hypocalcemia can also occur.

18. Which tumor carries the greatest risk for tumor lysis syndrome?

Burkitt lymphoma with disseminated intra-abdominal and retroperitoneal disease. Rarely, the tumor lysis syndrome occurs before the patient begins treatment, but most often it starts within 24 hours of beginning chemotherapy and may persist for 4–5 days. This syndrome can be fatal because of hyperkalemia or hypocalcemia; it can be lessened in severity or prevented by allopurinol, alkalinization, and aggressive hydration at 2–4 times maintenance rates.

Cohen LF, et al: Acute tumor lysis syndrome: A review of 37 patients with Burkitt's lymphoma. Am J Med 68:486–490, 1980.

19. What laboratory monitoring is needed in patients at risk for tumor lysis syndrome?

Monitoring should include serum sodium, potassium, calcium, phosphorus, BUN, creatinine, uric acid, and urine pH, specific gravity, and volume prior to initiating treatment. Blood pressure and sensorium should be followed. Chemotherapy should not be instituted until there is a urine specific gravity ≤ 1.010 and pH ≥ 7.0. These laboratory studies should be repeated 4–6 hours later and then every 4–12 hours, depending on the severity of the abnormalities that follow initiation of treatment.

Cohen LF, et al: Acute tumor lysis syndrome: A review of 37 patients with Burkitt's lymphoma. Am J Med 68:486–490, 1980.

20. Name the three mainstays of therapy to prevent tumor lysis syndrome.

1. **Hydration**—at 2–4 times maintenance levels to promote uric acid and phosphate excretion
2. **Alkalinization**—addition of 50–100 mEq $NaHCO_3$/L to maintain urine pH at 7.0–7.5 and thus lessen the likelihood of uric acid crystallization. Care should be taken not to overalkalinize because at pH > 7.5, hypoxanthine stones can form and at pH > 8.0, calcium phosphate crystallization is more likely.
3. **Allopurinol**—inhibits xanthine oxidase, which is involved in the formation of uric acid from hypoxanthine and xanthine (nucleic acid degradation products)

21. What factors can contribute to renal failure in tumor lysis syndrome?

Uric acid nephropathy: The degradation of nucleic acids leads to increases in serum uric acid, which is soluble at physiologic pH but can precipitate in the acid milieu of the collecting tubules.

Calcium-phosphate crystallization: Lymphoblasts (which contain four times the phosphate of lymphocytes) release phosphate, and if the calcium-phosphate product exceeds 60, crystals can form in the renal microvasculature.

Tumor burden: The tumor itself may contribute to preexisting renal problems by parenchymal involvement, obstructive uropathy, and venous stasis.

22. How do the superior vena cava (SVC) syndrome and superior mediastinal syndrome (SMS) differ?

SVC syndrome generally refers to symptoms that develop from obstruction of a major vessel, while SMS is the designation when tracheal impingement is also present. In adults, the respiratory problems are less common. In children, however, because vascular and tracheal problems frequently occur concurrently, the terms SVC syndrome and SMS are used synonymously. SVC syndrome is the more frequently used term.

23. What are the clinical features of a child with SVC syndrome?

Symptoms include cough, hoarseness, dyspnea, orthopnea, and chest pain. Patients with substantial obstruction may also show anxiety, confusion, and lethargy. They may have headaches, distorted vision, and a sense of fullness in the ears and head. Symptoms are aggravated by lying supine or flexing tightly. Signs of SVC syndrome include swelling of the face or neck and/or upper extremities, plethora, cyanosis, suffusion, conjunctival edema, diaphoresis, wheezing, and stridor.

24. Which tumors most commonly cause SVC syndrome?

In childhood, the most common is **non-Hodgkin lymphoma**. Less frequent causes are Hodgkin disease, neuroblastoma, and sarcomas. Nonmalignant infectious causes are unusual but can include histoplasmosis or tuberculosis. The **most frequent cause** in children, however, is **iatrogenic**, resulting from vascular thrombosis following surgeries for congenital heart disease, shunting procedures for hydrocephalus, or catheterization for venous access.

Janin Y, et al: Superior vena cava syndrome in children and adolescence: A review of the literature and report of three cases. J Pediatr Surg 17:219, 1982.

25. In a child receiving chemotherapy, what conditions can produce acute abdominal signs?

- Gastric or duodenal ulcer, especially due to corticosteroid use
- Small intestinal intussusception, primarily ileoileal, usually without intramural intestinal tumor involvement but may be led by tumor nodule
- Intestinal-wall tumor lysis with necrosis, perforation, or hemorrhage associated with chemotherapy response (common in NHL)
- Typhlitis, enterocolitis (nonspecific), leukemic cecal infiltration
- Aspergillosis or mucormycosis
- Lower-lobe pneumonia
- Hepatic or splenic abscesses; subdiaphragmatic, subhepatic, or pelvic septic collections; portal vein thrombosis
- Splenic infarcts
- Hemoperitoneum or retroperitoneal hematoma secondary to coagulation defects or tumor rupture
- Primary peritonitis
- Diseases common to children without neoplasms (e.g., acute appendicitis, abdominal manifestations of viremias)

Adapted from Hays DM, Atkinson JB: General principles of surgery. In Pizzo PA, Poplack DG (eds): Principles and Practice of Pediatric Oncology, 2nd ed. Philadelphia, J.B. Lippincott, 1993, p 266.

26. What can cause stroke in children with cancer?

Malignancy-related	**Radiation-related**
Leptomeningeal disease	Large-vessel occlusion
Metastatic disease	Mineralizing microangiopathy
Disseminated intravascular coagulation	**Infection-related**
Chemotherapy-related	Bacterial meningitis
L-Asparaginase	Fungal meningitis
Methotrexate	

Packer RJ, et al: Cerebrovascular accidents in children with cancer. Pediatrics 76:194–201, 1985.

27. Which neoplasms are associated with hemihypertrophy?

Wilms tumor, **hepatoblastoma**, and **adrenal cortical carcinoma** are associated with hemihypertrophy either as part of Beckwith-Wiedemann syndrome or in isolation. 1–3% of Wilms tumor patients have hemihypertrophy.

Breslow NE, Beckwith JB: Epidemiological features of Wilms tumor: Results of the National Wilms Tumor Study. JNCI 68:429–436, 1982.

28. Virilization may be associated with which childhood cancer?

Tumors that cause virilism are most commonly those producing large quantities of dehydroepiandrosterone (DHEA), a 17-ketosteroid. Tumors producing testosterone may also cause virilization. Most commonly these are benign tumors of the adrenal; rarely they are malignant. However, the distinction between carcinoma and benign adenoma frequently is difficult.

Occasionally males with primary hepatic neoplasms may become virilized because of production of androgens by the tumor.

Burr IM, et al: A testosterone-secreting tumor of the adrenal producing virilization in a female infant. Lancet 2:643, 1973.

29. Which childhood cancers commonly metastasize to the lungs?

Wilms tumor, osteosarcoma, Ewing sarcoma, rhabdomyosarcoma, and low-grade soft-tissue sarcomas such as fibrosarcoma and synovial sarcoma. Wilms tumor and Hodgkin disease can have lung metastases at diagnosis. Neuroblastoma and non-Hodgkin lymphoma rarely cause pulmonary parenchymal disease.

30. Which cancers are often associated with splenomegaly?

Acute leukemia, chronic myeloid leukemia, chronic myelomonocytic leukemia, Hodgkin disease, and non-Hodgkin lymphoma. Solid tumors rarely metastasize to the spleen to the point of causing splenomegaly.

31. Which cancers and chemotherapeutic agents are associated with the syndrome of inappropriate secretion of antidiuretic hormone (SIADH)?

SIADH occurs with CNS tumors, lung tumors (especially small cell carcinoma in adults), lymphoma, or GI carcinoma. It is also associated with vincristine or cyclophosphamide therapy.

32. A patient receiving chemotherapy has known bone marrow failure and a platelet count of 15,000/mm³ but no symptoms. Should prophylactic platelet transfusions be given?

A controversial matter. Many institutions empirically give platelets when the count falls below 20,000/mm³.

Reasons for	Reasons against
Hemorrhage from all sites reduced by maintaining platelet count > 20,000/mm³	Unnecessary since life-threatening bleeding rarely occurs without warning in a stable afebrile thrombocytopenic host
Risk of fatal intracranial hemorrhage practically eliminated	Fatal intracranial hemorrhage is extremely rare unless platelet count is < 5,000/mm³
Psychological benefit of preventing minor hemorrhage rather than treating it after it occurs	Platelets administered therapeutically for mucosal or internal bleeding just as effective as platelets given prophylactically
Alloimmunization, hepatitis, and other side effects not increased appreciably because most affected patients are heavily transfused anyway; leukocyte depletion filters and improved donor screening have reduced frequency of these complications	Greater likelihood of alloimmunization and allergic reactions
	Increased incidence of infectious complications, especially viral hepatitis
	Lack of controlled studies proving efficacy
	Expense

From Buchanan GR: Hematologic supportive care of the pediatric cancer patient. In Pizzo PA, Poplack DG (eds): Principles and Practice of Pediatric Oncology, 2nd ed. Philadelphia, J.B. Lippincott, 1993, p 978; with permission.

33. In a granulocytopenic patient receiving antibiotics who develops symptoms of esophagitis, what are the two most common infectious causes?

Candidiasis and **herpes simplex**. If examination of the oropharynx does not reveal signs of infection, this does not exclude the diagnosis because 50% of patients can have esophageal candidiasis without oral lesions. Controversy exists about whether to treat empirically (e.g., amphotericin, acyclovir, or both) or to perform esophagoscopy for a more definitive diagnosis (but with the risk of inducing bacteremia).

34. Is Langerhans cell histiocytosis a malignancy?

Formerly called histiocytosis X (the X tag was attached in 1953 because of the unknown nature of the entity), this condition is not considered a neoplasm but a disease of abnormal physiologic proliferation. The Langerhans cell is a tissue macrophage most commonly found in the skin. It functions as an antigen-presenting or dendritic cell. Excessive immune stimulation of unknown origin triggers growth of multiple cells rather than a clonal proliferation as is seen in a neoplasm. There is also a disorder designated malignant histiocytosis, which is histologically quite different from Langerhans cell histiocytosis.

35. Describe the clinical presentations of Langerhans cell histiocytosis.
The clinical presentation varies depending on the organs involved. This can range from solitary lytic bone lesions (in the skull, long bones, ribs, pelvis, and vertebral bodies) to more diffuse disease (bone lesions, proptosis, pituitary involvement with diabetes insipidus) to very disseminated disease (bone lesions, hepatosplenomegaly, lymphadenopathy, seborrheic skin lesions, pulmonary infiltration, and gastrointestinal involvement with subsequent failure to thrive). These three types of involvement were previously called eosinophilic granuloma, Hand-Schüller-Christian disease, and Letterer-Siwe disease, respectively.

EPIDEMIOLOGY

36. Is cancer the most common cause of death in children < age 15?
Cancer ranks a distant second, accounting for 10% of deaths in children < age 15. Accidents account for nearly 45% of deaths. Congenital anomalies rank third with 8%, and homicide ranks fourth with 5%.

37. What is the most common neoplasm of childhood?
Acute lymphoblastic leukemia. Approximately 4/100,00 children aged < 15 years develop this neoplasm annually, or about 2000 cases/year in the United States.
Pui C: Childhood leukemias. N Engl J Med 332:1618–1630, 1995.

38. What are the relative risks for children to develop leukemia?

Population at Risk	Estimate Risk	Time Interval (yrs)
U.S. white children	1:2800	10
Siblings of child with leukemia	1:700	10
Identical twin of child with leukemia	1:5	Wks to mos
Children with		
Down syndrome	1:75	10
Fanconi syndrome	1:12	21
Bloom syndrome	1:8	26
Ataxia-telangiectasia	1:8	25
Exposures		
Atom bomb within 1000 m	1:60	12
Ionizing radiation	?	10–25
Benzene	1:960	12
Alkylating agents	1:2000?	10–20

From Fernbach DJ: Neoplastic diseases. In Oski FA, et al (eds): Principles and Practice of Pediatrics, 2nd ed. Philadelphia, J.B. Lippincott, 1994, p 1702; with permission.

39. What is the relative incidence of the childhood cancers?

Leukemias	30%	Wilms tumor	6%
CNS tumors	19%	Bone tumors	5%
Lymphomas	13%	Retinoblastoma	1%
Neuroblastoma	8%	Other tumors	9%
Soft-tissue sarcomas	7%		

40. How does the type of cancer in pediatric patients vary by age?

Tumor Type	Newborns (%)	Infants (%)	Children < 15 yrs (%)
Leukemia	13	18	31
ALL	—	8	20
Other	—	10	10
CNS	3	8	18
Neuroblastoma	54	35	8
Lymphoma	0.3	1	14
Wilms tumor	13	11	6
Sarcoma (soft tissue and bone)	11	10	11
Liver	—	4	1.3
Teratoma	—	2	0.4
Retinoblastoma	—	9	4
Other	5.7	2	6.3

From Reaman GH: Special considerations for the infant with cancer. In Pizzo PA, Poplack DG (eds): Principles and Practice of Pediatric Oncology, 2nd ed. Philadelphia, J.B. Lippincott, 1993, p 304; with permission.

41. Which childhood cancers can be congenital?

In a 30-year period at the M.D. Anderson Hospital, there were 423 infant neoplasms, of which 24 (5%) occurred in neonates and could be considered congenital. These included 8 fibrosarcomas, 6 neuroblastomas, 3 CNS tumors, 3 leukemias, 2 retinoblastomas, 1 Langerhans cell histiocytosis, and 1 malignant melanoma.

Cangir A, et al: Malignant neoplasms in the neonatal period. Proc Am Soc Clin Oncol 6:A847, 1987.

42. Which childhood tumors are hereditary?

Retinoblastoma is familial in about 40% of cases. All patients with bilateral disease should be considered to have the hereditary form. Rarely, neuroblastoma and Wilms tumor are associated with familial occurrence. The hereditary basis for the Li-Fraumeni syndrome (in which there is cancer at an early age in two first-degree relatives of a proband with a sarcoma in childhood) involves a mutated tumor suppressor gene, p53.

Knudson AG Jr: Hereditary cancer, oncogenes and antioncogenes. Cancer Res 45:1437, 1985.

43. Which cancers have a significant racial predilection?

Wilms tumor has a higher incidence in black female infants. Ewing tumor is about 30 times more common in whites than in blacks. Hodgkin disease is rare in those of East Asian descent.

44. Name the cancers that are most commonly associated with a second neoplasm.

Primary Tumors	Secondary Tumors
Retinoblastoma	Osteosarcoma Pinealoblastoma
Hodgkin disease	Acute nonlymphoblastic leukemia Non-Hodgkin lymphoma Sarcoma in radiation field Thyroid carcinoma
Acute lymphoblastic leukemia	Brain tumors Non-Hodgkin lymphoma
Sarcomas	Sarcomas

45. Are any childhood cancers associated with an increased alpha-fetoprotein?

Increased alpha-fetoprotein is associated with germ cell tumors, including endodermal sinus tumors of the ovary and testicular yolk sac carcinoma, hepatocellular tumors, and retinoblastoma. Normally, alpha-fetoprotein is synthesized in the liver, yolk sac, and GI tract of the fetus. Synthesis usually stops at birth; it disappears with a half-life of 3.5 days. Elevated serum levels are most commonly seen with nonmalignant liver disease. Levels remain elevated for 5–7 weeks after resection of the tumor but persistence beyond that time is suggestive of residual disease.

46. Are there any known transplacental carcinogens?

Diethylstilbestrol, which was used to prevent spontaneous abortion, has been associated with an increased risk of vaginal cancer in the female offspring. It has also been reported that there is a 10-fold increased risk of monoblastic leukemia in the infants of mothers who smoke marijuana. It has been suggested that sedatives and a number of nonhormonal drugs are transplacental carcinogens, but this is not proven. It also has not been proved that cigarette smoke or the use of oral contraceptives are transplacental carcinogens.

47. Over the past 35 years, how has the 5-year survival rate changed for children aged < 15 with cancer?

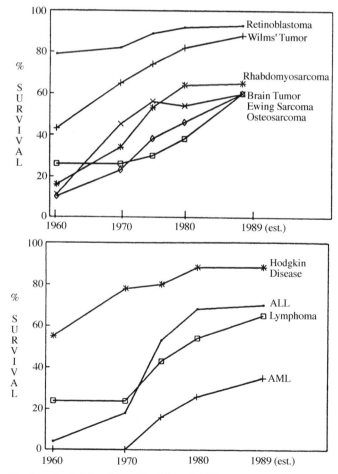

From Robison LL: General principles of the epidemiology of childhood cancer. In Pizzo PA, Poplack DG (eds): Principles and Practice of Pediatric Oncology, 2nd ed. Philadelphia, J.B. Lippincott, 1993, p 9; with permission.

LEUKEMIA

48. What is the normal lymphoblast concentration in bone marrow?

5%. At least 25% of the bone marrow should be occupied by lymphoblasts to confirm the diagnosis of leukemia. In most cases, the marrow is very hypercellular, with 60–100% of the contents being lymphoblastic.

49. What are the most common clinical findings in the initial presentation of acute lymphoblastic leukemia (ALL)?

Hepatosplenomegaly—70% (10–15% of children have marked enlargement of the liver or
   spleen to a level below the umbilicus).
Fever—40–60%
Lymphadenopathy—25–50% with moderate or marked enlargement
Bleeding—25–50% with petechiae or purpura
Bone/joint pain—25–40%
Fatigue—30%
Anorexia—20–35%

50. What are the typical hematologic findings noted on presentation of ALL?

Leukocyte count (mm³)
   <10,000   45–55%
   10,000–50,000   30–35%
   > 50,000   20%
Hemoglobin (gm/dl)
   < 7.5   45%
   7.5–10.0   30%
   > 10   25%
Platelet count (mm³)
   < 20,000   25%
   20,000–99,000   50%
   > 100,000   25%

51. What is the single most important prognostic factor in leukemia at the time of diagnosis?

The **total WBC count**. The greater the total WBCs (particularly counts > 50,000), the worse the prognosis.

52. List the other prognostic indicators in ALL.

Prognostic Factors in Acute Lymphoblastic Leukemia

FACTOR	FAVORABLE	UNFAVORABLE
WBC	< 10,000/mm³	> 10,000/mm³
Age	2–10 yrs	<1 or > 10 yrs
Immunophenotype	CALLA⁺, non-T cell	CALLA⁻, SIg⁺, Cyμ⁺, T cell
Morphology	L1	L2, L3
Chromosomes	Normal	Translocations: t9;22, t4;11, t8;14, t2;8, t8;22, t1;19
DNA content	Normal or hyperdiploid	Hypodiploid, haploid
Bulky disease	Absent	Present
Sex	Female	Male

Bleyer WA, et al: The staging of childhood acute lymphoblastic leukemia: Strategies of the Children's Cancer Study Group and a three-dimensional technic of multivariate analysis. Med Pediatr Oncol 14:271–280, 1986.

53. Which factors are important in the prognosis of acute myelogenous leukemia (AML)?

Prognostic Factors in Acute Myelogenous Leukemia

FACTOR	FAVORABLE	UNFAVORABLE
WBC	< 100,000/mm³	> 100,000/mm³
Age	< 17 yrs	> 60 yrs
Morphology	Myelocytic	Monocytic
Chromosomes	Normal, t8;21, 47 + 8	–x, –y, –7, –5
Onset	Abrupt	Preleukemia, myelodysplasia, secondary leukemia

Grier HE, et al: Prognostic factors in childhood acute myelogenous leukemia. J Clin Oncol 5:1026–1032, 1987.

54. Why do children with acute leukemia under 1 year of age have a worse prognosis?

The great majority of infants with ALL under age 1 year often have a full complement of unfavorable features: high WBC count, CNS leukemia, bulky extramedullary disease, and t4;11 (a translocation associated with poor response to therapy). In contrast, the prognosis for infants with AML is not necessarily less favorable than for older children (except for those with monoblastic leukemia, who fare poorly).

Reamon G, et al: Acute lymphoblastic leukemia in infants less than one year of age. J Clin Oncol 3:1513–1521, 1985.

55. Why do boys with ALL fare more poorly than girls?

The precise answer is unclear, but two factors may be important:

1. In boys who are in remission after a full course of chemotherapy, testicular involvement is the most common site of relapse, occurring in up to 10% of cases. In girls, ovarian relapse is very rare, though difficult to diagnose after bone marrow relapse.

2. In older boys and teenage males, there is a higher incidence of T-cell disease than in girls. T-cell disease is associated with adverse prognostic factors (high WBC count, hepatosplenomegaly, and mediastinal masses) and alone carries a poor prognosis.

56. What bony changes are seen in leukemia?

1. Osteopenia
2. Metaphyseal lucency
3. Pathologic fractures
4. Periosteal elevation

57. What percentage of children with ALL can successfully achieve a first remission?

Almost all children (98%) with ALL achieve remission with combination chemotherapy. Some require only vincristine, prednisone, and L-asparaginase; others with unfavorable features may require additional therapy such as daunorubicin.

58. Why is CNS preventive therapy important in the treatment of leukemia?

At the time of diagnosis, < 5% of pediatric patients diagnosed with leukemia have evidence of overt CNS involvement. Before the institution of cranial irradiation and intrathecal chemotherapy, as many as 75% of patients demonstrated a CNS relapse. With the advent of CNS prophylaxis, that relapse rate has been reduced to < 5%. However, the preventive treatment (especially radiation) has been associated with multiple long-term effects, particularly injury to the hypothalamic-pituitary axis. Alternative experimental methods which avoid the use of radiation include the use of triple intrathecal chemotherapeutic agents and high-dose systemic methotrexate (which can penetrate the CNS).

59. What is the optimal duration for maintenance chemotherapy in ALL?

While this may ultimately be shown to vary by prognostic factors (e.g., sex), most centers treat between 2.5–3 years. The optimal duration remains a question for ongoing study.

60. How is ALL distinguished from AML?

A variety of techniques are used to make the distinction. The primary basis for the distinction involves the findings seen on light microscopy. Morphologically, compared with AML, ALL has a high nuclear/cytoplasmic ratio, clumped (rather than spongy) nuclear chromatin, fewer nucleoli (< 2 vs 2–5), and no Auer rods. With histochemical staining, AML (unlike ALL) usually stains positive with peroxidase and Sudan black. ALL (except FAB L3) is positive for terminal deoxynucleotidyl transferase (TdT), whereas AML is not. Through the use of monoclonal antibodies, immunophenotyping may also be done. Cytogenetic chromosomal studies may be helpful, as abnormalities are found in > 80% of patients with AML.

61. What factors are associated with an increased incidence of AML?

- Down syndrome
- Fanconi anemia
- Bloom syndrome
- Kostmann syndrome
- Diamond-Blackfan anemia
- Ionizing radiation
- Myelodysplastic syndromes
- Aplastic anemia (after immunosuppressive therapy)
- Benzene exposure
- Drugs (alkylating agents and epipodophyllotoxins)

From Grier HE, Weinstein HJ: Acute myelogenous leukemia. In Pizzo PA, Poplack DG (eds): Principles and Practice of Pediatric Oncology, 2nd ed. Philadelphia, J.B. Lippincott, 1993, p 484; with permission.

62. How do adult and juvenile types of chronic myelogenous leukemia (CML) differ?

	Adult CML	Juvenile CML
General health	Well	Ill
Splenomegaly	Marked	Moderate
Hepatomegaly	Usually absent	Usually present
WBC	> 100,000/μm^3	< 100,000/μm^3
Differential	Mostly granulocytes	Monocytosis
Platelets	> 400,000/mm^3	< 150,000/mm^3
LAP[A]	Decreased or absent	Normal
Chromosomes	Ph^1	Normal or –7
Growth in vitro	Granulocytic colonies	Monocytic colonies or increased clusters
Median survival	3 yr	9 mo–1 yr, but variable
Therapy	Stem cell transplantation	Stem cell transplantation

LAP[A] = leukocyte alkaline phosphatase; Ph^1 = Philadelphia chromosome (t9;22)
Cao A: Juvenile chronic myelogenous leukemia. Lancet 1:1002, 1970.
Chessels JM, et al: The Ph chromosome in childhood leukemia. Br J Haematol 41:25–41, 1979.
Nix WL, Ferbach DJ: Myeloproliferative diseases of childhood. Am J Pediatr Hematol Oncol 3:397–407, 1981.

63. In children who have very elevated WBC counts, why are CNS hemorrhagic complications more likely in AML than ALL?

Compared with lymphocytes, leukocytes (especially promyelocytes and monoblasts) contain compounds with procoagulant activity that are released as the cells lyse and may led to microthrombi formation, disseminated intravascular coagulation, and hemorrhage.

64. In what setting does the Philadelphia chromosome (Ph^1) occur?

Ph^1 is the result of a balanced translocation between chromosomes 9 and 22 [specifically, t(9;22) (q34;q11)]. The result is a new fusion gene that codes for a tyrosine kinase with increased enzymatic activity. Ph^1 is seen in > 90% of patients with CML, but also in up to 5% of children with ALL and in up to 2% with AML.

65. How do remission and relapse rates vary in ALL and AML?

Most children with ALL survive relapse-free, and so the median duration of first remission has not been reached. If relapse occurs in the CNS or testes, many children can still be cured with irradiation and additional chemotherapy. If relapse occurs in the marrow within 18 months of diagnosis, the chance of cure with either chemotherapy or stem cell transplant is < 10%. If marrow relapse occur > 18 months from diagnosis, and especially if it occurs after treatment has been stopped, intense chemotherapy or stem cell transplant may offer prolonged second remission and possible cure in > 25% of patients.

Between 75–80% of children with AML achieve remission, with median remission duration of about 14 months. About 10% of the patients die from infectious or hemorrhagic complications during induction, and another 10–20% fail to respond to the initial therapy. Of the children who achieve remission, between 40–50% survive 5 years. If disease recurs, it is usually fatal. Transplant may cure some patients who relapse.

66. How do survival rates in children vary by leukemia type?

- Chemotherapeutic regimens cure as many as 70% of children with ALL, ranging from approximately 40% with multiple high-risk factors to 85% with lower risk.
- AML is associated with a cure rate of 30–40%.
- CML requires allogenic stem cell transplantation and has a 5-year survival rate of 80–90% for the adult form of the disease and 40–50% for the juvenile form.

Pui C-H: Childhood leukemias. N Engl J Med 332:1618–1630, 1995.

67. What distinguishes leukemia from lymphoma?

The distinction is often difficult because ALL can resemble non-Hodgkin lymphoma. Cytomorphologically, there is little difference between T-cell lymphoblastic lymphoma and ALL or between the B-cells of Burkitt lymphoma and mature B-cell ALL. As a rule, the presence of a significant number of blasts cells in the bone marrow (in most centers, > 25%) indicates leukemia.

68. Besides leukemia, what childhood malignancies can present with significant bone marrow involvement?

Neuroblastoma, rhabdomyosarcoma, retinoblastoma, non-Hodgkin lymphoma

LYMPHOMA

69. What is the age distribution of children with Hodgkin lymphoma?

Hodgkin disease is uncommon before 5 years of age, but rare cases occur under 3 years. In North America, the peak incidence occurs in the second decade of life with a slight male predominance. It continues into young adulthood and then decreases in frequency until the sixth decade. The sex ratio changes from male predominance to female predominance after 12 years of age.

70. How is Hodgkin disease clinically staged?

Ann Arbor Staging

Stage I	Single lymph node region (I) or single extralymphatic organ or site (I_E)
Stage II	Two or more lymph node regions on the same side of diaphragm (II)
Stage III	Involvement of lymph node regions on both sides of diaphragm (III), which may also be accompanied by localized involvement of extralymphatic organ or site (III_E) or by involvement of spleen (III_S)
Stage IV	Diffuse or disseminated involvement of one or more extralymphatic organs or tissues with or without associated lymph node enlargement

Hodgkin lymphoma, like non-Hodgkin lymphoma, is classified according to stage of disease and histology, as in the Ann Arbor System. It is also staged according to whether there are symptoms. Patients with no symptoms are referred to as having *A* disease. Patients with documented fever, involuntary weight loss > 10%, or night sweats are considered to have *B* disease. Intractable pruritus may also be a symptom but is not among the B symptoms used for staging.

Stage is determined both clinically and pathologically. Clinical staging refers to staging that is done without histologic proof. Pathologic staging refers to biopsy-proven disease in a given region and usually involves a staging laparotomy and splenectomy to determine the extent of disease. For example, a patient who is symptom-free and who has a positive node in his neck and a mass in the mediastinum but nothing else detectable on physical examination or radiologic studies is said to have *clinical stage* IIA disease. If the patient goes on to have a staging laparotomy and splenectomy, and no disease is found, he would then be considered to have *pathologic stage* IIA disease.

71. What is the histologic classification of Hodgkin disease?

*The Rye, New York, Histologic Classification**

	LYMPHOCYTES	R/S CELLS	OTHER	INCIDENCE
Lymphocyte predominant	Many	Few	Histiocytes	5%
Nodular sclerosing	Many	Few or many	Bands of refractile fibrosis	70%
Mixed cellularity	Many	Few or many	Eosinophils, histiocytes	20–30%
Lymphocyte depletion	Few	Many	No refractile fibrosis	< 5%

* Based on the relative number of lymphocytes and Reed-Sternberg (R/S) cells.

72. What is the prognosis for the various stages of Hodgkin disease?

The prognosis for children with Hodgkin disease is excellent in that most are cured. For stages I and IIA, the 5-year relapse-free survival is > 80% for patients treated with radiation only and may be > 90% for patients given radiation and chemotherapy. For stage IIB, prognosis is less good, especially if there is a massive mediastinal tumor, but 5-year survival is still > 80%. The same survival figures pertain to stage IIIA disease, but treatment generally is more extensive than that for a limited stage II disease. For stage IV disease, 5-year relapse-free survival is > 60–70%.

73. How are non-Hodgkin lymphomas classified?

Non-Hodgkin lymphomas (NHLs) include a heterogeneous group of malignant solid tumors that are of lymphoid origin. Their classification is still disputed. In general, NHLs are divided according to the extent of spread in the body and histology. The disease is either localized or disseminated. Localized tumors are limited to either a node or an area, such as the appendix or a tonsil, and may include some regional surrounding nodes. It can also originate in bone. The tumor cells may spread to the bone marrow or spinal fluid much like leukemia or disseminate throughout the abdomen and pleural space.

Histology is divided into lymphoblastic and nonlymphoblastic types. The most common type of lymphoblastic lymphoma occurs in the mediastinum and probably originates in the thymus. Disease is virtually always disseminated at diagnosis. Nonlymphoblastic lymphomas include Burkitt lymphoma or peripheral T-cell lymphomas. Burkitt lymphoma often occurs in the retroperitoneum and is usually disseminated. The classification of NHLs of childhood is very different from that of adults.

Sandlund JT, et al: Non-Hodgkin's lymphoma in childhood. N Engl J Med 334:1238–1248, 1996.

74. Which tumor has the shortest doubling time?

Burkitt lymphoma. The generation time of the Burkitt cell is 24–36 hours. However, the actual doubling time is less than that because there is a very high spontaneous cell death rate. Some T-lymphoblastic leukemia/lymphomas have a doubling time similar to that of Burkitt cells.

NERVOUS SYSTEM TUMORS

75. How do pediatric brain tumors differ from those of adults?

In adults, most tumors are supratentorial with the vast majority being astrocytomas. In children, most tumors are infratentorial, of which up to 40% may be primitive neuroepithelial neoplasms. Meningiomas, Schwann-cell tumors, pituitary tumors, and metastatic intracranial disease are relatively common in adults but rare in children. However, in children, histologic types vary more widely than in adults.

76. What is the relative distribution of the most common brain tumors in children?

Infratentorial	(45–60%)
Primitive neuroectodermal tumor (i.e., medulloblastoma)	20–25%
Low-grade cerebellar astrocytoma	12–18%
Ependymoma	4–8%
Malignant glioma, brainstem	3–9%
Supratentorial, hemispheric	(25–40%)
Low-grade astrocytoma	8–20%
Malignant glioma	6–12%
Supratentorial, midline	(15–20%)
Craniopharyngioma	6–9%
Low-grade hypothalamic glioma	4–8%
Pineal tumors	2–6%

Pollack IF: Brain tumors in children. N Engl J Med 331:1500–1507, 1994.

77. What are the advantages and disadvantages of MRI (compared to CT) in the diagnosis of pediatric brain tumors?

Advantages	Disadvantages
• No radiation exposure	• Longer scanning time
• Images in multiple planes	• Increased movement artifact
• Minimal bone artifacts	• Difficulties in separating tumor from edema or scar
	• Poor visualization of subarachnoid space

These disadvantages are being minimized by newer technologies with shorter scanning times.

78. Where do brain tumors metastasize?

Most brain tumors do not metastasize. They are fatal because of local invasion. Some may disseminate through the cerebrospinal fluid or "drop" metastases to the spinal cord or cauda equina. Medulloblastoma may metastasize to bone or bone marrow. Rarely, lymph nodes, liver, or pancreas may be involved.

79. Which CNS tumors are associated with a favorable or unfavorable prognosis?

Tumor Type	Treatment	Prognosis (5-Year Survival)
Posterior fossa		
Cerebellar astrocytoma	Surgical resection	> 90%
Medulloblastoma	Surgery + craniospinal radiation therapy ± chemotherapy	Good risk, 70% Poor risk, 30–40%
Brainstem glioma	Biopsy ± local radiation (hyperfractionation)	< 20%
Midline tumors		
Craniopharyngioma	Surgery, total or partial resection ± radiation therapy	50–90%
Hypothalamic glioma	Biopsy + local radiation	50–70%
Germinoma	Surgery + radiation + chemotherapy	70–90%
Supratentorial		
Oligodendroglioma	Surgery ± local radiation therapy	70%
Glioblastoma multiforme	Surgery + wide-field radiation therapy (consider chemotherapy)	0–20%
Low-grade astrocytoma	Surgery ± local radiation	50–70%

From Duffner PK, Cohen ME: Brain tumors in children. In Kaufman DM, et al (eds): Child and Adolescent Neurology for Psychiatrists. Baltimore, Williams & Wilkins, 1992, p 123; with permission.

80. How is the DNA content useful in assessing the prognosis of tumors?

With flow cytometric analysis, the content of DNA per cell (i.e., tumor DNA index) can be calculated. The DNA index correlates with cell ploidy (i.e., the number of chromosome sets in a cell) and can be compared with that of normal cells. In various neoplasms (e.g., leukemia, neuroblastoma) DNA indexes > 1 are associated with a better prognosis.

81. Which posterior fossa tumor is commonly associated with erythrocytosis?

Cerebellar hemangioblastoma. This tumor can secrete erythropoietin.

82. How does the pathophysiology of spinal cord compression differ in children compared with adults?

In children, spinal cord compression most commonly is due to primary or metastatic disease in the epidural space, especially with sarcoma, neuroblastoma, lymphoma, and leukemia. In adults, metastatic disease is likely to involve the vertebral body, with compression caused by tumor growth extending through the intervertebral foramina. This event rarely occurs in children.

83. How can the site of spinal cord compression be clinically localized?

Spinal tenderness on percussion correlates with localization in up to 80% of patients. In addition, neurologic evaluation of strength, sensory level changes, reflexes, and anal tone can help to pinpoint the location in the spinal cord, conus medullaris (terminal neural portion of the spinal cord), or cauda equina.

Clinical Localization of Site of Spinal Cord Compression

SIGN	SPINAL CORD	CONUS MEDULLARIS	CAUDA EQUINA
Weakness	Symmetric, profound	Symmetric, variable	Asymmetric, may be mild
Tendon reflexes	Increased or absent	Increased knee, decreased ankle	Decreased, asymmetric
Babinski reflex	Extensor	Extensor	Plantar
Sensory	Symmetric, sensory level	Symmetric, saddle	Asymmetric, radicular
Sphincter abnormality	Spared until late	Early involvement	May be spared
Progression	Rapid	Variable, may be rapid	Variable, may be rapid

From Lange B, et al: Oncologic emergencies. In Pizzo PA, Poplack DG (eds): Principles and Practice of Pediatric Oncology, 2nd ed. Philadelphia, J.B. Lippincott, 1993, p 964; with permission.

84. Should all infants be screened for neuroblastoma?

Urinary vanillylmandelic acid (VMA) is often elevated in children with neuroblastoma. Screening of infants using urinary VMA has been investigated in Japan, Canada, and the United States, and initial studies indicated that patients might be identified earlier in the course of disease and cured at a higher rate. However, subsequent analyses showed that screening may identify a group of patients with tumors that are destined for spontaneous regression or a benign course.

Carlsen LT: Neuroblastoma: Epidemiology and pattern of regression: Problems in interpreting results of mass screening. Am J Pediatr Hematol Oncol 14:103–109, 1992.

85. How can neuroblastoma be distinguished from other "small round blue cell" tumors in children?

Certain tumors—neuroblastoma, non-Hodgkin lymphoma, Ewing sarcoma, rhabdomyosarcoma, retinoblastoma, and primitive neuroectodermal tumors (i.e., medulloblastoma)—appear very similar when stained with hematoxylin-eosin and examined with light microscopy. **Immunohistochemical staining** can help to distinguish between them. For example, neuroblastoma stains with monoclonal antibodies that recognize neurofilaments, synaptophysin, and neuron-specific enolase, and the other tumors do not. Other distinguishing features are the elevation of urinary catecholamine metabolites and the amplification of the N-*myc* gene.

86. What are the most common presentations of neuroblastoma?

The most common presentation is generalized disease in a child < 5 years of age (88%). 55% of children with generalized disease are under age 2. Most children with neuroblastoma are irritable and ill, and they often have exquisite bone pain, proptosis, and periorbital ecchymoses. 70% of neuroblastomas arise in the abdomen; half of these arise in the adrenal, and the other half in the parasympathetic ganglia distributed throughout the retroperitoneum and the paravertebral area in the chest and neck. The tumor produces and excretes catecholamines, which can cause systemic symptoms such as sweating, hypertension, diarrhea, and irritability. Children with localized neuroblastoma may have symptoms referable to a mass such as Horner syndrome. Some may have no symptoms, but the condition may be detected on a routine newborn examination when an adrenal mass is felt, or on a chest radiograph taken for other reasons where an incidental posterior mediastinal mass is seen.

87. What percentage of neuroblastoma tumors do not produce catecholamines?

5–10%. About 70% of the neuroblastomas secrete vanillylmandelic acid (VMA) which is excreted in the urine. If all catecholamines and their metabolites (e.g,. norepinephrine, epinephrine, dopamine, homovanillic acid [HVA], and VMA) are measured, 90–95% of patients will have elevated values. A high ratio of HVA to VMA and the absence of any catecholamine excretion are considered unfavorable prognostic factors.

Siegel SE, et al: Patterns of urinary catecholamine metabolite excretion. In Neuroblastoma Research. New York, Raven Press, 1990.

88. How is neuroblastoma classified?

International Classification of Neuroblastoma

Stage I	Localized tumor grossly excised with or without microscopic residual disease; lymph nodes negative microscopically
Stage IIA	Unilateral tumor incompletely excised with lymph nodes negative microscopically
Stage IIB	Unilateral tumor completely or incompletely excised with positive ipsilateral regional lymph nodes; identifiable contralateral lymph nodes negative microscopically
Stage III	Tumor infiltrating across the midline incompletely excised with or without lymph node involvement; or unilateral tumor with contralateral regional lymph node involvement
Stage IV	Dissemination of tumor to distant lymph nodes; bone marrow, bone, liver, and/or other organs
Stage IVS	Localized primary tumor as defined for Stage I or IIA with dissemination limited to liver, skin, or bone marrow in an infant ≤ 12 months of age

89. How does the prognosis for neuroblastoma vary by stage?

Patients with **Stage I or II** disease have nearly a 90% chance of cure with surgery alone. Children whose disease is not controlled with surgery frequently have unfavorable biologic features, such as unfavorable histology (i.e., many mitotic figures and/or karyorrhexis) and elevated serum ferritin, amplified N-*myc* cellular oncogene, or both.

Patients with **Stage III** disease have a 50% chance of cure with surgery, radiation, and chemotherapy. Their prognosis is also determined by biologic features at diagnosis.

Patients with **Stage IV** disease have about a 20% chance of long-term survival. Age is an especially important prognostic variable in that those < 1 year have a considerably better outlook.

Patients with **Stage IVS** disease have a > 80% chance of long-term survival with supportive care alone. Infants under age 6 weeks may die of liver failure or mechanical problems related to a big liver. Few patients with stage IVS disease actually progress to typical Stage IV disease with bone and extensive marrow involvement.

Brodeur GM, et al: International criteria for diagnosis, staging and response to treatment in patients with neuroblastoma. J Clin Oncol 6:1874–1881, 1990.

90. How does N-*myc* gene affect the prognosis of neuroblastoma?

N-*myc* is a proto-oncogene which, upon activation, may be important in the development and aggressiveness of neuroblastoma. The number of copies of N-*myc* per cell has been shown to be important in prognosis: < 3 indicates a more favorable prognosis and > 10 suggests a poorer prognosis.

Look T, et al: Clinical relevance of tumor cell ploidy and N-*myc* gene amplification in childhood neuroblastoma: A Pediatric Oncology Group study. J Clin Oncol 9:581–591, 1991.

91. In addition to retinoblastoma, what diseases can present with leukokoria?

Leukokoria, or white pupil, can be obvious or can be a subtle asymmetry on pupillary red reflex evaluation. Of note, 20–30% of cases of retinoblastoma are bilateral. A pediatric ophthalmologist familiar with the disease is usually able to distinguish retinoblastoma from other causes of leukokoria, which include:

- *Toxocara canis* infection
- Persistent hyperplastic primary vitreous
- Coats disease
- Large chorioretinal coloboma
- Retinopathy of prematurity (retrolental fibroplasia)
- Congenital cataract
- Retinal dysplasia
- Medulloepithelioma (dictyoma)
- Congenital retinal fold
- Uveitis

French-Howard GL, Ellsworth RM: Differential diagnosis of retinoblastoma: A statistical survey of 500 children: I. Relative frequency of lesions which simulate retinoblastoma. Am J Ophthalmol 60:610, 1965.

92. What role does genetic evaluation have in patients with retinoblastoma?

Patients with retinoblastoma and their families should have genetic counseling. Patients or parents who are suspected to be gene carriers include those with bilateral disease or multiple tumors in one eye, those with a family history of retinoblastoma, and those with one or more affected offspring. With familial retinoblastoma, the risk of disease in subsequent offspring is 30–50%. Among these offspring, half will have bilateral tumors. In counseling parents of a child with familial retinoblastoma, it is important to discuss the increased risk of other tumors (e.g., osteosarcoma) in patients who are gene carriers. Cure rates for retinoblastoma are excellent; however, osteosarcoma is a more sinister and less curable disease. The risk to the offspring of the patient with unilateral sporadic retinoblastoma or to subsequent offspring of unaffected parents with a negative family history and one affected offspring is relatively low.

Vogel F: Genetics of retinoblastoma. Hum Genet 52:1, 1979.

93. How are tumor-suppressor genes involved in retinoblastoma?

Tumor-suppressor genes encode for proteins necessary in the control of cell growth and differentiation. The *RB1* gene belongs to a group of tumor-suppressor genes located on chromosome 13. In some cases of retinoblastoma, there appears to be loss of one allele of the *RB1* gene in the germline followed by the loss of the other allele in the tumor. This loss of heterozygosity leaves the tumor cells without the regulatory function of the gene and is thought to contribute to oncogenesis. A similar situation is thought to occur with the p53 tumor-suppressor gene in the Li-Fraumeni syndrome (cancer at an early age in two first-degree relatives of a proband with sarcoma in childhood).

94. What is the most common secondary tumor in patients with bilateral retinoblastoma?

Osteogenic sarcoma. In the past, when the primary tumor was treated with radiation therapy in high doses, the incidence of osteosarcomas was as high as 33%, and the tumors were often in the orbit. Without any radiation therapy, only 5% of children with bilateral retinoblastoma develop osteosarcoma, and the osteosarcoma usually occurs at the femur.

95. What are the sequelae of treatments for brain tumors?

In the effort to achieve a cure, therapies can disrupt normal brain function. **Surgery** can result in abnormal cognitive and motor function, because it is often impossible to excise the malignant tissue without some normal brain. Surgery involving the hypothalamus or pituitary axis may result in SIADH or diabetes insipidus. The placement of a ventricular shunt device increases the infection of risk and the risk of subsequent shunt malfunction. There is also an increased risk of bleeding into the tumor bed.

Radiation therapy can affect cognitive functioning and may result in microangiopathic vasculitis or large-vessel disease. Postirradiation edema is usually transient but may cause seizures or signs and symptoms of increased intracranial pressure.

Chemotherapy may result in hearing impairment (platinum derivatives) and leukoencephalopathy (methotrexate). Seizures are a common problem during and after **multimodal therapy**.

Bloom HG, et al: The treatment and long-term prognosis of children with intracranial tumors: A study of 610 cases, 1950–1981. Int J Radiat Oncol Biol Phys 18:722–745, 1990.

96. In what setting does the "somnolence syndrome" occur?

About 3–12 weeks after receiving cranial irradiation (most commonly CNS prophylaxis for ALL), children can develop symptoms of lethargy, irritability, nausea and vomiting, cerebellar ataxia, dysarthria, dysphagia, anorexia, low-grade fever, and headache that last for about 2 weeks. CT and CSF studies are usually normal, but an EEG will often reveal a slow-wave activity consistent with diffuse cerebral disturbance. The use of steroids during irradiation appears to minimize the occurrence of the syndrome.

Mandell LR, et al: Reduced incidence of the somnolence syndrome in leukemic children with steroid coverage during prophylactic cranial radiation therapy. Cancer 63:1975, 1989.

SOLID TUMORS

97. What is the most common solid malignancy of childhood?

As a group, **brain tumors** are most common. Medulloblastoma, a primitive neuroectodermal tumor arising in the cerebellum or vermis, is the single most common type of this tumor.

98. What is the 5-year survival for the common solid tumors of childhood?

Survival from solid tumors in childhood has increased dramatically over the last three decades. For all diagnoses, the survival rate has increased from 28% for 1960–63 to 65% for 1980–85. One of the most dramatic successes has been in the treatment of Wilms tumor: survival increased from 33% in the 1960s to 80% in the 1980s.

Crist WM, Kun LE: Common solid tumors of childhood. N Engl J Med 324:461–471, 1991.

99. What are the factors contributing to relapse of solid tumors?

Even in the best centers, and despite treatment delivered in an optimal manner for very curable tumors, relapses occur for reasons that remain unexplained and are probably intrinsic to the biology of the tumor. However, the following variables may contribute to treatment failure:

1. Suboptimal treatment not according to a recognized protocol or administered by an inexperienced physician
2. Failure to control the primary tumor with surgery and irradiation
3. Metastatic spread of tumor at presentation
4. Tumor resistant to chemotherapy

Poor patient compliance with the treatment regimen has been documented, but its contribution to outcome remains unclear.

100. How is Wilms tumor distinguished radiographically from neuroblastoma?

In Wilms tumor, CT images will show intrinsic distortion of the kidney parenchyma and collecting system. Neuroblastoma is almost always extrarenal and causes displacement, not distortion, of the renal parenchyma and collecting system. In addition, calcifications are seen in > 50% of children with abdominal neuroblastoma, but in only 10% of children with Wilms tumor.

101. Which congenital anomalies are associated with Wilms tumor?

Congenital abnormalities include genitourinary anomalies (4.4%), hemihypertrophy (2.9%), and aniridia (1.1%). The genitourinary anomalies include hypoplasia of the kidney, fusion or ectopia of the kidney, duplication of the collecting system, and hypospadias. Multiple pigmented nevi and hemangiomas are also associated with hemihypertrophy and Wilms tumor. Patients with aniridia may have associated eye lesions, mental retardation, or deformities of the skull or face. Wilms tumor has also been described in patients with neurofibromatosis.

Pendergrass TW: Congenital anomalies in children with Wilms' tumor. Cancer 37:403, 1976.

102. Why can congestive heart failure develop in some patients with Wilms tumor?

Heart failure in uncommon in this disease, but if it develops, it is usually iatrogenic and most commonly caused by a combination of irradiation and radiomimetic antitumor drugs, such as doxorubicin and dactinomycin. Radiation alone is unlikely to cause heart failure, but the addition of the cardiotoxic doxorubicin may add to myocardial damage. Dactinomycin is not cardiotoxic but can contribute to heart damage by its radiomimetic affect. Heart failure can also be caused by the upward spread of a renal vein tumor thrombus to the heart, causing tamponade. Rarely, long-standing hypertension may result in dilated cardiomyopathy and congestive heart failure.

103. What are unfavorable prognostic factors in Wilms tumor?

The most important prognostic factors include the presence of metastases and tumor histology. In the National Wilms Tumor Study, patients with no metastatic disease had an actuarial survival of 83%, but only 31% of those with liver metastases and 5% of children with pulmonary metastases survived. Anaplastic, sarcomatous, or clear cell histology are all unfavorable prognostic factors. Additional unfavorable factors include age > 2 years, positive regional lymph nodes, operative spillage of tumor, large tumor size, direct extension within the abdomen, and invasion of extrarenal vessels.

104. At what ages do the common bony tumors occur?

The two common primary tumors of bone in children are osteogenic sarcoma and Ewing sarcoma. **Osteogenic sarcoma** most commonly occurs during the adolescent growth spurt. It rarely occurs in young children. **Ewing sarcoma** has a peak incidence in adolescents but may be seen in patients as young as 2–4 years of age. Its incidence increases progressively in the first two decades of life.

105. Osteosarcoma is generally located in which part of the bone?

The **metaphyses** of long bones of the extremities. Sixty percent of tumors are located in the metaphyses of the knee, i.e., the proximal tibia or distal femur.

106. What is the prognosis for children with osteosarcoma?

Between 40–70% of children with osteosarcoma will be alive without evidence of metastatic disease 2 years after diagnosis if they are treated with amputation or limb-salvage procedure plus multiagent chemotherapy. Some of these children will develop pulmonary metastases at a later time, and a proportion of these can be saved with thoracotomy. Without the use of chemotherapy, only 20% of the children will be free of metastatic disease 1 year after diagnosis.

107. Why is surgical intervention (i.e., amputation) alone insufficient in the treatment of osteosarcoma?

Up to 80–90% of patients have silent pulmonary micrometastases at the time of diagnosis. The micrometastases are not apparent on imaging studies but will become radiographically evident in 6–9 months if not treated with adjuvant chemotherapy. Surgical treatment alone is associated with only a 10–20% survival rate.

108. What is the cell of origin of Ewing sarcoma?

Until the 1980s, it was believed that this tumor was of endothelial origin. More recently, evidence suggests that it arises from **postganglionic parasympathetic cholinergic neurons** (in contrast to classic neuroblastoma, which arises from adrenergic or mixed neurons of the adrenal medulla and sympathetic nervous system).

109. Where do rhabdomyosarcomas usually develop?

The four most common areas are the **head** and **neck, genitourinary region, extremities**, and **orbit**. Survival of patients with orbital disease is nearly 100%. The survival rate for those with tumors in other areas is dependent on the amount, if any, of tumor left after resection and the presence or absence of metastatic disease.

110. What is the most common ovarian tumor of childhood?

Germ cell tumors in girls (in contrast, women develop stromal tumors most commonly). The most frequent ovarian germ cell tumors are dysgerminomas, followed by endodermal sinus tumors, teratomas, and mixed germ cell tumors. Stromal tumors are rare.

111. Which germ cell tumors occur in children?

The most common germ cell tumor is a histologically benign, mature cystic teratoma occurring in the sacrococcygeal area. Germ cell tumors can occur outside the gonads in brain, kidneys, mediastinum, lung, liver, or stomach. Malignant germ cell tumors include embryocarcinomas, choriocarcinomas, teratocarcinomas, endodermal sinus tumors (yolk sac tumors), dysgerminomas, seminomas, and mixed germ cell tumors.

112. List the risk factors for testicular cancer.

Cryptorchidism, atrophic testes, prenatal exposure to diethylstilbestrol (DES), history of viral orchitis, and positive family history of testicular cancer. Because testicular cancer is the most common solid tumor in males aged 15–34 years and because prognosis is clearly related to early diagnosis, testicular self-examination should be taught to all male adolescents.

113. How great is the risk of malignant transformation in undescended testes?

The risk of malignancy may be 5–10 times higher in the undescended testis than in a normal testis. The risk in the contralateral testis may also be increased. Orchidopexy decreases, but does not eliminate, the risk of subsequent malignant transformation.

114. In evaluating an 8-month-old with constipation, you feel a firm, discrete mass on rectal exam. What is the likely diagnosis?

If the mass is posterior in the presacral area, it is most likely a sacrococcygeal germ cell tumor or a neuroblastoma. If the mass is anterior, a rhabdomyosarcoma is likely.

STEM CELL TRANSPLANTATION

115. Identify the three types of stem cell transplantation.

1. **Allogenic:** transfer of bone marrow, peripheral blood stem cells, or umbilical cord blood from a donor to another individual
2. **Autologous:** use of a person's own bone marrow or peripheral blood stem cells
3. **Syngeneic:** transfer of bone marrow, peripheral blood stem cells, or umbilical cord blood from a genetically identical donor (i.e., identical twins)

116. What is the chance of siblings having the same HLA type?

The human leukocyte antigens (HLA), located on chromosome 6, approximate simple mendelian inheritance, with two siblings having a 1:4 chance of same typing. A 1% crossover of material may also occur during meiosis. The larger the family, the more likely a match becomes, as shown by the formula $[1 - (0.75)^n]$, with n being the number of siblings. Thus, a child with five brothers and sisters has a 76% chance of having a sibling with an HLA match.

117. What is the chance of finding an HLA-matched unrelated donor?

Although in theory the number of possibilities would equal or even exceed the world's population, making a match astonishingly unlikely, HLA types cluster in individuals of similar genetic and racial backgrounds. In one estimate of persons of European ancestry, approximately 200,000 individuals would need to be screened to reach a 50% chance of finding a match.

Gahrton G: Bone marrow transplantation with unrelated volunteer donors. Eur J Cancer 27:1537–1539, 1991.

118. Which childhood cancers can be successfully treated with stem cell transplantation?

1. Chronic myelogenous leukemia (adult and juvenile types in first remission)
2. Myelodysplastic syndrome (i.e., preleukemia)
3. Acute myeloid leukemia
4. Acute lymphoblastic leukemia (failed induction, second or third remission, or high-risk patients in first remission)
5. Non-Hodgkin lymphoma (recurrent or refractory)
6. Neuroblastoma (stage III or stage IV in first remission)
7. Hodgkin disease (recurrent)

Armitage JO: Bone marrow transplantation. N Engl J Med 330:827–838, 1994.

119. What is the survival rate for children with solid tumors receiving autologous stem cell transplantation?

The cure rate for most solid tumors is still well below 50% because stem cell transplantation is being used for patients with relapsed or high-risk disease. The best results in children are in those with otherwise fatal neuroblastoma, in whom a cure rate of about 30% has been achieved.

120. How are tumor cells purged from a marrow or peripheral blood stem cell specimen?

1. Immunologic methods using monoclonal antibodies
2. Ex vivo use of chemotherapy
3. Selective binding of tumor cells to lectins
4. Treatment of marrow with anti-sense cDNA
5. Selective culture of normal cells
6. Selection of normal hematopoietic progenitor cells (e.g., CD34+ cells)

121. What are the indications for G-CSF and GM-CSF in stem cell transplant and cancer patients?

Granulocyte–colony-stimulating factor (G-CSF) and granulocyte/macrophage–colony-stimulating factor (GM-CSF) are used to shorten the period of neutropenia, and hence the associated risk of infection, after stem cell transplantation and myelosuppressive chemotherapy. They have been effective at shortening the period of isolation after transplantation and in allowing for more intensive chemotherapy regimens. Thus far, no effect on disease progression or survival has been demonstrated. The use of these growth factors in patients with myeloid leukemia is controversial because receptors for these factors are present on the surface of myeloid leukemia cells.

Lieschke GJ, Burgess AW: Granulocyte colony-stimulating factor and granulocyte-macrophage colony-stimulating factor: pts I and II. N Engl J Med 327:28–35, 99–106, 1989.

122. What are the most common symptoms and signs of acute graft-versus-host disease (GVHD)?

In GVHD, the newly transplanted lymphocytes recognize portions of the skin, liver, and GI tract in the recipient as foreign tissue, and a T-cell-mediated inflammatory reaction develops, leading to the following manifestations:

Skin—maculopapular rash, erythroderma, desquamation, bullae

Hepatic—jaundice (secondary to cholestasis rather than hepatitis)

GI—diarrhea, abdominal pain, nausea, vomiting, anorexia

123. How does chronic GVHD differ from the acute form?

Chronic GVHD, which usually develops after day 100, has different dermatologic features (e.g., hyperpigmented, thickened skin; nail changes) and eye problems (e.g., dry eyes, photophobia, eye pain). Additionally, dysphagia (secondary to esophageal strictures), vaginal strictures, obstructive lung disease, and oral ulcerations may develop. Weight loss is common. The hepatic dysfunction, which is prevalent in the acute form, often persists and worsens in chronic GVHD. Severe immunosuppression is the manifestation of chronic GVHD that most often leads to the death of patients with this complication.

124. How is GVHD prevented?

The best means of prevention is use of identical HLA-matched stem cells, but this is often not possible. Multiple immunosuppressive regimens are utilized involving cyclosporine, methotrexate, corticosteroids, and antithymocyte globulin. One promising method had been the removal of T cells from the stem cell product by various means (e.g., lectins, sheep RBC agglutination, monoclonal antibodies) prior to transplant. However, for reasons unclear, T-cell-depleted marrow has resulted in increased rates of nonengraftment of the marrow and increased relapse rates in patients with CML. The best method(s) of prevention of GVHD remains under investigation.

16. ORTHOPEDICS

John P. Dormans, M.D., Richard S. Davidson, M.D., and Mark Magnusson, M.D.

CLINICAL ISSUES

1. What is the differential diagnosis for torticollis?

Infection: cervical adenitis, retropharyngeal abscess, meningitis, tonsillitis (Grisel syndrome), post-tonsillectomy

Trauma: rotary subluxation, atlantoaxial subluxation (especially in Down syndrome), soft tissue trauma, birth trauma with hematoma of sternocleidomastoid muscle

Congenital conditions: congenital muscular torticollis, Klippel-Feil syndrome (fusion of cervical vertebrae), strabismus, vascular ring, abnormal skin webs (pterygium colli)

Miscellaneous: oculogyric crisis, tumor, Sandifer syndrome (severe gastroesophageal reflux and esophagitis)

2. When does the mass of congenital muscular torticollis disappear?

In the presence of congenital muscular torticollis, a soft nontender mass may appear in the sternocleidomastoid muscle on the affected side. The mass reaches its maximal size at 1 month and usually disappears by 4–6 months. Histologically, it consists of dense fibrous tissue and may represent prenatal venous obstruction and muscle damage to the sternocleidomastoid muscle. Congenital muscular torticollis may be associated with developmental dysplasia of the hips.

3. Which tests can be used to distinguish between ocular and orthopedic torticollis?

Abnormal head tilt caused by extraocular muscle imbalance is **ocular** torticollis, while that caused by sternocleidomastoid muscle imbalance is **orthopedic** torticollis. If the torticollis vanishes when one of the patient's eyes is covered (i.e., changing from binocular to monocular vision), the likely culprit is ocular. If the torticollis vanishes when the patient goes from sitting to supine, ocular pathology is also likely. If the cause remains uncertain, ophthalmologic testing of ocular deviation in various fields of gaze may be needed.

Caputo AR: The sit-up test: Alternate clinical tests for evaluating pediatric torticollis. Pediatrics 90:612–615, 1992.

4. What is infantile cortical hyperostosis?

Caffey disease (or syndrome), which usually occurs before 6 months of age, is a condition of unknown etiology that consists of tender, nonsuppurative, cortical swellings of the shafts of bone, most commonly the mandible and clavicle. It remits spontaneously, but exacerbations may persist for several years. In severe cases, corticosteroids may be helpful. Infantile cortical hyperostosis is a rare condition. The presence of periosteal reaction, especially if asymmetric, should raise the suspicion of battered child syndrome.

5. Name four entities associated with an absent or hypoplastic radius.

1. Congenital thrombocytopenia–absent radius (TAR) syndrome
2. VACTERL (formerly VATER) syndrome (anomalies of vertebrae, imperforate anus, cardiac origin, tracheoesophageal fistula, absent radii, renal origin and limbs)
3. Fanconi anemia
4. Holt-Oram syndrome (associated with a secundum atrioseptal defect)

6. What causes Sprengel's deformity?

Sprengel's deformity (congenital elevation of the scapula) is a failure of normal scapular descent during fetal life, resulting in an elevated, hypoplastic scapula. The affected side of the neck appears shorter and broader and may give the appearance of torticollis. A fibrocartilaginous band or omovertebral bone may bridge the space between the medial upper scapula and the spinous process of a cervical vertebra. Abduction of the ipsilateral arm is usually limited, but this limitation may not be clinically significant. Sprengel's deformity may be associated with congenital scoliosis and renal anomalies.

7. What are the causes of osteoporosis in children?

In osteoporosis bone is normal in structure and appearance but reduced in quantity. Susceptibility to fractures may result. Osteopenia is a nonspecific term indicating a reduction in bone mass, usually noted radiographically. Inability to mineralize osteoid for whatever reason is termed osteomalacia or rickets in children. Osteoporosis is fortunately rare in children. It is usually secondary to other problems, such as immobilization, chronic renal or liver failure, renal tubular acidosis, malabsorption, or medications (e.g., steroids, heparin). Osteoporosis may be associated with Turner syndrome, osteogenesis imperfecta, or homocystinuria and may also be seen in a primary juvenile idiopathic form. The vertebrae and ends of long bones are usually affected.

8. Describe the physical signs suggestive of rickets.

The anatomic abnormalities of rickets result primarily from the inability to normally mineralize osteoid. The bones become weak and subsequently distorted. Signs of rickets include:

- Craniotabes
- Delayed suture and fontanel closure
- Frontal thickening and bossing
- Defective tooth enamel
- Palpably widened physes at wrists and ankles
- Femoral and tibial bowing
- "Pigeon breast," or sternal protrusion secondary to use of accessory muscles
- Harrison's groove, a rim of rib indentation at insertion of the diaphragm
- "Rachitic rosary" (enlarged costochondral junctions)

9. Which growth sites are known to develop aseptic necrosis?

The **osteochondroses** are a group of disorders in which aseptic necrosis of growth centers (epiphyses and apophyses) occurs with subsequent fragmentation and repair. The exact cause is unknown. The patient usually presents with pain at the affected site.

Location	Eponym	Typical Age of Onset (yrs)
Tarsal navicular bone	Köhler disease	6
Capitellum of distal humerus	Panner disease	9–11
Carpal lunate	Keinböck disease	16–20
Distal lunar epiphysis	Burn disease	13–20
Head of femur	Legg-Calvé-Perthes disease	3–5
Second metatarsal head	Freiberg disease	12–14
Calcaneal Achilles tendon insertion	Sever disease	8–9

10. Discuss the inheritance pattern and clinical features of osteogenesis imperfecta (OI).

Of the several types of OI, the most common is type IV, which occurs in 1:30,000 live births. The clinical features vary and depend on the severity of the condition.

Type	Inheritance	Clinical Features
I	Autosomal dominant	Bone fragility, blue sclerae, onset of fractures after birth (most at preschool age) Type A, without dentinogenesis imperfecta Type B, with dentinogenesis imperfecta
II	Autosomal recessive	Lethal in perinatal period, dark blue sclerae, concertina femurs, beaded ribs
III	Autosomal recessive	Fractures at birth, progressive deformity, normal sclerae and hearing
IV	Autosomal dominant	Bone fragility, normal sclerae, normal hearing Type A, without dentinogenesis imperfecta Type B, with dentinogenesis imperfecta

11. McCune-Albright syndrome is associated with what skeletal abnormalities?

Polyostotic fibrous dysplasia (i.e., fibrous tissue replacing bones). The fibrous dysplasia occurs most commonly in long bones and pelvis and may result in deformity and/or increased thickness of bone. There is associated precocious puberty and café-au-lait spots.

12. What are the causes of in-toeing gait (pigeon-toeing)?

The condition may be due to problems anywhere in the lower extremity.

Foot:	metatarsus adductus
	talipes equinovarus (clubfoot)
	pes planus (flat feet)
Leg:	tibial torsion (internal)
	genu valgum (knock knees)
	tibia vara (Blount disease)
	bow legs
Hip:	femoral anteversion (medial femoral torsion)
	paralysis (polio, myelomeningocele)
	spasticity (cerebral palsy)
	maldirected acetabulum

Tunnessen W: Signs and Symptoms in Pediatrics, 3rd ed. Philadelphia, J.B. Lippincott, 1987.

13. A 15-year-old with tibial pain (which is worse at night and relieved by aspirin) has a small hypodense area surrounded by reactive bone formation on x-ray. What is the likely diagnosis?

Osteoid osteoma, which is a benign bone-forming tumor. It is typically seen in older children and adolescents and exhibits a male predominance (M:F 2:1). Most children complain of localized pain, usually in the femur and tibia; however, arms and vertebrae may also be involved. Radiographs and CT scans demonstrate an osteolytic area surrounded by densely sclerotic reactive bone. Bone scans reveal "hot spots." The site is usually < 1 cm in diameter and arises at the junction of old and new cortex. Pathologically, the lesion is highly vascularized fibrous tissue with an osteoid matrix and poorly calcified bone spicules surrounded by a dense zone of sclerotic bone. Treatment is surgical excision.

14. What is the clinical significance of leg-length discrepancy?

A significant portion of the population has mild leg-length discrepancy. Leg-length discrepancies of < 2 cm in a skeletally mature individual usually require no treatment. In addition to quantitating leg discrepancy in a skeletally immature child, it is important to estimate what the leg-length discrepancy will be at skeletal maturity. This can be done by periodically measuring leg-length discrepancy radiographically and using charts, such as the Green and Anderson "growth remaining graph" or the Moseley "straight line graph," to calculate anticipated leg-length discrepancy at skeletal maturity. Assessment of skeletal age is based on the bone age from an anteroposterior hand and wrist radiograph,

15. What are the long-term effects of uncorrected leg-length discrepancy?

Equinus contracture of the ankle, scoliosis, low-back problems, and late degenerative arthritis of the hip. Discrepancy < 2cm can be ignored or treated by a lift worn in the shoe. If the discrepancy is > 2 cm, one should consider equalization by epiphysiodesis, acute shortening, or a limb-lengthening procedure.

Guidera KJ, et al: Management of pediatric limb length inequality. Adv Pediatr 42:501–543, 1995.

16. How does nursemaid's elbow typically occur?

Nursemaid's elbow is subluxation of the radial head caused by a rapid pull or jerk on the forearm in toddlers and preschoolers, such as when a child is suddenly lifted by one arm. The annular ligament surrounding the radial head is torn or subluxated. The child presents with an extended, painful elbow with forearm pronated and arm guardedly held at the side. The examiner should look for other injuries. Pain, if localized, is usually at the posterolateral aspect of the radial head. Radiographs may be indicated to rule out fracture or dislocation, particularly if manipulation does not relieve the pain and abnormal positioning.

17. How is nursemaid's elbow reduced?

The subluxation can be reduced by manipulation. On the involved side, traction is applied to the forearm, which is then supinated and flexed at the elbow. A thumb placed anterolaterally over the radial head, pushing posteriorly, will often feel a "click." The child usually cries or protects the arm afterwards but, within 15 minutes, starts to move the arm spontaneously. If symptoms persist, the child should be reassessed for a possible fracture. Nursemaid's elbow may occur repeatedly throughout childhood and may occur bilaterally. The parents should learn the reduction maneuver. No long-term sequelae have been reported.

18. Why have many Little Leagues banned the throwing of a curve ball?

To minimize the cases of Little League elbow, which is a medial epicondylitis that results from overuse and flexor-pronator strain. The throwing of a curve ball puts extra stress on the ulnar collateral ligament of the medial aspect of the elbow. Severe strain can result in partial separation of the apophysis. Occasionally bony avulsions can occur.

19. What signs and symptoms suggest a serious cause of back pain in children that warrants further evaluation?

Symptoms: Pain in children < 4 years of age; interference with daily activities in school, play, or athletics; pain persistence > 4 weeks

Signs: Concurrent fever; postural changes; neurologic abnormalities; reproducible point tenderness; limitation of motion on forward bending

Thompson GH: Back pain in children. J Bone Joint Surg Am 75:928–937, 1993.

20. Give the differential diagnosis of back pain in children.

Congenital	Neoplastic
Tethered cord	Bony
Inflammatory	Osteoid osteoma, osteoblastoma
Ankylosing spondylitis	Eosinophilic granuloma
Enteropathic arthritis	Leukemia, lymphoma
Infectious	Osteosarcoma
Tuberculosis	Ewing's sarcoma
Discitis	Neurogenic
Traumatic	Glioma
Spondylolysis	Neuroblastoma
Spondylolisthesis	Developmental
"Musculoligamentous"	Scheuermann disease
Herniated nucleus pulposus	Painful scoliosis
Herniated apophysis	Psychogenic

Sponseller PD: Back pain in children. Curr Opin Pediatr 6:99–103, 1994; with permission.

21. Which sports injuries are the most common in school-aged children and adolescents?

Some 75% of injuries in school-aged children involve the lower extremities, and a majority of injuries to the knee and ankle are reinjuries due to incomplete healing from a previous problem. Contusions and sprains are the most common types of injury, with fractures and dislocations accounting for an additional 10–20%. Cranial injuries are the most common cause of sports fatality.

Adolescent boys who participate in contact team sports, particularly football and wrestling, are at highest risk for injuries. Among girls, softball and gymnastics have the highest injury rate.

Only 10% of sports injuries are caused by an opponent. Most injuries are caused by stumbling, falling, or misstepping. The latter finding suggests that improving intrinsic factors, such as raising the level of physical fitness, avoidance of overuse, and strengthening joint stability, may be more important factors in prevention of injuries than external factors such as the choice of equipment.

Committee on Sports Medicine and Fitness: Epidemiology and prevention of sports injuries. In Health Care for Young Athletes, 2nd ed. Elk Grove Village, IL, American Academy of Pediatrics, 1991, pp 146–171.

FOOT DISORDERS

22. Name the most common congenital foot abnormality.

Metatarsus adductus. In this condition, the front part of the foot (forefoot) is turned inward. Most cases are mild and flexible, with the foot easily dorsiflexed and the lateral aspect easily straightened by passive stretching. A simple test to determine if the kidney-shaped curvature is within normal limits is to draw a line that bisects the heel. When extended, this line normally falls between the second and third toe space. If it falls more laterally, metatarsus adductus is present. Improvement usually occurs within 2 months with passive stretching exercises.

23. How do congenital metatarsus adductus and congenital metatarsus varus differ?

Both deformities are types of kidney-shaped feet in which the forefoot becomes adducted secondary to varying degrees of intrauterine compression. In metatarsus adductus, there is no bone abnormality, and the curvature can be readily corrected by passive stretch. In metatarsus varus, there is subluxation of the tarsometatarsal joints when the foot is dorsiflexed. Physical exam usually reveals a deep medial cleft, prominence of the base of the fifth metatarsal, and an inability to correct the forefoot passively to align with the heel. Making the distinction is important because metatarsus adductus usually resolves spontaneously while metatarsus varus gradually worsens without treatment.

Craig CL, Goldberg MJ: Foot and leg problems. Pediatr Rev 14:395–400, 1993.

24. How is clubfoot distinguished from severe metatarsus varus?

Clubfoot, or talipes equinovarus congenita, is distinguished pathologically by forefoot and hindfoot abnormalities (e.g., malrotation of the talus under the calcaneus and plantar flexion or equinus of the ankle). As a rule, clubfoot is a rigid deformity, while metatarsus is more flexible. If the ankle can be dorsiflexed to neutral or beyond, metatarsus is a much more likely diagnosis.

25. Clubfoot is associated with which syndromes?

- Arthrogryposis
- Caudal regression syndrome
- Cerebral palsy
- Craniocarpotarsal dystrophy
- Diastrophic dwarfism
- Larsen syndrome
- Meningomyelocele
- Progressive muscle atrophy (peroneal type)
- Spinal cord tumor
- Myotonic dystrophy

26. What foot abnormality results in the appearance of a "Persian slipper" foot?

Also called "rocker bottom foot," this abnormality is due to **congenital vertical talus**. Lateral radiographs reveal a vertically oriented talus with dislocation of the talonavicular joint. On exam, the forefoot is markedly dorsiflexed, and the heel is rigid and points downward, giving the sole the characteristic convex or boat-shaped appearance. Serial casting and subsequent surgical reversion are the usual treatments. The syndrome most commonly associated with this deformity is trisomy 18.

27. What should be suspected when pes cavus is noted on exam?

Pes cavus, or high-arched feet (often associated with claw toes), can result from contractures or disturbed muscle balance. A neurologic cause should be suspected. The differential diagnosis includes normal familial variant, Charcot-Marie-Tooth disease, spina bifida, cauda equina lesion, peroneal muscle atrophy, Friedreich ataxia, Hurler syndrome, and polio.

28. Should children with flexible flat feet be given corrective shoes?

Flexible flat feet (pes plenovalgus) is a common finding in infants and children and up to 15% of adults. On weight-bearing, the arch shows very poor formation, and the heel is in valgus (outward) position. It is felt to be a normal variant due to ligamentous laxity. When there is no weight-bearing, the arch appears more normal. This condition is distinguished from pathologic flat feet in which lack of weight-bearing does not lessen the flatness and rigidity is present on physical examination. Prospective studies have shown that corrective shoes or plastic insets (orthotics) are not necessary in children with flexible flat feet, as the arch spontaneously develops during the first 8 years of life.

Wenger DR, et al: Corrective shoes and inserts as treatment for flexible flat feet in infants and children. J Bone Joint Surg 71:800–810, 1989.

29. How does the cause of foot pain vary by age?

Probable Causes of Foot Pain by Age

0–6 YEARS	6–12 YEARS	12–19 YEARS
Ill-fitting shoes	Ill-fitting shoes	Ill-fitting shoes
Foreign body	Foreign body	Foreign body
Occult fracture	Accessory navicular bone	Ingrown toenail
Osteomyelitis	Occult fracture	Pes cavus
JRA (if other joints involved)	Tarsal coalition (peroneal spastic	Hypermobile flat foot with tight
Rheumatic fever	flat foot)	Achilles tendon
(Hypermobile flat foot)	Ingrown toenail	Ankle sprains
	Ewing sarcoma	Stress fracture
	(Hypermobile flat foot)	Ewing sarcoma
		Synovial sarcoma

From Gross RH: Foot pain in children. Pediatr Clin North Am 33:1397, 1986; with permission.

30. A 10-year-old boy with recurrent ankle sprains and painful flat feet should be evaluated for what possible diagnosis?

Tarsal coalition. Fusion of various tarsal bones via fibrous or bony bridges can result in a stiff foot which inverts with difficulty. When inversion of the foot is done during an exam, tenderness occurs on the lateral aspect of the foot, and peroneal tendons become very prominent. Thus, the condition is also referred to as "peroneal spastic flat foot." Unless the condition is very severe warranting surgery, corrective shoes are usually adequate treatment.

FRACTURES

31. What are the most common types of fractures in children?

Physeal (growth plate) and **metaphyseal** (ends of long bones) fractures are the most common in children. These are sites where children's bones are weakest and ossification is not yet complete. Buckle (compression) and greenstick (incomplete) fractures are also common.

32. Where are the most frequent sites for fractures in children?

1. The clavicle
2. Distal radius
3. Distal ulna

33. How are growth plate fractures classified?

The *Salter-Harris classification* of growth plate (physis) injuries was devised in 1963:

Type I   Epiphysis and metaphysis separate; usually no displacement occurs due to the strong periosteum; radiograph may be normal; tenderness over the physis may be the only sign; normal growth after 2–3 week cast immobilization.

Type II	Fragment of metaphysis splits with epiphysis; usually closed reduction; casting is for 3–6 weeks (longer for lower extremity than upper extremity); growth usually not affected, except distal femur and tibia
Type III	Partial plate fracture involving a physeal and epiphyseal fracture to the joint surface; occurs when growth plate is partially fused; closed reduction more difficult to achieve
Type IV	Extensive fracture involving epiphysis, physis, metaphysis, and joint surface; high risk for growth disruption unless proper reduction (usually done operatively) is obtained
Type V	Crush injury to the physis; high risk for growth disruption

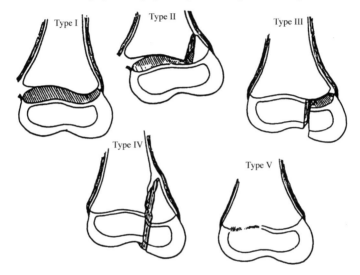

From Bachman D, Santora S: Orthopedic trauma. In Fleisher G, Ludwig S (eds): Textbook of Pediatric Emergency Medicine, 3rd ed. Baltimore, Williams & Wilkins, 1993, p 1237; with permission.

34. What is the Thurston-Holland sign?
The small section of metaphyseal bone that remains attached to the epiphysis in a type II fracture. It is diagnostic of injury to the growth plate.

35. What is the difference between subluxation and dislocation?
Subluxation is an incomplete or partial dislocation.

36. What is the most common cause of a pathologic fracture?
Also called secondary fractures, these are fractures through a bone that is weakened by a pathologic process. The most common such fracture is through unicameral bone cysts (simple bone cysts). These cysts usually occur in the metaphysis of a long bone, most frequently the humerus. They occur predominantly in males, are usually asymptomatic (until a fracture occurs), are centrally located in the bone, and are often quite large.

37. In a patient with a suspected fracture, what are the key points on physical examination?
Assess "the five P's" in the affected extremity:
1. **P**ain and point tenderness
2. **P**ulse (distal to the fracture)
3. **P**allor
4. **P**aresthesia (distal to the fracture)
5. **P**aralysis (distal to the fracture)

The involved extremity also should be carefully examined for deformity, swelling, crepitus, discoloration, and open wounds. A primary concern in any evaluation is a distal neurovascular compromise, which may require immediate surgical intervention.

38. How do you treat a simple clavicular fracture?

Place the child in a figure-of-eight strap or triangular sling for comfort. Complete union occurs in 10–14 days in infants and in 3–5 weeks in toddlers and young children, but the splint can be removed when spontaneous and painless motion occurs. The resulting callus of healing (the bump) takes about 2 years to disappear through bone remodeling.

39. A teenager who punches a wall in anger typically incurs what fracture?

Boxer's fracture. This is a a fracture of the distal fifth metacarpal, usually with apical dorsal angulation. Up to 35% of dorsal angulation can be accepted without compromise of function. Reduction often requires pin fixation.

40. Children who fall on outstretched arms often suffer what type of fracture?

Colles' fractures. This is a group of complete fractures of the distal radius with varying displacement of the distal fragment. The fall, with the hand outstretched, wrist dorsiflexed, and forearm pronated, often results in a classic "dinner-fork" deformity of the wrist on exam.

41. Compare Monteggia and Galleazzi fractures.

These fractures occur at opposite ends of the lower arm. In the various types of Monteggia fractures, there is dislocation of the radial head with an angulated diaphyseal fracture of the ulna. In Galleazzi fractures, the distal radioulnar joint is dislocated with a distal radial diaphyseal fracture.

42. How is the anterior humeral line helpful in evaluating an elbow fracture?

On a lateral x-ray, a line drawn along the anterior edge of the humerus ordinarily intersects the middle third of the capitellum. In acute elbow trauma, especially with hyperextension, the distal humerus can be displaced posteriorly when a fracture occurs. On an x-ray in this setting, the anterior line will intersect the capitellum in the anterior third or beyond. If this occurs, a fracture should be suspected. In children < 2½ years of age, this sign becomes less helpful because of variations in the rates of ossification of the capitellum.

43. What does the presence of the posterior fat pad on an elbow x-ray suggest?

Of the two fat pads that overlie the elbow joint, only the anterior one is visible on a lateral x-ray. If fluid accumulates in the joint space, as in bleeding, inflammation, or fracture, the fat pads are displaced upward and outward. The position of the anterior pad changes, and the posterior pad becomes visible. If acute trauma has occurred, a fracture should be suspected, and immobilization continued with follow-up studies as needed.

44. In a teenager with wrist trauma, why is palpation of the anatomic "snuff box" a critical part of the physical sign?

The anatomic snuff box, the inpouching formed by the tendons of the abductor pollicis longus and extensor pollicis longus when the thumb is abducted (in hitchhiker fashion), sits just above the scaphoid (carpal navicular) bone. The scaphoid is the carpal bone most commonly fractured, and these fractures are at higher risk for nonunion or avascular necrosis. Snuff box tenderness, pain on supination with resistance, and pain on longitudinal compression of the thumb should increase suspicion for fracture of the scaphoid bone. Even when an x-ray is negative, if there is significant snuff box tenderness, a fracture should be suspected and the wrist and thumb immobilized. A repeat x-ray in 2–3 weeks may better reveal a fracture. If very high clinical suspicion exists, MRI can identify a fracture when the plain film is negative.

45. Name the eight carpal bones of the wrist.

Disdaining some of the classic (mostly obscene) mnemonics, remember what will happen if a wrist fracture is missed:

Sinister Lawyers Take Physicians To The Court House

In order of proximal to distal, lateral to medial: scaphoid, lunate, triquetrum, pisiform, trapezium, trapezoid, capitate, hamate

46. In pediatric fractures, what amount of angulation is acceptable before reduction is recommended?

Acceptable angulation or displacement varies with a child's age. Younger children have remarkable healing potential even with complete translocation (e.g., bayonet apposition). As a rule, in children up to 6 years, as much as 15° of angulation will heal satisfactorily without reduction. In older children, 10° is acceptable.

47. In which fractures will remodeling of bone *not* occur?

Bony deformities in children (angulation, displacement, or shortening) can remodel as bone is removed from the tension side and placed on the compression side of the deformity by redirection of physeal growth. Factors that favor remodeling include young age, proximity of the fracture to the physis, and angulation in the plane of motion of the adjacent joint. The following fractures have a low chance of remodeling and may require closed or open reduction: intra-articular fractures; fractures with excessive shortening, angulation, or rotation; displaced epiphyseal plate fractures; and midshaft or diaphyseal fractures.

48. How long should fractures be immobilized?

Children's fractures generally heal more quickly than their counterparts in adults. The length of immobilization, however, depends on several variables, including the child's age, location of fracture, type of treatment, etc. As a rule of thumb, physeal, epiphyseal, and metaphyseal fractures heal more rapidly than diaphyseal fractures. On average, epiphyseal, physeal, and metaphyseal fractures heal in children within 3–5 weeks, whereas diaphyseal fractures may heal in 4–6 weeks.

49. How long do fractured clavicles and femurs take to heal?

	Newborn	16-Year-Old
Clavicle	10–14 days	6 wks
Femur	3 wks	6–10 wks

50. When is open reduction of a fracture indicated?

An open reduction is an operative reduction of a fracture. Open reduction may be combined with internal fixation with pins, plates, or screws. Indications include:
1. Failed closed reduction (often in older children with displaced fractures)
2. Displaced intra-articular fractures
3. Displaced Salter-Harris III and IV fractures (to prevent premature growth plate closure)
4. Unstable fractures in patients with head trauma
5. Open fractures (for irrigation and debridement)

HIP DISORDERS

51. Why has DDH replaced CHD?

The term developmental dysplasia of the hips (DDH) has replaced congenital hip dislocation (CHD) to reflect the evolutionary nature of hip problems in infants in the first months of life. About 2.5–6.5 infants per 1000 livebirths develop problems, and a significant percentage of these are not present on neonatal screening examinations. Clearly, the overt pathologic process may not be present at birth, and periodic examination of the infant's hip is recommended at each routine well-baby exam until the age of 1 year.

52. What signs are indicative of DDH in the newborn?

The most reliable clinical methods of detection remain the Ortolani reduction and the Barlow provocative maneuvers. The infant should be lying quietly supine. The examiner then flexes the hip and thigh to 90°. The **Ortolani test** is done by lifting the greater trochanter toward the acetabulum as the leg is abducted in an attempt to palpate and reduce a dislocated femoral head. The **Barlow test** is an effort to dislocate the hip by adduction of the thigh and gentle downward pressure.

53. What is the significance of a "hip click" in a newborn?

A hip click is the high-pitched sensation felt at the very end of abduction when testing for development dysplasia of the hip with Barlow and Ortolani maneuvers. It occurs in up to 10% of newborns. Classically, it is differentiated from a hip "clunk" which is heard and felt as the hip goes in and out of joint. Although a debatable point, the hip click is felt to be benign. Its cause is unclear and may be due to movement of the ligamentum teres between the femoral head and acetabulum or the hip adductors as they slide over the cartilaginous greater trochanter. Worrisome features that might warrant evaluation (e.g., hip ultrasound, hip x-ray) include late-onset of click, associated orthopedic abnormalities, or other clinical features suggestive of developmental dysplasia (e.g., asymmetric skin folds/creases, unequal leg length).

54. What other diagnostic signs are suggestive of DDH?

1. Asymmetry of thigh and gluteal folds. However, these may be present in up to 10% of normal infants.

2. Galleazzi test. With the hips flexed at 90°, the knees may be at different levels due to apparent femoral shortening on one side in asymmetrical dislocation.

3. Allis test. With the hips flexed and the heels on the table, uneven knee level suggests hip dislocation.

4. Limited hip abduction. This is usually a later sign.

Aronsson DD, et al: Developmental dysplasia of the hip. Pediatrics 94:201–208, 1994.

55. Why are hip x-rays for DDH often difficult to interpret in the newborn period?

The femoral head and acetabulum are cartilaginous at birth, and significant calcification to permit adequate visualization on x-ray does not occur until 3–4 months of age.

56. Who is at higher risk for DDH?

Dislocated, dislocatable, and subluxable hip problems occur in about 1–5% of infants. However, 70% of dislocated hips occur in girls, and 20% occur in infants born in breech position. Other risk associations include:

- Congenital torticollis
- Skull or facial abnormalities
- First pregnancy
- Positive family history of dislocation
- Metatarsus adductus
- Calcaneovalgus foot deformities in infants < 2500 gm
- Amniotic fluid abnormalities (especially oligohydramnios)
- Prolonged rupture of membranes
- Large birthweight

MacEwen GD: Congenital dislocation of the hip. Pediatr Rev 11:249–252, 1990.

57. How is DDH treated?

The recommended treatment is to keep the legs abducted and the hips and knees flexed, so that the developing head of the femur is kept within the acetabulum. Two commonly used devices are the Pavlik harness and the Frejka splint. Use of two or three diapers to keep the hip adducted generally is not recommended for DDH, as this method does not provide reliable stabilization.

58. What is the significance of a positive Trendelenburg test?

If a normal individual stands on one leg, ipsilateral hip abductors (primarily the gluteus medius) prevent the pelvis from tilting, and balance is maintained. Children over 4 years of age can usually stand this way for at least 30 seconds. If the opposite side of the pelvis does tilt or the trunk lurches to maintain balance, this is a positive Trendelenburg sign. It may be an indicator of muscle weakness (due to muscular or neurologic pathology) or of hip instability (such as acetabular dysplasia).

59. What is the most common cause of a painful hip in a child less than age 10 years?

Transient synovitis is a self-limiting, mild inflammation of the hip joint of unclear etiology. It is also called toxic synovitis, irritable hip, and coxitis fugax. It must be differentiated from infection, Legg-Calvé-Perthes disease, and slipped capital femoral epiphysis.

60. How can transient synovitis be differentiated from septic arthritis?

	Transient Synovitis	Septic Arthritis
History	Preceding URI ± low-grade fever Hip or referred knee pain Limp	Fever Usually large joint involvement (hip, ankle, knee, shoulder, elbow)
Physical	Refusal to bear weight Can delicately elicit range of motion in affected hip joint	Exquisite pain, swelling, warmth Marked resistance to mobility
Laboratory	ESR normal or mildly elevated Mild peripheral leukocytosis Negative blood culture Joint fluid cloudy Negative Gram stain	ESR markedly elevated Leukocytosis with "left shift" Often positive blood culture Joint fluid purulent Often positive Gram stain
Radiographs	Occasionally shows fluid in joint space	Widening of joint space Possible associated bony findings (early osteomyelitis)

61. What are the pathologic stages in Legg-Calvé-Perthes (LCP) disease?

LCP is a condition of aseptic necrosis of the femoral head involving children primarily ages 4–10.

1. Incipient or synovitis stage. Lasting 1–3 weeks, this first stage is characterized by an increase in hip-joint fluid and a swollen synovium associated with reduced movement.

2. Avascular necrosis. Lasting 6 months to 1 year, the blood supply stops to part (or all) of the head of the femur. That portion of the bone essentially dies, but the contour of the femoral head remains unchanged.

3. Fragmentation or regeneration and revascularization. In the last and longest pathologic stage of LCP, lasting 1–3 years, the blood supply returns and causes both resorption of necrotic bone and laying down of new immature bone. Permanent hip deformity can occur in this last stage.

It is important to note that plain radiographs may lag behind the progression of the disorder by as much as 3–6 months. Radionuclide bone scans are much better because early ischemia and avascular necrosis are depicted as decreased localizations of isotope.

62. What is the prognosis for children with Legg-Calvé-Perthes disease?

The two main prognostic factors for LCP disease include the age of the child and the amount of epiphyseal involvement. Children < 6 years of age tend to have a more favorable prognosis.

Those with less epiphyseal involvement also tend to have a better prognosis. Epiphyseal involvement has been classified by Salter into Type A (those with < 50% epiphyseal involvement) and Type B (those with > 50% head involvement).

63. What condition does this child have?

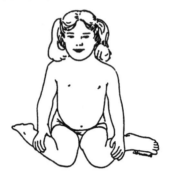

This is **femoral anteversion** (or medial femoral torsion), which is a common cause of intoeing in younger children. The child is demonstrating the reverse tailor position, a sign of the internally rotated hip.

From Staheli LT: Torsional deformity. Pediatr Clin North Am 33:1382, 1986; with permission.

64. How is the extent of femoral anteversion measured?

With the child lying prone and knees flexed at 90°, the hip normally cannot be rotated internally (i.e., feet pushed outward) more than 60° (angle *A* in diagram A). In addition, external rotation (angle *B* in diagram B) should exceed 20°. A normal child averages approximately 35°. Abnormal results indicate that the cause of in-toeing is likely due to physiologic femoral anteversion (or less commonly, hip capsular contractions such as in cerebral palsy).

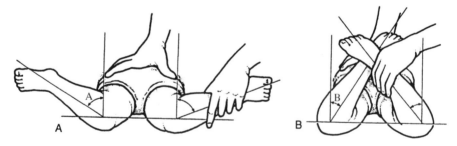

From Dormans JP: Orthopedic management of children with cerebral palsy. Pediatr Clin North Am 40:650, 1993; with permission.

65. How do children with slipped capital femoral epiphysis (SCFE) present?

SCFE involves progressive displacement with external rotation of the femur on the epiphyseal growth plate. The patient presents with intermittent or constant hip, thigh, or knee pain which has often lasted weeks to months. In 25%, the pain is bilateral. A limp, lack of internal rotation, and a hip flexion contracture may be noted. If the patient's hip is flexed, the thigh tends to fall into external rotation. It is important to realize that any patient presenting with knee pain may have underlying hip pathology.

66. What systemic conditions are associated with SCFE?

Children with SCFE tend to have delayed skeletal maturation and obesity and usually present between the ages of 8–14 years. This suggests that hormonal factors may lessen the bone's ability to resist shearing forces, resulting in a pathologic fracture through the proximal femoral physis. Systemic factors associated with SCFE include hypothyroidism, panhypopituitarism, hypogonadism, rickets, and irradiation.

INFECTIOUS DISEASES

67. Which patients with septic arthritis warrant open drainage?

There is debate as to the relative merits of open surgical drainage versus repeated needle aspiration. At present, three settings warrant surgical intervention:

1. Septic arthritis of the hip (and possibly shoulder)
2. Large amounts of fibrin, debris, or loculation within the involved joint space
3. Lack of improvement in 3 days by medical treatment alone

Dagan R: Management of acute hematogenous osteomyelitis and septic arthritis in the pediatric patient. Pediatr Infect Dis J 12:88–93, 1993.

68. Where does acute hematogenous osteomyelitis most commonly localize in children?

Lower extremity (femur, tibia, fibula)	70%
Upper extremity (humerus, radius, ulna)	15%
Foot	4%
Pelvis	4%
Vertebrae, skull, ribs, sternum, scapulae	2%

Gold R: Diagnosis of osteomyelitis. Pediatr Rev 12:293, 1991.

69. What are the most common bacterial agents in osteomyelitis?

Neonates	Children
1. *Staphylococcus aureus*	1. *Staphylococcus aureus*
2. Group B streptococci	2. Group A streptococci
3. Enterobacteriaceae (*Salmonella, Escherichia coli, Pseudomonas, Klebsiella*)	3. *Haemophilus influenzae*

The incidence of *H. influenzae* osteomyelitis is declining due to immunization.

70. How helpful is a screening white blood count (WBC) in the diagnosis of osteomyelitis?

Not very. In two-thirds of patients, the total WBC is normal (although in half of these, the differential is left-shifted). In the other one-third, the WBC is elevated, usually with a left shift. The erythrocyte sedimentation rate (ESR) is more sensitive, as 95% of cases have an ESR > 15 mm/hr with an average rate of 70 mm/hr.

71. How often are blood cultures positive in osteomyelitis?

Only 50%. Because this rate is relatively low, direct bone aspiration should be strongly considered. Aspiration raises the yield to 70–80% and greatly facilitates antibiotic therapy.

72. As osteomyelitis progresses, how soon do x-ray changes occur?

3–4 days: deep-muscle plane shifted away from periosteal surface
4–10 days: blurring of deep tissue muscle planes
10–15 days: changes in bone occur (e.g, osseous lucencies, punched-out lytic lesions, periosteal elevation)

73. In treatment of osteomyelitis, which serum bactericidal level is a better indicator of successful outcome: peak or trough?

Both may be important. Peak titers (approx. 20–30 min after infusion) are associated with successful treatment in acute osteomyelitis if ≥ 1:8 and in chronic osteomyelitis if ≥ 1:16. Trough titers are predictive of a good outcome if ≥ 1:2 in acute osteomyelitis and if ≥ 1:4 in chronic osteomyelitis.

74. When is treatment of osteomyelitis with oral antibiotic agents appropriate?

1. An identified organism
2. Available oral antibiotic against the organism
3. Adequate surgical debridement
4. Improving clinical course on IV antibiotics
5. Patient without vomiting or diarrhea
6. Adequate serum levels can be obtained on oral therapy
7. Reliable parents and/or patient

Nelson J: Skeletal infections in children. Adv Pediatr Infect Dis 6:59, 1991.

75. How long should antibiotics be continued in osteomyelitis and septic arthritis?

The precise answer is unclear, but infections caused by *Staphylococcus aureus* or enteric gram-negative bacteria must be treated for longer periods than those caused by *Haemophilus influenzae, Neisseria meningitidis,* or *Streptococcus pneumoniae.* A minimum of 4–6 weeks is likely necessary for the former group and 2–3 weeks for the latter. If diagnosis has been delayed, initial clinical response is poor, or ESR remains elevated, longer durations may be needed.

76. When is open surgical drainage indicated in cases of osteomyelitis?

1. Abscess formation in the bone, subperiosteum, or adjacent soft tissue
2. Bacteremia persisting > 49–72 hours after initiation of antibiotic treatment
3. Continued clinical symptoms (e.g., fever, pain, swelling) after 72 hours of therapy
4. Development of a sinus tract
5. Presence of a sequestrum (i.e., detached piece of necrotic bone)

Dagan R: Management of acute hematogenous osteomyelitis and septic arthritis in the pediatric patient. Pediatr Infect Dis J 12:88–93, 1993.

77. Why are treatment failures more common in osteomyelitis than in septic arthritis?

1. Antibiotic concentrations are much greater in joint fluid than in inflamed bone. Concentration in joint fluid may actually exceed peak serum concentrations, while those in bone may be significantly less than serum concentration.
2. Devitalized bone may serve as an ongoing nidus for infection.
3. Diagnosis of osteomyelitis is more likely to be delayed than that of septic arthritis.

78. How do the features of osteomyelitis in the neonate differ from those in the older child and adult?

1. Neonatal osteomyelitis almost invariably follows hematogenous dissemination.
2. Multiple foci of infection are frequently seen.
3. Septic arthritis is a frequent association, probably reflecting the spread of infection via blood vessels penetrating the epiphyseal plates.
4. Chronic osteomyelitis is infrequent.
5. The pathogens causing neonatal osteomyelitis are the same as those responsible for sepsis neonatorum.

79. Why are young children more susceptible to infectious discitis than adolescents or adults?

Increased susceptibility in younger children is due to the differing anatomy of the spine. In children < 12, blood vessels extend from the vertebral body through hyaline cartilage to supply nutrition directly to the intervertebral disc and nucleus pulposus. These vessels slowly regress until the adult picture is reached (age 12), at which time nutrition to the nucleus pulposus is supplied primarily by diffusion. The extra blood vessels in early life may facilitate hematogenous spread of infection or direct extension of early vertebral osteomyelitis.

80. How is the diagnosis of discitis established?

Discitis, which is infection and/or inflammation of the intervertebral disc, most commonly occurs in children between ages 4–10. The etiology is often unclear, but a bacterial cause, particularly *Staphylococcus aureus*, is identified by blood cultures in about 50% of cases. The diagnosis can be difficult because of varied presentations, including generalized back pain with or without localized tenderness, refusal to stand or walk, back stiffness with loss of lumbar lordosis, abdominal pain, and unexplained low-grade fever.

As with osteomyelitis, the most helpful laboratory test is an elevated ESR. WBC counts may often be normal, and early x-rays (< 2–4 weeks of symptoms) may not show changes. Technetium-99 bone scans will demonstrate abnormalities early in the course of illness.

Treatment consists of 3–6 weeks of antistaphylococcal antibiotics, with variable amounts of immobilization and bracing depending on severity of symptoms. Persistent or atypical cases may require biopsy to identify the etiology.

Cushing AH: Diskitis in children. Clin Infect Dis 17:126, 1993.

81. When is bone scintigraphy used in the evaluation of children with obscure skeletal pain?

When correlated with clinical findings, the results of bone scintigraphy can help localize an abnormality in the bones, joints, or soft tissues. Additional unrelated asymptomatic lesions also may be identified. The bone scan is very sensitive but not very specific. Often, other diagnostic tests are needed to establish the exact etiology of the pain. A bone scan should only be considered after a careful history and physical exam have been performed and plain x-rays of the abnormal area are obtained. The scan is most useful in establishing or ruling out occult infection or bone tumor.

82. What are the three phases of a bone scan?

The phases are generally demarcated by the time elapsed since injection of the radionuclide dye.

Phase I—angiographic phase. In the first few seconds, the dye passes through the large blood vessels and provides early assessment of regional vascularity and perfusion.

Phase II—blood pool phase. Usually obtained in the first minutes after an injection, this phase highlights the movement of the dye into extracellular spaces of soft tissue and bone.

Phase III—delayed phase. By 1.5–3 hours after injection, the dye localizes in the bone with minimal soft tissue imaging.

The three-phase process is used to differentiate soft tissue from bony abnormalities. At times a Phase IV study may be done by rescanning for the same dye at 24 hours, which further minimizes soft tissue background activity.

KNEE, TIBIA, AND ANKLE DISORDERS

83. What is the difference between valgus and varus deformities?

Some things seem to be destined to be learned, forgotten, and relearned many times as a rite of passage. The Krebs cycle is one. This is another. The terms refer to angular deformities in the musculoskeletal system. If the distal part of the deformity points toward the midline, the term is **varus**. If the distal part points away from the midline, it is **valgus**. For example, in knock-knees, the lower portion of the deformity points away, so the term is genu valgum.

Another method is to consider the body in the supine (anatomic) position. Draw a circle around the body. All angles conforming to the curve of the circle are varus; all angles going against the circle are valgus. Bowleggedness conforms to the circle around the body and is, therefore, genu varum.

84. Are children normally knock-kneed or bowlegged?

It varies by age. If you use the angle formed by the tibia and femur as a guide, most children at birth are bowlegged (genu varum) up to 20°, but this tendency progressively diminishes until about 24 months, when the trend toward knock-knees (genu valgum) begins. Knock-knees continue to age 3 (up to 15°) and then begin to diminish. At about age 8, most children are, and will remain, knock-kneed at about 7–9°.

85. Which bowlegged infants or toddlers require evaluation?

Radiographs should be considered if bowleggedness is:
• Present after 24 months (the time of normal progression to physiologic genu valgum)
• Worse after age 1 as the infant begins to bear weight and walk
• Unilateral
• Visually > 20° (tibiofemoral angle)

86. Which children are more likely to develop Blount disease?

Tibia vara, or Blount disease, is a medial angulation of the tibia in the proximal metaphyseal region due to a growth disturbance in the medial aspect of the proximal tibial epiphysis. In the infantile type, the child is usually obese and an early walker and develops pronounced bowlegs during the first year of life. Black females are particularly at risk for severe deformity. In the adolescent variety, the onset occurs during late childhood or early adolescence, and the deformity is usually unilateral and mild. Correction of severe deformity often requires surgical intervention.

87. How does tibial torsion change with age?

Tibial torsion, the most common cause of in-toeing in children aged 1–3, gradually rotates externally with age. For excessive internal rotation, bracing was used extensively in the past, but its efficacy is questionable as the natural history of the condition is self-resolution. Measurement is done by noting the thigh–foot angle with the knee flexed to 90°.

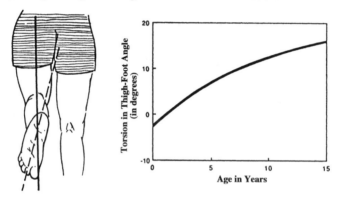

From Sponseller PD: Bone, joint, and muscle problems. In Oski FA, et al (eds): Principles and Practice of Pediatrics, 2nd ed. Philadelphia, J.B. Lippincott, 1994, p 1026; with permission.

88. How effective is the Denis Browne splint in the treatment of tibial torsion?

The splint consists of a metal bar connected to shoes or strings about the feet. The bar provides varying degrees of external rotation. The splint has been used in children with tibial torsion in whom spontaneous correction is not occurring. However, there is no scientific evidence that this device alters the natural history of tibial torsion.

89. What is the most common diagnosis if a 15-year-old basketball player presents with painful swelling below both knees?

Osgood-Schlatter disease. Clinically, this entity consists of painful swelling of one or both tibial tubercles (tibial tubercle apophyses) at the insertion of the patellar ligament. It is very common in adolescents, usually beginning between ages 11–15. Vigorous exercise results in traction apophysitis and repeated stress fractures at the tibial tubercle insertion of the patellar ligament. The tubercle may enlarge from repetitive injury and subsequent new bone formation at the apophysis. Restriction of activity for 2–3 weeks and gradual resumption of activity usually diminish the symptoms, which may recur intermittently until maturity. In mature patients with persistent pain in the tibial tubercle, ossicles have been found in the patellar ligament, and their removal may provide relief of pain. The year 1903 was a banner one for the tibial tubercle, as Osgood and Schlatter, working independently, both described the phenomenon.

90. What painful condition is snowshoeing likely to produce?

Shin splints. This term describes the pain and cramping felt in the compartments of the lower leg after strenuous exercise. It is rare in children but may be seen in teenagers who exercise (especially running on hard surfaces) after extended periods of inactivity. The pain results from muscle strain and inflammation of the musculotendinous units. Swelling and cramping occur, particularly in the flexor digitorum longus muscle, which flexes the lateral four toes and plantar-flexes the foot at the ankle joint. The muscle swelling may contribute to ischemia. Snowshoeing may be the ultimate test of the anterior tibial muscles.

91. Which long bone is most frequently absent congenitally?

The **fibula**. Absence of the fibula may be partial or complete and is usually unilateral. The involved leg is shortened and commonly demonstrates bowing of the tibia and slight shortening of the femur. The foot usually shows a severe deformity with equinus and valgus deformities with absence or abnormal development of lateral phalanges.

92. Why are sprained ligaments uncommon in children?

Growth plates are weaker than ligaments in a child, and thus disruption will occur in the growth plate (such as a Salter-Harris epiphyseal fracture) prior to ligamentous disruption.

93. How are ankle sprains graded?

80–90% of ankle sprains are the result of excessive inversion and/or plantar-flexion resulting in injury to the lateral ligaments (anterior talofibular and calcaneofibular). The anterior ankle drawer sign is a test of ankle stability (particularly the anterior talofibular ligament). It is accomplished by immobilizing the lower tibia with one hand and, with the ankle at 90°, moving the heel and foot forward with the other hand. If there is marked laxity with a poor endpoint, a complete tear or **third-degree sprain** is likely. Moderately increased laxity compared with the other ankle indicates a partial tear or **second-degree sprain**. No laxity indicates a **first-degree sprain**.

94. Which ankle sprains should be evaluated with an x-ray?

More than 5 million radiographs are estimated to be taken annually in children and adults for ankle injuries, yet there are no widely accepted guidelines. One set of guidelines suggests obtaining an x-ray if there is malleolar pain and one or both of the following conditions is present: (1) inability to bear weight for 4 steps immediately following the injury and on office or ER evaluation, and/or (2) bone tenderness at the posterior edge or tip of either malleolus. When these simple criteria were used in studies involving children and adults, no fractures were missed and unnecessary x-rays were reduced by 25%.

Stiell IG, et al: Decision rules for the use of radiography in acute ankle injuries. JAMA 269:1127–1132, 1993.
Chande VT: Decision rules for roentgenography of children with acute ankle injuries. Arch Pediatr Adolesc Med 149:255–258, 1995.

95. Should ankle sprains be casted?

If inversion ankle sprains are not complicated by a fracture or peroneal tendon dislocation, casting is not warranted. It has no benefit over early immobilization with a wrap, such as a commercially available air stirrups. Additionally, complete immobilization may delay rehabilitation.

Hergenroeder AC: Diagnosis and treatment of ankle sprains. Am J Dis Child 144:809–814, 1990.

96. A ninth-grade soccer player with knee swelling "felt a pop" while scoring a goal. He or she has one of what three possible diagnoses?

A pop or snap sensation in the setting of acute knee injury is usually associated with:
1. Anterior cruciate ligament injury
2. Meniscal injury
3. Patellar subluxation

97. In acute injury, what are the main causes of blood in the knee joint?

Acute hemarthrosis is most commonly due to:
1. Rupture of the anterior or posterior cruciate ligaments
2. Peripheral meniscal tears
3. Intratrabecular fracture
4. Major disruption or tear in the joint capsule

98. A teenager presents with chronic knee pain, swelling, and occasional "locking" of the knee joint, and his x-ray reveals increased density and fragmentation at the medial femoral condyle. What condition does he likely have?

Osteochondritis dissecans. In this avascular necrosis syndrome, focal necrosis of articular cartilage and underlying bone occurs. The cause is unknown, but antecedent trauma is common. The section of bone may detach and lodge in the contiguous joint. Males are more commonly affected, and pain occurs especially with strenuous activity. Associated findings may include stiffness, swelling, clicking, and occasional locking. A plain radiograph can reveal the diagnosis, but MRI is more sensitive when findings are equivocal. Extended immobilization is the primary treatment. Continued pain or locking of the joint warrants consideration of arthroscopy to search for intra-articular fragments. Long-term complications can include degenerative arthritis.

99. What predisposes a child or teenager to recurrent dislocation of the kneecap?

Orthopedic conditions: genu valgum, patella alta, hypoplasia of the lateral femoral condyle, laterally located tibial tubercle, vastus medialis insufficiency, abnormal attachment of the iliotibial tract

Syndromes of generalized ligamentous laxity: Down syndrome, Ehlers-Danlos syndrome, Marfan syndrome, Turner syndrome

Mizuta H, et al: Recurrent dislocation of the patella in Turner syndrome. J Pediatr Orthop 14:74–77, 1994.

100. Who manifests the "apprehension sign"?

Individuals with acute or subacute **subluxation** or **dislocation of the patella.** With the patient's knee supported at 30°, the examiner applies pressure to the medial border of the patella. If the patient displays impending distress or apprehension, the test is positive. No discomfort makes patellar pathology less likely. The apprehension sign is also seen in individuals with **shoulder instability** (especially glenohumeral problems) who fear dislocation when certain maneuvers are performed. For anterior instability, the arm is placed in maximal external rotation and abduction (similar to an overhand throw position). For posterior instability, the shoulder is placed at 90° of forward flexion and internal rotation.

101. How does patellofemoral stress syndrome occur?

This major cause of chronic knee pain in teenagers results from malalignment of the extensor mechanism of the knee due to a variety of causes. It is most commonly seen as an "overuse" entity in sports that involve running and full-knee flexion, such as track or soccer. It has been inappropriately called chondromalacia patella, which is a specific pathologic diagnosis of an abnormal articular surface that occurs in a minority of these patients. The patella serves as the fulcrum on which the various muscles of the quadriceps extend the knee. Forces may act asymmetrically, causing greater stress on lateral aspect of the patella, especially in individuals with anteversion of the femur, external torsion of the patella, high (alta) patella, abnormally developed quadriceps, excessive flattening of the femoral groove, or wide Q angle. Treatment consists of ice, rest, nonsteroidal anti-inflammatory drugs, quadriceps strengthening, hamstring stretching, and possibly patellar-stabilizing braces.

102. What is the Q angle?

Draw a line from the anterior-superior iliac spine through the center of the patella, and then draw a line from the center of the patella to the tibial tubercle. The resultant angle is the Q angle, or quadriceps angle. For teenage males, the average Q angle is 14°, and for females, 17°. Angles > 20° predispose to chronic knee pain (particularly in runners) because of patellar strain.

SPINAL DISORDERS

103. How is screening for spinal deformity performed?

The child should be undressed or dressed only in underwear or a gown (open from the back). From the back and side, the child is examined standing, flexed forward at the hips, and sitting (to eliminate leg-length inequality). The following signs suggest scoliosis:

1. Shoulder or scapular asymmetry.
2. Visible deformity of spinous processes.
3. Asymmetry of paraspinal muscles or rib cage in the thoracic spine while bending (> 0.5 cm in lumbar region and > 1.0 cm in thoracic region). A scoliometer may be used for this determination.
4. Sagittal plane deformity when viewed from the side.
5. Waist crease asymmetry that does not disappear on sitting. Most waist crease asymmetries are due to minor leg-length discrepancies.
6. Excessive thoracic kyphosis in forward-bending when viewed from the side.

104. What constitutes an abnormal scoliometric measurement?

The scoliometer, also called an inclinometer, is a type of protractor used to measure the vertebral rotation and rib-humping that is seen in scoliosis with the forward-bending test. An angle of 5° or less is usually insignificant; 7° or more warrants consideration of standing posteroanterior and lateral radiographs for more precise assessment of curvature.

105. Are males or females more likely to have scoliosis?

Females are 5 times more likely than males.

106. What is the differential diagnosis for scoliosis?

Scoliosis is a lateral curvature of the spine (i.e., coronal plane deformity). **Kyphosis** and **lordosis** are posterior and anterior curvatures, respectively (i.e., sagittal plane deformity). About 1–2% of the pediatric population have a spinal deformity, but very few are severe enough to require treatment: 85% of cases are idiopathic; 5% are congenital (including hemivertebrae and vertebral fusions); 5% neuromuscular (cerebral palsy, polio, spinal muscular atrophy, muscular dystrophy); and 5% miscellaneous (Marfan syndrome, Ehlers-Danlos syndrome, tumors).

107. How is scoliosis measured by the Cobb method?

This is the standard technique used to quantify scoliosis in posteroanterior or lateral radiographs. One line is drawn along the vertebra tilted the most at the top of the curve, and another at the bottom of the curve. The curvature is represented by angle a, which can be measured in the two ways illustrated:

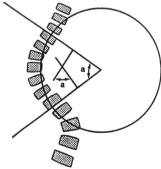

From Tolo VT, Wood B: Pediatric Orthopaedics in Primary Care. Baltimore, Williams & Wilkins, 1993, p 88; with permission.

108. Why is Risser staging important in following patients with scoliosis?

Risser staging is a method of estimating bone growth potential based on the appearance of the iliac crest on radiographs taken for scoliosis. Scoliosis progresses most during the rapid growth phase of adolescence. The **iliac apophysis** is the secondary ossification center which develops laterally to the iliac crest and can be used to quantify the remaining growth potential. Stage I begins shortly after puberty, and stage IV indicates spinal growth is nearly complete. Stage V, seen in adults, indicates complete fusion. If a patient has entered stage IV or V, progression of scoliosis is unlikely. Earlier stages indicate that careful follow-up must be done because of increased risk of progression.

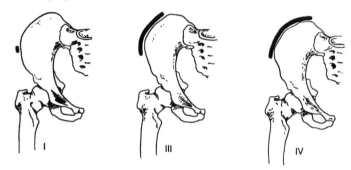

From Tolo VT, Wood B: Pediatric Orthopaedics in Primary Care. Baltimore, Williams & Wilkins, 1993, p 90; with permission.

109. What is the recommended treatment for scoliosis?
- Observation if the patient is mature and the curvature is < 25°.
- Bracing if the curvature is 25–40° with > 2 years of growth remaining.
- Surgery if the curvature is > 40°.

110. What is the differential diagnosis of disc space narrowing seen on a radiograph?

Disc space infection, posttraumatic changes, congenital abnormalities, and tumor. If the patient presents with disc space narrowing and a history of pain, the diagnosis of acute disc space infection is likely. Asymptomatic patients with isolated findings of disc space infection may have congenital abnormalities (such as congenital kyphosis or a failure of segmentation).

111. What diagnosis should you consider in a teenage male with very poor posture that is not self-correctable?

Scheuermann kyphosis. This is a wedge-shaped deformity of vertebral bodies of unclear etiology that causes juvenile kyphosis (abnormally large dorsal thoracic or lumber curves). Common in teenagers (up to 5–8%), it is distinguished from simple bad posture ("postural round-back deformity") by its sharp angulation and lack of correction by active or passive maneuvers. X-ray studies reveal anterior vertebral body wedging and irregular erosions of the vertebral endplate. Treatment consists of exercise, bracing, and, rarely, surgical correction (for severe deformities).

112. How does spondylolysis differ from spondylolisthesis?

Spondylolysis is a condition in which there is a break in the pars interarticularis (vertebral arch) of a vertebra. **Spondylolisthesis** is a condition (usually resulting from spondylolysis) characterized by slippage of one vertebra forward on the lower vertebra. Spondylolisthesis in children is usually due to a fracture that occurs with repetitive hyperextension of the back (isthmic) or a congenital defect in the pars (dysplastic). Spondylolisthesis is graded according to severity of slip into Grades I (0–25%), II (25–50%), III (50–75%), and IV (75–100%). Patients usually present with low-back pain. The most commonly affected vertebra is L5.

17. PULMONOLOGY

Robert W. Wilmott, M.D., Ellen B. Kaplan, M.D., and Carlos R. Perez, M.D.

ALLERGIC RHINITIS

1. What conditions should be considered in the differential diagnosis of chronic nasal stuffiness in children?

Allergic rhinitis, infection (e.g., sinusitis), anatomic obstruction (e.g, adenoidal hypertrophy, nasal polyps, deviated nasal septum), nonallergic rhinitis with eosinophilia (more often seen in older children), vasomotor rhinitis, rhinitis medicamentosa, illicit drug use (e.g., sniffing cocaine), foreign body, pregnancy, hypothyroidism, tumor, and cerebrospinal rhinorrhea.

2. How does the time of year help identify the potential cause of allergic rhinitis?

Perennial: house dust mites, animal dander, molds (in damp areas or areas where humidifiers are in continual use)
Early spring: trees
Mid-summer: grasses
Late summer, early fall: ragweed
Winter: molds (in colder climates)

3. Why might you examine the nasal secretions from children with chronic nasal stuffiness?

Nasal secretions, when examined after Wright or Hansel staining, can reveal eosinophils, neutrophils, basophils, and bacteria. In conjunction with a positive clinical history and physical examination, a patient with > 10% eosinophils on nasal smear is likely to have allergic rhinitis. These patients will also have allergen-specific IgE.

A small group of children have perennial symptoms, > 10% eosinophils, but no allergen-specific IgE (nonallergic rhinitis with eosinophilia, or NARES). Rhinitis with neutrophilic predominance and few eosinophils is more suggestive of infection or irritation, such as smoke exposure. It should be noted that there is considerable overlap. An elevation of nasal smear eosinophils may be normal in infants < 3 months of age.

4. How do the RAST and ELISA tests differ?

RAST (radioallergosorbent test): An in vitro laboratory method to quantify the amount of allergen-specific IgE. The test allergen is bound to solid-phase particles, with which the patient's serum is then incubated. If the patient's serum contains the allergic-specific IgE, then the RAST allergen will bind to the patient IgE. Nonspecific IgE is removed by washing. Radiolabeled anti-IgE is then added and binds to the IgE–allergen complex. Quantification of radioactivity (which correlates with the quantity of allergen-specific IgE) is done using a gamma counter.

ELISA (enzyme-linked immunosorbent assay): A variation of the RAST that uses enzyme-conjugated, rather than radiolabeled, anti-IgE. The amount of enzyme bound is verified by adding the appropriate substrate and measuring it with a spectrophotometer.

5. Discuss the pros and cons of skin testing versus in vitro (e.g., RAST) testing for allergies.

Both tests have their proponents in the diagnosis of allergen-specific IgE-mediated sensitivities, although skin tests are more commonly done.

In vitro tests:	No risk of anaphylaxis
	Results not influenced by medications, dermatographism, extensive dermatologic disease
	Limited number of available allergens
	More costly

Skin testing: Considered more sensitive than in vitro tests
                         Results immediately available
                         Contraindicated in pregnancy

6. Which variables affect allergy skin testing in children?

1. Patient age: Skin tests to inhalant allergens are rarely positive in children < 2 years of age
2. Test site: Upper back is more sensitive than the forearm
3. Medications: Inhibit responses for various lengths: astemizole (6 wks); hydroxyzine, terfenadine (5 days); other antihistamines (1–3 days)
4. Test technique: Prick skin tests more specific, intradermal skin tests more sensitive

Bush RK, Gern JE: Allergy evaluation: Who, what and how. In Schidlow DV, Smith DS (eds): A Practical Guide to Pediatric Respiratory Diseases. Philadelphia, Hanley & Belfus, 1994, pp 261—270.

7. What is the recommended treatment for children with chronic allergic rhinitis?

Chronic allergic rhinitis can be seasonal, perennial, or perennial with seasonal exacerbations.

1. After identification of the responsible allergen(s), therapy is directed, first and foremost, at avoidance measures.

2. As it is often difficult to eliminate the offending antigen(s) from the environment totally, adjunctive pharmacotherapy is frequently necessary. Intranasal anti-inflammatory agents (i.e., topical corticosteroids or cromolyn sodium) employed on an ongoing basis are very effective in many patients. A short course of oral corticosteroid therapy may also be needed at the initiation of intranasal therapy. Oral antihistamine treatment with or without a decongestant may also be helpful.

3. Allergen immunotherapy is third-line therapy in patients with chronic allergic rhinitis. Considerations for the use of immunomodulatory therapy include the severity of symptoms, the degree to which symptoms are controlled by allergen avoidance measures and pharmacotherapy, patient compliance, and cost.

Kaplan EB: Allergic disorders. In Friedman SB, Fisher M, Schonberg SK (eds): Comprehensive Adolescent Health Care. St. Louis, Quality Medical Publishing, 1992, pp 633–640.

8. How can you get rid of cat allergen?

Up to one-fourth of U.S. households have a cat as a pet and the principal allergen of cat dander, Fel d I, is a major contributor to allergic rhinitis and bronchial hyperreactivity. Because the allergen is so small, it remains airborne for hours. High-efficiency particulate air (HEPA) filters may help reduce the allergen level, and frequent cat washings are helpful (but hazardous to the owner!). Felinectomy is the ultimate solution.

9. How can house dust mite (HDM) concentrations be minimized?

Allergens from the house dust mites, *Dermatophagoides pteronyssinus* and *D. farinae*, are extremely important triggers of rhinitis and asthma. Unlike cat dander, they are not airborne except for a short time after dusting or vacuuming. Measures of control include:
- Completely encasing mattresses, pillows, and box springs with airtight covers
- Washing bedding at very high temperatures (> 130°F) weekly
- Removing carpeting if possible
- Minimizing or eliminating stuffed toys

Of note, if the removal of little purple Barney will be too traumatic, overnight freezing in a plastic bag helps to kill dust mites and their larvae. Commercially available acaricidal products (e.g., Acrosan) can be used on upholstered furniture and carpets.

10. Which children should be considered for immunotherapy?

Allergen immunotherapy can be helpful for many children with IgE-mediated sensitivities when allergen avoidance and adjunctive pharmacotherapy have produced suboptimal results. Immunotherapy to various allergens has been effective in the treatment of allergic rhinitis in controlled trials. Definitive data on its efficacy in the treatment of asthma are less clear, though some studies suggest that it is effective.

11. What serologic changes occur in a child receiving immunotherapy?

Three principal changes occur: a rise in serum antigen-specific IgG-blocking antibodies, a fall in antigen-specific IgE, and a reduction in basophil reactivity.

Virant FS: Allergic rhinitis. Pediatr Rev 13:323–328, 1992.

12. How common is exercise-induced bronchospasm in children with allergic rhinitis?

Up to 40% of patients with allergic rhinitis but no history of asthma may have abnormal pulmonary function tests in response to exercise.

Bierman EW: Incidence of exercise-induced asthma in children. Pediatrics 56:847–850, 1975.

ASTHMA

13. When does asthma usually have its onset of symptoms?

Approximately 50% of childhood asthma develops before 3 years of age and nearly all by age 7 years. The signs and symptoms of asthma, including chronic cough, may be evident much earlier than the actual diagnosis but may be erroneously attributed to recurrent pneumonia or "wheezy bronchitis."

14. Is asthma more common in males or females?

Asthma is two to three times more common in boys than girls until the onset of puberty. It becomes more common in females after puberty.

15. What historical points suggest that a child's asthma may have an allergic trigger?

1. Seasonal nature with concurrent rhinitis (suggesting pollen)
2. Symptoms worsen when visiting a family with pets (suggesting animal dander)
3. Wheezing occurs when carpets are vacuumed or bed is made (suggesting mites)
4. Symptoms develop in damp basements or barns (suggesting molds)

16. What types of challenge testing are given to children to test for airway hyperreactivity?

Pharmacologic:	Methacholine (stimulates muscarinic receptors on bronchial smooth muscle)
	Histamine (direct bronchoconstrictive effect and reflex vagal stimulation)
Physiologic:	Exercise
	Cold air hyperventilation
	Ultrasonically nebulized distilled water inhalation
Allergenic:	Cat dander or ragweed

17. What is the "88% saturation test"?

A test devised for younger children with lower cognitive function or developmental maturity who cannot adequately perform standard spirometry. The patient breathes a nonhumidified 12% oxygen and nitrogen mixture for 10 minutes or until oxygen saturation as measured by pulse oximetry falls to 88%. The dry, hypoxic air acts as a bronchial challenge, and the inability to complete 10 minutes may indicate reactive airways disease.

Wagner CL, et al: The "88% saturation test": A simple lung function test for young children. Pediatrics 93:63–67, 1994.

18. How common is exercise-induced bronchospasm (EIB)?

Very common, and often overlooked. In asthmatic children, significant symptoms (e.g., cough, chest tightness, wheezing, dyspnea) are noted following exercise in 70–90%, although abnormal pulmonary function tests can be found in nearly 100%. In atopic children, the incidence of EIB has been estimated to be as high as 40%.

19. How is exercise-induced bronchospasm diagnosed?

EIB is likely if the peak flow rate or FEV_1 drops by $\geq 15\%$ after 6 minutes of vigorous exercise. This exercise can include jogging on a motor-driven treadmill (15% grade at 3–4 mph), riding a stationary bicycle, or running up and down a hallway. Peak flow can then be measured with simple peak flow meters or a spirometer every 2–3 minutes. The greatest reduction in EIB is seen usually 5–10 minutes after exercise. As further verification of the diagnosis, if the patient has developed a decreased peak flow (and possibly wheezing), two puffs of a beta-agonist should be administered to reverse the bronchospasm.

20. What mechanisms lead to airway obstruction during an acute asthma attack?

The pathophysiology of airway obstruction in asthmatics and the sequence of events that leads to status asthmaticus are incompletely understood. It appears that an attack may be analogous to the late reaction noted after bronchial provocation with inhaled allergen. There are three main components to airway obstruction: bronchospasm, mucosal edema, and plugging of airways by thick secretions. These abnormalities are probably secondary to the release of mediators from mast cells and eosinophils. The mast cell mediators include histamine, leukotrienes, platelet-activating factor, and neutrophil chemotactic factor. Major basic protein and eosinophil cationic protein are released from the eosinophil.

21. Which other noninfectious diseases besides asthma should be considered in an infant who wheezes?

1. Aspiration pneumonitis, especially in a neurologically impaired infant because of the higher likelihood of gastroesophageal reflux. If there is a clear association with feedings, consider the possibility of tracheoesophageal fistula.

2. Bronchiolitis obliterans (chronic wheezing usually following adenoviral infection)

3. Bronchopulmonary dysplasia (especially if prolonged oxygen therapy/ventilatory requirement in the neonatal period)

4. Ciliary dyskinesia (especially if recurrent otitis media , sinusitis, or situs inversus is present)

5. Congenital malformations (including tracheobronchial anomalies and malacia, lung cysts, and mediastinal lesions)

6. Cystic fibrosis (if associated with recurrent wheezing, failure to thrive, chronic diarrhea, or recurrent pneumonia)

7. Congenital cardiac anomalies (especially lesions with large left-to-right shunts)

8. Foreign-body aspiration (if associated with acute choking episode in infant > 6 months old)

9. Vascular rings (especially if stridor present when supine)

22. What clinical signs correlate best with severity of respiratory disease during an acute asthmatic attack?

- Markedly increased respiratory rate
- Pronounced retractions (especially sternocleidomastoid retractions)
- Altered mental state (agitation, drowsiness)
- Diminished breath sounds (wheezing may be absent if flow rates are very low)
- Increased pulsus paraodoxus (This is performed by measuring the blood pressure and noting the difference in pressure between the point at which the systolic pressure is initially heard intermittently and the point at which the systolic pressure is heard with every heart beat. Normally, this is < 10 mmHg.)

23. What is the Hoover sign?

The paradoxical inward motion (retraction) of the costal margins with inspiration. It is seen in children with significant asthma, bronchiolitis, or other conditions in which peripheral airway obstruction results in overinflated lungs and a flattened diaphragm. This mechanical change results in costal margin retraction rather than elevation with diaphragmatic contraction.

Klein M: Hoover sign and peripheral airways obstruction. J Pediatr 120:495, 1992.

24. Is a chest x-ray necessary for all children who wheeze for the first time?

In children > 2 years of age who wheeze for the first time, the most likely diagnosis statistically is asthma. In children < 2, bronchiolitis is the most likely cause. While a chest x-ray is often recommended routinely for evaluation of an initial episode of wheezing to rule out other diagnoses (e.g., pneumonia, foreign-body aspiration), the vast majority will not add any new information for diagnosis or treatment if the clinical picture is consistent with bronchiolitis or asthma. A chest x-ray should be considered for a first-time wheezing patient in the following situations:

1. Features on physical exam that suggest other diagnoses (e.g, marked adenopathy suggesting mediastinal mass, clubbing suggesting chronic respiratory problem, hyperresonance to percussion suggesting pneumothorax, or supraclavicular crepitance suggesting pneumomediastinum)

2. Marked asymmetry of breath sounds

3. Suspected pneumonia (e.g., high fever, localized rales, or locally diminished breath sounds)

4. Suspected foreign-body aspiration

5. Hypoxemia or marked respiratory distress

6. Older child with no family history of asthma or atopy

Even though the necessity of a chest x-ray is far from clear, if you do not obtain a chest x-ray on a first-time wheezer, be prepared for stern questioning. The heartland of pediatrics is filled with anecdotes of the simple wheeze that turned out to be a multiloculated fascinoma.

25. What are the usual findings on arterial blood gas sampling during acute asthma attacks?

The most common finding is hypocapnea because of hyperventilation. Hypoxemia is also usually present unless the child is being treated with oxygen. Hypercapnia is therefore a serious sign which suggests that the child is tiring or becoming severely obstructed. This finding should prompt reevaluation and consideration of admission to a high acuity unit.

26. Which asthmatics should be admitted to the hospital?

After therapy, admission is advisable if a child has:

- Depressed level of consciousness
- Incomplete response with moderate retractions, wheezing, peak flow < 60% predicted, pulsus paradoxus ≥ 15 mmHg, $SaO_2 \leq 90\%$
- Breath sounds significantly diminished
- Evidence of dehydration
- Pneumothorax
- Residual symptoms and history of severe attacks involving prolonged hospitalization (especially if intubation was required)
- Parental unreliability

An equally difficult (and very unpredictable) challenge relates to which patients will relapse after responding to therapy and subsequently require hospitalization. This is a major problem as rates of relapse can approach 20–30%.

27. How has management for an acute asthma attack changed in the past decade?

While there remains variability in approach, certain trends have emerged:

1. Use of subcutaneous epinephrine and intravenous theophylline in initial management has greatly diminished.

2. Aerosolized β_2-adrenergic agents (especially albuterol), including frequent miniboluses or continuous aerosol therapy, have become the first-line therapy.

3. More aggressive use of oral and intravenous corticosteroids.

28. State the advantage of the "minibolus" aerosolized treatment of acute asthmatic exacerbations.

Although the most beneficial dosing regimen of β_2-agonists remains unclear, studies have shown that in acute exacerbations, the dose-response curve of bronchial smooth muscle is shifted to the right. Thus, higher doses may be needed to obtain a response. In addition, the duration of action of the aerosolized agent is significantly shorter in an acute episode compared with chronic asthma. Thus, a common recommendation is to administer nebulized albuterol, 0.15 mg/kg/dose (max 5 mg/dose) every 20 minutes up to 1 hour for initial management.

NHLBI National Asthma Education Program Expert Panel: Guidelines for the diagnosis and management of asthma. J Allergy Clin Immunol 88:425–534, 1991.

29. How much medication reaches the lungs in metered-dose inhaler or nebulizer therapy?
On average, about 10–15% of the total dose, if proper technique is used.

30. Is a nebulizer more effective than a metered-dose inhaler (MDI) with a spacer in the treatment of asthma?
In the treatment of exacerbations of asthma, nebulizers are used almost exclusively in children < 2 years because of the ease of administration. While they are also used more commonly in older children, some studies indicate that an MDI with spacer is equally effective. Furthermore, the MDI with spacer requires less treatment time and has fewer side effects.

Chou KJ, et al: Metered-dose inhalers with spacers vs. nebulizers for pediatric asthma. Arch Pediatr Adolesc Med 149:201–205, 1995.

31. List the possible acute side effects of albuterol.
General: hypoxemia, tachyphylaxis
Renal: hypokalemia
Cardiovascular: tachycardia, premature ventricular contractions, atrial fibrillation
Neurologic: headache, irritability, insomnia, tremor
Gastrointestinal: nausea

Committee on Drugs, American Academy of Allergy and Immunology: Position statement: Adverse effects and complications of treatment with beta-adrenergic agonist drugs. J Allergy Clin Immunol 75:443–449, 1985.

32. How significant is the risk of death with use of β-agonists?
Several investigators have reported increased bronchial hyperreactivity and a greater risk for death and near-death with chronic albuterol usage. However, this association remains controversial, as there is not a well-substantiated cause-and-effect relationship. One meta-analysis of six case-control studies found the risk to be extremely small. Heavy or increasing use of albuterol indicates poorly controlled asthma, and inhaled cromolyn or corticosteroids should be considered.

Mullen M, et al: The association between beta-agonist use and death from asthma. JAMA 270:1842, 1993.

33. Do inhaled steroids suppress the hypothalamic-pituitary axis?
Not to the same extent as systemic steroids, but they do impair cortisol secretion. However, in a carefully done study, the response to stimulation with ACTH was normal in children receiving up to 800 μg/day of beclomethasone or budesonide. It is likely that the suppression of natural cortisol secretion is of little clinical significance, with the possible exception of nocturnal suppression when diminished pulmonary function and asthmatic attacks are common. The effects of higher doses remain undetermined.

Law CM, et al: Nocturnal adrenal suppression in asthmatic children taking beclomethasone dipropionate. Lancet 1:941–944, 1986.

Bisgaard H, et al: Adrenal function in children with bronchial asthma treated with beclomethasone dipropionate or budesonide. J Allergy Clin Immunol 81:1088–1095, 1988.

34. Do inhaled steroids affect growth in children?
For children who require frequent courses of oral steroids, inhaled corticosteroids are indicated, particularly if inhaled cromolyn sodium has been of no benefit. The data on side effects continue to emerge. Results are conflicting but tend to indicate that growth suppression does not occur or is very minimal, particularly in more severe asthmatics. Longer-term studies will help to clarify that issue. It is important that accurate growth measurements, preferably with a stadiometer, be made on children requiring extended use of inhaled steroids.

Barnes PJ: Inhaled glucocorticoids for asthma. N Engl J Med 332:868–875, 1995.

35. Why has theophylline fallen from grace as a treatment for asthma?

Due to concerns about its potential toxicity (e.g., vomiting, tachycardia, seizures), side effects (e.g., behavioral changes, impaired school performance), and questionable efficacy, it is no longer considered part of routine therapy. Its use may be considered in an acute setting if a patient is becoming fatigued and developing respiratory failure. Some practitioners still use it in chronic settings, particularly for nocturnal asthma.

Szefler ST, et al: Evolving role theophylline for treatment of chronic childhood asthma. J Pediatr 127:176–185, 1995.

Weinberger M, Hendeles L: Drug therapy: Theophylline in asthma. N Engl J Med 334:1380–1388, 1996.

36. What factors affect theophylline clearance?

Increased Clearance
- Age (increased in children)
- Low-carbohydrate, high-protein diet
- Charcoal-broiled meat
- Cigarette smoking
- Marijuana smoking
- Chronic ethanol intake
- Cystic fibrosis

Decreased Clearance
- Age (decreased in infants)
- High-carbohydrate, low-protein diet
- Caffeine
- Antibiotics (e.g, erythromycin, ciprofloxacin)
- Cimetidine
- Viral infections
- Cor pulmonale
- Congestive heart failure
- Liver disease

Canny GJ, Levison H: The modern management of childhood asthma. Pediatr Rev Commun 1:123–162, 1978.

37. When is cromolyn sodium indicated in the treatment of asthma?

Cromolyn inhibits mast-cell degranulation (blocking mediator release) and reduces airway hyperreactivity by unknown mechanisms. It has no bronchodilator properties and is thus not useful in acute settings. However, when used by inhalation on a regular basis, it is helpful in treating allergic (extrinsic) asthma and exercise-induced bronchospasm. The role of nedocromil, a nonsteroidal anti-inflammatory medication with mechanisms of action similar to those of cromolyn, remains to be elucidated in children.

38. Are anticholinergics useful in the treatment of pediatric asthma?

The precise role of anticholinergics (including ipratropium bromide and atropine sulfate) in pediatrics remains ill-defined due to potential side effects and the paucity of studies on their efficacy in both acute and chronic asthma management.

39. In chronic asthma, how do mild, moderate, and severe types differ?

	Mild	Moderate	Severe
Episodes of cough or wheeze	Brief, < 2/wk	≥ 2/wk	Almost daily, continuous
Symptoms between episodes	No	Occasional	Present
Exercise tolerance	EIB with strenuous exercise	EIB with most exercise	Activity limited even with medication
Nocturnal cough or wheezing	< 2/mo	Weekly	Frequent
School loss	None	> 7 days/yr	> 21 days/yr
ER, office visits for acute asthma	None	≤ 3/yr	> 3/yr
Hospitalization	None	None	1/yr
PEFR % reference	≥ 80%	60–80%	< 60%
PEFR variability	20%	20–30%	> 30% episodes while medicated
Response to optimal medication	Symptoms controlled with prn inhaler	Regular medication required to control	Symptoms even with regular medication

EIB—exercise-induced bronchospasm; PEFR—peak expiratory flow rate.
From Eggleston PA: Asthma. In Oski FA, et al (eds): Principles and Practice of Pediatrics, 2nd ed. Philadelphia, J.B. Lippincott, 1994, p 220; with permission.

40. How useful are pulmonary function tests (PFTs) in evaluating and following children with asthma?

PFTs are very useful in the longitudinal evaluation of outpatients with asthma, in demonstrating a satisfactory response to therapy, and for identifying the severely obstructed, hyperinflated asymptomatic patient who has a poor prognosis if unrecognized. The use of home peak flow meters to measure the PEFR on a daily or as-needed basis can also be helpful. A baseline predicted or personal-best value can be obtained and home therapy initiated when the PEFR falls. PFTs may be particularly helpful in cough-variant asthma to distinguish between upper and lower airway disease.

41. What proportion of childhood asthmatics "outgrow" their symptoms?

Popular pediatric teaching has been that most children with asthma outgrow their symptoms. However, studies suggest that this is erroneous and that only 30–50% become symptom-free, primarily those with milder disease. Studies also indicate that most infants who wheeze (in whom a prime provocative factor is viral infection) tend to "outgrow" their asthma, but that children whose initial wheezing occurs later in life (with allergen sensitization as a major factor) tend to have more persistence of recurrent bronchospasm. Although the overall trend is for asthma to become more muted, a large percentage of adults have persistent obstructive disease, both recognized and unrecognized.

Silverman M: Out of the mouths of babes and sucklings: Lessons from early childhood asthma. Thorax 48:1200–1204, 1993.

Godden DJ, et al: Outcome of wheeze in childhood: Symptoms and pulmonary function 25 years later. Am J Respir Crit Care Med 149:106–112, 1994.

BRONCHIOLITIS

42. What is the most important cause of lower respiratory tract disease in infants and young children?

Respiratory syncytial virus (RSV). Up to 100,000 children are hospitalized annually in the U.S. due to this paramyxovirus. Disease most commonly occurs during outbreaks in winter or spring in the U.S. and in the winter months of July and August in the southern hemisphere.

43. What other agents cause bronchiolitis?

Although RSV is estimated to cause 50–90% of cases, other responsible agents include parainfluenza viruses (second most common cause), influenza virus types A and B, adenovirus, enterovirus, rhinovirus, and *Mycoplasma pneumoniae*.

44. What are the best predictors of the severity of bronchiolitis?

The single best predictor at an initial outpatient assessment appears to be oxygen saturation, which can be determined by pulse oximetry. $SaO_2 < 95\%$ correlates with more severe disease. Of note, low SaO_2 is often not clinically apparent, and objective measurements are necessary. An arterial blood gas with PaO_2 of ≤ 65 or $PaCO_2 > 40$ mmHg is particularly worrisome. Other predictors of more severe disease include:

1. An ill or "toxic" appearance
2. History of prematurity (gestational age < 34 wks)
3. Atelectasis on chest x-ray
4. Respiratory rate > 70/min
5. Infant < 3 months old

Shaw KN, et al: Outpatient assessment of infants with bronchiolitis. Am J Dis Child 145:151–155, 1991.

45. Describe the typical findings on chest x-ray in a child with bronchiolitis.

The picture is varied. Most commonly, there is hyperinflation of the lungs. Bilateral interstitial abnormalities with peribronchial thickening are common. Up to 20% of children may have lobar, segmental, or subsegmental consolidation which can mimic bacterial pneumonia. Of note, with the possible exception of atelectasis, the chest x-ray findings do not correlate well with the severity of the disease.

46. How common is apnea in RSV bronchiolitis?

About 20% of hospitalized infants develop apnea. Infants at highest risk include former premature infants, particularly those who are < 44 weeks postconception. The apnea tends to occur early in the course of the disease, and monitoring should be done for those hospitalized high-risk infants. Of note, SIDS has not been clearly associated with RSV infection.

Hall CB: Respiratory syncytial virus: What we know now. Contemp Pediatr 10:92–110, 1994.

47. Is the use of steroids justified for bronchiolitis?

Multiple controlled studies have shown no immediate or long-term advantage with the use of corticosteroids in acute bronchiolitis. However, their use remains debated.

Spinger C, et al: Corticosteroids do not affect the clinical or physiological status of infants with bronchiolitis. Pediatr Pulmonol 9:181, 1990.

48. Is albuterol or other bronchodilators effective as a therapy for bronchiolitis?

The house is divided. Many say no, but others argue that 30–50% of infants with RSV bronchiolitis will have a positive response to inhalation therapy. In most studies that show benefit, however, the response is minimal, with small (1–2%) increases in SaO_2. Infants with a strong family history of asthma may be most likely to respond. In infants with significant wheezing, a trial of albuterol (0.15 mg/kg every 20 min for 3–4 doses) may be indicated, with continuance if benefits are noted.

Gadomski AM, et al: Efficacy of albuterol in the management of bronchiolitis. Pediatrics 93:907–911, 1994.

49. What are the indications for ribavirin?

Ribavirin is a synthetic nucleoside analog used as an aerosolized antiviral agent for RSV infections. Because of high cost and conflicting data on clinical effectiveness, its precise use remains controversial. According to the AAP Committee on Infectious Diseases, infants hospitalized with lower respiratory tract disease caused by RSV who are in the following categories may be considered candidates for treatment with ribavirin:

1. Infants at high risk for severe or complicated RSV infection, including infants with congenital heart disease, bronchopulmonary dysplasia, and other chronic lung conditions; those with cystic fibrosis; and certain premature infants. In addition, children with immunodeficiency (especially those with severe combined immunodeficiency disease), those who are recent transplant recipients, and those undergoing chemotherapy for malignancy may be considered to be at high risk for complicated RSV infection.

2. Infants hospitalized with RSV lower respiratory tract disease who are severely ill. Severity of illness can be assessed by determination of arterial blood gas values. Infants with $PaO_2 < 65$ mmHg or increasing $PaCO_2$ concentrations may be considered candidates for ribavirin treatment.

Committee on Infectious Diseases: Reassessment of the indications for ribavirin therapy in respiratory syncytial virus infections. Pediatrics 97:137–140, 1996.

50. Does infection with RSV confer lifelong protection?

On the contrary, reinfection is very common, especially in day-care centers. In these settings, up to 75% of infants who acquire RSV infections in the first year of life are reinfected during the subsequent 2 years. The good news is that primary infections (especially those requiring hospitalization) tend to be the most severe episodes, with subsequent illnesses being more muted. In older children and adults, RSV infections present more as "colds," and reinfection is also common.

Of note, the use of prophylactic RSV immune globulin has been shown to reduce the incidence and duration of RSV hospitalization and the severity of illness in high-risk infants (e.g., bronchopulmonary dysplasia).

Groothuis JR, et al: Prophylactic administration of respiratory syncytial virus immune globulin to high-risk infants and young children. N Engl J Med 329:1524–1530, 1993.

51. If a 5-month-old is hospitalized due to RSV bronchiolitis, what should the parents be told about the likelihood of future episodes of wheezing?

In follow-up studies, 40–50% of these infants have subsequent recurrent episodes of wheezing, usually in the first year after illness. Subclinical pulmonary abnormalities may also persist. The question of whether the pulmonary sequelae are due to the bronchiolitis or a genetic predisposition to asthma remains unclear. Host factors, including pulmonary abnormalities prior to the illness, passive cigarette smoke exposure, atopic diathesis, and immunologic responses of virus-specific IgE, may be involved in recurrent problems.

52. How is bronchiolitis distinguished from asthma in a wheezing infant?

Asthma is a clinical diagnosis in all age groups that is characterized by reversible airway obstruction with hyperresponsiveness to various stimuli, including viral infections. Of course, the viral infections themselves, rather than underlying bronchial pathology, can be responsible for the wheezing in an infant with acute symptoms. Differentiating between the two diseases at the time of presentation can be virtually impossible. The infant wheezing from bronchiolitis generally has collateral symptoms, such as fever and rhinorrhea, and RSV antigen testing may be positive. If repeated episodes of reversible wheezing occur, especially during off-peak RSV season, asthma is likely. Other diagnoses, such as cystic fibrosis and gastroesophageal reflux, must also be considered. Two unanswered questions remain: (1) Does RSV infection cause asthma from postinfectious sequelae in those not otherwise predisposed to asthma? and (2) Are infants predisposed to asthma more prone to severe viral lower respiratory tract infections?

CLINICAL ISSUES

53. How is hemoptysis differentiated from hematemesis?

	Hemoptysis	*Hematemesis*
Color	Bright red and frothy	Dark red or brown
pH	Alkaline	Acid
Consistency	May be mixed with sputum	May contain food particles
Symptoms	Preceded by gurgling noise	Preceded by nausea
	Accompanied by coughing	Accompanied by retching

From Rosenstein BJ: Hemoptysis. In Hilman BC (ed): Pediatric Respiratory Disease. Philadelphia, W.B. Saunders, 1993, p 533; with permission.

54. What are the indications for surgical repair of pectus excavatum?

An area of considerable dispute. Children with pectus excavatum tend to have reduced total lung capacity, reduced vital capacity, increased residual volume, and decreased cardiac output with exercise. These abnormalities, in general, are mild, and most children are asymptomatic. The precise indications for surgery for children with more severe defects are unclear because of difficulties in predicting which level of deformity might have long-term adverse (particularly cardiovascular) consequences. Psychologic distress and embarrassment are often indications for surgery. Complicating the picture is the fact that the optimal patient age for surgery remains unclear.

Shamberger RC: Congenital chest wall deformities. Curr Probl Surg 33:478–498, 1996.

55. How is the "slipping rib syndrome" diagnosed?

The slipping rib syndrome is a cause of upper abdominal or chest pain during which a patient will often experience a slipping sensation of the ribs with a pop or click upon heavy lifting. Anatomically, the tip of one of the lower "floating" (not joined directly to the sternum) ribs overrides a rib above. This condition may follow trauma. Diagnosis is likely if the pain can be reproduced by grasping the affected rib and pulling it anteriorly.

Porter GE: Slipping rib syndrome: An infrequently recognized entity in children: A report of three cases and review of the literature. Pediatrics 76:810–813, 1985.

56. How do the possible causes of chronic cough vary by age group?

Infancy
- Aspiration/swallowing dysfunction
- Gastroesophageal reflux with or without aspiration
- Congenital malformations
- Cystic fibrosis
- Environmental tobacco smoke exposure
- Infection, especially chlamydia or pertussis
- Immunodeficiency

Toddlers and preschoolers
- Asthma, usually with atopy
- Other atopic diseases: rhinitis, possibly sinusitis
- Cystic fibrosis
- Foreign-body aspiration
- Community-acquired viral infections

Middle and later childhood
- Asthma
- Cystic fibrosis
- Infection, especially mycoplasma
- Psychogenic cough
- Smoking experimentation

Adolescence
- Asthma
- Cystic fibrosis
- Primary smoking
- Psychogenic cough

From Black P: Evaluation of chronic or recurrent cough. In Hilman BC (ed): Pediatric Respiratory Disease. Philadelphia, W.B. Saunders, 1993, p 150; with permission.

57. When should the diagnosis of psychogenic cough be considered?

Most children and adolescents with a psychogenic cough begin with a mild upper respiratory infection (URI) accompanied by a cough. However, the cough persists after the URI resolves. Typically, the cough is barky, harsh, and nonproductive. While it may occur every 5–10 minutes during the day, it subsides while the child is asleep. There are no other signs or symptoms of systemic or pulmonary pathology, and the cough is usually unresponsive to potent antitussive medications. Treatments for psychogenic cough (also called "cough tic syndrome") include overnight chest wrapping (effective possibly through a placebo effect), behavior management techniques, and, for severe cases, psychiatric intervention.

Lavigna JV, et al: Behavioral management of psychogenic cough: Alternative to the "bedsheet" and other aversive techniques. Pediatrics 87:532–537, 1991.

58. Which is more effective as a cough medicine in children, dextromethorphan or codeine?

Multiple studies have shown that neither agent is superior to placebo in the treatment of cough.

Taylor JA, et al: Efficacy of cough suppressants in children. J Pediatr 122:799–802, 1993.

59. What are the risks of passive smoking in children?

- Passive cigarette smoke exposure, which consists of the inhalation of both the smoker's exhalation (mainstream smoke, about 15% of total) and the more noxious sidestream (the unfiltered burning end of the cigarette, about 85% of total), has been the subject of much study. While the extent of effect is debated, risks include:
  - Decreased fetal growth
  - Increased incidence of SIDS
  - Increased incidence of middle ear effusions
  - Increased frequency of upper and lower respiratory tract infections
  - Presentation of asthma at an earlier age with more frequent exacerbations
  - Impaired lung function

Longer-term issues of increased cancer rates and cardiovascular disease remain under study. Of note, if a parent smokes, a child is twice as likely to become a smoker.

DiFranza JR, Lew RA: Morbidity and mortality in children associated with the use of tobacco products by other people. Pediatrics 97:560–568, 1996.

60. How is clubbing diagnosed?

Digital clubbing is caused by the presence of increased amounts of connective tissue under the base of the fingernail. This may be determined by:

1. Rocking the nail on its bed between the examiner's finger and thumb. In clubbing, the nails seems to be floating.

2. Visual inspection reveals that the distal phalangeal depth (DPD), which is the distance from the top of the base of the nail to the finger pad, exceeds the interphalangeal depth (IPD), which is the distance from the top of the distal phalangeal joint to the underside of the joint. Normally, the DPD/IPD ratio is < 1, but in clubbing it is > 1. If the abnormality is not readily apparent, precise measurements can be made from a plaster cast of the finger.

3. The diamond (or Scamroth) sign. Normally, if the nails of both index fingers or any other two identical fingers are opposed, there is a diamond-shaped window present between the nail bases (see figure). This window disappears in clubbing.

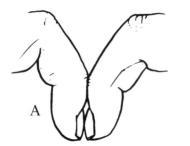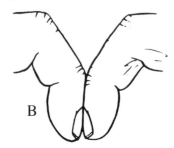

A, A normal child with a diamond-shaped window present between the nail bases when the fingers are opposed. *B,* The appearance of digital clubbing where the diamond-shaped window has been obliterated by the increased amount of soft tissue under the base of the nail.

61. Clubbing is associated with which diseases?

Pulmonary:	Bronchiectasis (as in cystic fibrosis, bronchiolitis obliterans, ciliary dyskinesia), pulmonary abscess, empyema, interstitial fibrosis, malignancy, pulmonary atrioventricular fistula
Cardiac:	Cyanotic congenital heart disease, chronic congestive heart failure, subacute bacterial endocarditis
Hepatic:	Biliary cirrhosis, biliary atresia, α_1-antitrypsin deficiency
Gastrointestinal:	Crohn's disease, ulcerative colitis, chronic amebic and bacillary diarrhea, multiple polyposis
Endocrine:	Thyrotoxicosis
Hematologic:	Thalassemia

Hilman BC: Clinical assessment of pulmonary disease in infants and children. In Hilman BC (ed): Pediatric Respiratory Disease. Philadelphia, W.B. Saunders, 1993, p 61.

62. What is the pathophysiology of clubbing?

The answer remains unclear. The increased soft tissue under the nailbeds that causes digital clubbing is thought to be vascular (possibly multiple arteriovenous connections). These might be caused by the presence of vasoactive substances that are increased either by hypoxia or by decreased lung clearance. Another theory postulates that digital clubbing is caused by local release of platelet-derived growth factor. Ordinarily, platelet-emboli containing this factor are trapped by the pulmonary circulation, but in cases of pulmonary shunting they may become trapped in the digital vessels.

63. Nasal polyps are associated with which conditions?

Pediatric: Nasal polyps are very rare in children except as a manifestation of cystic fibrosis. Approximately 3% of children with cystic fibrosis present with nasal polyps, which are often a recurrent problem. A sweat test is essential in these patients.

Adolescents: There is a wider range of possible diagnoses, including cystic fibrosis, allergic rhinitis, chronic sinusitis, malignancy, "triad asthma" (asthma, nasal polyps, aspirin sensitivity), and ciliary dyskinesia syndrome (e.g., Kartagener syndrome).

64. A 13-year-old with chronic sinusitis and recurrent pulmonary infections has a chest x-ray demonstrating a right-sided cardiac silhouette. What diagnostic test should be considered next?

Bronchial or **nasal turbinate biopsy** for electron microscopic evaluation of cilia. Kartagener syndrome is one of the ciliary dyskinesia (or immotile cilia) syndromes. It presents with a constellation of recurrent pulmonary infections, chronic sinusitis, recurrent otitis media, situs inversus, and infertility (in males). Structural ciliary abnormalities (most commonly absent dynein arms) result in decreased clearance of respiratory secretions, predisposing to infection. In addition, since spermatozoa have tails with the same ultrastructural abnormalities as respiratory cilia, they move less well. The cause of the situs inversus is not fully understood. It has been suggested that cilia are important for movement of the midgut into the coelomic cavity in the proper orientation during fetal life and that derangements of this process may lead to situs inversus.

65. If a teenager presents with hemoptysis, frequent nosebleeds, and mucosal telangiectasia (just like his father), what condition should you suspect?

Hereditary hemorrhagic telangiectasia (also called Osler-Weber-Rendu syndrome). This autosomal dominant condition is characterized by increasing numbers of telangiectasias as the patient ages (often on the lips, tongue, ears, fingers, and toes). The development of AV fistulas and AV malformations in multiple organs is common.

66. In which children who snore should obstructive sleep apnea (OSA) be suspected?

Progressive obstruction should be suspected if a parent notes a child is developing frequent nighttime awakenings, snoring with periods of silence, marked intercostal or substernal retractions, sleep with predominantly mouth breathing, or unusual sleeping postures, enuresis, or profuse sweating. In school, daytime hypersomnolence, learning problems, morning headache, and personality change may be noted. Many families have a video camera and will record their child's sleep if requested.

67. What evaluations should be done in a child with suspected OSA?

The sounds of snoring are due to structural upper airway narrowing (most commonly seen in children with adenoidal or tonsillar hypertrophy) or due to loss of pharyngeal muscle tone during sleep. OSA can also be complicated by central apnea (i.e., CNS respiratory center dysfunction). If history, physical examination or recordings of the child's snoring suggest OSA, referral for ENT evaluation and possible tonsillectomy and adenoidectomy is appropriate. Since lymphoid tissue continues to hypertrophy until approximately age 9–10 years, younger children with symptoms due to tonsillar or adenoidal enlargement are more likely to exhibit progression. However, most children who snore do not require surgery. If the clinical picture is less clear, additional evaluations can include overnight pulse oximetry, polysomnography, and/or upper airway evaluation by radiographic imaging (e.g., cinefluoroscopy, CT) or fiberoptic endoscopy.

68. What are the potential long-term consequences of OSA?

With repetitive episodes of apnea, a patient experiences periods of hypoxia and hypercapnia. Cumulatively, these can lead to right ventricular hypertrophy, hypertension, polycythemia, and a compensatory metabolic alkalosis. The most feared long-term complication is life-threatening cor pulmonale.

Strollo PJ Jr, Rogers RM: Obstructive sleep apnea. N Engl J Med 334:99–104, 1996.

69. What is the natural history of laryngomalacia?

Congenital laryngomalacia is the most common cause of infantile stridor and generally has an excellent prognosis. Even children with mild laryngomalacia have increased episodes of brief desaturation and hypercapnia, but they are usually otherwise asymptomatic and the symptoms resolve by 2 years of age. However, close follow-up is mandatory because an occasional child has failure to thrive, difficulty in feeding, and significant obstruction. This may require surgical correction or tracheostomy to relieve the obstruction.

Nussbaum E, Maggi JC: Laryngomalacia in children. Chest 98:942–944, 1990.

70. How can you clinically distinguish bilateral from unilateral vocal cord paralysis in an infant?

Normally, the vocal cords are tonically abducted, with voluntary adduction resulting in speech. With unilateral paralysis, one cord is ineffective in speech and hoarseness results. The infant's cry may be weak or absent. Stridor is usually minimal but may be positional (e.g., sleeping on the side with the paralyzed cord up may allow it to fall to midline and produce obstructive sounds). With bilateral paralysis, hoarseness is less apparent, the cry remains weak, but stridor (both inspiratory and expiratory) is usually quite prominent.

71. What is the most common cause of chronic hoarseness in children?

Screamer's nodes. These are vocal cord nodules caused by vocal abuse, such as repetitive screaming, throat-clearing, and coughing. They are the cause of a hoarse voice in > 50% of children when the hoarse voice persists for > 2 weeks.

72. A 3-month-old who wheezes loudly while active, but not while sleeping, should be suspected of having what condition?

Congenital intrathoracic tracheomalacia or **bronchomalacia**. In these infants, the underlying weakness of the airways may not be evident in the newborn period, but it becomes manifest later when the larger infant is able to generate greater expiratory pressure during periods of activity. This increased intrathoracic pressure results in airway collapse. Fluoroscopy or bronchoscopy will confirm the diagnosis.

73. Which clinical features are suggestive of foreign-body aspiration?

Symptoms and history	**Signs**
• Child < 4 years old	• Fixed, localized wheeze
• Boys twice as common as girls	• Generalized wheezing in child with no prior
• Coughing	history of asthma
• Hemoptysis	• Reduced breath sounds over one lung, one lobe,
• Respiratory infection not resolving	or one segment
with treatment	• Mediastinal shift
• History of choking	• One nipple higher than other
• Difficulty in breathing	• Stridor

74. Are chest x-rays useful in evaluating a foreign-body aspiration?

Unfortunately, only about 10–15% of aspirated foreign bodies are radiopaque. Thus, inspiratory films are often normal. Features suggesting a foreign-body aspiration are:

1. Expiratory chest x-ray showing asymmetry in lung aeration due to obstructive emphysema (the foreign body often acts as a ball-valve mechanism, allowing air in but not out)

2. Decubitus films that show the same asymmetry (these views are often used in uncooperative children who cannot or will not exhale on command)

3. Obstructive atelectasis

75. What characterizes the acute respiratory distress syndrome (ARDS)?

This entity was previously known as the adult respiratory distress syndrome, but it is a significant cause of morbidity in critically ill children. Most typically, a patient with previously normal lungs has an acute insult with subsequent deterioration in pulmonary function characterized by:

1. Hypoxemia, right-to-left pulmonary shunting and decreased lung compliance

2. Improved oxygenation only with high peak inspiratory pressure and positive end-expiratory pressure (PEEP)

3. Marked nonhydrostatic pulmonary edema with capillary leak in the early stages and with interstitial changes and even lung destruction in the later phases.

Its name derives in large part from histologic similarities to neonatal respiratory distress syndrome.

76. In what settings can children develop ARDS?

Direct pulmonary injury	Indirect pulmonary injury
• Smoke or chemical inhalation	• Septic or hypovolemic shock
• Gastric aspiration	• Burns
• Near-drowning	• Multiple trauma
• Fat embolism	• Pancreatitis
• Trauma	• Drug overdoses (e.g., aspirin,
• Infection	barbiturates, tricyclic antidepressants)

77. Is surfactant an efficacious therapy in ARDS?

An important clinical manifestation of ARDS is stiff lungs due to surfactant deficiency. The protein leak into the lungs of patients with ARDS inhibits the normal function of surfactant-associated proteins, with a resulting increase in surface tension of the alveolar air-liquid interface. This inhibition can be overcome by providing exogenous surfactant proteins and phospholipid. So far, only limited data address the role of surfactant in the clinical management of ARDS. Anecdotal reports of individualstreated with large doses of surfactant show a positive response in lung compliance and oxygenation. One potential drawback is the high cost of the large doses that would be required.

Paulson TE, et al: New concepts in the treatment of children with acute respiratory distress syndrome. J Pediatr 127:163–175, 1995.

78. What four types of disease can be produced by pulmonary aspergillosis?

Aspergillus fumigatus is a mold that produces four different types of disease in humans:

1. **Invasive infection** in immunocompromised hosts (e.g., chronic granulomatous disease, T-cell deficiencies, chemotherapy patients)

2. **Allergic disease**—sensitized individuals with asthma may simply react to *A. fumigatus* as an allergen in the same way that they might react to ragweed.

3. **Mycetoma**—the mold fills an old cavity in the lung (e.g., tuberculosis).

4. **Allergic bronchopulmonary aspergillosis**. This is a hypersensitivity response to saprophytic colonization of diseased airways. A significant component of the disease is produced by the immune response to *A. fumigatus* and not by the organism itself. This disease tends to affect children with abnormal airways, especially those with cystic fibrosis. In adults, it is usually associated with asthma, but this association is uncommon in childhood.

79. List the characteristic features of allergic bronchopulmonary aspergillosis.

• Hyphae in the sputum	• Positive serum precipitins
• Sputum eosinophilia	• Positive immediate and delayed skin tests
• Peripheral blood eosinophilia	• Transient infiltrates on chest x-ray
• Increased serum IgE	• Proximal, cylindrical bronchiectasis
• Positive IgE antibody test (RAST)	

80. When should bronchiolitis obliterans be suspected?

Bronchiolitis obliterans is a condition of diffuse fibrosis and scarring of the bronchioles and alveolar ducts following a lower respiratory insult (e.g., infection, aspiration, toxic inhalation). It has also been associated with connective tissue diseases and transplantation, but many times a cause is not determined. The diagnosis should be suspected in patients with prolonged respiratory symptoms (including exercise intolerance) or auscultatory findings following infection. Often, the radiographic findings are disproportionately minor compared with the severity of respiratory impairment and clinical findings. In some cases, a unilateral hyperlucent lung is noted (Swyer-James syndrome).

81. What are the possible mechanisms for the development of lung abscesses in children?

1. Following pneumonia, particularly *Staphylococcus aureus, Haemophilus influenzae, Streptococcus pneumoniae,* and *Klebsiella pneumoniae*

2. Hematogenous spread, especially if an indwelling central catheter or right-sided endocarditis is present
3. Direct extension from a liver abscess or rib osteomyelitis
4. Penetrating trauma
5. Aspiration, especially in neurologically compromised patients
6. Secondary to infection of an underlying pulmonary anomaly, such as a bronchogenic cyst
   Campbell PW: Lung abscess. In Hilman BC (ed): Pediatric Respiratory Disease. Philadelphia, W.B.
Saunders, 1993, pp 257–262.

82. Describe the typical clinical findings in bronchiectasis.

Bronchiectasis is the progressive dilation and possible eventual destruction of bronchi most
likely from acute and/or recurrent obstruction and infection. It may result from a variety of infections (e.g., adenoviral, rubeola, pertussis, tuberculosis) and is often associated with underlying
pulmonary susceptibility (e.g., cystic fibrosis, ciliary dyskinesia syndromes, immunodeficiencies). Clinical findings can be variable but usually include persistent cough, production of
purulent sputum, recurrent fevers, and digital clubbing. Inspiratory crackles and coarsening of
breath sounds are often heard over the affected area. Hemoptysis and wheezing can occur but are
uncommon.

83. Name the most common finding in childhood sarcoidosis.

Sarcoidosis, a systemic granulomatous disease of unknown etiology, is very rare in children. Nearly 100% of children with sarcoidosis have an **abnormal chest x-ray**, most commonly **hilar adenopathy**, although only half have respiratory symptoms. Weight loss, fatigue,
and peripheral adenopathy occur in ≥ 50%. A normal chest x-ray makes this diagnosis very
unlikely.

84. A novice teenage mountain-climber develops headache, marked cough, and orthopnea at the end of a rapid, second-day climb. What is the likely diagnosis?

Acute mountain sickness with high-altitude pulmonary edema. This condition results
from insufficient time to adapt to altitude changes with resultant alveolar and tissue hypoxia, increased pulmonary vascular permeability, and possible pulmonary hypertension. In severe cases,
cerebral edema can result. Treatment consists of returning to lower altitude, administration of
oxygen, and use of medications to lessen cerebral edema (e.g., diuretics, acetazolamide, corticosteroids). Unfortunately, the effectiveness of these medications is highly variable.

85. What are the two forms of pulmonary sequestration?

Pulmonary sequestration is a portion of lung tissue that has become isolated from the rest
of the lung during morphogenesis and has a systemic blood supply without the normal connections to the airways and pulmonary circulation. There are two forms: **Intralobar** forms, which
are the more common, often become infected and may be discovered during evaluation for recurrent pneumonia. **Extralobar** sequestrations, which are separated from the lung by a pleural
reflection, are often asymptomatic but may come to light because of associated congenital
malformations.

86. What is the likely diagnosis in a child with diffuse lung disease, microcytic anemia, and sputum containing hemosiderin-laden macrophages?

Pulmonary hemosiderosis. This condition, which can present with chronic respiratory
problems or acute hemoptysis, is characterized by alveolar hemorrhage and a microcytic hypochromic anemia with a low serum iron level. Hemosiderin is ingested by alveolar macrophages
that can often be detected in sputum or gastric aspirates after staining with Prussian blue. Most
commonly, the condition is idiopathic and isolated, but it can be associated with cow's milk sensitivity (Heiner syndrome), glomerulonephritis with basement membrane antibodies (Goodpasture syndrome), collagen vascular disease, or pancreatitis.

87. How should a child with a spontaneous pneumothorax be managed?

If the pneumothorax is small and the child asymptomatic, observation alone is appropriate. Administration of supplemental oxygen may speed resorption of the free air. If the pneumothorax is > 20% [as measured by the (diameter of pneumothorax)^3/(diameter of hemithorax)^3] and/or the patient has evolving respiratory symptoms, needle aspiration should be considered. More severe symptoms, discovery of underlying pathology, or the need for a subsequent surgical procedure would warrant placement of a chest tube. Signs of tension pneumothorax (e.g., marked dyspnea, tachypnea and tachycardia, unilateral thoracic hyperresonance with negligible breath sounds, tracheal shift) necessitate emergent aspiration and tube placement. Of note, children and adolescents with spontaneous pneumothoraces have a high recurrence rate because of the common association with subpleural blebs. Many authorities recommend chest CT with contrast as a follow-up, because significant blebs can be treated with surgical pleurodesis.

88. In children with pleural effusions, how are exudates distinguished from transudates?

Most exudates have a protein of > 2.6 gm/dl, protein ratio (pleural fluid:serum) > 0.5, lactate dehydrogenase (LDH) > 200 IU, and LDH ratio (pleural fluid:serum) > 0.6. Exudates are more common in parapneumonic effusions, malignancies (especially lymphoma), uremia, traumatic hemothorax, chylothorax, and tuberculosis. Transudates are seen more commonly in congestive heart failure, nephrotic syndrome, upper airway obstruction, and atelectasis.

Papastamelos C: Pleural effusions. In Schidlow DV, Smith DS (eds): A Practical Guide to Pediatric Respiratory Diseases. Philadelphia, Hanley & Belfus, 1994, pp 113–126.

89. Pleural effusions are most commonly associated with which infectious agents?

Staphylococcus aureus	*Mycobacterium tuberculosis*
Streptococcus pneumoniae	*Mycoplasma pneumoniae*
Haemophilus influenzae	Viruses (esp. coxsackieviruses, echoviruses)

90. Who was Ondine and what was her curse?

Ondine was a legendary water nymph who fell in love with a mortal and put a curse on him that, should he ever betray her, he would suffocate by not breathing when he fell asleep. Ondine's lover, Hans, unfortunately fell for the greater charms of Bertha, and he eventually succumbed while dozing. The term **Ondine's curse** has been used to describe the syndrome of sleep apnea secondary to reduced respiratory drive. This rare condition is often associated with other abnormalities of brainstem function. Ondine's curse may be idiopathic, or it may be a complication of an earlier insult to the developing brain. In some families, it is genetic. These children are treated by tracheostomy and mechanical ventilation during sleep. Recent results with phrenic nerve pacing have been good.

CYSTIC FIBROSIS

91. What is the importance of the CFTR protein in cystic fibrosis (CF)?

Cystic fibrosis transmembrane conductance regulator (CFTR) protein is a key ionic channel that regulates chloride transfer across the apical membrane of the respiratory epithelial cell. In CF patients, chloride (with the simultaneous passive movement of sodium and water) is poorly secreted, resulting in respiratory and pancreatic secretions that are relatively dehydrated and viscid. These hyperviscous secretions may obstruct pancreatic ducts as well as interfere with pulmonary mucociliary clearance. Steatorrhoea and chronic respiratory disease result.

92. What is the incidence of cystic fibrosis?

Whites	1:2000
Blacks (U.S.)	1:17,000
Native Americans (U.S.)	1:80,000
Orientals (Hawaii)	1:90,000

93. List the indications for sweat testing.

Pulmonary/Upper Respiratory	Gastrointestinal	Metabolic/Other
Atelectasis, chronic/recurrent (especially RUL)	Cirrhosis and portal hypertension	Acrodermatitis enteropathica
Bronchiectasis	Intestinal atresia	Aspermia/absent vas deferens
Bronchiolitis, chronic/recurrent	Meconium ileus	Edema, hypoproteinemia
Chronic cough	Meconium plug syndrome	Failure to thrive
Digital clubbing	Mucoid-impacted appendix	Hypoprothrombinemia beyond newborn period
Hemoptysis	Recurrent intussusception	Metabolic alkalosis, hypochloremia
Mucoid *Pseudomonas* colonization	Recurrent pancreatitis	Positive family history
Nasal polyps	Rectal prolapse	Salt depletion syndrome
Pansinusitis	Steatorrhea, malabsorption	Salty taste/salt crystals
Pneumonia, chronic/recurrent		Vitamin A deficiency (bulging fontanel)

Adapted from Rosenstein BJ: Cystic fibrosis. In Loughlin GM, Eigen H (eds): Respiratory Disease in Children. Baltimore, Williams & Wilkins, 1994, p 275; with permission.

94. What constitutes an abnormal sweat test?
When sweat gland secretions are obtained by pilocarpine iontophoresis, a level of sweat chloride > 60 mEq/L is abnormal, 40–60 mEq/L is borderline, and < 40 mEq/L is normal.

95. What are the causes of false-positive and false-negative sweat tests?
False-positive sweat tests

Malnutrition	Type I glycogen storage disease
Celiac disease	Hypoparathyroidism
Untreated adrenal insufficiency	Atopic dermatitis
Anorexia nervosa	Pupillotonia-areflexia and segmental hypohidrosis
Renal diabetes insipidus	Mucopolysaccharidosis
Ectodermal dysplasia	Klinefelter syndrome
Fucosidosis	Hypogammaglobulinemia
Familial cholestasis	Laboratory error
Untreated hypothyroidism	

False-negative tests
Peripheral edema
Administration of cloxacillin (not well-substantiated)
Laboratory error

Adapted from Ruddy RM, Scanlin TF: Abnormal sweat electrolytes in a case of celiac disease and a case of psychosocial failure to thrive. Clin Pediatr 26:83–89, 1987; with permission.

96. How does the spectrum of clinical manifestations of CF vary among infants, children, and adults?

Clinical Manifestations of Cystic Fibrosis by Age Group

	APPROXIMATE INCIDENCE (%)		
MANIFESTATION	INFANTS	CHILDREN	ADULTS
Respiratory			
Bronchiectasis	—	30–50	> 90
Pneumothorax	—	1–2	10–15
Hemoptysis	—	5–15	50–60
Pancreatic			
Insufficiency	80–85	85	90
Pancreatitis	—	1–2	2–4
Diabetes mellitus	—	2–4	5

(Table continued on following page.)

Clinical Manifestations of Cystic Fibrosis by Age Group (Cont.)

MANIFESTATION	INFANTS	CHILDREN	ADULTS
		APPROXIMATE INCIDENCE (%)	
Hepatobiliary			
Biliary cirrhosis	—	10–20	> 20
Cholelithiasis	—	5	5–10
Biliary obstruction	—	1–2	5
Intestinal			
Meconium ileus	10–15	—	—
Rectal prolapse	—	10–15	1–2
Intussusception	—	1–5	1–2
Esophageal reflux	—	1–5	> 10
Distal intestinal obstruction syndrome	—	1–5	10–20
Appendiceal abscess	—	0–1	1–2

From MacLusky I: Cystic fibrosis for the primary care pediatrician. Pediatr Ann 22:545, 1993; with permission.

97. What is the pathophysiology of rectal prolapse in CF?

Rectal prolapse is a common complication of CF—up to 20% of patients may be affected. Possible explanations include:
- Poor nutrition with defective connective tissue supporting structures
- Chronic coughing which raises intra-abdominal pressure
- Abnormal bowel movements (increased volume of stools with abnormal consistency)
- Redundant colonic mucosa

98. Explain the mechanisms of action of amiloride, recombinant human DNase, and α_1-antitrypsin in the treatment of CF.

1. Amiloride is a sodium channel blocker that has been shown to decrease sputum viscosity in patients with CF and delay the rate of respiratory deterioration. The use of medications that affect electrolyte transport at the membrane level is a major focus of current research.

2. The sputum of patients with CF has a very high DNA content due to degenerating host neutrophils, and this contributes greatly to increased viscosity. Aerosolized recombinant DNase (Dornase alpha) degrades this DNA, reduces viscosity, and has proven beneficial in clinical trials.

3. Recurrent pulmonary infections with marked neutrophil accumulation lead to lysosomal release of hydrolytic enzymes, such as elastase, often in excess of natural inhibitors such as α_1-antitrypsin. This imbalance can contribute to airway destruction and bronchiectasis. Aerosolized treatment with α_1-antitrypsin or other antiproteases may lessen the damage.

Wilmott RW, Fiedler MA: Recent advances in the treatment of cystic fibrosis. Pediatr Clin North Am 41:431–451, 1994.

99. How is hemoptysis managed in CF?

Minor hemoptysis (< 1 oz blood)
  See the patient if hemoptysis represents a new problem.
  Check coagulation studies, hemoglobin, sputum culture.
  Start antibiotics if the patient has infection.
  Stop irritating, inhaled medications (Mucomyst)
  Stop percussion temporarily and substitute vibration and postural drainage.
Moderate hemoptysis (1–6 oz blood)
  All of the above.
  Type and cross-match blood.
  Consider hospital admission for observation.

Major hemoptysis (> 6 oz blood)
   All of the above.
   Admit to hospital.
   Transfuse if indicated.
   Evaluate for GelFoam embolization of bleeding bronchial artery or for partial pneu-
     monectomy.

100. How are recurrent pneumothoraces in CF managed?

Medical treatment includes chemical pleurodesis with intrapleural instillation of tetracycline or quinacrine. Surgical treatment includes parietal pleurectomy (also known as pleural stripping) or pleural abrasion with dry gauze/abrasive pads. The morbidity and efficacy of medical
and surgical therapy appear to be similar. An extensive pleurodesis may make a CF patient ineli-
gible for heart-lung transplantation; therefore, the most appropriate therapy is a limited surgical
pleurodesis if the patient may become a candidate for a heart-lung transplant in the future.
Thoracoscopic evaluation and talc pleurodesis is a growing trend in adult pulmonology that may
have application in the treatment of CF.

101. What are the complications of pediatric lung transplantation?
   • Perioperative hemorrhage with multisystem organ failure
   • Severe, life-threatening infections with resistant organisms
   • Development of bronchiolitis obliterans
   • Development of post-transplant lymphoproliferative disorder
   • Rejection
   Noyes BE, et al: Experience with pediatric lung transplantation. J Pediatr 124:261–268, 1994.

102. Which features of CF have prognostic significance?
   1. **Gender.** Males have better survival rates than females, although the gap is narrowing.
   2. **Colonization with virulent bacteria.** *Pseudomonas aeruginosa* and *Burkholderia*
(formerly *Pseudomonas*) *cepacia* are more serious pathogens which are difficult to clear once the
patient is persistently infected. Patients who are chronically colonized with these organisms have
significantly poorer survival rates than other patients with CF.
   3. **Nasal polyps** appear to be a positive prognostic indicator. Patients with polyps appear
to have milder pulmonary disease. This is a surprising observation with no obvious explanation.
   4. **Cor pulmonale** is one of the late complications of CF because progressive obstructive
airway disease leads to the development of pulmonary hypertension and respiratory failure. The
prognosis after developing cor pulmonale is poor.
   5. **Pneumothorax** is associated with moderate to advanced lung disease in patients
with CF. Therefore, air leak has traditionally been regarded as a poor prognostic sign. The
prognosis has been improving now that pneumothoraces are being managed aggressively at
major centers.
   6. **Worsening pulmonary function tests**. Patients with an FEV_1 < 30% of predicted will
have a 2-year mortality rate of > 50%.
   Kerem E, et al: Predictions of mortality in patients with cystic fibrosis. N Engl J Med 326:1187–1191,
1992.

103. How has the survival rate for CF changed since the 1960s?

In 1965, the median survival was age 7 years. By the mid-1990s, the mean survival had increased to 30.5 years for males and 28 years for females.
   Fitzsimmons SC: The changing epidemiology of cystic fibrosis. J Pediatr 122:1–9, 1993.

104. What are the barriers to widespread prenatal screening for CF?

The CFTR gene was identified in 1989 on the long arm of chromosome 7. Although the
most common mutation was found to be a deletion of phenylalanine at position 508 (delta F508),
this mutation accounts for only 75% of the total mutations. More than 500 mutations to date have

been identified. Although the more common mutations could be included in screening, the potential for false-negative testing is significant. Other issues include cost-benefit uncertainties, as well as ethical issues regarding the rationale for screening for an illness with a life-expectancy that may soon approach 40 years.

PNEUMONIA

105. Which agents cause pneumonia in children?

Newborn	2–6 mos	6 mos–5 yrs	School age/teenager
Group B streptococci	RSV	RSV	*M. pneumoniae*
Gram-negative bacilli	Adenoviruses	Parainfluenza viruses	*S. pneumoniae*
S. aureus	Parainfluenza	Influenza viruses	*C. pneumoniae*
CMV	Influenza viruses	*S. pneumoniae*	Influenza viruses
	C. trachomatis	*H. influenzae*	
	U. urealyticum	*S. aureus*	
	S. pneumoniae		
	H. influenzae		

106. Are throat or nasopharyngeal cultures helpful in the diagnosis of pneumonia?

As a rule, the correlation between throat and nasopharyngeal bacterial cultures and lower respiratory tract pathogens is poor and of limited value. Healthy children may be colonized with a wide variety of potentially pathologic bacteria (e.g., *Staphylococcus aureus, Haemophilus influenzae*) which can be considered part of the normal flora. *Bordetella pertussis* is an exception. Cultures or antigen detection systems to identify respiratory viruses or chlamydia, however, are highly informative, because these organisms are rarely carried asymptomatically.

107. How often are blood cultures positive in children with suspected bacterial pneumonia?

10–15%. This number is an estimate because the true denominator in the equation (the number of true bacterial pneumonias) is difficult to ascertain due to the difficulty in making a definitive diagnosis. The low rate of positive blood cultures does suggest that most bacterial pneumonias are *not* acquired through hematogenous spread.

108. Can a chest x-ray reliably distinguish between viral and bacterial pneumonia?

No. Although viral infections more commonly have perihilar, peribronchial, or interstitial infiltrates, hyperinflation, segmental atelectasis, and hilar adenopathy, there can be considerable overlap with bacterial (and chlamydial and mycoplasmal) pneumonia. Bacterial pneumonia more commonly results in an alveolar infiltrate, but the sensitivity and specificity of this finding are not very high.

Korppi M, et al: Comparison of radiological findings and microbial aetiology of childhood pneumonia. Acta Pediatr 82:360–363, 1993.

109. Which children with pneumonia should be hospitalized?

1. All who appear toxic, dyspneic, or hypoxic
2. All with suspected staphylococcal pneumonia (e.g., pneumatocele on chest x-ray)
3. All with a significant pleural effusion
4. All with suspected aspiration pneumonia (because of the higher likelihood of progression)
5. All who cannot tolerate oral medications or are at significant risk for dehydration
6. Suspected bacterial pneumonia in infants < 12 months
7. Poor response to outpatient therapy after 48 hours
8. All whose family situation is of unclear stability

110. What clinical clues suggest atypical pneumonia?

These infections are characterized by minimal or nonproductive cough, headache, lack of consolidation on chest x-ray, and sometimes confusing extrapulmonary signs. The two most common causes in pediatric and adolescent populations are *Mycoplasma* and *Chlamydia pneumoniae*. *Chlamydia* is more commonly associated with pharyngitis and hoarseness.

111. What are the causes of "afebrile infant pneumonia" syndrome?

The syndrome is usually due to *Chlamydia trachomatis*, CMV, or the genital mycoplasmas (*Ureaplasma urealyticum, Mycoplasma hominis*). Affected infants develop progressive respiratory distress over several days (to a few weeks) along with failure to thrive. A maternal history of a sexually transmitted disease is commonly obtained. Chest x-rays reveal bilateral diffuse infiltrates with hyperinflation. There may be eosinophilia and elevated quantitative immunoglobulins (IgG, IgA, IgM). The causes overlap clinically, although a history of conjunctivitis suggests chlamydia.

Overall JC: Is it bacterial or viral? Laboratory differentiation. Pediatr Rev 14:251–261, 1993.

112. How likely is an infant to develop infection if born to a mother with positive cervical cultures for *Chlamydia trachomatis*?

Up to 50% of infants demonstrate an inclusion conjunctivitis, and approximately 20% develop pneumonia. Since the chlamydial infection rate during pregnancy is approximately 5% (and estimating an annual U.S. birth rate of 3 million), then up to 30,000 infants annually may develop chlamydial pneumonia, making it the most common cause of pneumonia in children under 6 months of age.

113. What are the clinical characteristics of chlamydial pneumonia in infants?

- Most infants (90% or more) present by 8 weeks of age
- Onset is gradual with upper respiratory prodromal symptoms lasting > 1 week
- Nearly 100% are afebrile
- Less than half have inclusion conjunctivitis
- Respiratory picture: staccato cough, diffuse rales, little wheezing
- Chest x-ray: bilateral hyperexpansion, symmetric interstitial infiltrates
- 70% have an elevated absolute eosinophil count (> $400/mm^3$)
- Over 90% have elevated quantitative immunoglobulins (IgG, IgM)

114. What is the best method for diagnosing chlamydial pneumonia?

The gold standard is culture of the organism, but at present this requires techniques not available in most hospital labs. Furthermore, the lability of the organism makes transport difficult. Antigen detection techniques (using direct fluorescent antibody or enzyme immunoassay) of respiratory secretions are the most commonly used devices. Serologic studies demonstrating a fourfold or greater rise in IgG titers or an elevated single IgM titer are also used.

115. What is the most common auscultatory finding in mycoplasmal pneumonia?

Dry rales (crackles)—80%. These may persist 2 weeks or more along with cough and sputum production. Wheezing is heard in < 50% of patients.

116. How characteristic is the radiologic picture of mycoplasmal pneumonia?

The chest x-ray is variable and nonspecific. Most findings are unilateral (up to 85%) and occur in the lower lobes. Early in the course of illness, the picture is one of increased interstitial markings with a reticulonodular pattern. Frequently, this progresses to patchy, segmental, or even lobar areas of consolidation. Hilar adenopathy occurs in up to one-third of patients. Pleural effusions, as demonstrated by lateral decubitus views, may occur in up to 20% of children.

Broughton RA: *Mycoplasma pneumoniae* infections in childhood. Pediatr Infect Dis J 5:71–84, 1986.

117. How helpful are cold agglutinins in the diagnosis of *Mycoplasma pneumoniae* infections?

Cold agglutinins are IgM autoantibodies that agglutinate red cells at 4°C by reacting with the I antigen. Up to 75% of patients with mycoplasmal infections will develop them, usually toward the end of the first week of illness with a peak at 4 weeks. A titer of 1:64 supports the diagnosis. Other infectious agents, including adenovirus, cytomegalovirus, Epstein-Barr virus, influenza, rubella, *Chlamydia*, and *Listeria*, can also give a positive result. A single cold agglutinin titer of ≥ 1:64 is therefore suggestive but not conclusive evidence of infection with *M. pneumoniae*.

118. How is the bedside test for cold agglutinins done?

In a tube containing sodium citrate, blood of equal volume (usually about 4–5 drops) is added. The tube is immersed in ice for 30–60 seconds, and the fluid is observed by rolling the tube on its side. Coarsely flocculating red blood cells constitute a positive test, which correlates with a cold agglutinin titer of ≥ 1:64.

119. When do the radiologic findings with pneumonia resolve?

Although there is a wide range, as a rule, most infiltrates due to *Streptococcus pneumoniae* resolve in 6–8 weeks and those due to RSV in 2–3 weeks. However, with some viral infections (e.g., adenovirus), it may take up to 1 year for x-rays to normalize. Unfortunately, in most instances, the underlying etiology is not known. If significant radiologic abnormalities persist > 6 weeks, there should be a high index of suspicion for a possible underlying problem (e.g., unusual infection, anatomic abnormality, immunologic deficiency).

Regelmann WE: Diagnosing the cause of recurrent and persistent pneumonia in children. Pediatr Ann 22:561–568, 1993.

120. Do children with pneumonia need follow-up x-rays to verify resolution?

In the absence of pleural effusion and in a child who is not immunocompromised, no repeat x-ray study is needed to verify resolution if there are no symptoms or signs of disease present at a 3–4-week follow-up. The clinical course of the illness is a sufficient and accurate guide in itself.

Gibson NA, et al: Value of radiological follow-up of childhood pneumonia. BMJ 307:1117–1120, 1993.

121. What factors can contribute to recurrent pneumonia?

1. Aspiration susceptibility (e.g., airway anomalies, swallowing dysfunction, gastroesophageal reflux)

2. Congenital pulmonary anomalies (e.g., pulmonary sequestration)

3. Abnormal secretions and clearance of secretions (e.g., cystic fibrosis, ciliary dyskinesia, postinfectious ciliary dysfunction)

4. Immunodeficiency

5. Congenital or acquired airway compression (e.g., vascular rings, enlarged lymph nodes, tumor)

122. How does the pH of a substance affect the severity of disease in aspiration pneumonia?

A low pH is more harmful than a slightly alkaline or neutral pH and is more likely to be associated with bronchospasm and pneumonia. The most severe form of pneumonia is seen when gastric contents are aspirated; symptoms may develop in a matter of seconds. If the volume of aspirate is sufficiently large and the pH is < 2.5, the mortality may exceed 70%. The radiographic picture may be that of an infiltrate or pulmonary edema. Unilateral pulmonary edema may occur if the child is lying on one side.

123. How should children with aspiration pneumonia be managed?

Aspiration pneumonia is best treated supportively and conservatively. Administration of antibiotics does not appear to improve the prognosis significantly, probably because the pathophysiology is that of a chemical pneumonitis. Cultures of blood and sputum (or tracheal aspirate) should be obtained. Penicillin is the antibiotic of choice for an aspiration pneumonia when secondary infection is suspected. Postural drainage is helpful to remove the inhaled fluid. If gastric acid has been inhaled, a short course of corticosteroids may be helpful if therapy is started within a few hours of the aspiration.

PULMONARY PRINCIPLES

124. In addition to underlying immunologic immaturity, why are infants more susceptible to an increased severity of respiratory disease?

1. High thoracic compliance (allows passage through birth canal, but limits inspiratory effort)
2. Respiratory muscles more easily fatigued due to decreased muscle mass
3. Elastic recoil is low in infancy and increases toward adolescence (airway closure occurs at a higher relative lung volume)
4. High airway compliance secondary to incomplete development of cartilage facilitates airway collapse and air trapping
5. Collateral ventilation poorly developed, increasing likelihood of atelectasis during illness
6. Higher airway mucous gland concentration in infants than adults

Black P: Evaluation of chronic or recurrent cough. In Hilman BC (ed): Pediatric Respiratory Disease. Philadelphia, W.B. Saunders, 1993, pp 146–147.

125. At what age do alveoli stop increasing in number?

Although the bronchial tree is fully formed by 16 weeks of gestation, a newborn has only about one-tenth of the eventual adult number of alveoli. These continue to increase in number throughout childhood, but there is uncertainty as to the cut-off age. The most widely quoted estimates are that alveolar numbers increase until approximately 8 years, at which point hypertrophy, rather than cell division, becomes the principal mechanism of growth.

126. What is the normal respiratory rate in a child?

Rates in awake children can be widely variable depending on the state of anxiety or agitation. Rates while sleeping are much more reliable. As a general rule, the sleeping rate in infants is usually < 35/min; in toddlers, < 30/min; in older children, < 25/min; and in adolescents, < 20/min.

127. What is the difference between Kussmaul, Cheyne-Stokes, and Biot types of breathing patterns?

Kussmaul:	Deep, slow, regular respirations with prolonged exhalation (most commonly seen in ketoacidosis)
Cheyne-Stokes:	Crescendo-decrescendo respirations alternating with periods of apnea (most commonly seen in deep hemispheric, thalamic, or hypothalamic lesions, CNS trauma, increased intracranial pressure, severe congestive heart failure)
Biot:	Very irregular breathing of varying rate and depth (most commonly seen in severe CNS damage)

128. How frequently does sighing occur?

A sigh is just a sigh in Casablanca, but it is also a very effective anti-atelectatic maneuver. By definition, it is a breath more than three times the tidal volume. Data on children are unclear, but women sigh more frequently than men (10 vs 9 times/hr).

129. Is there a respiratory basis for yawning?

Although a respiratory function for yawning is frequently suggested, support for this belief is minimal. Increasing the concentration of CO_2 in inspired air will increase the respiratory rate but does not change the rate of yawning. Relief of hypoxia and opening areas of microatelectasis also are not supported by scientific studies. Some studies hypothesize that yawning may be an arousal reflex.

130. What are "coarse" breath sounds?

In coarse breath sounds the loudness of expiration equals the loudness of inspiration on auscultation. In large airways, expiratory breath sounds are louder than inspiratory breath sounds due to turbulence. Coarse breath sounds can be physiologic (as when listening just below the center of the clavicle to primarily bronchial sounds) or pathologic (if interposed fluid allows transmission of large airway sounds or if airways are widened such as in bronchiectasis).

131. At what concentration is inspired oxygen toxic?

In addition to atelectasis, high oxygen concentration can cause alveolar injury with edema, inflammation, fibrin deposition, and hyalinization. The precise level of hyperoxia that results in injury is unclear and subject to variance by age and underlying lung pathology, but a reasonable rule is to assume that a concentration of $\geq 80\%$ for > 36 hours is likely to result in significant on-going damage; $60–80\%$ is likely to be associated with more slowly progressive injury. An inspired oxygen concentration of 50%, even when administered for extended periods of time, is unlikely to cause pulmonary toxicity.

Jenkinson SG: Oxygen toxicity. J Intens Care Med 3:137–152, 1988.

132. Why is a child receiving 100% oxygen more likely to develop atelectasis than one breathing room air?

Nitrogen is more slowly absorbed than oxygen by alveoli. In room air (with its 78% nitrogen), alveolar collapse is minimized by continued presence and pressure of nitrogen gas. In 100% oxygen, however, the more rapid absorption of oxygen can lead to absorption atelectasis with intrapulmonary shunting.

133. At what PaO_2 does cyanosis develop?

Cyanosis develops when the concentration of desaturated (i.e., reduced) hemoglobin is at least 3 gm/dl centrally or 5–6 gm/dl peripherally. However, multiple factors affect the likelihood that a given PaO_2 will result in clinically apparent cyanosis: anemia (less likely), polycythemia (more likely), reduced systemic perfusion or cardiac output (more likely), and hypothermia (more likely). Cyanosis is generally a sign of significant hypoxia. In a patient with adequate perfusion and a normal hemoglobin, central cyanosis is commonly noted when the PaO_2 is approximately 50 mmHg.

134. How is the A–a gradient calculated?

The alveolar–arterial oxygen difference or gradient ($A–aDO_2$) is as measure of the efficiency of gas exchange and can be especially useful in critical care settings to monitor changes in disease severity. It is the difference between the theoretical PO_2 in the alveoli (PAO_2) and the measured oxygen tension (PaO_2) and is calculated according to the following formula:

$$A–aDO_2 = FiO_2 (P_B – 47) – (PaCO_2/RQ) – PaO_2$$

where P_B = barometric pressure, FiO_2 = inspiratory oxygen concentration, 47 = saturated water vapor pressure at 37°C, RQ = respiratory quotient (usually 0.8), and $PaCO_2$ = measured arterial CO_2 tension. The normal $A–aDO_2$ is usually < 15 mmHg, rising up to 30 mmHg in older adults. Of note, in a healthy individual breathing 100% oxygen, the $A-aDO_2$ increases significantly (up to 100 mmHg) for reasons that are not fully understood.

135. What are the causes of a reduced PaO_2 associated with an increased $A–aDO_2$?

1. **Right-to-left shunting:** intracardiac, abnormal arteriovenous connections; intrapulmonary shunts which result from perfusion of airless alveoli (e.g., pneumonia, atelectasis), often referred to as ventilation-perfusion mismatching

2. **Maldistribution of ventilation:** as in asthma, bronchiolitis, atelectasis

3. **Impaired diffusion:** an uncommon mechanism, as many of the conditions previously thought to have a "diffusion block," such as respiratory distress syndrome, also have a major component of shunting; may be seen when interstitial edema affects the septal walls (e.g., in early pulmonary edema and interstitial pneumonia)

4. **Decreased central venous oxygen content:** secondary to a sluggish circulation (e.g., shock) or increased tissue oxygen demands (e.g., sepsis)

136. What are the causes of hypoxemia with a normal A–aDO$_2$?

Hypoxemia can occur in the absence of any lung or cardiac disease from:

1. Hypoventilation (e.g., narcotic overdose, neuromuscular disease)
2. Increased altitude
3. Inspiration of hypoxic gas mixtures (e.g., iatrogenic errors)

137. How does the pulse oximeter work?

The key principle behind pulse oximetry is that oxygenated hemoglobin allows more transmission of red light than does reduced hemoglobin. In contrast, transmission of infrared light is unaffected by the amount of oxyhemoglobin present. In oximetry, pulses of red and infrared light (emitted by diodes) pass through tissue and are verified using a photodetector. During systole, when more oxygenated arterial blood is present in tissues, the amount of red light that is detected by the photoreceptor increases. The pulse oximeter measures the peak absorption of both red and infrared light during systole, subtracts the amounts from diastole and calculates a red:infrared absorption ratio. This ratio, in turn, is used to determine the arterial saturation, which is calculated according to a complex formula.

138. What are the disadvantages or limitations of pulse oximetry?

1. Patient movement disturbs measurements
2. Poor perfusion states affect accuracy
3. Fluorescent or high-intensity light (as in phototherapy for hyperbilirubinemia) or sunlight can interfere with results
4. Unreliable if abnormal hemoglobins present (e.g., methemoglobin)
5. Unable to detect hypoxia. Until the PaO$_2$ decreases below 80 mmHg, the saturation will not fall below 100%. Thus, the pulse oximeter is unable to distinguish between a PaO$_2$ of 80 mmHg and a PaO$_2$ of 130 mmHg.
6. Reliability diminishes with arterial saturations below 70–80%
7. Pressure necrosis possible in very small, ill neonates

Pramanik AK, Diaz-Blanco J: Continuous noninvasive monitoring of blood gases. In Hilman BC (ed): Pediatric Respiratory Disease. Philadelphia, W.B. Saunders, 1993, pp 172–183.

139. What are the advantages of rigid versus flexible bronchoscopy in children?

Flexible

No requirement for general anesthesia; may be done with sedation and topical anesthetics

Minimal risk to upper airway in patients who are awake

Possible to examine more distal airways

Assessment of airway dynamics is better

Rigid

Easier removal of foreign bodies

Better airway control, allowing patient to be ventilated through the bronchoscope

Superior optics

Larsen GL, et al: Respiratory tract and mediastinum In Hay WW, et al (eds): Current Pediatric Diagnosis and Treatment, 12th ed. Norwalk, CT, Appleton & Lange, 1995, p 497.

140. Why is the determination of "leak pressure" important in intubated children?

Excessive pressure from an endotracheal tube may result in ischemic injury, particularly at the level of the cricoid cartilage which is the narrowest portion of the airway. "Leak pressure" is an estimate of the snugness of the tube. It is determined by auscultation of the neck and notation of the pressure at which air escapes around the endotracheal tube. The exact point at which injury is most likely is unclear, but leak pressure > 35 cm H$_2$0 has been associated with airway complications.

DiCarlo JV, Steven JM: Respiratory failure in congenital heart disease. Pediatr Clin North Am 41: 525–542, 1994.

141. What features on pulmonary function testing distinguish obstructive from restrictive lung disease?

Obstructive

Impaired airflow during expiration with decreased flow rates (decreased FEV_1, decreased $FEF_{25-75\%}$)

Air trapping with increased residual volume (RV) and decreased forced vital capacity (FVC)

FEV_1/FVC ratio is decreased

Total lung capacity (TLC) increased in children with severe disease

Restrictive

Decreased FVC and TLC

Decreased expiratory flow rates; however, the FEV_1/FVC ratio is normal or slightly increased

142. In infants with unilateral lung disease, should the good lung be up or down?

The good lung should be up. This is another example of why children are not simply small adults. It is well established that adults with unilateral lung disease treated in a decubitus position will have an increase in oxygen saturation when the good lung is placed down; this occurs because of an increase in ventilation to the dependent lung. Studies have shown that the opposite occurs in infants and children because ventilation is preferentially distributed toward the uppermost lung. This positional redistribution of ventilation seems to change to an adult pattern during the late teenage years.

Davies H, et al: Effect of posture on regional ventilation in children. Pediatr Pulmonol 12:227–232, 1992.

143. Are home vaporizers of proven scientific value for treatment of respiratory tract infections?

Home vaporizers are one of the most frequently prescribed home remedies by grandmothers and physicians alike. One small problem: There are few data to support their utility for most of their currently prescribed indications. First, deposition data show that only 5% of the actively nebulized fluid in a mist tent enters the body. The percentage from a home vaporizer would be significantly less, and most of the mist is trapped in the nasopharynx or GI tract. Thus, vaporizing liquid to help with lower airway secretions is of dubious value. However, warmed mist does help improve nasal patency in adults with colds or allergic rhinitis. In young infants, where respiration is primarily nasal, any improvement in nasal patency during colds is likely to produce some symptomatic relief. With regards to laryngotracheitis, no prospective, placebo-controlled trial evaluating the benefit of mist therapy has ever documented an improvement in obstruction. As always, the benefits from warmed mist need to be weighed against the risk of burns, infections, and mold allergy from improper cleaning of humidifiers. Now, what are the data on chicken soup?

Szilagyi PG: Humidifiers and other symptomatic therapy for children with respiratory tract infections. Pediatr Infect Dis J 10:478–479, 1991.

144. What is the longest word in the English language?

Pneumonoultramicroscopicsilicovolcanoconiosis. As the saying goes, all that wheezes is not asthma, especially if one lives close to Mount St. Helen's.

18. RHEUMATOLOGY

Andrew H. Eichenfield, M.D.

CLINICAL ISSUES

1. List the common ocular manifestations seen in the pediatric connective tissue diseases.
When it comes to pediatric rheumatic diseases, the eyes have it. Eye problems (especially chronic uveitis) are particularly common in children with type I pauciarticular JRA, especially those with a positive ANA.

Ocular Manifestations of Pediatric Rheumatic Diseases

OCULAR MANIFESTATION	DISEASE
Uveitis—acute	Pauciarticular JRA (type II)
	Ankylosing spondylitis
	Arthritis of inflammatory bowel disease
Uveitis—chronic (± band keratopathy)	Pauciarticular JRA (type I)
Keratoconjunctivitis sicca	Sjögren's syndrome
Retinopathy (cotton wool spots)	Systemic lupus erythematosus
	Polyarteritis nodosa
	Dermatomyositis

2. What is the significance of a positive ANA?
Chudwin and colleagues reviewed the clinical and laboratory findings of 138 children with positive tests for antinuclear antibodies (ANA) over a 10-year period and found it to be a very sensitive but not a very specific test. The likelihood of rheumatic or autoimmune disease is high in pediatric patients with a positive ANA, and these children should be carefully followed with further clinical and laboratory evaluation.
Chudwin DS, et al: Significance of a positive ANA test in a pediatric population. Am J Dis Child 137:1103–1106, 1983.

3. What distinguishes dermatomyositis and polymyositis in children?
The clinical criteria of Bohan and Peter were developed to aid in diagnosis. A definitive diagnosis of dermatomyositis or polymyositis is made in the presence of 4 criteria:
1. Symmetrical proximal muscle weakness (Gowers sign, etc.)
2. Elevated serum enzymes in muscle (CK, LDH, AST, and/or aldolase)
3. Abnormal EMG (increased insertional activity; bizarre high-frequency discharges)
4. Inflammation and/or necrosis on muscle biopsy
5. Characteristic skin eruption

Presence of the rash distinguishes dermatomyositis from polymyositis. Thus, a child who has the rash and 3 of the other 4 criteria (biopsy is not necessary if you know what the rash looks like) has definite juvenile dermatomyositis and if the rash and 2 criteria are fulfilled, possible dermatomyositis. If there is no rash, there is no dermatomyositis, so definite polymyositis requires a muscle biopsy for diagnosis.
Bohan A, Peter JB: Polymyositis and dermatomyositis. N Engl J Med 292:344–347, 1975.

4. What skin changes are pathognomonic for dermatomyositis?
Gottron's papules. They begin as inflammatory papules over the dorsal interphalangeal joints. The papules become violaceous and flat-topped. Atrophy, telangiectasia, and hypopigmentation eventually result.

5. Describe the other classic cutaneous findings in dermatomyositis.
   1. Periorbital edema and erythema, with a violaceous (heliotrope) color. It can mimic the butterfly eruption of SLE and may extend down to the upper chest in a "shawl" distribution.
   2. Periungual changes: abnormal nailfold capillaries with thickening, clustering, and tortuosity.
   3. Photosensitivity in up to one-third of patients.
   4. Rarely, cutaneous vasculitis with purpura and ulceration.

6. What is the prognosis for children with juvenile dermatomyositis?
   The advent of corticosteroid therapy has greatly changed the prognosis. Before steroids, 1 in 3 children died. Now, the mortality rate is 5–10%. Up to 80% of patients will have minimal physical limitations.

7. Which infectious agents are known to cause myositis?
   Viruses (notably influenza A and B, echoviruses, and coxsackieviruses) can cause acute myositis. Viral myositis is characterized by severe pain (unusual in dermatomyositis), predilection for the calf muscles, and resolution within 1–4 weeks. Toxoplasmosis and trichinosis should also be considered in the differential diagnosis. *Staphylococcus aureus* and *Yersinia enterocolitica* have been implicated in acute episodes of more localized pyomyositis, especially after local traumatic injury.

8. Which drugs can be associated with myopathies?
   Corticosteroids, diuretics, hydroxychloroquine, amphotericin B, alcohol, vincristine, D-penicillamine, cimetidine, clofibrate.
   Zucker J: Drug-induced myopathies. Semin Arthritis Rheum 19:259, 1990.

9. What comprises the mix in mixed connective tissue disease?
   Mixed connective tissue disease is what it sounds like: a mish-mash of scleroderma, dermatomyositis, rheumatoid arthritis, and SLE. Common signs and symptoms include Raynaud syndrome, esophageal dysmotility, diffuse puffiness of the hands, as well as myositis. Studies in adults emphasize the relative rarity of renal and CNS involvement, but children do not appear to be so spared. Severe vasculitis and thrombocytopenia have been reported in children. The serologic markers which confirm the diagnosis are high-titer speckled ANA (1:1,000–1:1,000,000) and antibodies to the extractable nuclear antigen RNP.
   Cassidy JT, et al: Clinical outcome of children with mixed connective tissue disease. J Rheumatol 19(suppl 33):121, 1992.

10. Is Raynaud's a phenomenon, disease, or syndrome?
   Maurice Raynaud, while still a medical student in 1874, described a triad of episodic pallor, cyanosis following exposure to cold or physical stress, and subsequent erythema and hyperemia. The term Raynaud **phenomenon** is used to describe this clinical situation. The Raynaud **syndrome** occurs when the phenomenon is associated with a disease (e.g., scleroderma, SLE). Raynaud **disease** is the phenomenon occurring in isolation (present for several years without apparent association).

11. How are children with Raynaud phenomenon managed?
   Children are cautioned to avoid cold exposure and to protect their hands and feet. Many can learn to control the temperature of their extremities through biofeedback. Those who cannot and who are progressing to trophic changes may benefit from pharmacotherapy, particularly nifedipine.

12. Name the varieties of localized scleroderma.
   Localized scleroderma involves all layers of skin and can cause abnormalities of underlying tissue down to bone. Localized scleroderma embraces several confusing terms:

Morphea: patches of plaque-like, hidebound skin, which may start as a violaceous or erythematous discoloration before hardening and becoming waxy.

Linear scleroderma: like morphea, but in bands.

Scleroderma "en coup de sabre": involvement of the upper face, forehead, and scalp; may lead to hemifacial atrophy (Parry-Romberg syndrome).

13. In children with systemic scleroderma, which organ systems are most commonly affected?

Systemic scleroderma, also called progressive systemic sclerosis, is a condition of fibrous and degenerative changes in the skin and multiple organ systems. Visceral involvement most commonly includes the GI tract (motility abnormalities), lung (interstitial pneumonitis), kidney (vasculopathy leading to hypertension), and, less commonly, heart (conduction abnormalities and cardiomyopathy secondary to fibrosis). Of note, 90% of patients with systemic scleroderma have Raynaud syndrome.

14. Which conditions can mimic scleroderma?

Conditions associated with thickened skin include vinyl chloride poisoning, bleomycin toxicity, silicon-induced skin changes, eosinophilic fasciitis (idiopathic and associated with adulterated tryptophan), phenylketonuria, chronic graft-versus-host disease, and Werner syndrome (progeria).

15. How does scleredema differ from scleroderma?

Classically, scleredema is the post-streptococcal development of indurative edema of the face, neck, shoulders, and proximal extremities. Unlike scleroderma, it usually spares the hands and feet. Histologically, it is distinct from scleroderma in having minimal inflammatory changes, little dermal hydrophilic glycosaminoglycan infiltration, and scant endothelial hyalinization. It is a self-limited condition but can take up to a year to resolve.

16. What is CREST syndrome?

C—Calcinosis
R—Raynaud phenomenon
E—Esophageal dysmotility
S—Sclerodactyly
T—Telangiectasis

CREST is a subset of scleroderma. It is associated with the presence of anti-centromere antibodies. CREST syndrome is rare in children and, while less severe than progressive systemic sclerosis, can be quite debilitating.

17. When is a child considered to have hypermobile joints?

A child with hypermobile joints can:

1. Passively appose the thumbs to the flexor aspect of the forearm
2. Passively hyperextend the fingers to that they lie parallel to the extensor aspect of the forearms
3. Hyperextend the elbows at least 10°
4. Hyperextend the knees at least 10°
5. Touch the floor with palms from a standing position with the knees extended

18. Do hypermobile joints have any clinical significance?

Gedalia and colleagues found that hyperextensibility was more common among children with intermittent joint complaints than in controls. They termed this entity **juvenile episodic arthritis/arthralgia** if 3 of the hyperextensible features were present (see Question 17). The condition is generally benign, although predisposition to injury in scholastic athletics is likely. Hypermobile joints can also be found in multiple other conditions, including Ehlers-Danlos syndrome (secondary to collagen abnormality), Marfan syndrome, osteogenesis imperfecta (type I),

522 Rheumatology

and Down syndrome. However, hypermobility is a common entity, and most children have no associated abnormalities.

Gedalia A, et al: Hypermobility of the joints in juvenile episodic arthritis/arthralgia. J Pediatr 107:873–876, 1985.

19. Which children can demonstrate a positive Gorlin sign?

This is the ability to touch the tip of the nose with the tongue. It is seen in conditions of connective tissue hypermobility, such as Ehlers-Danlos syndrome.

20. Describe the articular manifestations of parvovirus B19 infection in children.

Although joint symptoms are present in up to 80% of adults with **erythema infectiosum**, they are rarely present in children. Nocton and colleagues identified 22 children with joint complaints associated with parvovirus infection, 20 of whom had arthritis and 2 arthralgia. Ten cases presented with polyarthralgia/arthritis, and 12 had a pauciarticular course (2 monarticular). Large joints were affected more often than small joints, and the knee was most commonly involved. While the duration of symptoms was usually brief, 8 children had persistent symptoms and fulfilled the criteria for juvenile rheumatoid arthritis.

Nocton JJ, et al: Human parvovirus B19-associated arthritis in children. J Pediatr 122:186–190, 1993.

21. Which joints are classically involved in psoriatic arthritis?

The **distal interphalangeal joints** of the hands and feet. Juvenile psoriatic arthritis (< 16 years old) often presents as an acute monarthritis. Joint changes often precede the skin changes. Psoriatic arthritis is more common in patients who have severe psoriasis. Flares are unrelated to the skin condition.

22. How is reactive arthritis diagnosed?

Reactive arthritis in its broadest sense refers to joint inflammation associated with a nonarticular infection and presumably is mediated by immune complexes. By definition, an organism cannot be isolated from synovial fluid or biopsies. Examples of reactive arthritis include rheumatic fever and Reiter syndrome (which can follow nongonococcal urethritis or bacterial enteritis). Some cases of polyarthritis associated with gonococcal and meningococcal infections are also likely to be reactive in origin, as is polyarthritis associated with *Mycoplasma* infection and tuberculosis (Poncet disease). A more restrictive definition of reactive arthritis embodies arthritis following infections with enteric bacteria, including *Salmonella*, *Shigella flexneri*, *Yersinia enterocolitica*, and *Campylobacter jejuni*. It often occurs in individuals who are HLA-B27 positive.

23. What is the prognosis for reactive arthritis following viral or bacterial infections?

It generally lasts for days to weeks, responds readily to nonsteroidal antiinflammatory medications, and leaves no sequelae.

24. What conditions are associated with gastroenteritis and arthritis?

Noninfectious etiologies	Infectious etiologies
Ulcerative colitis	*Salmonella*
Regional enteritis (Crohn disease)	*Shigella*
Behçet's syndrome	*Yersinia*
Henoch-Schönlein syndrome	Tuberculosis
	Adenovirus

25. A visiting bun-loving East Siberian teenager with arthritic knees and ankles likely has what condition?

Kashin-Beck disease. This is a zebra in the United States, but a definite horse in the Far East. It is a destructive arthropathy endemic to northern China and Siberia and affecting over 2 million people there, often beginning in adolescence. It appears to be caused by chronic ingestion of bread baked from grain infected with the fungus *Fusarium oxysporum*.

26. How do synovial fluid characteristics help in determining the diagnosis of arthritis?

Synovial Fluid Characteristics in Various Arthridites

GROUP/CONDITION	SYNOVIAL COMPLE-MENT	COLOR/ CLARITY	VIS-COSITY	MUCIN CLOT	WBC COUNT (μl)	PMN (%)	MISCELLA-NEOUS FINDINGS
Noninflammatory							
Normal	N	Yellow Clear	↑↑	G	< 200	< 25	
Traumatic arthritis	N	Yellow Turbid	↑	F–G	< 2,000	< 25	Debris
Osteoarthritis	N	Yellow Clear	↑	F–G	1,000	< 25	
Inflammatory							
SLE	↓	Yellow Clear	N	N	5,000	10	LE cells
Rheumatic fever	N–↑	Yellow Cloudy	↓	F	5,000	10–50	
JRA	N–↓	Yellow Cloudy	↓	Poor	15,000–20,000	75	
Reiter syndrome	↑	Yellow Opaque	↓	Poor	20,000	80	Reiter cells
Pyogenic							
Tuberculous arthritis	N–↑	Yellow-white Cloudy	↓	Poor	25,000	50–60	Acid-fast bacteria
Septic arthritis	↑	Serosanguinous Turbid	↓	Poor	50,000–300,000	> 75	Low glucose, bacteria

N = normal; G = good; F = fair; ↓ = decreased; ↑ = increased.
From Cassidy JT, Petty RE: Textbook of Pediatric Rheumatology, 3rd ed. Philadelphia, W.B. Saunders, 1995, p 585; with permission.

27. An afebrile 8-year-old child presents 1 week after mild trauma with swelling and exquisite tenderness of a cool and mottled foot. What is the likely diagnosis?

Reflex sympathetic dystrophy (RSD). This poorly understood entity, often confused with arthritis, is characterized by severe pain, loss of function, and dysautonomic changes in a distal extremity. Marked cutaneous hyperesthesia is common. Antecedent trauma is usually minimal or nonexistent. Laboratory findings are normal. Autonomic dysfunction can be confirmed by thermography or by decreased flow/blood pool phases on technetium bone scan. Regional osteopenia secondary to disuse can develop.

28. How is RSD managed?

Although many children are casted in emergency rooms for suspected "hairline fractures," immobilization is contraindicated in RSD. Treatment is aimed at providing some relief of pain (difficult at best) through the use of analgesics and transcutaneous nerve stimulation. Physical therapy is begun immediately and consists of desensitization of the skin and passive and active range of motion. Every effort should be made to have the child become an active participant in his or her care, so that the child can be the person effecting the improvement. If pain cannot otherwise be controlled, sympathetic blockade may be necessary.

There is a peculiar psychological set in affected children which is not described in adults. They are often highly motivated, overachieving individuals who are involved in an extensive array of school and extracurricular activities. Psychotherapy may be required if the RSD is prolonged or recurrent.

29. Do children develop fibromyalgia?

Fibromyalgia, a diffuse pain syndrome well-described in adults, consists of vague musculoskeletal aching, fatigue, disturbed sleep patterns, and characteristic trigger points, elicitable by pressure (e.g., iliac crests, scapula, spine). The cause is unknown and laboratory findings are normal. Children as young as 9 years have been described with the condition. However, the differentiation of chronic musculoskeletal pain of nonorganic origin can be difficult in children and adolescents.

Malleson PN, et al: Idiopathic musculoskeletal pain syndromes in children. J Rheumatol 19:1786, 1992.

30. How is serum sickness diagnosed?

Serum sickness is a clinical diagnosis, based on the appearance of fever, urticaria, arthralgia, and lymphadenopathy, developing approximately 1–3 weeks after primary antigen exposure. Visceral involvement is unusual. Associated laboratory findings include mild leukocytosis, normal or elevated ESR, eosinophilia, hypergammaglobulinemia, and IgG antibodies against heterologous proteins ("reverse heterophile"). Plasma cells noted on a peripheral blood smear are highly suggestive of serum sickness.

JUVENILE RHEUMATOID ARTHRITIS

31. What is the relative frequency of the major pediatric rheumatic diseases?

Juvenile rheumatoid arthritis (JRA) is far and away the most common with an incidence of 1/10,000.

JRA	65–85%	Spondyloarthritis	5%
SLE	10%	Scleroderma	3%
Dermatomyositis	5%	Vasculitis	1%

32. List the criteria for the diagnosis and classification of the major subgroups of juvenile rheumatoid arthritis (JRA).

JRA is a diagnosis of exclusion. Features include:
1. Onset < 16 years of age
2. Clinical arthritis with joint swelling or effusion, increased heat, and limitation of range of motion with tenderness
3. Duration of disease ≥ 6 weeks
4. Major subgroups (systemic-onset, pauciarticular or oligoarticular, polyarticular) determined by:
   a. Presence or absence of fever at presentation
   b. Number of joints involved in the first 6 months of illness
5. No other known etiology for arthritis

33. What is the most common age of onset of JRA?

When all types are considered, ages 1–3 years are the most common times for JRA to present. In this age group, girls usually present with pauciarticular disease. Polyarticular disease and disease in boys generally occur later.

34. Describe the pattern of fever and rash in systemic JRA.

Systemic-onset JRA (Still disease) accounts for approximately 20% of children with JRA. Affected individuals typically present with fevers of unknown origin with single or twice-daily (i.e., quotidian) spikes, often > 40°C. The fever is often preceded by shaking chills. The temperature characteristically returns to 37° or lower. Continuous fever should suggest other diagnoses.

A blotchy, light pink, evanescent rash, which blanches on compression and which may show perimacular pallor, accompanies the fever in over 90% of cases. The rash of systemic JRA is diagnostic only *after* the diagnosis is made (by exclusion). Of note, arthritis may not be present for the first several weeks of illness.

Pinals RS: Polyarthritis and fever. N Engl J Med 330:769–774, 1994.

35. How can acute leukemia clinically mimic systemic JRA?

Some cases of leukemia with primarily musculoskeletal findings and minimal hematologic abnormalities can mimic JRA, resulting in diagnostic delay, misdiagnosis, or inappropriate use of steroids. Distinguishing clinical features in this setting include:

1. Only 10–20% of patients with leukemia have high spiking fevers, morning stiffness, and rash, compared with 80–90% of children with JRA.

2. Leukemia is more likely to awaken the patient at night with musculoskeletal pain.

3. Nonarticular bone pain is more common in leukemia than JRA.

4. Serum lactate dehydrogenase levels are usually elevated in children with leukemia, but slightly below normal in those with JRA.

Of note, both entities commonly have lymphadenopathy and hepatosplenomegaly. Plain films (demonstrating periosteal elevation in leukemia but not in JRA), technetium bone scans, and bone marrow biopsy can distinguish the two.

Ostrov BE, et al: Differentiation of systemic juvenile rheumatoid arthritis from acute leukemia near the onset of disease. J Pediatr 122:595–598, 1993.

Wallendal M, et al: The discriminating role of serum lactate dehydrogenase levels in children with malignant neoplasms presenting as joint pain. Arch Pediatr Adolesc Med 150:70–73, 1996.

36. Is the measurement of rheumatoid factor (RF) a good screening test for JRA?

RF, as measured by the classic latex-fixation test, is an anti-IgG antibody of the IgM class. It is present in the sera of 80% of adults with rheumatoid arthritis but in only 5–10% of children with JRA (primarily older girls with polyarticular disease). Because JRA has a relatively low prevalence rate, about 1/10,000, one would have to screen 10,000 children to identify 1 child with JRA and positive RF (assuming 10% sensitivity and 100% specificity). False-positives can be seen in SLE, Sjögren's syndrome, mixed connective tissue disease, viral infections, parasitic infections, malignancies, subacute bacterial endocarditis, and sarcoidosis. The measurement of RF is of no benefit in ruling JRA in or out.

Eichenfield AH, et al: Utility of rheumatoid factor in the diagnosis of JRA. Pediatrics 78:480–484, 1986.

37. Describe the features of the various subgroups of JRA.

Clinical Features of JRA Subgroups

JRA SUBGROUP (% AFFECTED)	GENDER	NUMBER AND DISTRIBUTION OF JOINTS INVOLVED	HLA	EYE FINDINGS	JOINT DISABILITY
Pauciarticular					
Type I (35%)	F > M	≤ 4, asymmetrical; knee, wrist, ankle	DR5	Chronic uveitis (associated with ANA)	10%
Type II (15%?)	M > F	≤ 4, asymmetrical; knee, wrist, ankle, hip, sacroiliac	B27	Acute uveitis	10%
Polyarticular					
RF-positive (5–10%)	F > M	≥ 5, symmetrical; small and large joints	DR4	Rare	50%
RF-negative (20–30%)	F > M	≥ 5, symmetrical; small and large joints	?	Rare	15%
Systemic-onset (15–20%)	F = M	40% pauciarticular, 60% polyarticular	?	Rare	25%

38. In the initial workup of a child with suspected JRA, what serologic studies and other laboratory tests should be ordered?

Laboratory tests are helpful primarily in excluding other (reactive, infectious, rheumatic, paraneoplastic) causes of arthritis in childhood but cannot establish a diagnosis of JRA. In a prospective analysis of 278 Finnish children with arthritis, Kunnamo et al. examined the utility of 22 laboratory tests and concluded that 5 are indicated in all children with joint symptoms:

- Complete blood count with platelets and differential
- Erythrocyte sedimentation rate
- C-reactive protein
- Urinalysis
- Throat culture

Their recommendations for evaluation of children with symptoms lasting > 2 weeks include ANA and quantitative immunoglobulins. In selected cases, determinations of RF, antistreptolysin O, and Lyme antibodies may be indicated.

Kunnamo I, et al: Clinical signs and laboratory tests in the differential diagnosis of arthritis in children. Am J Dis Child 141:34–40, 1987.

39. What is the recommended first-line therapy in suspected JRA?

For years, the "gold standard" for antiinflammatory therapy in JRA was not gold, but aspirin. Most pediatric rheumatologists no longer initiate therapy with aspirin, as other nonsteroidal antiinflammatory drugs (NSAIDs) offer greater ease of administration and fewer side effects. The most commonly used nonsalicylates are ibuprofen, naproxen, and tolmetin sodium. Adverse reactions are similar among all the NSAIDs and include, most often, GI upset and bleeding and, less often, elevation of hepatic transaminases, headaches, and nephrotoxicity (e.g., interstitial nephritis, papillary necrosis). Patients will experience relief of pain and stiffness within 7–10 days of institution of therapy, and joint swelling will decrease within 2–3 weeks. Continued improvement can be expected for up to 6 weeks.

There is a strong association between Reye syndrome and salicylate therapy during episodes of varicella and influenza, and therefore, patients on therapy should receive the influenza and varicella vaccines (if previously uninfected). Prudence suggests discontinuing aspirin during such illnesses.

Lindsley CB: Uses of nonsteroidal anti-inflammatory drugs in pediatrics. Am J Dis Child 147:229–236, 1993.

Giannini EH, Cawkell GD: Drug treatment in children with juvenile rheumatoid arthritis: Past, present, and future. Pediatr Clin North Am 42:1099–1126, 1995.

40. What if the child is unresponsive to NSAIDs?

Second-line therapies for JRA include corticosteroids, disease-modifying antirheumatic drugs (gold salts, hydroxychloroquine, D-penicillamine, sulfasalazine), and immunosuppressive drugs (methotrexate). The use of steroids is limited due to their side effects. Parental gold salts may be helpful in up to 50% of patients, but up to 25% of children cannot remain on chrysotherapy because of reversible toxic effects (e.g., proteinuria, bone marrow suppression, rashes). Auranofin (an oral gold compound), D-penicillamine, and hydroxychloroquine have been less than satisfactory in placebo-controlled multicenter trials, though sulfasalazine has shown promise. Significant improvement has been well-documented in children treated with weekly oral methotrexate.

Difficulties lie in determining which subgroups will most benefit, as spontaneous remissions do occur in children with seemingly horrific arthritis. Even more controversial is the suggestion that multiple antirheumatic agents be used concurrently at the onset of disease and successively withdrawn as the patient responds, rather than the current practice of stepwise escalation of therapy.

Giannini E, et al: Methotrexate in resistant juvenile rheumatoid arthritis: Results of the U.S.A.–U.S.S.R. double-blind, placebo-controlled trial. N Engl J Med 326:1043, 1992.

Lehman T: Aggressive therapy for childhood rheumatic diseases: When are immunosuppressives appropriate? Arthritis Rheum 36:71, 1993.

41. When are corticosteroids indicated in children with JRA?

1. Life-threatening disease (e.g., carditis or myocarditis)
2. Unremitting fever unresponsive to NSAIDs
3. Unrelenting polyarthritis with severe limitations requiring intensive physical therapy to achieve ambulatory status

4. Topical therapy for uveitis (rarely, systemic steroids are needed for children with aggressive uveitis unresponsive to topicals)

5. Intra-articular administration for a single severely symptomatic joint

42. What are the most common side effects of prolonged corticosteroid therapy?

A trip to Oslo awaits the individual who can synthesize an antiinflammatory steroid without untoward side effects. These effects can be minimized by alternate-day therapy, but sometimes the treatment is worse than the disease. Commonly encountered problems associated with high-dose corticosteroid use in children can be remembered by referring to the "Cushingoid map":

C Cataracts
U Ulcers
S Striae
H Hypertension
I Infectious complications
N Necrosis of bone (avascular)
G Growth retardation
O Osteoporosis
I Increased intracranial pressure (pseudotumor cerebri)
D Diabetes mellitus

M Myopathy
A Adipose tissue hypertrophy (obesity, "buffalo hump")
P Pancreatitis

43. Which children with JRA require the most frequent monitoring for uveitis?

Uveitis (also called iridocyclitis) is inflammation of the iris and ciliary body. It occurs on average in 20% of patients with pauciarticular JRA and in 5% with polyarticular disease, but those in either group with positive ANA are at higher risk. Patients age < 7 with ANA-positivity should be seen every 3–4 months for ophthalmologic evaluation. Fewer than 2% of patients with systemic JRA will develop ocular inflammation. These children require eye exams only every 12 months. Periodic exams are critical, because most patients with ocular inflammation are asymptomatic.

Section on Rheumatology, Section of Ophthalmology: Guidelines for ophthalmologic examinations in children with juvenile rheumatoid arthritis. Pediatrics 92:295–296, 1993.

44. What is the earliest sign of uveitis in patients with JRA?

When the anterior chamber of the eye is examined with a slit lamp, a "flare" is the earliest sign. This is a hazy appearance due to an increased concentration of protein and inflammatory cells. Later signs can include a speckled appearance to the posterior cornea (secondary to keratic precipitates), an irregular or poorly reactive pupil (secondary to synechiae between the iris and lens), band keratopathy, and cataracts.

45. Is there any evidence that JRA has a hereditary, infectious, or traumatic basis?

Unlike SLE, JRA rarely affects other first-degree relatives. Sibling pairs with JRA are decidedly uncommon, with the exception of identical twins. However, there is clearly a genetic component to chronic arthritis in childhood, with some JRA subgroups showing associations with HLA types. JRA probably represents an abnormal immune response to any number of inciting antigens.

Infections may mimic JRA, notably Lyme disease and parvovirus infection. Reactive arthritides follow infections, but causative organisms cannot be isolated from affected joints. Organisms implicated as causes of reactive arthritis include group A streptococci, *Salmonella*, *Yersinia*, and meningococcus.

Occasionally, a history of antecedent trauma is elicited in a patient subsequently who has JRA. It is possible that a sprain may "uncover" antigens to which the patient then makes an abnormal immune response; this is more likely if the arthritis is polyarticular and does not involve only the traumatized joint. In most cases, however, the trauma probably calls attention to an otherwise unrecognized arthritis.

LYME DISEASE

46. Where do most cases of Lyme disease occur?

Lyme disease has been reported in 48 states, but the major focus of disease is in southern New England (Massachusetts, Connecticut, Rhode Island) and the Middle Atlantic states (New York, New Jersey, Pennsylvania, Delaware), extending as far south as Virginia. Another hotbed of Lyme activity is in the Midwest, most notably Wisconsin, Michigan, and Minnesota. The West coast is not immune from *Borrelia burgdorferi* infection, with an endemic focus in northern California, Oregon, and Washington. In Europe, most cases occur in the Scandinavian countries and the central continent (Germany, Austria, Switzerland).

47. How is the diagnosis of Lyme disease made?

The criteria for the diagnosis of Lyme disease require one of the following:
1. Erythema chronicum migrans
2. At least one late manifestation (dermatologic, rheumatologic, neurologic, cardiac)

in addition to laboratory confirmation of infection (isolation of *B. burgdorferi* from clinical material, diagnostic levels of IgM or IgG antibody in serum or CSF, significant change in antibody titers in paired sera).

48. What percentage of patients with Lyme disease can recall a tick bite?

Fewer than 40% of adults with erythema chronicum migrans can recall the tick bite responsible for the lesion. *Ixodes* ticks are tiny. The nymphal forms are the size of a poppy seed, and the adults are about the size of a sesame seed. The bite is painless. Unless one is specifically looking for ticks, they are easy to miss.

49. Describe the classic rash of Lyme disease.

Erythema chronicum migrans (ECM) is the distinctive cutaneous lesion of Lyme disease. The lesion begins as a small red macule or papule and enlarges in an annular centrifugal fashion to approximately 10–15 cm or more in diameter. The lesions may have varying intensities of redness within the plaque, partial central clearing, or a ring-within-a-ring configuration. Occasionally, the central area may become indurated, vesicular, or crusted. ECM lesions usually appear within 14 days of the bite of an infected ixodid tick (range 2–28 days). Multiple lesions are present in only about 20% of cases.

50. After a tick bite, what is the natural history of Lyme disease?

1–2 weeks: Following the bite of an infected *Ixodes* deer tick, ECM develops in two-thirds of cases. The skin lesion may be associated with constitutional symptoms (fever, arthralgia, myalgia, severe headache, profound fatigue), especially in patients in whom secondary lesions occur. The rash and other symptoms are self-limited, even without antibiotic treatment.

Weeks to months: If treatment has not been given, early disseminated Lyme disease occurs, characterized by neurologic and/or cardiac involvement. Neuroborreliosis occurs in up to 20% of patients and presents most commonly as facial palsy, lymphocytic meningitis, or peripheral radiculoneuropathy. Up to 8% of patients develop cardiac involvement (most commonly fluctuating atrioventricular block or, more rarely, myopericarditis).

Months to years: The most common late manifestation of Lyme disease is a large-joint, self-limited oligoarthritis, most often affecting the knees. Late neurologic disease does occur and, like tertiary syphilis, usually presents as a subacute encephalopathy, although it can mimic multiple sclerosis. In Europe, a morphea-like eruption termed acrodermatitis chronica atrophicans is a late dermatologic sequela.

Steere AC: Lyme disease. N Engl J Med 321:586–589, 1989.

51. Why is the laboratory diagnosis of Lyme disease often difficult?

1. It is extraordinarily difficult to culture the Lyme spirochete from clinical specimens.

2. False-negative serologic tests are the rule in early Lyme disease. Diagnostic levels of antibody do not develop in patients with ECM for at least 4–6 weeks.

3. Standardization of testing has been lacking among various laboratories, and interlaboratory variability is common.

4. Antibiotic treatment abrogates the humoral immune response, and convalescent titers may be misleadingly diminished.

5. Cross-reactivity (and thus false-positivity) occurs in patients with other treponemal infections, including syphilis and periodontal disease caused by *Treponema denticola*, as well as those with viral infections (e.g., HIV, EBV), rickettsioses, and severe bacterial infections such as subacute bacterial endocarditis. Autoimmune diseases (rheumatoid arthritis, SLE, dermatomyositis) are also associated with false-positive reactions.

Ostrov B, Athreya B: Lyme disease: Difficulties in diagnosis and management. Pediatr Clin North Am 38:535, 1991.

52. What should be suspected if a patient with Lyme disease develops fever and chills after starting antibiotic treatment?

The **Jarisch-Herxheimer reaction**. This reaction consists of fever, chills, arthralgia, myalgia, and vasodilation and follows the initiation of antibiotic therapy in certain illnesses, most typically syphilis. It is thought to be mediated by endotoxin release as the organism is destroyed. A similar reaction occurs in up to 40% of patients treated for Lyme disease and may be mistaken for an allergic reaction to the antibiotic.

53. Are prophylactic antibiotics indicated following a tick bite?

The risk of transmission of the spirochete varies according to the proportion of infected ticks in the area, life stage of the tick (adult ticks carry the spirochete more than nymphal ticks), and duration of attachment to the human host (infected adult ticks must be attached for 48–72 hours to transmit the spirochete).

If parents examine their children on a daily basis and remove ticks promptly, there should be no need for prophylactic antibiotics. Ticks should be removed with the aid of tweezers, grabbing them as closely as possible to the skin surface. Petroleum jelly or matches should not be applied. The tick may be saved in alcohol for later identification.

Management of tick bites of indeterminate duration is more controversial. Not all deer ticks are infected, making the likelihood of developing Lyme disease after a known tick bite in a given endemic area a matter of conjecture. Prospective, placebo-controlled studies of antibiotic prophylaxis of tick bites have failed to confirm the need for such therapy (although the power of such studies has been lacking). At present, "watchful waiting" is an appropriate course of action. The bite site should be observed for about 1 month for the development of ECM.

Shapiro ED, et al: A controlled trial of antimicrobial prophylaxis for Lyme disease after deer-tick bites. N Engl J Med 327:1769–1773, 1992.

RHEUMATIC FEVER

54. How is the diagnosis of acute rheumatic fever (ARF) established?

The criteria for the diagnosis of rheumatic fever were proposed in 1944 by T. Duckett Jones. They have been revised four times, most recently in 1992. A diagnosis of rheumatic fever is highly probable in the presence of 2 major criteria, or 1 major and 2 minor criteria, if supported by evidence of preceding streptococcal infection (positive throat culture or rapid streptococcal antigen test, or elevated or rising streptococcal antibody titer).

Major criteria	Minor criteria
• Carditis	• Polyarthralgia
• Polyarthritis	• Fever
• Chorea	• Elevated acute-phase reactants (ESR, CRP)
• Erythema marginatum	• Prolonged PR interval
• Subcutaneous nodules	• Previous rheumatic fever or rheumatic carditis

55. How is evidence of a preceding streptococcal infection established?

A history of sore throat or scarlet fever is not sufficient evidence of antecedent streptococcal infection without documentation of positive streptococcal culture, antigen, or antibody tests.

1. **Positive throat culture** or **antigen tests** do not distinguish between recent infection and a chronic carrier state. Although antigen tests are specific, they are not necessarily sensitive. A negative rapid streptococcal antigen test should be confirmed with a conventional throat culture.

2. **Streptococcal antibody tests** provide reliable evidence of recent group A streptococcal infection. An elevated antibody response to streptolysin O (ASO) is present in at least 80% of patients with streptococcal pharyngitis and is generally considered positive if > 320 Todd units in a school-aged child and > 240 Todd units in an adult. If the test is negative (approx. 20% of patients in the first 2 months of the attack and 40% of those with Sydenham chorea), antibodies to DNase B and hyaluronidase should be sought. Anti-DNase B levels of ≥ 240 units are diagnostic in children; the cut-off level in adults is 120 units.

The Streptozyme **slide agglutination test** for detection of antibodies to streptococcal antigens is less standardized and reproducible than the other antibody tests. The 1992 Jones criteria suggest that it not be used as definitive evidence of antecedent streptococcal infection.

El-Khateeb MS: Comparison of antibody titres to streptococcal extracellular antigens. J Trop Pediatr 35:159–162, 1989.

56. What are the most common manifestations of carditis in ARF?

Carditis is almost always associated with a murmur of valvulitis (e.g., mitral insufficiency, mid-diastolic murmur of relative mitral stenosis, aortic insufficiency), which can be a new or changing murmur. Myocarditis (with resting tachycardia out of proportion to fever, cardiomegaly, and congestive heart failure) and pericarditis may accompany the valvular involvement but rarely occur in isolation. Of note, the severity of carditis is often inversely proportional to the severity of the arthritis.

57. How quickly can valvular lesions occur in children with ARF?

In patients with valvular involvement, signs appear within the first 2 weeks of illness in 80% of patients and rarely appear after the second month of illness. The average duration of a rheumatic attack is < 3 months.

58. Describe the clinical characteristics of arthritis in ARF.

Polyarthritis is the most typical finding and is almost always migratory. The large joints (knees, ankles, elbows, wrists) are most frequently involved. Pain is usually severe and often out of proportion to the physical examination, which reveals marked warmth, erythema, and tenderness over the large joints. The arthritis of ARF is exquisitely sensitive to salicylates. Failure to respond to aspirin should suggest another diagnosis.

59. How long does the arthritis associated with ARF usually persist?

In the classic rheumatic attack, several joints become affected in succession. A given joint will remain inflamed for < 1 week and the entire sequence rarely lasts > 4 weeks. The arthritis never occurs > 35 days from the time of pharyngitis and is virtually always associated with positive streptococcal serology.

60. What is Jaccoud syndrome?

Jaccoud syndrome is a "post-rheumatic" periarticular fibrosis and not a synovitis. It results in subluxations of the metacarpophalangeal joints with ulnar deviation. It also occurs in SLE.

61. How common is erythema marginatum in rheumatic fever?

The rash is very uncommon, occurring in < 5% of cases. It is characterized by evanescent, coalescing large macules with pale centers and serpiginous borders. The rash is found primarily on the trunk and proximal extremities. It may be induced by the application of heat and always blanches on palpation.

62. Are steroids beneficial in the treatment of ARF?

Controlled studies have failed to show any beneficial effect of corticosteroids (or salicylates) in altering the course of rheumatic carditis or in preventing cardiac sequelae. They may be useful in providing symptomatic and supportive therapy, but they are not curative. Nonetheless, in life-threatening situations with pancarditis and severe congestive heart failure secondary to myocarditis, many authorities recommend a trial of corticosteroids in an effort to limit inflammatory edema.

63. What are appropriate regimens of prophylaxis for patients who have had ARF?

• Benzathine penicillin, IM, 0.6–1.2 million units every 3–4 wks
• Penicillin V, po, 125–250 mg twice daily
• Sulfadiazine, po, 500–1000 mg once daily
• Erythromycin, po, 250 mg twice daily, if allergic to above regimens

The cutoff for the larger doses is approximately 30 kg. Choice of regimen depends in large part on expected compliance.

64. Can prophylaxis for rheumatic fever ever be discontinued?

The optimal duration of antibiotic prophylaxis is unclear. Some experts recommend that chemoprophylaxis be continued for life. However, the risk for recurrence decreases with age and the years elapsed since the previous attack and correlates with the number of previous attacks and the presence and severity of preexisting rheumatic heart disease. Thus, the risk is very low in older adults without heart disease who are not in contact with school-age children. Therefore, it may make sense to discontinue prophylaxis in patients who have a low risk of recurrence (in some clinical trials as young as age 18).

Berrios X, et al: Discontinuing rheumatic fever prophylaxis in selected adolescents and young adults. Ann Intern Med 118:401–406, 1993.

65. Is the incidence of rheumatic fever increasing or decreasing?

In the mid- to late 1980s clusters of rheumatic fever developed in Salt Lake City, Pittsburgh, and portions of Ohio. These occurred in primarily middle-class suburban locales, in contrast to past outbreaks which occurred mainly in settings of overcrowding and poverty. These outbreaks appeared to be associated with possible "rheumatogenic" strains of group A streptococci, such as those heavily encapsulated and highly mucoid with particular capsular M-proteins. However, on nationwide surveys, the overall incidence of rheumatic fever declined from the early 1980s to 1990.

Shulman ST: Complications of streptococcal pharyngitis. Pediatr Infect Dis J 13:S70–S74, 1994.

66. Who was St. Vitus?

St. Vitus was a Sicilian youth martyred in the year 303 AD. In the middle ages, individuals with chorea felt that this saint had curative powers and would worship at the shrines of St. Vitus. Accordingly, the chorea associated with acute rheumatic fever has been called "St. Vitus' dance" (although more commonly it is known as Sydenham chorea).

SPONDYLOARTHROPATHIES

67. How are the spondyloarthropathies distinguished from juvenile rheumatoid arthritis?
The spondyloarthropathies (SA), which consist primarily of juvenile ankylosing spondylitis, juvenile psoriatic arthritis, and the arthritis of Reiter syndrome and inflammatory bowel disease, can be distinguished from JRA by the following features:
1. Back pain, stiffness, or limitation of motion are common symptoms in SA (peripheral arthritis may be observed early in disease)
2. Involvement of axial skeleton (spine and sacroiliac joints) is more common
3. Higher incidence of accompanying enthesitis
4. High likelihood of HLA-B27 positivity (up to 90% in SA vs only 15% in JRA)
5. Rheumatoid factor and ANA usually negative
6. Age of onset is typically later (> 10 years) in SA than JRA
7. Males more commonly affected than females (opposite in JRA)

68. How is enthesitis diagnosed clinically?
The enthesis is the area of attachment of ligaments, tendon, or fascia to bone. Enthesopathy is unique to the spondyloarthropathies. Knowledge of the attachment sites of various tendons is helpful in making the diagnosis. Painful localized swelling, exacerbated by motion, and marked tenderness on palpation of these areas is characteristic. Chronic inflammation results in cellular resorption, bony erosion, and ultimately calcification. The heel spurs and "bamboo spine" of juvenile ankylosing spondylitis are a consequence of this process.

69. What is the triad of Reiter syndrome?
Conjunctivitis, urethritis, arthritis.

70. With which infections is Reiter syndrome associated?
Although it is classified as a spondyloarthropathy (particularly because of the high association with HLA-B27 positivity), Reiter syndrome is also very much a postinfectious entity. It can appear in epidemic form following outbreaks of diarrheal diseases (especially due to *Shigella*, *Yersinia* and *Salmonella*). In adults, Reiter syndrome can follow episodes of sexually transmitted diseases, particularly gonorrhea or chlamydia.

71. Why is the diagnosis of ankylosing spondylitis difficult to make in children?
Various sets of criteria for diagnosis have been established that include clinical features (e.g., history of lumbar spine pain, limitation of lumbar motion, or thoracic expansion) and radiologic evidence of sacroiliitis, which is the sine qua non of the diagnosis. In adults, it take an average of 5 years from the first symptoms to make a diagnosis of ankylosing spondylitis, and so the criteria are rarely fulfilled in children. Children are more likely to present with a prodrome of oligoarticular asymmetrical arthritis (indistinguishable from pauciarticular JRA type II) and/or enthesitis. Sacroiliitis or spondylitic symptoms are uncommon early in the disease, and radiologic changes can take years to evolve.

72. What is the connection between young men and the SEA?
The syndrome of seronegative enthesopathy and arthropathy (SEA) was described in 1982 in a group (mainly boys) with enthesitis or arthralgia who lacked RF and ANA. Many were HLA-B27-positive but did not fulfill criteria for definite seronegative spondyloarthropathies. As with many rheumatic diseases, time did tell, and about half went on to develop more definitive ankylosing spondylitis.
Cabral DA, et al: SEA syndrome revisited: A long-term follow-up of children with a syndrome of seronegative enthesopathy and arthropathy. J Rheumatol 19:1282–1285, 1992.

73. Where are the dimples of Venus?
The dimples of Venus are the paravertebral indentations in the lower back prominent in some individuals while standing with feet together. A line joining these dimples represents the lumbosacral junction.

SYSTEMIC LUPUS ERYTHEMATOSUS

74. What are the most common manifestations of SLE in children?

SLE is the prototypical multisystem autoimmune disease. Its manifestations are protean and virtually any organ system can be involved.

Rash/fever	70%
Arthritis	70%
Renal (proteinuria/casts)*	60%
Anemia, leukopenia, thrombocytopenia	50–75%
Cardiac	25%
CNS (psychosis/seizures)	15%

* Every patient with SLE is likely to have some abnormality demonstrable on kidney biopsy.

75. Describe the neurologic manifestations of SLE.

Lupus cerebritis is a term that implies an inflammatory etiology of CNS disease. Microscopically, however, widely scattered areas of microinfarction and noninflammatory vasculopathy are seen in brain tissue; actual CNS vasculitis is rarely observed. The lumbar puncture may reveal CSF pleocytosis or an increased protein concentration but also can be normal. Neuropsychiatric manifestations (psychoses, behavioral changes, depression, emotional lability) are most commonly observed. An organic brain syndrome with progressive disorientation and intellectual deterioration is seen in severe cases. Seizures are also common. Less common are cranial neuropathies, peripheral neuropathies, chorea, and cerebellar ataxia.

Kovacs J, et al: Dilemmas in neuropsychiatric lupus. Rheum Dis Clin North Am 19:795, 1993.

76. Which laboratory tests should be ordered in a child suspected of having SLE?

The best screening study for SLE is the fluorescent antinuclear antibody (FANA) test. ANAs are immunoglobulins directed against a variety of nuclear antigens, including nucleic acids, histones, nonhistone proteins, and the nuclear matrix. Up to 97% of patients with SLE have positive ANAs at some point in their illness (not necessarily at diagnosis). In a patient with characteristic signs and symptoms, a FANA test may serve to confirm suspicions of SLE. Other antibodies considered to be more specific for the diagnosis of SLE include those to native DNA and the extractable nuclear antigen Sm. The finding of a low C3 and positive anti-native DNA antibody is *100% specific* for SLE.

77. Which diseases should be considered in the differential diagnosis of children with butterfly rash?

A malar rash is present in 50% of children with SLE and cutaneous involvement. In the typical butterfly rash, the malar areas are prominently involved, with the nasolabial folds being relatively spared. The rash crosses the nasal bridge in a "butterfly" distribution. Occasionally, it is difficult to distinguish from the rash of dermatomyositis (eruption on the extensor surfaces of the fingers is common in dermatomyositis and rare in SLE). Vesiculation should suggest a diagnosis of pemphigus erythematosus or contact dermatitis. A malar flush is clinically distinct and can be seen in individuals with mitral stenosis or hypothyroidism.

78. Should children with SLE undergo a renal biopsy?

This is an area of controversy as nearly all children with SLE will have some evidence of renal involvement. Usually, clinical disease (e.g., abnormal urine sediment, proteinuria, renal function changes) correlates with the severity of renal disease on biopsy, but this is not always the case. Extensive glomerular abnormalities can be found on biopsy with minimal concurrent clinical manifestations. For this reason, many authorities are aggressive with early biopsy. Three circumstances in particular warrant biopsy:

1. A child with SLE and the nephrotic syndrome, to distinguish membranous glomerulonephritis from diffuse proliferative glomerulonephritis (which requires more aggressive therapy)

2. Failure of high-dose corticosteroids to reverse deteriorating renal function, to determine the likelihood of benefits from cytotoxic agents

3. A prerequisite to entry into clinical therapeutic trials

Cassidy JT, Petty RE: Textbook of Pediatric Rheumatology, 3rd ed. Philadelphia, W.B. Saunders, 1995, pp 260–322.

79. How can the result of renal biopsy affect treatment in SLE?

Biopsy can reveal a spectrum of renal pathology, ranging from a normal kidney to mesangial nephritis to glomerulonephritis (focal or diffuse, proliferative or membranous). Histologic transformation from one group to another over time is not unusual. Treatment of lupus nephritis is based on the severity of the lesion. Patients with membranous nephropathy commonly present with nephrotic syndrome, respond to prednisone, and seem less likely to develop renal failure. Mesangial disease may require little or no intervention. Focal proliferative nephritis can be controlled with corticosteroids alone. Diffuse proliferative glomerulonephritis is best managed with corticosteroids and intermittent intravenous cyclophosphamide.

Steinberg AD, Steinberg SC: Long-term preservation of renal function in patients with lupus nephritis receiving treatment that includes cyclophosphamide versus those treated with prednisone alone. Arthritis Rheum 34:945–950, 1991.

80. When should high-dose corticosteroid therapy be considered in SLE management?

High-dose corticosteroid (2 mg/kg prednisone-equivalent up to 80–100 mg/day) should be considered for:

• Lupus crisis (widespread acute multisystem vasculitic involvement)
• Worsening CNS disease (in conjunction with antiepileptic and psychotropic medications)
• Acute hemolytic anemia
• Severe lupus nephritis
• Acute pleuropulmonary disease (e.g., lupus pleuritis, pneumonitis)

It is important that evaluations include other possible causes of a worsening clinical condition (e.g., subarachnoid hemorrhage, infection).

81. What is the prognosis for children with confirmed SLE?

The prognosis for survival has improved remarkably in the last 20 years. Survival rates at 10 years in excess of 85% can be expected. However, it is not clear that the improved outcome is a function of aggressive treatment with corticosteroids and/or immunosuppressive agents. It may well reflect earlier diagnosis of milder forms of disease and improved general supportive care of those with end-stage renal disease.

Mills JA: Systemic lupus erythematosus. N Engl J Med 330:1871–1879, 1994.

82. What is the association of false-positive tests for syphilis and an increased susceptibility to clotting in some patients with SLE?

Some patients with SLE develop antibodies against phospholipids, including cardiolipin (the substrate in many reagin tests), which can result in a falsely-positive VDRL test. One of these antibodies is the lupus anticoagulant, which in vitro interferes with the ability of normal blood to clot but in vivo results in increased potential for recurrent arterial or venous thromboses (e.g., stroke, phlebitis, retinal vein thrombosis, placental thrombosis). Patients with lupus anticoagulants and/or false-positive tests for syphilis generally have anticardiolipin antibodies, although there is not a one-to-one correspondence.

83. In addition to SLE, which other clinical conditions are associated with the presence of antiphospholipid antibodies?

• Primary antiphospholipid syndrome (patients prone to recurrent first trimester miscarriages, thrombophlebitis, strokes, early heart attacks, livedo reticularis)
• Idiopathic thrombocytopenic purpura
• Addison disease
• Rheumatic fever

84. Which laboratory tests are most useful in the monitoring of the effectiveness of anti-lupus therapy?

Serologic studies can provide useful information regarding the activity of SLE and the effect of therapy on the disease process. The titer of ANA does not correlate well with disease activity, but antibodies to double-stranded DNA are helpful in this regard. Complement levels (C3, C4, CH_{50}) are inversely related to levels of anti-DNA antibody and are also useful in gauging response to therapy.

85. In infants born to mothers with SLE, what are the most common manifestations during the neonatal period?

Although relatively rare, this situation is the most common reason to call a rheumatologist to the nursery, but (s)he will no doubt have been beaten to the consult by a dermatologist or cardiologist. The syndrome of neonatal lupus (NLE) was first described in babies born to mothers with overt SLE or Sjögren's syndrome, but it has since been found that 70–80% of mothers are asymptomatic. The **cutaneous manifestations** of NLE include erythematous macules, papules, and annular plaques, usually on areas exposed to light. These can be present at birth or develop within the first 2 months of life, usually resolving by 6 months of age. The other major clinical feature, occurring in 50% of infants with NLE, is **complete heart block**. Although usually an isolated finding, affected infants may also have congenital anomalies. Conduction defects other than complete heart block have also been described. Thrombocytopenia or neutropenia may occur in up to 5% of cases.

86. What is the pathophysiology of the congenital heart block in the neonatal lupus syndrome?

You can look like a star the next time you encounter a newborn infant with complete heart block (1 in 20,000 deliveries) by casually inquiring about symptoms of SLE in the baby's mother and sending off her serum for ANA and anti-Ro antibodies. Ro is a non-DNA nuclear antigen. Although the mother is likely to be asymptomatic, the anti-Ro antibody will be positive 80% of the time. It is not yet clear how intimately involved the Ro antibody is in the pathophysiology of the heart block, but Ro antigen has been demonstrated in fetal myocardium. Mothers of babies with heart block can go on to have normal pregnancies subsequently, despite the persistence of the antibody. Therefore, anti-Ro is unlikely to be the only cause of heart block in these infants.

87. What are the common features of drug-related lupus?

Abrupt onset of symptoms, fever, myalgia/arthralgia ± serositis, resolution of symptoms within weeks of discontinuation, and anti-histone antibodies. The following are *not* associated: multisystem involvement, CNS or renal involvement, low complement levels, antibodies to native DNA, malar rash, alopecia, or oral ulcers.

88. What are the most common causes of drug-induced lupus in children?

Antiepileptic medications (especially ethosuximide, phenytoin, primidone) are most commonly implicated. Of note, up to 20% of children receiving antiepileptic medications may develop a positive ANA. Hydralazine, isoniazid, procainamide, alpha-methyldopa, and chlorpromazine are also associated with drug-induced lupus. A variety of beta-blockers and antithyroid agents have a tentative association.

VASCULITIS

89. What clinical features suggest a vasculitic syndrome?
- Fever of unknown origin
- Palpable purpura, vasculitic urticaria, dermal necrosis
- Mononeuritis multiplex (a severe sensorimotor peripheral neuropathy)
- Unexplained arthritis, myositis, serositis

• Unexplained pulmonary, cardiovascular, or renal disease
• Accompanying lab features include leukocytosis, eosinophilia, hypocomplementemia, cryoglobulinemia, circulating immune complexes, increased ESR or C-reactive protein.
Cassidy JT, Petty RE: Textbook of Pediatric Rheumatology, 3rd ed. Philadelphia, W.B. Saunders, 1995, p 366.

90. How are the primary systemic vasculitides classified?
Attempts have been made to classify the vasculitic diseases by clinical presentation, by the size of the blood vessel involved, and by pathologic findings. A useful scheme follows:

Polyarteritis

Classic polyarteritis nodosa	Kawasaki syndrome
Cutaneous polyarteritis nodosa	

Leukocytoclastic vasculitis

Hypersensitivity vasculitis (serum sickness-like)	Hypocomplementemic urticarial vasculitis
	Essential mixed cryoglobulinemia
Henoch-Schönlein purpura	

Granulomatous vasculitis

Wegener granulomatosis	Lymphomatoid granulomatosis
Churg-Strauss syndrome	Isolated angiitis of the CNS

Giant cell arteritis

Takayasu arteritis	Temporal arteritis (exceedingly rare in children)

Miscellaneous

Behçet disease	HIV-related vasculitis
Cogan syndrome	

91. What is the clinical triad of Behçet disease?
Aphthous stomatitis, genital ulcerations, uveitis. Behçet disease is a vasculitis of unclear etiology. In two-thirds of cases in children, polyarthritis and inflammatory GI lesions occur, which can confuse the diagnosis with inflammatory bowel disease.

92. Who first described what would later become known as Henoch-Schönlein purpura?
People who have nothing better to do will argue that this syndrome should be called Schönlein-Henoch purpura, as Schönlein described the association of purpura and arthralgia in 1837, to which Henoch added associated GI symptoms in 1874 and renal involvement in 1899. Actually these Viennese Meisters were preempted by William Heberden in 1806 in his *Commentaries on the History and Cure of Disease*, in which he described a 5-year-old boy with joint and abdominal pains, petechiae, hematochezia, and gross hematuria. You can avoid this eponymic boggle if you call it anaphylactoid purpura, and you will remember that the rash starts out looking urticarial.

93. What are the characteristic laboratory findings in Henoch-Schönlein purpura (HSP)?
Acute phase reactants, including the ESR, are commonly elevated and there is frequently a mild leukocytosis. Thrombocytopenia is *never* seen. Microscopic hematuria and proteinuria are indicators of renal involvement. HSP appears to be an IgA-mediated illness, so elevated serum IgA has been noted and has been demonstrated by immunofluorescence in skin and renal biopsies. (The latter are indistinguishable from Berger disease, which some people feel is HSP without the P.) Circulating immune complexes and cryoglobulins containing IgA are also found with some regularity.

94. What kind of skin lesions are noted in HSP?
HSP is one of the hypersensitivity vasculitides and, as such, is characterized by leukocytoclastic inflammation of arterioles, capillaries, and venules. Initially, urticarial lesions predominate, which may itch or burn. These develop into pink maculopapules. With damage to vessel walls, there is bleeding into the skin, resulting in nonthrombocytopenic petechiae and palpable purpura.

95. In addition to the skin, what other organ systems are typically involved in HSP?

Classically, HSP involves the skeletal system, GI tract, and/or kidneys.

- The most common abdominal finding is GI colic (70%), frequently associated with nausea, vomiting, and GI bleeding. These findings may precede the skin rash in up to 30% of cases. Intussusception can occur in up to 5% of cases.
- Renal involvement occurs in about one-half of reported cases and is usually apparent early in the course of HSP, ranging in severity from microscopic hematuria to nephrotic syndrome.
- Joint involvement often results in periarticular swelling of the knees, ankles, wrists, and elbows, rather than a true arthritis.
- Up to 15% of males can have scrotal involvement with epididymitis, orchitis, testicular torsion, and scrotal bleeding.

96. How commonly does chronic renal disease develop in children with HSP?

The long-term prognosis depends in large part on the initial renal involvement. In patients with severe cresentic glomerulonephritis documented by biopsy, up to two-thirds may develop terminal renal failure within 1 year. Of those with the onset of nephritis and/or nephrotic syndrome, up to 45% may have long-term problems with hypertension or impaired renal function as adults. Microscopic hematuria as the sole renal manifestation is associated with a good long-term outcome. Overall, < 5% of all patients with HSP progress to end-stage renal failure.

Goldstein A, et al: Long-term follow-up of childhood Henoch-Schönlein nephritis. Lancet 339:280, 1992.

97. Why is the diagnosis of intussusception often difficult in patients with HSP?

1. Intussusception can occur suddenly without preceding abdominal symptoms.

2. Nearly half of cases of HSP intussusception are ileoileal (compared with non-HSP intussusceptions of which 75% are ileocolic). This increases the likelihood of a false-negative barium enema.

3. The variety of possible GI complications in HSP (e.g., pancreatitis, cholecystitis, gastritis) can confuse the clinical picture.

4. The common occurrence (50–75%) of melena, guaiac-positive stools, and abdominal pain in cases of HSP without intussusception may lead to a lowered index of suspicion.

98. When are corticosteroids indicated in the treatment of HSP?

The precise indications for corticosteroids in HSP remain controversial. Prednisone, 1–2 mg/kg/day for 5–7 days, is most often used for severe intestinal symptoms to decrease the likelihood of intussusception. Corticosteroids may be helpful in settings of significant pulmonary, scrotal, or CNS manifestations to minimize vasculitic inflammation. They are sometimes used when severe joint pain is present if salicylates or NSAIDs are contraindicated (e.g., severe abdominal pain). Most studies indicate that the early initiation of corticosteroids will not diminish the likelihood of long-term renal complications, but the debate is ongoing.

99. Which etiologic agents are thought to cause HSP?

HSP is probably mediated by immune complexes that require the participation of an inciting antigen. Any number of infectious agents or drugs can fit the bill. The vast majority of children with HSP have a history of prodromal illness, usually an upper respiratory infection. Serologic evidence of antecedent streptococcal infection is present in up to 50% of cases. Drugs associated with HSP include penicillin, tetracycline, sulfonamides, thiazides, and aspirin.

100. What is the triad of Wegener granulomatosis?

Sinusitis, pneumonitis, and **glomerulonephritis.** This necrotizing granulomatous vasculitis can be suspected by the presence of indirect immunofluorescent antibodies to neutrophil cytoplasm (c-ANCA, or cytoplasmic antineutrophil cytoplasmic antibodies) and confirmed by biopsy of the upper or lower respiratory tract.

101. In addition to Wegener granulomatosis, what other diseases are associated with "pulmonary-renal" involvement?
- Goodpasture syndrome
- Churg-Strauss disease
- Henoch-Schönlein purpura
- Systemic lupus erythematosus
- Lymphomatoid granulomatosis

102. A 7-year-old boy with a history of chronic asthma develops fever, eosinophilia, and palpable purpura. A biopsy reveals necrotizing vasculitis with eosinophils and granulomas. What is the probable diagnosis?
   Churg-Strauss disease. Also called allergic granulomatosis, it is decidedly rare in children.

103. Which infections can be associated with vasculitis?

Viral	HIV, hepatitis, CMV
	EBV, herpes zoster/varicella
	Parvovirus B19
Bacterial/fungal	Subacute bacterial endocarditis
	Disseminated sepsis due to *Staphylococcus, Pseudomonas,* etc.
	Immunocompromised host
Mycobacterial	Tuberculosis
Spirochetal	Syphilis
Rickettsial	Rocky Mountain spotted fever
	Typhus
	Rickettsial pox

From Athreya BH: Vasculitis in children. Pediatr Clin North Am 42:1252, 1995; with permission.

INDEX

Page numbers in **boldface type** indicate complete chapters.